PREFACE.

THIS work was originally intended as an introductory chapter to a treatise I have for some time been preparing for publication on "Softening, and other types of Organic Disease of the Brain."

In consequence of the great and unexpected length to which the contemplated prefatory essay extended, it occurred to me that it would be more consistent with a scientific analysis of the subject to continue my researches, and publish them in a distinct and separate volume, " On the Incipient Symptoms of Obscure Diseases of the Brain, and Disorders of the Mind," as an *avant courier*, or introduction to the work which is exclusively to relate to the specific and individual types of encephalic disease. Such briefly is the origin of the present treatise.

I have anticipated in the first chapter what, strictly speaking, should have been reserved for prefatory observation. The general design of this work, as well as my estimate of the great importance of the subject analyzed, will be found there fully detailed.

The reader will perceive that I have endeavored to confine myself to a *resumé* of the more prominent incipient symptoms of the various forms of cerebral and mental disorder. I could not enter more minutely into an investigation of these subjects without trenching upon *matériel* which will constitute the bases of two succeeding works, viz., one on Organic Affections of the Brain, and the second on Disorders of the Intelligence, Cerebro-Psychical in their nature.

In justice to the reader as well as to myself, I make this explanation, as an apology for the somewhat cursory manner in which I have been obliged to treat the more practical portions of my subject. I refer particularly to those sections of the treatise that relate to the medical treatment of incipient paralysis, apoplexy, softening, as well as other forms of organic cerebral disease and functional mental disorder.

It was impossible for me, without greatly enlarging this already too bulky volume, to enter, except in general terms, upon the consideration of the subject of therapeutics. If I had attempted to do otherwise, it would have been necessary for me to have excluded from the work much salient, illustrative, and relevant matter having a direct bearing upon the class of morbid phenomena under analytical investigation.

I am bound to confess that I fully and sensitively appreciate the many shortcomings and defects to be found in the

ON OBSCURE DISEASES

OF THE BRAIN AND MIND.

ON OBSCURE

DISEASES OF THE BRAIN,

AND

DISORDERS OF THE MIND:

THEIR INCIPIENT SYMPTOMS, PATHOLOGY, DIAGNOSIS,
TREATMENT, AND PROPHYLAXIS.

BY

FORBES WINSLOW, M.D., D.C.L., Oxon.

&c. &c. &c.

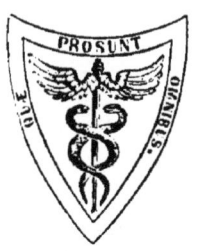

PHILADELPHIA:

BLANCHARD & LEA.

1860.

C. SHERMAN & SON, PRINTERS,
Southwest corner Seventh and Cherry Streets, Philadelphia.

following pages. It is not my duty, however, to point them out to the reader. His critical eye will no doubt soon detect all signs of omission and commission, and will, considering the vast extent of ground over which I have had to travel, make every allowance for them.

I sincerely trust that I shall not be exposing myself to the imputation of egotism, if I were to repeat what Goldsmith said in his preface to the " Vicar of Wakefield,"— " There are an hundred faults in this thing, and an hundred things might be said to prove them beauties. But it is needless. A book may be amusing with numerous errors, or it may be dull without a single absurdity."

23 CAVENDISH SQUARE, LONDON,
    April, 1860.

CONTENTS.

CHAPTER IV.

CHAPTER V.

CHAPTER VI.

CHAPTER VII.

THE STAGE OF CONSCIOUSNESS.

CHAPTER VIII.

STAGE OF EXALTATION.

CHAPTER IX.

STAGE OF MENTAL DEPRESSION.

CHAPTER X.

STAGE OF ABERRATION.

CHAPTER XVI.

PERVERSION AND EXALTATION OF MEMORY—MEMORY OF THE INSANE.

CHAPTER XVII.

PSYCHOLOGY AND PATHOLOGY OF MEMORY.

CHAPTER XVIII.

MORBID PHENOMENA OF MOTION.

CHAPTER XIX.

MORBID PHENOMENA OF SPEECH.

CHAPTER XX.

MORBID PHENOMENA OF SENSATION.

CHAPTER XXI.

MORBID PHENOMENA OF THE SPECIAL SENSES.

CHAPTER XXII.

MORBID PHENOMENA OF VISION, HEARING, TASTE, TOUCH, AND SMELL.

CHAPTER XXIII.

MORBID PHENOMENA OF SLEEP AND DREAMING.

CHAPTER XXIV.

MORBID PHENOMENA OF ORGANIC AND NUTRITIVE LIFE.

CHAPTER XXV.

GENERAL PRINCIPLES OF PATHOLOGY, DIAGNOSIS, TREATMENT, AND PROPHYLAXIS.

ON

OBSCURE DISEASES

OF

THE BRAIN AND MIND.

CHAPTER I.

INTRODUCTION.

THERE is not in the whole range of medical literature, ancient or modern, a passage that transcends in grandeur of conception, majesty of diction, and sublimity of truth, the exordium with which *Hippocrates* introduces to the reader his celebrated aphorisms: 1. ‘Ο βιος βραχὺς (*Life is short*); 2. ‘Η δὲ τέχνη μακρὴ (*Art long*); 3. ‘Ο δὲ καιρὸς ὀξὺς (*The occasion fleeting*); 4. ‘Η δὲ πείρα σφαλερὴ (*Experience fallacious*); 5. ‘Η δὲ κρίσις χαλεπὴ (*Judgment difficult*).

"‘Ο δὲ καιρὸς ὀξὺς." How important it is, to fully appreciate, when considering the treatment of the diseases of all vital structures, the practical significance of this great medical apophthegm.

"*The occasion fleeting!*" Let this profoundly wise axiom ever be present to the mind, and engraven in imperishable materials, and in indestructible characters, upon the memory.

If these "fleeting" moments of inestimable, incalculable, and precious value, are neglected or trifled with; if serious morbid states of brain are overlooked, or, if recognized, not immediately subjected to proper treatment, chronic, irreparable, and incurable organic alterations in its structure may be the result, succeeded, when it is too late to remedy the mischief, by the bitterness of

2

self-accusation, or the unceasing lamentations and regrets of those who ought to have been the first to observe and attack the fatal disease!

How often is the physician called upon to witness the melancholy consequences, to health of body and mind, life and reason, of a neglect of well-marked premonitory symptoms of cerebral disease! It is frequently his painful duty to hear both relatives and friends reproach themselves, when the time for action has, alas! passed away, for their criminal negligence in wilfully closing their eyes to the long-existing evidence of positive disease of the brain.

The late Dr. Marshall Hall, when addressing himself to the consideration of head affections, remarks: "A useful work might be written on the subject of insidious and impending diseases, with the view of making their first or antecedent symptoms known to the public, and of thus suggesting the care and means necessary for their prevention."[1]

No one was better qualified, by habits of thought, educational attainments, practical sagacity, and enlarged experience, to form a right estimate of the importance of an accurate acquaintance with the incipient symptoms of the diseases of the brain and nervous system, than this justly distinguished and accomplished physician.

It was his painful province, in the course of a long and brilliant career, to witness the sad consequences of the non-recognition of the precursory or premonitory symptoms of those organic affections of the brain, for the relief of which his great skill and extensive knowledge was so often called into requisition.

This able physiologist fully appreciated, that many of the fatal cases of brain disease with which he had to grapple formed so many sad illustrations of the neglect of premonitory symptoms.

Upon investigating the history of the diseases of the encephalon, how frequently does the medical man discover that positive and unequivocal symptoms of brain affection have existed, and perhaps, during the early stage, been observed for months, and in some cases for years, without exciting any apprehension on the part of the patient, his family, or his friends!

[1] "On Diagnosis," sect. iv. "Diseases of the Head." By Marshall Hall, M.D., F.R.S. 1817

In the majority of these instances, clearly manifested head symptoms were entirely overlooked, and, if noticed, no right estimation was made of their value. My attention has been called to cases, in which serious mischief to the delicate structure of the brain and its investing membranes, has been thus allowed by the patient's friends to proceed uninterruptedly for years, no treatment being adopted to arrest the progress of the fatal disorganization!

The brain, the most important, and exquisitely organized, of all the structures of the human body,

"The Dome of Thought; the Palace of the Soul,"

the material instrument of the intelligence, the centre of sensation, the source of volition, is permitted to be in a state of positive disorder, in fact disease, without exciting any attention, until some frightfully urgent, alarming, and dangerous symptoms have been manifested, and then, and not till then, has the actual extent of the mischief been appreciated, the condition of the patient recognized, and advice obtained for his relief!

Other deviations from organic conditions do not, as a general rule, meet with similar systematic neglect. In affections of the stomach, liver, bowels, lungs, and skin, &c., the first symptoms of approaching disease, or departure from a healthy condition of those organs, are observed, and the patient, without loss of time, seeks the aid of his physician.

Under such circumstances, he does not hesitate to place himself under curative treatment; he feels no delicacy in describing his physical sensations; is not ashamed at being thought ill, and readily adopts the treatment suggested for his recovery. But when the brain is affected, and the patient is troubled with persistent headache, associated with some slight derangement of the intelligence, disorder of the sensibility, illusions of the senses, depression of spirits, loss of mental power, or modification of motility, his condition is, in many cases, entirely overlooked, or studiously ignored, as if such abnormal symptoms were signs of robust health, instead of being, as they undoubtedly are, indications of cerebral disorder, requiring the most grave and serious attention, prompt, energetic, and skilful treatment!

It will be well to consider, briefly, the cause of the neglect to which the brain is subjected when under the influence of disease. It is a notion too commonly entertained, that many fatal cerebral diseases are *suddenly* developed affections, presenting no evidence of any antecedent encephalic organic change, and unaccompanied by a premonitory stage, or incipient symptoms.

It is indeed natural that such an idea should be entertained, even by educated professional men, whose attention has not been specially directed to a study of this class of disease, or whose opportunities of watching the progress of such affections have been limited and circumscribed.

A man, apparently in vigorous health, mixing daily with his family, going to his counting-house, engaging in the active pursuits of commerce, or occupying his attention in professional or literary duties, whilst stepping into his carriage, or when entertaining his friends at the festive board, falls down either at his door in a state of unconsciousness, or quietly bows his head on his plate at the dinner table and dies, surrounded by his family, in a fit of cerebral hemorrhage!

A midwife, whilst sitting by the bed of a patient whom she is attending, suddenly exclaims, "I am gone," and immediately falls down in a state of apoplectic coma!

A gentleman, during dinner, complains suddenly of giddiness and sickness. He retires to another room, where he is found a minute afterwards supporting himself by a bed-post, confused and pale. Being put to bed, he soon becomes comatose, and dies.

A person in good health, after using rather violent exercise in the forenoon, returns home to dinner, and whilst sitting near the fire, without any warning starts up, pushes his chair backwards with violence, exclaiming, "Oh, my head!" Immediately afterwards he falls on the floor in a state of apoplectic insensibility.

A literary man, whilst speaking at a public meeting, is suddenly seized with an uneasy sensation in his head. He says it feels "as if it would burst," "as if the brain was too big for the skull." He returns home, becomes apoplectic, and dies on the evening of that day.

A clergyman, whilst preaching, is observed to stop, and put his hand to his head. He then attempts to proceed with his sermon, but talks indistinctly, and has evidently lost his recollection. He keeps himself from falling by grasping the side of the pulpit. He is immediately removed from the church, and is found cold, pale, speechless, and paralytic. He dies in a few days after the attack.[1]

A young lad who had not previously complained of ill-health, or of any uneasy head symptoms, suddenly awakes from an apparent state of profound slumber, and begins screaming, "Oh, my head! my head! my head!" Before his parents could be summoned into the room he becomes insensible, and dies without being restored to a state of consciousness![2]

A lady, apparently in excellent health, is riding with her brother in Rotten Row. Whilst engaged in active and cheerful conversation, she suddenly complains of giddiness and sickness, and becomes deadly pale. A few minutes afterwards it is found that she could not articulate. She is carried home, soon becomes unconscious, and dies on the following day!

A gentleman who had formerly been in Parliament, and who had been for many years engaged in electioneering contests, is in the act of getting into a railway carriage. He complains of vertigo, mental confusion, and defective power of articulation. He, however, takes his seat apparently restored to his usual health. Once, during a three hours' journey, he has a slight recurrence of these symptoms, but they again pass away. On his arrival home he complains of nausea, and an indisposition to take food. He has no headache, and can speak clearly and distinctly. As he resides some distance from a medical man, and as the symptoms are not such as to create any grave apprehension as to his state of health, nothing is done medically for the case. The gentleman, after partaking of a light dinner, retires in a cheerful state of mind to bed. About two o'clock in the morning his wife is suddenly roused from sleep by her husband's loud stertorous breathing. She finds him in a state of profound coma. He dies before the surgeon, who is immediately summoned, could arrive. The brain exhibits symptoms, of what was assumed to be, organic disease of long existence.

---

[1] After death there was found in this case extensive extravasation of blood in the left ventricle, which had passed partly into the right, by laceration of the septum. *All the arteries of the brain were extensively ossified.*—ABERCROMBIE.

[2] All the ventricles were completely filled with coagulated blood. In the substance of the left hemisphere there was a cavity formed by laceration of the cerebral substance, filled also by the coagulum, and communicating with the ventricle. There was no other morbid appearance.—ABERCROMBIE.

A medical gentleman of known reputation, and great personal worth, having been to one of her Majesty's levees, visits on the evening of that day the home of a friend in the environs of town. He appears, during dinner and afterwards, in excellent health and spirits. After playing a rubber of whist, he retires, with his wife, to bed, complaining only of general lassitude, but exhibiting no other sign of bodily indisposition. In the middle of the night he is found by his wife in a state of apoplectic coma. In the attempt made by her to place him on his back, he heaves a deep sigh, and instantly expires!

The history of these sad cases is carefully investigated, without, it is alleged, affording satisfactory evidence of any decided precursory symptoms that would have justified the suspicion of the presence of any latent and dormant mischief within the head. It is possible there may have been headache, defective articulation, dimness and loss of vision, giddiness, cerebral lassitude, and evanescent attacks of mental depression and confusion, but of so trivial and unimportant a character, as not to awaken apprehension, or excite attention.

In many instances of this kind it is affirmed, that no appreciable precursory stage could be discovered. The attack, whether it be one of apoplexy, acute softening, paralysis, epilepsy, meningitis, cerebritis, or mania, had all the characteristics of a *sudden* seizure, which no prudence could have anticipated or foresight prevented, had the patient's state of brain and general health been made the subject of careful and anxious analysis.

It occasionally happens, that in some cases, what *à priori* would be considered as the most important symptoms of serious brain disorder, are represented to be altogether absent. For example: attacks of apoplexy and paralysis are alleged to occur without being preceded by any *observable* cerebral symptoms! There have been no headache, alienation of mind, lesion of the sensorial or motor power, to warn the unhappy patient or his friends of the approach of the enemy. The fatal, obscure, and insidious disease, has crept quietly and stealthily on its victim, giving no sign of its advent, no indication of its advance, no notice of its presence, until it has surprised the sentinels, boldly seized upon the outposts, effected a breach in, or scaled, the ramparts, and by an act of pathological *coup de main*, taken possession of the citadel!

It is generally an object of physiological, as well as of practical

importance, for the physician, when consulted in a case of sud-
denly-developed brain disease, to make himself acquainted with
the past condition of his patient. With this view he institutes
diligent inquiries into the invalid's pathological antecedents. To
the often repeated interrogatories, "Have there been observed any
previously manifested symptoms of disorder of the encephalon and
nervous system?" how commonly is the response, "No, none
whatever; the patient has not known a day's illness; his brain has
never shown the slightest indication of any kind of disorder!" It
is singular, in some cases, how pertinaciously and obstinately all
idea of past, and even existing cerebral indisposition, is emphatically ignored, and zealously repudiated by the relations of the
patient! But how often does the physician detect, before he concludes his investigation of the history of the case, that his patient
has exhibited, it may be, in the far distant horizon, some time
previously to his attack, evidences of the threatening and approaching storm, which, if seen, had not been made matter of
observation, reflection, anxiety, or treatment! The headache has
been attributed to derangement of the stomach, or to bilious disorder; the vacillation of temper,—feebleness of purpose,—flightiness of manner,—paroxysms of irritability or passion,—inaptitude
for business,—depression, or exaltation of spirits,—the loss of
sensibility, even manifest lesion of motility, have all (if made the
subject of comment) been attributed to some trifling and transient
bodily ailment, connected with the digestive, hepatic, or renal
organs. Epileptic vertigo, cerebral headache, and disordered conditions of vision, caused by the pressure of a tumor in the immediate neighborhood of the optic thalami, have existed for some
time without exciting a suspicion as to the presence of serious disease affecting the brain! The attacks of epileptic vertigo have
occurred, unobserved, at night, and with little or no convulsive
movement, or loss of consciousness; the headache has been considered to be of a bilious, rheumatic, or nervous character; the
impairment of visual power has been treated as an affection of the
eye, unconnected with disease in the neighborhood of the *thalami
optici*, for the relief of which the *optician*, instead of the *physician*,
has been consulted, and thus have all the salient, important, and
significant symptoms of encephalic organic mischief been permitted
to undermine the bodily health, damage and impair the intellect,
even threaten the extinction of reason, and destruction of life,

without any remedial or palliative treatment being adopted to arrest the steady and onward advancing progress of the fearfully destructive cerebral disorganization!

Fully recognizing the obscurity in which this subject is involved, I would ask, whether the affections of the brain, in the majority of cases, are not preceded by a well-marked, clearly defined, but often undetected and unobserved precursory stage? Is it possible for a person to be suddenly laid prostate in the arms of death by an attack of apoplexy, cerebritis, meningitis, paralysis, acute softening, or mania, evidencing, after death, long-existing chronic alterations in the cerebral structure, without having exhibited, for some time previously, faint and transitory they may be, but nevertheless decidedly characteristic symptoms, pointing unmistakably to the *brain*, as the *fons et origo mali?*[1]

Is not the alleged absence of all premonitory symptoms more *apparent* than *real?* Would not the history of the antecedents, the pre-existing pathological state of these cases, if carefully unravelled and cautiously analyzed, afford conclusive, if not demonstrative evidence of a prior state, of undetected and unrecognized brain disorder?

A man dies of what is termed a *sudden* attack of cerebral hemorrhage, or acute softening of the brain. The *post-mortem* examination reveals a state of serious organic change in the structure of the brain, which, from its anatomical character, must have been of long duration, and of slow and progressive growth![2] The

---

[1] I freely realize the fact, that in many cases of sudden death the heart is *primarily*, and the brain *secondarily*, affected. This will account for the absence of all morbid conditions of the brain in many cases of death from what is termed apoplexy, associated with appreciable organic diseases of the heart.

It is often a difficulty to decide, in cases of sudden death, conjoined with head symptoms, what proportion of the fatal issue is attributable to the heart and what to the brain. If the former organ be examined after death, and the slightest alteration is detected in its structure, the conclusion drawn is, that this is the cause of death, even although the vessels of the brain may be discovered in a condition of great turgescence. Under such circumstances, we have no right to infer, that the brain has had nothing to do with the death, merely because the heart is found either in a partial state of disease, or weak, small, and flabby in its condition. It would be safer, under such circumstances, to conclude, that death has been caused by the combined effect of disorder in both organs.

[2] In another work will be detailed several remarkable illustrations of fatal disease of the brain, the origin of which could be traced back for long periods, in one case for *forty* years!

bloodvessels in the head are found in a state of fatty degeneration, or the seat of atheromatous deposits. A scirrhous tumor of some magnitude is discovered imbedded in the substance of the cerebral mass, the consequence of an injury inflicted· upon the cranium some years previously. An encysted abscess is detected in the head, evidently not of recent origin. There may exist an aneurismal tumor connected with one of the cerebral arteries, a considerable thickening and opacity of the membranes enveloping the encephalon, or dipping down between its *sulci*, or, an extensive pulpy disorganization of the brain, involving a large portion of one of its hemispheres.

It is not logical, upon *à priori* reasoning, to conclude, that such a degree of fatal organic lesion, so serious an amount of positive structural disease of the brain, could have been developing itself for *months*, and, in some cases, for *years*, without impairing, deranging, disturbing, or modifying the recognized and admitted psychical, motorial,·and sensorial functions, of the cerebro-spinal system. Has the intelligence in such cases been intact, the volition unenfeebled, the emotional powers in a sound state, the brain free from all symptoms of *physical* as well as *psychical* disturbance, the cerebral circulation (as respects the *quantity*, *quality*, and *momentum* of the blood sent to the brain) proceeding in healthy integrity; the sensibility natural, the organs of special sense, viz., *sight*, *smell*, *hearing*, *taste*, and *touch*, in a normal state of activity; the life of relation, as well as the phenomena of nutritive and organic life, free from all signs of morbid derangement?

It is generally admitted, that no structural changes can originate in the heart, lungs, liver, stomach, uterus, kidneys, or bladder, without presenting, prior to death, obvious symptoms of their existence.

Tubercular disease of the lungs, hydatids of the liver, cancer of the uterus, calculus of the bladder, fatty degeneration of the kidneys, hypertrophy and valvular disease of the heart, cannot (in the majority of cases) exist without manifestly, and often seriously, disturbing the special functions of these organs. Upon what principle should the brain be an exception to the general pathological and physiological laws, regulating other organic structures?

The affections of the brain have, I maintain, undoubtedly a premonitory and precursory stage. In the majority of cases, the mischief established within the cranium, disorganizing the delicate tissue of the brain, may, upon careful examination, be detected.

There are pathognomonic and diagnostic precursory signs, which serve to guide the inquiring, diligent, observant, and intelligent eye of the practical physician, and enable him, with some degree of certainty, to discover the first scintillations of brain disease, even when the patient and those about him repudiate all idea of cerebral ill-health, and refuse to acknowledge the necessity for medical advice or treatment.

I do not affirm, that in all cases of incipient disease of the brain, the physician, even if his attention were closely riveted to the existing pathological condition, could satisfactorily diagnose its exact nature, or point out its precise locality; but he will have little or no difficulty, after carefully analyzing the case, in deciding the *general* question, whether the brain is the *seat* of disease, and the disorder, apparently referable to that organ, is of a sympathetic, or an idiopathic character?

Structural alterations may, undoubtedly, to a considerable extent; be developed in the material instrument of the mind, without, for a period, in a marked manner, interfering with the *mental, sensorial*, or *motorial* functions. This admits of a satisfactory explanation.

This disorder of the functions of the brain, in the early period of its manifestation, is of so slight and transient a character, that it is easily overlooked by the patient, as well as by his physician. An apparently unimportant knitting of the brows,—a trifling sensation of numbness in some part of the body,—a condition of general or local muscular weakness,—a state of *ennui*,—mental peevishness, irritability, and physical restlessness,—an almost inappreciable depression or exaltation of the animal spirits,—an impairment and disorder of the sense of sight,—loss, aberration, or confusion of memory,—defect in, or acute manifestation of the sense of hearing,—an inaptitude for mental work,—an inability to concentrate the attention continuously on any subject,—a state of sleeplessness, or condition of lethargy,—a trivial deviation from the usual mode of talking, such as suddenly pausing in the conversation, as if to regain a lost train of ideas,—a slight defect in the articulation, associated with a transposition of words, and inability to pronounce certain letters, *are all characteristic symptoms, frequently diagnostic of disease having commenced in the brain.*[1]

---

[1] *Vide* the interesting case of the late King of Sweden, detailed in the chapter on "The Morbid Phenomena of Attention."

How often do we discover, when the history of a serious case of brain disease is investigated, that years prior to its *apparent* development, the patient has exhibited symptoms of cerebral disorder, somewhat similar to those just detailed, which have entirely escaped observation!

Slight epileptiform seizures,—marked deviations from healthy thought,—obvious impairment of the intelligence,—occasional either *anæsthesia*, or exaltation of sensation in some part of the body,—trifling loss of motor power, and headache of an acute type, have existed for some time previously to the *supposed* commencement of the disease, and yet have entirely escaped observation, and, if recognized, been soon forgotten by the patient and his friends.

The alterations of structure so frequently observed after death on the internal table of the skull, *dura mater, pia mater, tunica arachnoidea*, and in the fibrous, as well as in the vesicular structure of the brain, are commonly the results of long-continued irritation, capillary congestion, inflammation (causing depositions of adventitious matter), *toxic* agents circulating in the blood producing modifications of cerebral nutrition, morbid changes in the coats of the bloodvessels of the brain (fatty degeneration), which have, in many cases, commenced years anteriorly to the attention being awakened to the state of this organ, and before death has revealed to the eye of the pathologist the sad extent of fatal structural disorganization that has been progressing, almost unrecognized and untreated, within the cranium.

In considering this subject, we are bound not to ignore the fact, that the brain has great powers of accommodation, and is facile to the existence of a considerable degree of organic pressure, if equally diffused, and of structural lesion, provided it be restricted to the medullary matter, and has been of slow and progressive growth; but the smallest appreciable amount of sudden extravasation of blood, the effect of the rupture of one of the minute cerebral vessels on the surface of one of the hemispheres, or on the *corpus striatum, thalami optici, pons varolii*, or *medulla oblongata*, is immediately followed either by *paralysis* or *convulsions*, and often by death itself. A considerable extent of pulpy disorganization, or softening of the cerebral structure, a large amount of fluid effused into the ventricles, a great extent of thickening and opacity of the membranes investing the encephalon, as well as large collections of encysted pus, in the shape of abscesses, may, however, exist embedded in the substance of the brain, without apparently, for a period, disordering to any marked, palpable, and serious extent, its functions. It is necessary, for a right appreciation of this subject, that we should fully recognize one of the laws regulating and governing the physiological action of the brain.

The encephalon, although admitted to be the material instrument of the mind, the seat and fountain head of sensation, the organ which takes cognizance of impressions, made either upon the peripheral extremities of the nerves, remote from the encephalon, or of those conveyed through the special senses directly to the sensorial ganglia, is, when in a state of health, insensible to any kind of stimulus, or even laceration of its substance. The brain, whilst destined to perceive acutely the painful impressions of other organs, is itself not conscious, in the incipient stage of disease, of the lesions of its own structure. Its sensibility, however, becomes most acute when its structure is diseased. Large portions of the hemispherical ganglia have been removed by the knife, and have even sloughed away, without giving rise to any appreciable disturbance of cerebral phenomena, pain, or obvious inconvenience; but any injury, however, inflicted upon the *sensorial ganglia*, whether the result of a morbid process, or artificial irritation, is invariably followed by great cerebral disorder, and unequivocal disturbance of their special functions.[1]

---

[1] As to the sensibility in those parts of the brain supposed to be the seat of the intellectual faculties, Sir Charles Bell observes, that we ought not to expect the same phenomena to result from the cutting or tearing of the brain as from injury done to the nerves. The function of the latter is to transmit sensation; that of the former is higher, and this is inferred from its being insensible. "If, on examining the structure of the brain," says this eminent physiologist, "we find a part consisting of white medullary striæ, and fasciculated like a nerve, we should conclude that, as the use of the nerve is to transmit sensation, such tracts of matter are media of communication connecting parts of the brain. If masses are found in the brain unlike the matter of the nerves, and which yet occupy a place guarded as an organ of importance, and holding evidently important relations, we may presume that such parts have uses different from that of merely conveying sensation; we may rather look upon such as the seat of the higher powers. I have found," continues the same authority, "at different times all the internal parts of the brain diseased, without loss of sense, but I have never seen disease general on the *surface of the hemispheres without derangement of the mind.* If I be correct in this view of the subject, then the experiments made upon the brain tend to confirm the conclusions which I should be inclined to draw from anatomy, viz., that the cineritious and superficial parts of the brain are the seat of the intellectual functions."

The physiological physician has no difficulty in predicating the immediate effect of an alteration in the structure of, or mechanical pressure upon the *thalami optici, pons varolii, corpora quadrigemina,* or *medulla oblongata.* The functions, as well as pathology of these and other ganglia, are well ascertained, and fully established.

When referring to this subject, a distinguished physiologist says: "Considered theoretically, we should expect that the sentient fibres, which proceed from the *medulla oblongata,* and expand themselves in all parts of the greater and lesser brain, would bestow on these formations, as well as upon the *medulla oblongata,* a high degree of sensibility. But experience gives results for which a satisfactory explanation is still entirely deficient; thus, if the cerebral hemispheres be laid bare in a mammal or bird, an operation which in itself in no degree destroys the capability of perceiving pain, we find that they can be touched and even transfixed without in the least disturbing the animal; it only struggles and cries out when the trifacial nerve, the crura cerebri, the optic thalami, or the medulla oblongata, are accidentally touched. Again, if the hemispheres be removed by slices down to the centrum ovale, or to the cavity of the lateral ventricle, the animal remains as indifferent as if we were cutting a hair or a nail. The same phenomena have also been repeatedly observed in man; thus, a portion of the hemisphere projecting through a wound of the skull has been removed without producing any action; and, again, parts of the substance of the hemisphere have been taken away by the surgeon in removing pus or foreign bodies without the patient's consciousness."[1]

This sad neglect of well-marked symptoms of brain disorder may, to a degree, arise from the fact, that the abnormal mental state of the patient is, in many cases, viewed in the light of healthy exaggerations, eccentricities, or extravagances of natural conditions of thought. It is difficult for some to understand the important physiological principle, that disturbed intelligence has the same relation to the brain that disordered respiration has to the lungs, pleura, and heart. The importance of detecting the earliest symptoms of approaching or existing disease of the brain cannot,

[1] "Lehrbuch der Physiologie des Menschen." Band 11. Von Dr. G. Valentin. P. 743.

in a practical point of view, be over-estimated or exaggerated.
Considering the peculiar and special functions of this organ, and
the close sympathy established between the sensorium, and other
organic tissues; appreciating how slight, minute, and infinitesimal
a degree of structural change in the nerve vesicle paralyzes both
body and mind, we can have no difficulty in estimating the value
which should attach to the detection, at the earliest possible
period, of the faintest scintillation of any actual disease existing
in the delicate nervous organization.

How cautiously, zealously, and closely should the physician
watch for the incipient dawnings of cerebral mischief! Who can
guarantee the integrity of the intelligence, normal condition of the
sensibility, and healthy action of the motor power, if the delicate
vesicular structure is the seat of morbid action? Is it not possible
to predicate with certainty the result of neglected inflammation of
the periphery of the brain? We should never lose sight of the
fact, that no irritation or inflammatory action can exist for any
length of time in the more important tissues, or ganglia of the
brain, without seriously perilling the reason, and endangering life!

How forcibly do these observations apply to the detection of the
incipient symptoms of all types and degrees of mental disorder!
It is a well-established fact, that *seventy*, if not *eighty*, per cent.
of cases of insanity admit of easy and speedy cure, if treated in
the early stage, provided there be no strong constitutional predisposition to cerebral and mental affections, or existing cranial mal-
formation; and even when an hereditary taint exists, derangement
of mind generally yields to the steady and persevering administration of therapeutic agents, combined with judicious moral measures, provided the first scintillations of the malady are fully
recognized, and, without loss of time, grappled with, by remedial
treatment.

A vast and frightful amount of chronic and incurable insanity
exists at this moment, within the precincts of our county and
private asylums, which can be clearly traced to the criminal neglect
of the disease in the first or incipient stage. It is at this period
when so much may be effected in preventing those destructive
alterations in the structure and membranes of the brain, so often
witnessed after death, in those who die of chronic mental alienation.

In the third report of the *Hanwell County Lunatic Asylum for*

1833, *Sir William Ellis*, the then resident Superintending Physician of the institution, thus speaks of the sad consequences that result from the neglect of recognizing and treating insanity in its early stage :—

"It is a melancholy fact, that, on a most careful personal examination of each of the 558 cases now in the house, there do not appear more than 50 who, under the most favorable point of view, can be considered curable. *This is to be attributed almost entirely to the neglect of proper remedies in the early stages of the disease.* To become acquainted with the symptoms first indicating it, not only requires much care and attention, but much experience; for a diseased action of the brain, or some part of the nervous system, may be gradually undermining the health, and still be scarcely suspected by common observers to exist, from the insidious manner in which it steals upon the constitution at first: it manifests itself by some trifling aberration of intellect, and that very generally on one point only; such aberration, if unaccompanied by bodily pain, is not only neglected by the sufferers, but disregarded by those around them. This, however, is precisely the time when medical aid is the most capable of being beneficial; and could the patients but be placed under proper care then, certainly three-fourths of them would be cured. But, unfortunately, the golden opportunity is too often neglected. DISEASED ACTION *is allowed to proceed unchecked until* DISEASED ORGANIZATION *has taken place, and the patient has become incurable;* and it is only in consequence of the commission of some violent outrage that he is at last sent to an asylum. Until something serious has occurred, the friends hope in a few days the mind will recover its tone.

"Unfortunately, this unwillingness to consider the patient sufficiently insane to be sent to an asylum is not confined to the friends of the patient. There have been instances of the magistrates themselves, from the kindest motives, refusing to grant warrants for the admission of a patient, even after he has been examined by a medical gentleman, who has given a certificate of his insanity, because when brought before them he has been able to answer certain questions correctly. The consequence is, that from this delay, instead of returning to his friends in a few weeks, which, in all probability, would have been the case if proper medical and moral remedies had at once been applied, he becomes incurable, and remains in the asylum for life, a burden to the parish. In some instances similar delay has been attended with fatal consequences.

" It is sincerely hoped that the knowledge of these circumstances will induce an early application to be made for the admission of patients ; as, even if the neglect does not prove fatal, it is contrary to every principle of justice and humanity that a fellow-creature deranged, perhaps only on one point, should, from the want of the early attention of those whose duty it is to watch over him, linger out his existence separated from all who are dear to him, and condemned, without any crime, to be a prisoner for life."

In the premonitory stage of insanity, the gray portion of the hemispherical ganglia is frequently in a state of capillary congestion. This pathological condition I may remark, without anticipating what I have to say on the subject of the medical treatment of the incipient symptoms of cerebral and mental affections, is easily dealt with, and the further progress of the disease arrested by therapeutic measures. A few leeches and cold applications to the head, particularly in young persons of plethoric habit, active purgation, quietude, and freedom from all excitement, physical and mental ; counter-irritation to the head, the administration of the tartrate of antimony, and the judicious exhibition of opium after the local congestion has been relieved, and the secretions brought into a healthy condition, will, in eighty per cent. of cases, cure the patient, and arrest the further progress of the mischief.

In a certain type of case, the brain, in the early stages of insanity, is in an *anæmic* condition, and the vital and nerve force but feebly manifested. In these cases, our sheet-anchor is undoubtedly opium in its various formulæ, generous diet, and blood tonics. But I must not anticipate what I have to advise in its proper place for the medical treatment of insanity.

" The importance or rather necessity of recognizing disorders of the head in their *early* stage," says Dr. F. Hawkins, "is obvious from the consideration that they can then alone be attacked with any chance of success. In acute cases, the period is brief indeed in which the power of art is available. But whether the case be acute or chronic, it is only in the early stage that its precise nature admits of being distinguished with accuracy. In its further progress, from the extensive sympathies of the brain with all parts of the body, so many functions become implicated, and so various are the symptoms which arise, as to preclude arrangement or classification, and defy the art of diagnosis. The aid which in most other cases the sensations of the patient are capable of affording us is lost to us too soon in disorders of the head, until in their advanced state they all resemble one another, and present alike a dreary abolition of the powers of animal life. The period therefore is highly precious in which these affections admit of being distinguished with precision or treated with any hope of advantage."[1]

Let the physician then estimate, in all its vital importance, the grave necessity for prompt treatment and decisive remedial measures, when satisfied that the enemy is at the gates, and has attacked, or, is on the eve of assaulting, the citadel! Under these circumstances, hesitation, delay, or procrastination in bringing the patient within the range of curative measures, is fraught with the direst results, and with the saddest consequences. Let us not wilfully close our eyes to the premonitory signs, however apparently insignificant, slight, transient, and fugitive they may appear, of actual mental disorder and brain disease, for it is in this early stage when so much may be effected by judicious medical treatment to obstruct the advance of the fatal cerebral mischief.

Having dwelt at some length on the existence of a precursory stage in all affections of the brain, and on the importance of watching for the first threatenings of incipient cerebral disorder, I propose to investigate, in detail, the general character of the premonitory symptoms of encephalic, and mental disease. It will be well, however, to premise, that I cannot, in this work, do more than generalize on this wide and expansive subject.

When I address myself, in the succeeding volume, to the consideration of *specific types* of brain disease, it will be my object to enter more elaborately into detail, and to point out, as far as practicable, the diagnostic premonitory signs of the various organic affections of the encephalon. Many of the symptoms to which I shall refer as valid evidences of incipient brain disorder will be found common to several lesions of this organ, each presenting an essentially different aggregate group of symptoms, as well as distinctive anatomical, and pathological phenomena.

Nevertheless, I am of opinion, that a *general* description or

[1] Croonian Lectures, delivered before the College of Physicians, May, 1829, by Francis Hawkins, M.D.

resumé of the incipient signs of morbid conditions of the brain, before considering individual forms of cerebral disease, will not be without its practical value and importance. Agreeably to this arrangement, I propose to analyze the subject in the following order :—

1. *Morbid Phenomena of Intelligence.*
2. *Morbid States of Motion.*
3. *Morbid Conditions of Sensation.*

This classification of the subject fully recognizes the three physiological functions of the cerebro-spinal system, *viz. :—*

α. Thought.   *β. Motion.*   *γ. Sensation.*

4. *Morbid Phenomena of the Special Senses.*

Viz.: δ. Sight.   *η. Touch.*
    ε. Hearing.   *θ. Smell.*
    ζ. Taste.

5. *Morbid Phenomena of Sleep, and Dreaming.*

6. *Morbid Phenomena of Organic, or Nutritive Life.*

Viz.: α. Digestion and Assimilation.   *γ. Respiration.*
    β. Circulation.   *δ. Generation.*

7. *General Principles of Pathology, Treatment, and Prophylaxis.*

CHAPTER II.

MORBID PHENOMENA OF INTELLIGENCE.

THE brain, being the material instrument of the intelligence, the physical media through which the mind manifests its varied powers, it is in conformity with the rules of logic, and, in obedience to the laws of inductive reasoning, to infer, that no changes in its structure or investing membranes can take place, no alteration in the quality of the vital fluid, or anatomical character or calibre of the numerous bloodvessels that circulate and ramify through its substance can exist, without, to some extent, interfering with, or modifying its *psychical* functions.   Cases, however, are on record, in which serious injury has been done to the brain during life without damaging the intelligence, and considerable encephalic disorganization (as the result of disease) has taken place, no aberration, exaltation, depression, or impairment of the mind, having been observed, previously to death.   If such cases have occurred, they must be considered either of a rare and exceptional character, or, as pathological curiosities, unless in every instance, the alteration of structure is strictly confined to one hemisphere, or restricted to the fibrous, or *conducting* part of the nervous structure, the *vesicular* matter, and its minute vessels remaining intact, and entirely free from all morbid change, or abnormal modification.   Is it possible to conceive any great extent of disorganization, even in the medullary portion of the cerebral mass, to exist, without implicating, to some degree, the gray matter of the brain, and, as a consequence, deranging the phenomena of thought?

It is not my intention to discuss in this work the complex questions (physiological and metaphysical) involved in an analysis of the psycho-somatic relation or union between mind and matter, life and organization.   It is sufficient for my purpose to affirm, as a general *postulate*, that all structural lesions of the encephalon, its investing membranes and bloodvessels, are associated with some derangement, modification, or altered action of the *psychical, motorial*, or *sensorial* functions of the great cerebral ganglion (πρῶτον Αισθήτηριον) the *sensorium commune*.

Softening of the brain, abscesses, tumors, atrophy, induration, and other forms of cerebral disorganization, have, it is alleged, been discovered in the brain after death, without having disordered, or even impaired the intelligence during life.   But are not these unusual and anomalous cases?

If the mental and cerebral condition of those who have been represented to have died of organic disease of the brain, apparently in full possession of their intellectual, sensorial, and motorial powers, had been subjected to a close and rigid analysis, some degree of disorder, or impairment of these functions would, I believe, in many cases have been detected.   We are too much disposed to form hasty generalizations in these cases, and to infer, that because the patient talks rationally for a time, on ordinary subjects, is under the influence of no appreciable illusion, hallucination, or aberration, that, therefore, the intellect is unclouded, and the brain in a perfectly sound and normal state.   Such apparently healthy psychical, and cerebral manifestations, are quite consistent with the existence of encephalic disease, impairment, and even of actual latent, and concealed mental aberration.   These conditions of the brain, and mind, would, I believe, be more frequently detected, if sufficient time were devoted to their analytical investigation, and, accurate, pathological, and psychical diagnostic tests, were sufficiently employed by experts, practically acquainted with the art of examining the subtle phenomena of insanity.

It has been observed, "that could we see the interior workings of such intellects, they would be found altered, limited, perverted, or changed in some way from their normal condition, although it may not be discovered in their *external* manifestations.   It should be recollected that there are many oddities which are dependent upon cerebral conditions, but which pass for mental peculiarities; and in this way the disordered actions escape notice.   Yet *the rule* will be found logically true, that wherever there has been found the trace of organic cerebral change, there also will have been disturbed mental manifestations."

I affirm, that in every case of disease of the encephalon, particularly if the organic change or pressure be established in the vesicular matter, or in the membranes immediately investing the brain, a disordered, or abnormal state of cerebro-psychical phenomena may, in the incipient stage, on careful examination, be detected.

Having made these preliminary remarks, I proceed to the investigation of the first, or *psychical* section of the subject.

The mind may be in a state of morbid—

1. *Exaltation.*
2. *Depression.*
3. *Aberration.*
4. *Impairment.*

These conditions of unhealthy intelligence, exhibit in their origin, progress, and termination, a variety of shades and degrees of disturbance, and disease, commensurate with the nature, extent, and position of the cerebral lesion.

The state of mind, included under the head exaltation, often resembles, in its earlier manifestations, a trifling exuberance, excessive buoyancy, an unnatural elasticity, extravagance, or exhilaration of the spirits.   The patient is unusually cheerful, indulges in great volubility and violence of speech, is boisterously loquacious, and manifests phases of hysterical, emotional, and pleasurable *psychical*, as well as *physical* exaltation, rarely considered, in the early stages of diseases of the brain, and alienation of mind, to be symptomatic of morbid *cerebral*, or disordered *mental* conditions.

> " E ai volti troppo alti e repentini
> Sogliono i precipitii esser vicini."[1]—TASSO.

This unnatural, and, often *suddenly* developed flow of animal spirits, frequently merges into a state of unhealthy mental exaltation, and morbid cerebral excitement, clearly indicative of organic disease of the brain, irritation, congestion, or inflammation of its investing membranes, unhealthy blood poisoning the encephalic mass, disordered states of nerve nutrition, retained excretions, or, disturbed conditions of the cerebral circulation.

[1] Our own illustrious poet thus gives expression to the same idea :—

> " These violent delights have violent ends,
> And in their triumph die."

When considering the second division of the subject, *viz.*, that of mental depression, it will be apparent that this phase of mental disorder often ranges, from mere listlessness, slight degrees of depression of spirits, tædium vitæ (the "*atra cura*" of Horace), and ennui, to profound conditions of despondency, despair, and acute melancholia, frequently urging its unhappy victim to the commission of suicide.[1]

It is in this state of insane thought, that a terrible struggle occasionally ensues, between an intensely morbid, and often, irresistible impulse to suicide, and the natural instinct of love of life, and self-preservation, as well as antagonistic principles of worldly prudence, religion, and morality, that are occasionally happily seen to retain a mastery, and exercise a controlling influence over the mind, goaded on by disease, to self-destruction.

In the morbid mental affections included under the heads of, aberration and impairment, are observed various gradations (blending almost imperceptibly with each other) of psychical disorder,

---

[1] It is a fallacy to suppose, a state of *ennui* to be one of *brain* rest, and *psychical* inactivity. It is, in many cases, an active condition of the mind, unaccompanied by the pleasurable, and, consequently, healthy gratification, usually associated with ordinary phases of intellectual labor, and emotional excitement. "In life," says Pascal, "we always believe that we are seeking repose, while, in reality, all that we seek is agitation." "Is," says Sir W. Hamilton, "the '*far niente*'—is that doing nothing in which so many find so sincere a gratification, in reality a negation of activity, and not in truth itself an activity intense and varied? To do nothing in this sense is simply to do nothing irksome, nothing difficult, nothing fatiguing, especially to do no outward work. But is the mind internally the while unoccupied and inert? This, on the contrary, may be vividly alive; may be intently engaged in the spontaneous play of imagination; and so far, therefore, in this case, from pleasure being the concomitant of inactivity, the activity is, on the contrary, at once vigorous and unimpeded. * * * * Ennui is a state in which we find nothing on which to exercise our powers; but ennui is a state of pain. All energy, all occupation, is either play or labor. In the former, the energy appears as free and spontaneous; in the latter, as either compulsorily put forth, or its exertion so impeded by difficulties that it is only continued by a forced and painful effort, in order to accomplish certain ulterior ends. Under certain circumstances, play may become a labor, and labor may become play."

A mind *ennuyed*, may unconsciously be occupied in the contemplation of mentally distressing, and physically laborious and depressing thoughts. Let us, therefore, not flatter ourselves with the illusion, that a life of idleness and inactivity is necessarily one of repose, rest, and freedom from painfully-perturbed thoughts. How true it is—

"A want of occupation gives no rest;
A mind quite vacant, is a mind distressed."

and weakness, extending from the shadowy forms of false perception, erroneous judgment, paralyzed volition, perversions of the
moral sense, derangement and confusion of thought, to positive
hallucinations, and clearly manifested insane delusions ; and from
brain-fag, cerebral lassitude, loss of mental stamina, tone, weakened memory (*dysmnesia*), actual loss of memory (*amnesia*), and
flagging powers of attention, to obvious states of imbecility and
idiocy.

In analyzing the precursory symptoms of cerebro-psychical disease, it will be important to remember, that the earliest signs of
appreciable deviation from mental health, often resemble, in a remarkable degree, temporary and transient exaggerations of natural and healthy conditions, or states of mind, the first symptoms
of the psychical affection being recognized by certain marked deviations from ordinary phases of *thouyht*, and normal modes of
action, or *conduct*.

CHAPTER III.

PREMONITORY SYMPTOMS OF INSANITY.

This subject is too important and comprehensive to be analyzed at any length in a work which professes to embody only an *outline* of incipient morbid *cerebral* and *psychical* phenomena.

This section will be considered in the following order :—

1. *Anomalous and masked affections of the mind.*
2. *Stage of consciousness.*
3. *Exaltation of mind.*
4. *Depression of mind.*
5. *Aberration of mind.*
6. *Impairment and loss of mind.*

This classification of the phenomena of disordered thought will embrace the more prominent and salient points connected with the subject of incipient insanity.

Previously, however, to my considering any one of the preceding sections, I propose to discuss cursorily,

1. *The present limited knowledge of the physiology of the nervous system, and ignorance of the phenomena of mind and life.*
2. *Analogy between insanity and dreaming.*
3. *State of the mind, when passing into a condition of alienation, as deduced from the written confessions of patients after recovery.*
4. *Morbid phenomena of thought, as manifested during the states of transition and convalescence from attacks of insanity.*

In order to obtain a right appreciation of the mind in its incipient, as well as matured conditions of disorder, it will be requisite for the psychological physician to analyze with metaphysical exactness, and scientific, medical precision, the intellect, when in the

preceding states of unhealthy manifestation. These are four philosophical *points d'appui* in this important inquiry, and if elaborately
and faithfully investigated, a clearer insight may yet be obtained
of morbid psychical phenomena, hitherto deemed very obscure, if
not altogether inexplicable.

Before proceeding to an analysis of the premonitory symptoms
of the various types and phases of mental and cerebral disorder,
it will be well to refer to the following important preliminary interrogatories : they suggest themselves as prefatory or starting-
points in this inquiry. What is insanity ? Is its nature known ;
its essence discovered ; the laws governing its phenomena understood ? What is the constitution of its *materies morbi ;* the exact
condition of the moral and intellectual faculties, emotions, instincts,
or passions, during, to use the significantly suggestive language of
Coleridge, "the mind's own revolt upon itself ?" In what does
mental derangement consist ? Is it an affection of the moral, intellectual, emotional, or perceptive faculties, and are the reason,
judgment, comparison, memory, and imagination most implicated
in the malady ? Is there a type of insanity manifesting itself more
in *conduct* than in the *ideas ?* What is the nature, where the seat
of the alienation of mind ? In which of the mental faculties does the
disease commence its ravages, and where is the precise position, in
the brain, of the latent insane *nidus* or germ ?[1]

---

[1] The subjoined poetical description of insanity was written by a lunatic confined
in the State Asylum, *Utica,* U.S.A. It is interesting as proceeding from the pen of a
man in an unquestionable state of mental derangement.

> "A maniac !
> Know ye the meaning of that word,
> Ye who of health and reason art possessed ?
>   Can ye scan
> The tumult raging in the inner man ?
> Couldst thou draw aside the curtain
> That doth envelope his distracted soul,
> And see behind it, what he doth conceive is real,
> Then mightst thou see him scorched
> 'Pon bars of iron, heated red by fire,
> Enkindled 'neath them. On every side
> Are those, whose office 'tis (it so doth seem to him)
> To see it is not quenched. Should this delusion leave him,
> His poor distracted soul will, by some new fear,
> Be tempest tossed. Then will he fancy
> Everything that he doth see or hear,

Has insanity a *centrifugal* or a *centripetal*, a subjective or an objective origin? In less technical phraseology, do the disordered ideas of the insane depend upon *centric* causes of irritation and disease, operating from within to without, or are they the consequences of *eccentric* or objective influences, acting from without to within; in other words, are we to consider the symptoms of mental alienation, as emanations from the brain, similar in character (to borrow an appropriate image) to the "rays of light proceeding from a body which is itself ignited," or are they analogous to the rays reflected from a polished surface, in intimate organic sympathy with disordered action established in a remote part of the body?

Is insanity an affection of the mind *per se?* Has the disease a psychical or a somatic origin? Is it possible for thought, in the abstract, to be diseased, independently of images occupying the consciousness? Does alienation of mind depend not exclusively upon a psychical or somatic cause, but upon a disturbance in the normal *relations* existing (in states of cerebral and mental health) between the mental and physical functions of the brain?

Before endeavoring to solve these subtle and abstruse psychological problems, it will be necessary to ask what is mind? Have we any knowledge of its *nature*, clue to its *seat*, accurate idea as to its mode of *action*, or anything approximating to a right conception of its essence? What are the modifications, the metamorphoses, organic or functional, which the vital principle and nerve-force undergo, during their passage through the exquisitely organized, and highly vascular cineritious, or vesicular brain structure?

How does the occult mental principle, believed by physiologists to be evolved or eliminated in the *gray* matter of the brain, become so mysteriously and marvellously changed from *nerve* to *mental* force, and *vice versa*, in the hemispherical ganglia? Is the

> And cannot comprehend, is but some method
> To destroy or harm him.
> Thou canst not know nor feel,
> O ye, whom God hath blessed with reason,
> A tithe of what he suffers:
> For thus to know or feel,
> Thou must become, like him,
>   A maniac!"

Asylum, Utica, N. Y.   J. M. B.

development of psychical phenomena the result of what is termed a correlation of the two preceding modes of dynamical action, or is mind a new creation, essence, principle, or power, organized or elaborated in the vesicular portions of the cerebral mass ?

What is the nature of the *vis nervosa* of Haller ? Is the brain a galvanic battery, and are the nerves constituted, for the transmission of impressions, like electric wires ? Is the mysterious and undefinable "fluid," or " force," circulating in the nerve tubes, a voltaic current ? in other words, a principle identical with that of electricity, or one in its essence, origin, and operations, entirely *sui generis ?* What is the *vis vitæ*, and how is it associated with and dependent upon organized structures ? What are the relations between the intellectual and vital manifestations ? Are not all these great problems of organic and psychical life still, with physiologists, *sub judice ?*[1] Have we arrived at any exact knowledge of the substratum of nervous matter ? Are we not obliged to confess our ignorance of the ultimate principles of vitality, as well as of intelligence ? Do we know anything of their nature or essence ? Is not our knowledge of mental as well as of vital phenomena, entirely confined to an acquaintance with these powers, as *manifested* during life ?[2] If our ignorance of healthy psychical

---

[1] Speaking of the mysterious union of mind and matter, St. Austin says :—

" Materium spiritumque cognoscendo ignorari et ignorando cognosci."

" Man is to himself the mightiest prodigy in nature, for he is unable to conceive what is body, still less what is mind; but least of all is he able to conceive how a body can be united to a mind ; yet this is his proper being."—(Pascal.) " A contented ignorance," says Sir W. Hamilton, when referring to this subject, " is indeed wiser than a presumptuous knowledge ; but this is a lesson which seems the last that philosophers are willing to learn. In the words of one of the acutest of modern thinkers, ' Magna immo maxima pars sapientiæ est quædam æquo nescire velle.' "

[2] " The notion we annex to the words matter and mind," says Reid, " is merely relative. If I am asked what I mean by matter, I can only explain myself by saying it is that which is extended, figured, colored, movable, hard, rough and smooth, hot or cold—that is, I can define it in no other way than by enumerating its sensible qualities. It is not matter or body which I perceive by my senses, but only extension, figure, color, and certain other qualities which the constitution of my nature leads me to refer to something which is extended, figured, and colored. The case is precisely similar with respect to mind. We are not immediately conscious of its existence, but we are of sensation, thought, volition—operations which imply the existence of something which feels, thinks, wills."

Sir Isaac Newton was asked why he stepped forward when he was so inclined, and from what cause his arm obeyed his will ? He honestly replied that he knew

conditions is so profound, is it practicable for the psychological inquirer to arrive at an accurate acquaintance of mind when disturbed and disordered by disease? Have not all the efforts that have hitherto been made to solve the mystery connected with alienation of thought, proved utterly unproductive of any scientific results? Is there any theory of insanity yet propounded from the bench, taught in the schools, or registered in our textbooks, which will bear the test of metaphysical analysis, or stand the ordeal of strict medical or legal criticism? Distinguished philosophers, experienced psychological physicians, accurate and profound logicians, have in vain attempted to analyze, unveil, and penetrate into the hidden nature of this disease, with a view of discovering a key to its accurate definition. The pursuit, it must be admitted, has hitherto signally failed. Let us then, with a spirit of humility, fully acknowledge the extent of our ignorance of subtle abnormal mental phenomena, as well as our limited knowledge of the healthy constitution of the human mind.

" We sometimes," says an eminent philosophical writer, "repine at the narrow limits prescribed to human capacity: 'hitherto shalt thou come and no further,' seems a hard prohibition, when applied to the operations of the mind. But, as in the material world, it is to this prohibition man owes his security and existence, so, in the immaterial system, it is to this we owe our dignity, our virtue, and our happiness. A beacon blazing from a well-known promontory is a welcome object to the bewildered mariner, who is so far from repining that he has not the beneficial light in his own keeping, that he is sensible its utility depends on its being placed on the firm land, and committed to the care of others."[1]

nothing about the matter. If we were to follow the example of this great philosopher, and modestly admit our ignorance of those subjects about which we really have no knowledge, we should have a just conception of the shallow pretensions of man. No undertaking would, perhaps, prove more beneficial to mankind, than that which endeavored to draw a correct line of demarcation between what is really known and that which is merely conjecture.

Our notion of the nature of mind is as limited as our knowledge of material substances. " When we wish to have a rude knowledge of a piece of metal," says a great French philosopher, " we put it on the fire in a crucible; but have we any crucible wherein to put the soul? Is it spirit? says one; but what is spirit? Assuredly no one knows. This is a word so void of meaning, that, to tell what spirit is, you are obliged to say what it is not. The soul is matter, says another; but what is matter? We know nothing of it but a few appearances and properties; and not one of these properties, not one of these appearances, bear the least affinity to thought."

[1] " Essay on the Nature and Immutability of Truth," p 79, by James Beattie, LL.D.

Dr. Reid, when referring to the limited nature of our knowledge, and the difficulties attendant upon the investigation of psychical, as well as somatic phenomena, observes: "The labyrinth may be too intricate, and the thread too fine to be traced through all its windings, but if we stop where we can trace it no farther, and secure the ground we have gained, there is no harm done: a quicker eye may in time trace it farther."

It would be foreign to the design of this work, were I to institute a psychological and pathological investigation of the mind, when in a state of fully-developed insanity. This is a profound and intricate subject. Its vast importance entitles it to separate and undivided consideration. I propose, therefore, to reserve any exposition I have to make in reference to it for another occasion. It will then be my duty to analyze in detail the mind, in its simple and complex morbid types of alienation, and to consider, as far as practicable, the nature of those deviations, from normal psychosomatic conditions, observed in certain forms of mental disorder. Important as I consider this section of the subject, it does not exceed in interest or value, the careful study of the points which I have suggested for further psychological examination.

I refer to the condition of the mind in the incipient stage of disorder, when *passing into* one of its numerous phases of disease, and to its state when *emerging out* of a *morbid*, into one of *healthy* thought. It is by pursuing a *deductive* as well as an *inductive* course of psychological inquiry; in other words, proceeding from the consideration of universals to particulars, and particulars to universals, thus ascertaining (to use the technical language of the schools) the relation in which the antecedent stands to the subsequent, and *vice versa ;* it is by the adoption of a rigid process of analysis, as well as of synthesis, in relation to the insane *element*, or *germ* evolved during the stage of incubation, as well as by a careful study of the laws governing the general operations of the mind, at the approach of convalescence, and during the process of cure, that we shall be enabled to appreciate (if such a result be at all practicable) the character and state of the intellect when reduced to an automatic condition, and deprived by disease of its powers of healthy co-ordination.[1]

[1] The laws governing the operations of thought, or which produce that co-ordination of the various states of mind, so essential to a healthy equilibrium of the understanding, are supposed by Cousin, after Aristotle, to be in their nature *impersonal*.

Without attempting to elaborate a special theory of insanity, I cannot refrain from directing attention, *en passant*, to the close resemblance that obtains, between many forms of mental alienation, and the state of the brain and mind, during the conditions of sleep and dreaming.

The many singular facts recorded in this volume, with a view of elucidating the subject of incipient insanity, as well as of obscure diseases of the brain, constitute, according to my apprehension, striking illustrations, good and valid evidence, of the remarkable analogy existing between these psychical phenomena.

How accurately does Sir W. Hamilton describe the transition state of the mind, between sleeping and waking, and how closely does it correspond with the condition of the intellect, during the

They are considered by metaphysicians, to act independently of the knowledge acquired by experience, and are designated, by Sir W. Hamilton and other authorities, as native mental cognitions, and primary conditions of intelligence. This constitutes what the same authority terms the " regulative" or " legislative" faculty, and is said to correspond with the Aristotelian phrases Noῦς—ιοῦς (*intellectus, mens*), as well as the term " reason," as used by the early English philosophers, and *vernunft*, as adopted by Kant, Jacobi, and other German metaphysicians. . The Regulative faculty is analogous in its effects to that subtle principle or force evolved in the cerebellum, which establishes a unity of action in, and adjusts, harmonizes, and co-ordinates the varied muscular movements of the body. There is a *psychical* as well as a *physical* chorea, or St. Vitus's dance, in which the patient is not under the influence of any fixed or transient delusion. In these cases the insanity appears to depend upon a *disordered state of the psychical co-ordinating power* (eliminated, in all probability, in the *cerebrum*), and paralysis of what may be designated the *executive*, or, to adopt the phraseology of Sir William Hamilton, " regulative" and " legislative" faculties of the mind.

The patients so affected deal in the most inexplicably absurd combinations of ideas. Filthy ejaculations, horrible oaths, blasphemous expressions, wild denunciations of hatred, revenge, and contempt, allusions the most obscene, are often singularly intermingled with the most exalted sentiments of love, affection, virtue, purity, and religion. United to the impassioned, fervent, and pious appeals to the Deity, clothed in appropriate, eloquent, and unexceptionable language, are phrases of a truly diabolical character, and frantic imprecations that cannot be listened to without exciting a feeling allied to terror in the breasts of those whose painful duty it is to observe such sad exhibitions of poor fallen and degraded human nature. I have known patients whilst suffering from this *choreic* type of insanity, alternately to spit, coax, bite, caress, beat, kiss, vilify, and praise those near them ; and to utter one moment sentiments that would do honor to the most orthodox of divines, and immediately afterwards use language only expected to proceed from the mouths of the most depraved of human beings ! This phase of mental alienation is often seen unassociated with any form of delusion, hallucination, or illusion. It is generally (in women) connected with some obscure irritation and disease of the uterine system.

stage of incubation, when the mind, losing its sane consciousness of objects, approaches the confines of mental alienation? When roused from the transition state (intermediate between sleeping and waking), we find, says Sir W. Hamilton, " ourselves conscious of being in the commencement of a dream; the mind is occupied with a train of thought, and this train we are still able to follow out to a point when it connects itself with certain actual perceptions. We can still trace imagination to sense, and show how, departing from the last sensible impressions of real objects, the fancy proceeds in its work of distorting, falsifying, and perplexing these, in order to construct out of their ruins its own grotesque edifices."

In dreaming, as in certain forms of disordered mind, phases of intellectual vigor, and states of mental acuteness are developed, which were not normal manifestations during the waking hours, and were not known to exist, in conditions of healthy thought. The most exquisite creations of the poetic fancy have been engendered under these circumstances, and conceptions suggested to the dreamy consciousness, which have paved the road to fame and fortune. During the hours of sleep, the intellect has, with rapid facility, solved subtle questions, which had puzzled and perplexed the mind when in full and unfettered exercise of its waking faculties. Difficult mathematical problems; knotty and disputed questions in the science of morals; abstruse points of philosophy, have (according to accredited testimony) found their right solution during the solemn darkness of night, and periods of profound sleep.[1]

---

[1] " Strictly speaking," says Rosenkrantz, " intellectual problems are not solved in dreams, because intense thought is without images, whereas dreaming is a creation of images. I perfectly recollect having dreamt of such problems, and, being happy in their solution, endeavored to retain them in my memory. I succeeded, but on awaking discovered that they were quite unmeaning, and could only have imposed upon a sleeping imagination."

Insanity is said to be a " waking dream," with this difference, the madman's conduct (as a general principle) is in correspondence with the delirious suggestions of his disordered, unbridled, and uncontrolled fancy. If every person were, as Cicero says, to carry practically into operation the ideas that enter the mind during the act of dreaming, it would be necessary, before going to sleep, mechanically to restrain all power of motion. " Majores enim quam ulli insani efficerent motus somniantes."— (" De Divinatione," 59.)

" If," says Pascal, " we dreamt every night the same things, it would perhaps affect us as powerfully as the objects which we perceive every day. And if an artisan

Sir Isaac Newton is alleged to have solved a subtle mathematical problem whilst sleeping, and Condorcet recognized in his dreams the final steps in a difficult calculation which had puzzled him during the day.

Condillac says, that when engaged in his " *Cours d'Etude*" he frequently developed and finished a subject in his dreams which he had broken off before retiring to rest.

Coleridge's poetical fragment, " Kubla Khan," was composed during sleep which had come upon him whilst reading the passage in " Purchas's Pilgrim," on which the poetical description was founded, and was written down immediately on awaking ; " the images rising up before him as things with a parallel production of the correspondent expressions without any sensation or consciousness of effort."[1]

In dreaming, the mind is occupied with the incongruous conceptions and fantastic combinations of images, so characteristic of many conditions of disordered intellect. There is also a similar want in the coherence of ideas, one conception following another, and this succeeded rapidly by a *series* of mental impressions, in opposition to all the legitimate laws governing associated thought. There is also a complete paralysis of the will, or subjective phenomena, this faculty exercising no controlling influence over the train of suggested ideas.[2]   In the act of dreaming, the most trivial

---

were certain of dreaming every night for twelve hours that he was a king, I am convinced that he would be almost as happy as a king who dreamt for twelve hours that he was an artisan.   If we dreamt every night that we were pursued by enemies, and harassed by horrible phantoms, we should suffer almost as much as if that were true, and we should stand in as great dread of sleep as we should be of waking, had we real cause to apprehend these misfortunes.   It is only because dreams are different and inconsistent, that we can say when we awake, that we have dreamt, for life is a dream a little less inconsistent."—(As quoted by Sir William Hamilton, in his " Lectures on Metaphysics.")

[1] " Carpenter's Physiology," p. 643.

[2] In states of imperfect sleep—conditions existing midway between wakefulness and profound cerebral and psychical repose—the will does not appear altogether to be suspended in its operations.   DUGALD STEWART has commented upon this fact. He observes, when referring to the phenomenon, " It may be proper to remark, that, if the suspension of our voluntary operations in sleep is admitted as a fact, there are only two suppositions which can be formed concerning its cause.   The one is, that the power of volition is suspended; the other, that the will loses its influence over those faculties of the mind, and those members of the body, which during our waking hours are subject to its authority.   If it can be shown that the former supposition is

circumstances give a decided character and direction to the current of thought. The application of a bottle of hot water to the feet of a person whilst sleeping, has given origin to the impression that he was walking on the crater of a volcano; and upon a blister being applied to the head, under similar states of mind, it suggested to the person an idea that he was being scalped by Indians. Any sudden noise occurring in the immediate neighborhood, or within hearing of the dreamer, will in many cases originate in the mind an idea of being exposed to the crushing effect of a terrible avalanche, or suggest the notion that he is wandering over some dreary moor during a fearful hurricane. In many instances, in a dream that has not continued beyond a minute, or even a second, the events of a long and chequered life have elaborately, and in their minutest relation, occurred to the mind, and in the smallest appreciable period of time, an eventful history, full of remarkable incidents, has, in the imagination of the person, taken place.

The rapidity of mental action occurring in dreams, where events, which in their actual development would occupy hours, days, nay, even years, are compressed and comprehended sometimes in a few minutes, or even seconds, is finely illustrated in the dream of Count Lavalette. "One night," he says, "while I was asleep, the clock of the Palais de Justice struck twelve, and awoke me. I heard the gate open to relieve the sentry, but I fell asleep again immediately. In this sleep I dreamed that I was standing in the Rue St. Honoré, at the corner of the Rue de l'Echelle. A melancholy darkness spread around; all was still. Nevertheless, a low and uncertain sound soon arose. All of a sudden I perceived, at the bottom of the street, and advancing towards me, a troop of cavalry; the men and horses, however, all flayed. The men held torches in their hands, the flames of which illuminated

not agreeable to the fact, the truth of the latter seems to follow as a necessary consequence.

"That the power of volition is not suspended during sleep appears from the efforts which we are conscious of making while in that situation. We dream, for example, that we are in danger; and we call out for assistance. The attempt, indeed, is in general unsuccessful, and the sounds which we emit are feeble and indistinct; but this only confirms, or rather is a necessary consequence of, the supposition, that in sleep the connection between the will and our voluntary operations is disturbed or interrupted. The continuance of the power of volition is demonstrated by the effort, however ineffectual."—("Philosophy of the Human Mind.")

4

faces without skin, and with bloody muscles. Their hollow eyes rolled in their large sockets, their mouths opened from ear to ear, and helmets of hanging flesh covered their hideous heads. The horses dragged along their own skins in the kennels, which over-flowed with blood on both sides. Pale and dishevelled women appeared and disappeared alternately at the windows in dismal silence; low, inarticulate groans filled the air, and I remained in the street alone, petrified with horror, and deprived of strength sufficient to seek my safety in flight. This horrible troop con-tinued passing in full gallop, and casting frightful looks on me. Their march, I thought, continued for five hours, and they were followed by an immense number of artillery wagons, full of bleed-ing corpses, whose limbs still quivered. A disgusting smell of blood and bitumen almost choked me. At length the iron gate of the prison, shutting with great force, awoke me again. I made my repeater strike; it was little more than midnight, so that the horrible phantasmagoria had lasted no longer than *ten minutes:* that is to say, the time necessary for relieving the sentry and shutting the gate. The cold was severe, and the watchword short. The next day the turnkey confirmed my calculations. I, nevertheless, do not remember one single event in my life the dura-tion of which I have been able more exactly to calculate."

How closely do these phenomena, resemble those automatic operations of the intellect, observed in insanity? In the latter condition, the rapidity of, as well as the loss of volitional power over, certain trains of thought, are significant and characteristic symptoms. How distressing is this lesion of the *will*,—how pain-ful are these insane, uncontrollable *impulses*,—how agonizing is this madness of the *emotions*, aberration of the *ideas*, exaltation, and perversion of the *passions!* The melancholy sound of the wind whistling among the trees, or through the lattice of the window, has originated in an insane mind, the idea of the bois-terous and wild revellings of infernal spirits, or wailing anguish, and bitter tortures, of lost souls in hell![1] The sound of thunder

---

[1] A person became insane, after listening to a sermon, in which an itinerant prea-cher thundered forth, in forcible Saxon phraseology, the fearful terrors of the law, drawing at the same time a terrible picture of the physical sufferings of the lost souls in hell. The patient, during his ravings, imagined that he was enveloped in fire and brimstone. On a dreary winter's night he was found squatting in a chimney-corner. As the wind howled over a neighboring heath, he vociferously exclaimed to those

has been suggestive to the actively morbid imagination, of the descent of a fearful avalanche, or of that awful crisis in the world's history when, to use the sublime language of Scripture, " *The heavens shall pass away with a great noise, and the elements shall melt with fervent heat, the earth also, and the works that are therein, shall be burned up.*"

Again, how often (as is established by the illustrations to be found in this work) all idea of *duration* appears to be obliterated from the mind of the insane, during the continuance of the disease, the patient appearing, after many months, and sometimes years, of sad illness, and distressing isolation, to awaken, as it were, out of a fanciful and troubled dream; the healthy ideas that had occupied the mind, a short period previously to the accession of the insanity, suggesting themselves to the consciousness, with all the freshness, vividness, and force of recently received sane impressions, contemporaneously with the restoration of reason, to its healthy supremacy.

In dreaming, as well as in some forms of mental aberration, the mind has, occasionally, a clear apprehension of its morbidly automatic condition.   A person, whilst under the influence of a series of fanciful occurrences, created by dreaming, or insanity, will, occasionally, acutely reason with himself as to the *reality of the images* occupying the attention, and be fully conscious that he is insane, or dreaming.   Dr. Johnson says, "I was often during sleep engaged in controversial discussions, and whilst recognizing that my antagonist occasionally had the best of the contest, I entirely forgot that my own arguments, as well as those advanced by my opponent, were supplied by myself!"

Even in cases of fully formed insanity, the mind has occasional gleams of healthy lucidity, and scintillations of sane consciousness, during which conditions (in accordance with the confession

---

near him, " Hark! there is the Devil, coming in his chariot to fetch me! Don't you hear his horses neigh?"

The military were in the habit, many years back, of performing their various evolutions in the immediate neighborhood of the *Salpêtrière* Lunatic Asylum, Paris. A female patient in one of the wards heard the repeated discharge of musketry. She immediately began, with great eagerness, to tear up her linen into bandages. Upon being asked, for what purpose she was destroying her clothes, she replied, " I am preparing bandages for the poor wounded soldiers."   The lunatic believed, that she was the queen, and that her right to the throne was about to be established by a battle, which was being fought near the hospital.

of patients) the lunatic fully recognizes the disordered state of his ideas, and abnormal condition of the emotions, and instincts, and makes a repeated effort to crush or dissipate the predominant morbid impression. I have often been informed by patients (after recovering from long and distressing attacks of mental derange-ment) that they have had, at varying intervals, a perfectly clear conviction of the insane character of their thoughts. These lucid moments, and transitorily sane conditions of mind, were, however, of an evanescent character, appearing like a flash of lightning across a dark and dreary heath.

In some cases of insanity, of long duration, and apparently of a chronic character, the reason has been known suddenly to be re-stored to its sovereignty, not only during the course of the malady, but immediately before death. I have witnessed some remarkable illustrations of the kind. When referring to this phenomenon, an accomplished writer observes :—

" There are few cases of mania or melancholy where the light of reason does not now and then shine between the clouds. In fevers of the mind, as well as those of the body, there occur frequent intermissions. But the mere interruption of a disorder is not to be mistaken for its cure or its ultimate conclusion. Little stress ought to be laid upon those occasional and uncertain disentangle-ments of intellect, in which the patient is for a time only extri-cated from the labyrinth of his morbid hallucinations. Madmen may show, at starts, more sense than ordinary men. There is, perhaps, as much genius confined as at large ; and he who should court coruscations of talent, might be as likely to meet with them in a receptacle for lunatics as in almost any other theatre of intel-lectual exhibition. But the flashes of wit betray too often the ruins of wisdom, and the mind which is conspicuous for the bril-liancy, will frequently be found deficient in the steadiness of its lustre.[1]

A young woman, who was employed as a domestic servant, be-came insane, and at length sunk into a state of apparently perfect dementia. In this condition, she continued many years. Late in life she had an attack of typhus fever. The physician who was in attendance upon her, was surprised to observe, that as the fever advanced, a development of the mental powers took place. During

[1] Dr. Reid's " Essays on Hypochondriasis."

the height of the fever, when delirium generally exists, this patient was entirely rational. She recognized, in the face of her medical attendant, the son of her old master, whom she had known so many years before, and she related many circumstances respecting his family, and others that had happened to herself in earlier days! But, alas! the reign of reason was but of short duration. It came like a flash of lightning across the intellectual desert, leaving behind a hopeless state of mental obscurity, and obliviousness! As the fever abated, and her bodily health returned, dark clouds again enshrouded her mind, and she sank into her former deplorable state of idiocy, and continued so for many years, until death terminated her sufferings.

CHAPTER IV.

CONFESSIONS OF PATIENTS AFTER RECOVERING FROM IN-
SANITY; OR, THE CONDITION OF THE MIND WHEN IN A
STATE OF ABERRATION.

THE autobiography of the insane, embodying a faithful record
of the state of the intellect, emotions, and instincts, whilst fading
into a condition of alienation, as well as an accurate account of
the condition of the mind after its complete subjugation by disease, proceeding from the pens of persons who have passed through
the terrible ordeal of insanity, opens a new, and profoundly interesting page, in the history of the pathology, as well as philosophy
of the human mind.

It may be asked, is it possible for the insane, accurately to describe the state of their mind, during a paroxysm of mania? Can
they have any recollection of their incoherent ramblings, wild and
fanciful imaginations, horrible and frightful hallucinations? In
many cases, such is the fact. Insanity does not invariably over-
throw, and alienate, *all* the powers of the understanding. It is
often a mixed condition, a combined state of reason and insanity.
This idea does not at all militate against the view, that I have elsewhere propounded, respecting partial insanity, using this phrase in
its strictly legal acceptation. The mind is "one and indivisible."
A part of the intellect cannot be affected, without, to a certain
extent, influencing and modifying the whole of the operations of
thought; nevertheless, there are in derangement of the mind occasional lucid moments, when the patient is conscious of his state
of disorder, and is able to describe his sensations clearly to those
about him. Again, after recovery, patients who have passed
through acute attacks of insanity, are occasionally able to recollect, with remarkable clearness, everything that occurred during
their long and painful illness. Patients, however, have frequently

very confused and incorrect notions of events that have transpired, in connection with themselves as well as with others, whilst insane. We are bound, therefore, to exercise extreme caution in admitting and acting upon evidence of this character, particularly if it materially affects the motives, and compromises the actions, of others.

With a view of analyzing the phenomena of morbid thought, I have often requested patients to detail the actual operations of the mind during the incipient, as well as advanced stages of its disorders. In many cases, I have not been able to obtain any trustworthy representation of facts; in other instances the patients could not, without considerable and painful revulsion of feeling, revert, even for a single moment, to the past. In a few instances I have had no difficulty in persuading patients not only to talk about their past condition, but to write, with great minuteness, an account of their sensations, mental and bodily, whilst insane.

I cannot, without a violation of good faith, and a breach of professional confidence, publish some of these remarkable confessions. I may, however, revert to them in general terms. Before doing so, I would briefly refer to the fallacy pervading all the poetic, dramatic, and artistic descriptions of insanity, save and excepting our own illustrious, and immortal Shakspeare, whose wonderfully truthful delineations of the different types of disordered mind, embodied in passages of rare and matchless beauty, must ever entitle him to the distinction of holding the foremost rank among the most eminent psychologists that have conferred lustre on the annals of this, or any other country.

The descriptions of insanity proceeding from the pens of novelists, as well as of poets, constitute, unquestionably, strikingly clever and graphic melodramatic sketches; but I hope the accomplished writers to whom I refer, will not be offended by my suggesting, that their portraits of insanity do not exactly correspond with the character of the disease, as exhibited in modern times. Thanks to the immortal PINEL, who effected a great revolution in the moral treatment of the insane, a lunatic asylum no longer resembles a Bastile surrounded by high serrated walls, and protected by iron-barred windows. We are not shocked at the sight of the straw bed upon which "Poor Tom" of former days was in the habit, like a wild animal, of crouching, with little or no covering to protect him from the cold, during the most inclement seasons of the year. We cease to observe the dens in which lunatics were formerly caged like ferocious beasts; we no longer witness the iron chains with which their attenuated and palsied limbs were frequently manacled. The sense of hearing is not pained by the wild and unearthly wailings of bitter anguish, caused by the whip of the keeper, as it fell unmercifully across the back of the unruly and excited patient. Thank God! Pinel, and those who have followed humbly in his wake, have given the deathblow to such brutal proceedings, and to such horrible barbarities. *Pari passû* with a liberal and enlightened recognition of the great principles of treatment which the genius of the illustrious Frenchman conceived, and boldly carried into effect, has the character of insanity been altogether deprived of many of its most painful and repulsive features. The modern principles of moral treatment, based upon kindness, gentleness, and soothing tenderness, have very materially modified the manifestations of insanity.

In estimating the circumstances that have led to the great improvement that has taken place in the condition of the insane in modern times, I am bound to refer, not only to the abolition, thanks to Dr. Conolly, of the severer forms of mechanical restraint, but to the progress made in the *pathology* as well as *therapeutics* of insanity. Compare for one moment the opinion entertained by medical men of great distinction, and of high professional eminence, who flourished and ruled despotic about sixty years ago, with the enlightened views that are, in the present day, almost universally adopted and acted upon. I refer to the principles of treatment as enunciated by the celebrated Dr. Brown (author of the "Brunonian theory" of medicine), who, for a short period, entered the arena, and successfully contested with the illustrious Dr. Cullen the sovereignty of the medical republic. Dr. Brown, when speaking of his method of curing mania, observes: "The patient should be struck with fear and terror, and driven in his state of insanity to despair. As a remedy against the great excitement of the organs of voluntary motion, the labor of draft cattle should be imposed upon him, and assiduously continued. The diet should be the poorest possible, and his drink only water. In water, as cold as possible, the patient should be immersed, and kept under it, covered all over, for a long time, till he is near killed!"

It is evident that Dr. Cullen himself entertained the most unenlightened views with regard to the treatment of insanity, for he says, when speaking of the management of lunatics, " In most cases it has appeared to be necessary to employ a very constant impression of fear to inspire them with the awe and dread of some particular persons; this awe and dread is therefore by one means or other to be acquired, sometimes it may be necessary to acquire it by STRIPES and BLOWS."[1] It is clear, that these notions were at that time generally prevalent, for I find in *Burns*[2] the following passage : " Any person may justify confining and beating his friend, *being mad*, in such manner as is proper in such circumstances." But COLLINS[3] ventures to expound much more monstrous views, in regard to the insane, than the three authorities previously mentioned, for he asserts, that "furious madmen may be legally *dispatched* by private men!" Whilst contemplating such barbarous and inhumane principles, we are not astonished to hear the solemn protest which the illustrious Lord Erskine, when Lord Chancellor, considered it necessary to make in behalf of the insane. " I consider," says this renowned judge, "the various trusts with which I am invested, in a manner, as nothing, when compared with the *sacred duty* of protecting those who are visited with mania. It is as much a disease as any other with which it pleases GOD to afflict mankind; and I am sure it is always exasperated in its symptoms, and frequently rendered incurable, by *unkind* and *rigorous* treatment."

How different are the modern views, with regard to the medical and moral treatment of insanity ! To these humanizing and enlightened principles (so successful in the cure of the malady) we may undoubtedly, in a measure, trace the great alteration that has happily been effected in the features of the disease. Kind, gentle, considerate, and affectionate treatment has disarmed insanity of many of its repulsive and most odious characteristics.

With these preliminary remarks, I proceed to a consideration of the incipient symptoms of insanity, as described by persons who have passed through the various phases of the disease.

A lady, who had been eighteen months insane, detailed to me, after her recovery, the symptoms that characterized the approach of her derangement. She informed me, that for nine months previously to her being considered mentally afflicted she was fully

[1] Dr. Cullen's " First Lines."
[2] Burns's " Justice," vol. iii, p. 311.
[3] " Essay on Human Liberty," p. 64.

aware that she was not "quite herself." She manifested extreme irritability at the most trifling circumstances. She had great difficulty in directing her attention to, and steadily occupying her mind with, any train of thought. She, to a morbid degree, secluded herself from the society of her old friends, and, to avoid all intimacy with her former associates (with whom she had never quarrelled), she left England, and resided for several months in a continental town, having little or no communication with her relatives and friends. She, however, found change of country effect no radical alteration in her feelings. Occasionally, she had sad, depressing, and melancholy forebodings as to approaching insanity. With this conviction she consulted, when in Paris, an eminent French psychological physician. At this time, she was quite able to conduct herself with great propriety, and to manage with prudence her own affairs. She was not then the subject of any insane delusion, although, at times, she had serious doubts as to her personal identity. This was the first sign of threatening alienation of intellect. On her return to England, she says: "I felt my mind much less disturbed by morbid apprehensions of insanity, and, for a period, all the absurd impressions, as to whether I was actually myself, or representing some one else, ceased to trouble me. My general health then became much out of order, and I had a severe attack of English cholera, followed by great debility, which confined me to my bed for several weeks. It was during this illness that my foolish fancies began to annoy me. At this time I used to talk out loudly to myself, a thing I never did before. This was irresistible. I ejaculated the most foolish remarks, and at times, too, with wonderful volubility of speech. I did my best to control myself, in this particular, but found it difficult to do so. I was quite conscious that my mind must be affected, and yet no delusion had taken possession of my intellect. For several days I succeeded, by strong efforts of thought, in checking this ridiculous inclination to utter absurd expressions, but I awoke one night in an excited state from a troublesome dream, and I then began to vociferate a number of most incoherent expressions, to this effect: 'You shall do it;' 'No you shan't;' 'He is like Satan;' 'Why don't you say the devil;' 'Ah! ah! ah!' 'It is beautiful;' 'No he-devils;' 'I can't be saved;' 'You have no hope;' 'Suicide;' 'Poison;' 'Hang yourself;' 'They are after you.' These strange remarks continued for nearly two hours, when I fell asleep, and arose much relieved. My mind, however, was for some time afterwards not in a right state, although I had intermissions from the misery I suffered. Eventually, I became quite insane, and, I am informed, remained so for nearly eleven months. During the whole of that time I fancied I was in hell, and tormented by evil spirits. I thought every person near me to be a devil. My mind was gradually restored to a healthy state. I cannot say when I first began to feel that I was recovering."

A gentleman, who for nine years had the command of an East Indiaman, encountered, during a voyage from Calcutta, great anxiety of mind, in consequence of a quarrel that had taken place among the passengers, and apprehensions he entertained of a mutiny occurring among the crew. A few weeks after his arrival in England he suffered from attacks of agonizing headache, and one day, whilst getting out of bed, he fell down in a fit of syncope. About a month after the attack of fainting, he became greatly depressed in spirits. This depression continued for nearly a fortnight. It was associated with a great weariness of life, and intense longing for death. He left home late one night, with the full determination of throwing himself into the London Docks, and thus putting an end to a miserable existence. When near the East India House he met an old friend, also a captain of a vessel. They recognized each other, and stood for some time in close conversation. The friend then proposed that they should adjourn to a hotel, and take some refreshment. To this suggestion an objection was raised, but upon the question being asked, as to where the gentleman was going, he became confused, and incoherent in his replies, and being pressed upon the point, burst into tears, and made a full confession of his contemplated commission of suicide. His friend then insisted upon taking him in tow, and they both proceeded to a neighboring hotel, and he subsequently saw him safely deposited in his own lodgings with his family. This mental depression continued, without any intermission, for several weeks. During this time he had no delusion. The case was, at this period, simply one of acute suicidal melancholia, accompanied by an overwhelming and apparently irresistible desire for eternal destruction.

Eventually this patient fancied that he was the subject of general remark. He arrived home one day in an unusual state of excitement, affirming that he knew certain parties were watching him in the street, and that a policeman had followed him for some distance. He then imagined that particular paragraphs in the *Times*, and skits in *Punch*, were directed against him. In about a week from this time he was acutely insane.

A professional gentleman stated, after his recovery, that for *nine* months before his wife noticed anything wrong with his mind, he was under an impression that everything he eat and drank was either drugged or poisoned. He was occasionally able to master this delusion, and then eat and drank heartily ; but he frequently subsisted on the minimum amount of nutriment. When engaged in the city he was in the habit of taking, almost daily, for luncheon a basin of mock-turtle soup. For a long period he never, for one moment, suspected that the soup contained any injurious matter ; but one morning he left home feeling physically very indisposed, and mentally more than ordinarily depressed. He went into *Birch's* (Cornhill) at one o'clock, and had his usual basin of soup. He eat one spoonful, and whilst in the act of taking another, the idea of its containing arsenic forcibly suggested itself to his mind, and he would eat no more. He tried at the time to reason himself out of this delusion, but without effect. Eventually the idea of his food being poisoned took complete possession of his mind, and he nearly starved himself to death ! For many months it was found necessary to administer nourishment by means of the stomach-pump. This patient ultimately recovered, and has continued well for many years.

A lady informed me (after her recovery), that her insanity commenced by her morbid fancy suggesting to her mind a number of lewd images. Being naturally of chaste feelings, and refined intellect, she was perfectly horror-stricken at the ideas that occurred to her. Everything she saw and heard appeared to be associated with physically impure notions. So acute were her mental sufferings that she endeavored to escape from her horrible thoughts by an act of suicide. For this purpose she threw herself into the water, but was fortunately observed, and dragged out of the pond before life was extinguished. This state of mind appeared inexplicable to her, because she had never indulged in any improper ideas ; and having a literary taste for a high class of books, she was not in the habit of reading anything that could have laid the foundation for so fearful a perversion of the animal instincts.

A clergyman, remarkable for sweetness of disposition, and·purity of thought, suffered severely from the same distressing symptoms.

At an early period of an attack of insanity his unhappy mind was tortured by the most obscene and blasphemous suggestions. Such was his condition more than twelve months previously to an attack of acute mental derangement. Two years before (so he informs me) he had experienced, but in a somewhat modified form, similar symptoms. For about two months he never could engage in family prayers, read the lessons in church, or preach a sermon, without having the most dreadful thoughts enter his mind. It appeared as if he were under the influence of "*double* consciousness," or, as if he had, to use his own phrase, "*two selfs*," one (or the *evil* self) urging him to utter certain impure expressions, and the words—actual words—were, as he thought, plainly spoken; the second (or *good* self), begging and beseeching him to resist the machinations of the devil, and to refuse compliance with his horrible suggestions.

On my advice he left England and went abroad, residing some short time at Spa. He then visited Baden-Baden, and remained on the Continent for six months, returning home apparently quite free from all nervous symptoms. For four months, previously to the recurrence of the peculiar morbid thought referred to, he had been greatly overworking himself in attempting to establish a new school in connection with his parish. He was also much annoyed and irritated by an unkind and unexpected opposition that had been raised by some neighbors upon whom he relied for support. This gentleman's insanity, in course of time, became so obvious that it was necessary to place him under control. In less than twelve months he appeared to recover, but was strongly advised not to return to ministerial duty for eighteen months. However, in defiance of such instructions, and in direct opposition to the wishes of his wife and friends, he insisted upon resuming clerical work. In less than three months from this time his mind again became deranged, and, whilst under the fearful dominion of a most horrible hallucination, he committed suicide by cutting his throat!

"For more than four years," writes a patient, "I was the subject of the most inexplicable and curious mental sensations. They commenced by attacks of what I thought to be, sick headache. These feelings were associated with depression of spirits. I began to lose all interest in matters, that had previously pleased, and occupied my mind. I carefully avoided the society of my relations, and friends, having a morbid craving for solitude, and yet, when so isolated, I was truly unhappy. I could not understand what possessed me. I was unable to account for the strange ideas, that often suggested themselves to my mind. I felt, at times, very wretched. These symptoms continued, in varying degrees of severity, for nearly two years. By this time I was quite estranged from all my friends, and many of my relations. I awoke one night, as I thought, out of a frightful dream. I felt much alarm, and yet I knew not why. I got out of bed, lighted a candle, and sat in a chair in a state of extreme mental, and muscular agitation. On the following morning I first began to hear voices speaking to me. Occasionally, the words they uttered were those of comfort and consolation; then texts of Scripture were repeated; verses from hymns, that were familiar to me; favorite pieces of poetry— all, happily, of a consoling character. I was certain, that the voices were *internal*—that is, originating within, and did not proceed from persons external to myself. But, alas! the character of the voices changed in about a week. They then gave expression to the most foul, coarse, and abusive epithets. I was charged with having committed the most abominable sins, and the most repulsive and morally degrading crimes. At other periods, I was told I had better cut my throat, hang myself, take prussic acid, and thus save myself from some dreadful punishment; and, strange to say, particular instructions were given to me *how* I could best destroy myself, without detection—*where* I could procure the fatal poison, mentioning the name of the chemist, as well as street, in which he resided. Now and then I appeared to be better, and my mind was quite free from such distressing illusions. For several days, to my great delight, the happy voices returned, and again passages from the Bible were repeated, and comforting hymns were sweetly and melodiously sung to me. During the whole of this time, I was fully persuaded, that the voices were only suggestions of my own mind, and did not proceed from other persons, nevertheless they gave rise, at times, particularly during what I term my 'bad days,' to great mental suffering. This state of mind existed for three years and eleven months. At the termination of this time, I heard of the brutal murder of a near relative. This was a great mental shock, and produced severe distress of mind, ending in an attack of jaundice. The voices then came back to me in great force, and the suggestions made by them were too horrible to narrate. In about a fortnight, I became extremely nervous, fancying that I was to be sacrificed ('crucified,' the voices said) in order to bring my poor murdered relative back again to life. I then conceived that I heard strange noises in the house at night, and on more than one occasion, I imagined I saw an assassin enter my bed-room and point a knife, covered with blood, directly at me. I then began to believe that a number of persons, dressed in the garb of priests, were actually speaking to me. I replied to them, and prayed that they would leave the room, but the more I ex-postulated with these spectral images, the louder they talked, and the more violently they gesticulated. It is impossible for me to repeat the filthy, obscene, and blasphemous language they used. Then some women appeared among the priests, and they com-menced to dance most lasciviously; men and women trying to outdo each other, in the most gross and sensual attitudes. My mind at this period was in a state of wild delirium. I remember two or three gentlemen coming in to see me, and a strange man, I recollect, always sat in my room. The gentlemen I refer to, were two surgeons, and the man was a respectable person, from the village, who acted as an attendant. I remember being driven away from home in a carriage, and entering a large house (an asylum), where I saw a number of singular men (patients). I then fancied that I was dead, and refused to eat. In consequence of this delusion, I had food forced into my stomach. My mind continued, in a fearful state of derangement, for more than sixteen months. I then began to recover, and at the end of two years from my being placed under treatment, I was discharged cured. I have now been well for more than seven years. My mind has been, ever since, quite free from all symptoms of insanity. I am not, however, in intellect as I was before I became subject to the illusions. I find it difficult to fix my attention to any subject requiring for its comprehension an effort of mind. If I attempt to read a book on an argumentative and philosophical subject, I am obliged to put it aside in about ten or fifteen minutes. This was not the case before my mental indisposition, for then I in-dulged freely in most abstruse reading, rarely looking at the light literature of the day. My head aches, and the mind gets con-fused, if I try to follow a complex train of reasoning, and I, there-fore, now do not read any work that is likely to produce tension of thought."

The following letters were addressed to Dr. Awl, superintendent physician of an American asylum. They were written by patients who had formerly been under his care in the institution. They illustrate the subject under consideration.

"I am now engaged (says the patient when addressing Dr. Awl), in writing to some of my friends at the asylum; and though you may not be expecting a letter from me, yet. I must ever consider myself under obligations to you, as the instrument, in the hands of Providence, in restoring me to health, reason, and my family. Of course you do not rank least in my affections, when I remember my friends at that truly benevolent institution, for I am fully confident, that had I not been placed there, I should never have recovered from the torments of a deranged mind.

"Should I undertake to describe to you the anguish which I suffered before, and for several weeks after I became your patient, my language would fall so far short, that I should convey no idea of it; but in our hall I found those that were under the same delusions that I was. One would say her children were murdered, and she had eaten them. Another would say, she was to be burned alive, and she was brought there to be boiled, and the doctors were to make an anatomy of her, &c. All these, together with hundreds more of the most horrid delusions that can possibly enter the imagination of the crazed brain, had haunted me for months. My brother, my husband, and even my own son, a child of ten years, I was afraid of. I thought everybody on earth knew my thoughts, and that I was not a human being; that I was the Devil! and that I ought to kill myself and children. I once told my husband that I would kill my boy, for he had already been murdered, and *he* was only the ghost of my child. The poor boy cried, and came to me, and said: 'Yes, mother, I am your boy;' so I could not do it then; but myself I was fully determined to murder before I got to the asylum; for I believed the people of —— had called a meeting on my account, and had resolved to send me to Columbus to be burned, and made an anatomy of; but when I found others in the asylum, who seemed to suffer in a degree the same fears and torments as myself, I was led to try to think I might be wrong in some things, until gradually reason returned, and with it the affections of the heart.

"When I entered the asylum, my sufferings cannot be described; and though I do not believe that any being on earth ever suffered anything to be compared with my anguish and torments, yet, if persons who are deranged do suffer even a thousandth part as much as I did, I am sure I pity them from my very soul."

After recovery this lady says:

"I arrived safe home, and found my children and friends well, and not a little astonished to see me so soon—and so well, too; I could scarcely make them know me. Before I left them and since last February, I scarcely ever spoke to any one of them, and they seemed surprised to hear me tell how much I suffered; and they wonder when I try to convey to them some faint idea of the many awful and horrid delusions I was under. What a dreadful thing it is to have had my children afraid of me! Now they are so happy, and say to the neighbors, 'My mother has come home, and she is not crazy at all.'"

Another patient writes, "As you desired me to give you some account of the manner in which I was taken sick, and the circumstances attending my long affliction, I will now endeavor to state them as near as my recollection of things will permit.

"In the fall of 1839, I was much exposed and labored exceedingly hard, which brought on an attack of fever that seemed to spend its force principally in my head. I also had a severe cough, and at one time spit blood. As the fever increased, I experienced a kind of stupor and derangement of mind. In this state, I had the most singular dreams or visions of things. One peculiar thought that entered my mind was, that my body was divided into four parts, the legs being cut off at the knees, and my head and breast severed from the body, which appeared to be real and true; and I suffered great anxiety as to how the parts of my body should be reunited, and made to grow together again. A physician was employed, and he ordered plasters to be applied to my ankles and a blister to my breast, and one on the top of my head, and gave me several emetics; and the pain of all these, and the distress of the fever in my head, was enough to render the strongest man, with the best constitution in the world, senseless and delirious.

"I continued in this condition some time, sometimes pretty sensible and others indifferent to what presented itself before me. At length, through the advice of some friends, I believe I was taken to your asylum. As near as I can recollect, I was taken twice. The first time there was no room for me, and my father had to take me home again. I remember on my first visit, seeing the four round pillars in front of the building, and walking up the

5

steps into your room. At this time I entertained the opinion of having just landed in the city of Rome; and from the circumstance of noticing these pillars and the immense size of the building, I was induced to entertain the belief of its being a house used by the Roman Catholics for their religious services. I thought it was a monastery. I also thought the piece of ground in front of the building was holy and consecrated ground, used by them for the interment of the dead. I suppose the reason why I thought so, was, because the ground between the gate and the house had been fresh ploughed, and it looked yellow. I had an idea that the Romans, and some other denominations, were exercising their authority upon young and old; and I thought I was brought here to be scourged, and taken through purgatory. After I arrived the second time, I thought that the building was used for a medical college, and the inmates were going through a certain preparation, or process of experiments, rendering them fit subjects for dissection and investigation. After that, I concluded it was a kind of a fort for the protection of the people of the country, for I expected that France had united with the southern parts of the United States, and we were suffering the unpleasant consequences of a war. These, and a great many other curious and singular notions, not necessary to mention, I entertained through the winter and spring, and until I began to get better.

"My greatest trouble was as to the place in which I was, and the true use made of it. I made various inquiries of my companions (*the other patients*) for correct information. I asked them often where I was, but the answers which they gave induced me to disbelieve every word they said; and it was a long time before I could credit anything I was told. When I reflect on the many incidents connected with my sickness and recovery, I am amazed."

"I was born," writes another patient, "in the State of Maryland, and am forty-four years of age. From my earliest recollection, I was of a quiet and steady turn of mind, and have seen nothing but hardship and trouble all my days. I was married in my twenty-fourth year, in opposition to the will of my parents, but was devotedly attached to the man of my choice. He received an injury in his shoulder, some time after our marriage, and I was in the habit of assisting him with his work on the farm. I worked uncommonly hard at making fence, burning brush, and clearing up the land. The stooping, heat of the sun, and hot fires of the burning brush, appeared to affect my head very much. On a certain day, while engaged in the field, I was suddenly struck almost blind, and felt an uncommon stiffness in the back of my neck, accompanied with a drawing down of the skin over my eyes and forehead, and the sensation of tight cords passing through my head. It was some time before I felt able to return to the house, and attend to my domestic duties. I had lost much sleep for two or three weeks previous to this attack, and felt troubled in my mind on account of our difficulties in getting along in the world. On the following night, I was greatly distressed, and thought somebody was coming to kill me. I could not go to sleep, and by morning I believe I was completely deranged. I continued out of my head for three or four months, and suffered much distress and anxiety of mind, from the apprehension that I was to be killed; but through the attention of the physicians and kindness of my husband, I began to recover by degrees, and eventually got entirely well.

"After I got well, we concluded to come out to the State of Ohio. We were very poor, and the journey was accomplished on foot. It was in March, and the three children and myself suffered greatly from cold and fatigue. Husband had taken to drink, and we had hard work to get along; and in the month of November following, I had another attack of derangement. I forgot to tell you that my health began to fail previous to my first attack, and I think this brought on the second attack also. I continued ill for several months, during which time we removed to the northwest part of the State. I did not know what was to become of me; my distress was so great that I longed to make my escape, and hide where no mortal could find me. We again had to make our journey on foot, and I cried and fretted most of the road. I wished I never had been born, and often said to my husband, 'There's my poor children, and I've got to go to hell for having them;' he would scold me for talking so, but I could not help it, such dreadful thoughts would come into my head, in spite of all I could do. I sometimes tried to drive it out of my head, by beating it against the'fence. Frequently it appeared to my mind as if it would rain hail and fire upon my head, and I should be beaten to pieces with thunder and lightning; and when I did, once in a great while, fall into a troubled sleep, I would suddenly start up in a fright, with my hands before my face, to keep the awful danger off. It was

all, however, respecting myself and the children : I did not think
that anything was to happen to their father.

"At this time husband was sometimes a little crabbed, but he
could not get any liquor in them parts, and did not get drunk. I
was as much attached to him as ever, for he was a kind and good
man to me. I don't think two persons could be fonder of each
other. At last, however, I took it into my poor head that *he* was
going to kill me! This painful idea continued to torment my
mind for two or three weeks. It was dreadful. We had lived
together so many years, and why should he want to kill poor me ?

" One Sunday, I was full of this idea the whole morning, and
about twelve o'clock ran off on to the wild prairie, where I wandered about during the whole afternoon, and did not think of returning until near night. I met husband coming after me, with
one of the children, and we all returned to the house together. I
got the supper, and the family went to bed as usual. I could not
sleep. It was a terrible night to me. About daybreak, I got up
and built a fire. Something appeared to tell me there was dreadful
work to be done. I was very much agitated when the thought
came into my head that I must kill him ; but my mind was so
much excited, I cannot tell anybody exactly how I felt. The
same thought came into my head in the night, but I succeeded in
putting it down. I had a confused notion that I was born to be
lost ; it appeared like a hidden mystery ; but the thought that I
was born to be lost was uppermost. At the same time, I supposed
he would be saved. I often thought that everybody was made
righteous beside myself.

" I stood alone by the fire. All were sound asleep. Husband
partly wakened when I first got out of bed ; he merely opened his
eyes, and then went to sleep again immediately: I knew he was
sound asleep, and I felt that I must kill him to save myself. I
accordingly went to where the children lay, and drew out a broad
axe from under their bed, that he had borrowed from a neighbor.
I went right to his bed, with the axe in my hand, trembling like a
leaf. He was laying on his right side, with his neck bare, and I
immediately struck him the one fatal lick across his neck ! He kind
o' struggled, and partly raised himself to his knees, and wakened
the children, a dying. My daughter came running to me in a
fright, and took the axe out of my hands, screaming that I had

murdered father! and sprang to him, and kissed him on his forehead, crying, 'Oh! he's my poor, poor father!'

"As quick as they could get their clothes on, the children ran off to the neighbors. I sat down, and stayed in the house alone, until the neighbors came. A gentleman first looked in at the door, and asked me what I had done. I said (*evasively*) that I had not done anything; that I had to go to hell, and that I would have something to go there for. He came in, and said he must tie me. I told him I did not want to run away, and would go along with him without tying. He first took me to the next house, and in three days they sent me to jail. I was as distracted as ever: and what I had done gave me no relief nor satisfaction. I think it was as much as three months before I began to come to myself. I was not tried for the murder, which I never attempted to deny, but sent here to the lunatic asylum. I supposed they would hang me, and did not expect anything else for a long time. My mind now appears to be entirely clear, and I want to go home to my children. I feel much better, though very weak. I am thankful they brought me here. My mind is altered now about going to hell; I have hopes, and think, when I die, I will go to rest. I like to go to your evening worship very much, when I am able to walk up stairs," &c.

"To our question, 'Well, Mrs. S., you say your mind is now clear; don't you know it was wrong for you to kill your husband?' 'Yes, doctor, I know it was wrong.' 'And are you sorry that you did it?'—This question appeared to touch the very chord that had been so long diseased. Her eyes flashed; the pupils contracted; and her whole frame shook, as she raised herself up and emphatically replied—'No, doctor, no! I'm not sorry for it! It was God's will—why should I be sorry? He made me do it to show me His power—and I was willing to do something to go to hell for!' It was but the flash of a moment, and all was calm as before.'"[1]

The writer of the following narrative was for some period an inmate of Bethlehem Hospital. After his recovery he wrote to Dr. Hood the following account of his case:

"Previous to the year 1851, I never for one moment suffered from mental derangement, although, I must confess, that I com-

---

[1] Extracted from "The American Journal of Insanity."

menced to take strong drinks with excess, at a period so far back
as the latter end of 1849; until that time the only complaint I
was subject to was accidental constipation, accompanied by fever
and loss of appetite.

" As my disease first made its appearance in Londonderry, I
shall take the liberty of giving you an account of my way of living
there, from the time of my arrival to the day when illness, despair,
and want of pecuniary resources, compelled me to leave it.

" In August, 1848, on my return from France, whither I had
gone to spend my vacation, I was, on the most pressing recommendation of the manager of the bank at Larne, who knew me,
appointed French master at Foyle College, Londonderry.   The
Reverend Mr. Henderson, who was and still is the head-master,
after the trial of a few days to put my qualifications to the test,
agreed with me that I should receive my board and lodging in the
establishment, in return for French tuition imparted to a limited
number of pupils; my lessons were to be given four times a week,
and to last two hours every time.

" For three months I lived in the college, attending my classes
there according to the agreement, and also other young gentlemen
and ladies in town; but finding that I could not meet every one's
wishes without interfering with the meal-hours at college, I resolved
on taking up my residence in the city.   The principal, to whom I
communicated my determination, gave me his full approval, and
desired me to continue my attendance in his establishment for the
salary of one pound per quarter for each pupil.

" I therefore removed on the 1st of December, and got lodgings
in a most respectable family, consisting of four sisters.   They
were elderly ladies, and nearly related to a gentleman whose
daughters I attended.

" There I spent, until June, the most happy months I ever enjoyed.   My health was excellent, I had as many scholars as I
could wish; the ladies of the house were more like sisters than
strangers to me, and the steadiness of my conduct as a teacher
caused the best families in and about Derry to honor me with their
esteem.   In a word, I saw before me most encouraging prospects,
but there was in me, steady, sober as I was, the seed of many sins,
—a profound disrespect for religion.

" Like many of my countrymen, and though brought up by a
most pious mother, I was a Christian only by name.   The college

life in Paris had almost rooted out from me all notion of God.
Thus, whilst in the sight of men my conduct was irreproachable,
I shamefully forgot that the discharge of our duties towards our
Creator is alone calculated to render our conduct irreproachable.
Never did I once go either to church or to chapel during upwards
of two years.

"I returned to France, as usual, in June, 1849, and came back
in August next, after a stay of a few weeks with my family and
friends; but there too I was so obstinate in my refusing any attendance at church, on Sundays, that I left my poor mother quite
dissatisfied at what she called my *déplorable esprit fort*. Many,
many a time did she prophesy to me that I should one day weep
on my impiety.

"I was soon to experience the realization of that prediction.
When I came back, I found on my arrival, a new servant occupied
in my sitting-room. She had been engaged, during my absence,
to replace the elderly woman who used to wait on me at table, and
to do whatever I might require. I was very much satisfied with
her attendance, and sincerely regretted her discharge. On my
asking why she had been dismissed, I was answered that she could
not do all the work, and that a young, active girl was by far
preferable.

"The new servant was young indeed, and possessed of some
attractions, which I was foolish and imprudent enough not to resist; but for my attention to which I have since been severely
punished. Let it suffice to say that I yielded to temptation.
From that time, I can assert it, may be traced all my troubles
and misfortunes. The girl, though young, was knowing enough
to perceive that I was in her power more than she was in mine.
She openly told me so more than once. In the mean time, she
took great care to obtain from me as much money as she could.
I then commenced to drink whiskey mixed with water, first in small
quantity and only at night, after my business was over. The
libations became by degrees more frequent and copious, especially
when she apprised me that she was with child, and consequently
expected that I should marry her.

"I cannot describe to you, Monsieur le Docteur, the state into
which that unpleasant news, expected as it might have been,
threw my mind. I saw that my ruin was unavoidable, whatever
plan I might adopt. If I do not marry her, said I, she will make

a scandal, and I shall be obliged to leave the town. If, on the other hand, I marry her, I am sure to fall into discredit, and to lose most of my pupils.

"This happened at the latter end of March, 1850. Instead of returning to better sentiments, and praying to God that he would inspire me with the means of averting the catastrophe, by sending the girl out of town, with a sufficient maintenance, until I should be able to atone for my fault in the only honest way, that is, in marrying her, but so as to keep our marriage secret, I became the more reckless of the time to come, went on drinking whiskey, and hoped in *chance*, the providence of those who have none.

"Despite my endeavors to drive remorse away, the thought of what I had done did not cease to pursue me. My nights were restless, or troubled with painful dreams; I could no longer indulge in reading or in walks, as before; my appetite, too, was lost. The tuitions to which I had fortunately to devote a considerable portion of the day, were alone able to afford me a little tranquillity, by temporarily removing the annoying idea from my mind.

"An incident which I little anticipated caused the girl to be removed from the house, and led me to hope that she would not object to leave the town, where her presence was a permanent danger for me. She, either on purpose (as she told me), or otherwise, got drunk, and received her immediate discharge. It was in May, two months before her quarter was over. In the precipitation of her dismissal, I found only time to direct her to go home, and to wait for me, on the next Sunday, at an appointed place, when I should see what was best to be done. The ladies of the house consented to accept, for the two remaining months, of the services of her sister, who was then out of employment. The girl had always assured me that no one had the slightest suspicion of her state. I was, therefore, not a little surprised and annoyed when I learned from the new comer that *she* had not made her pregnancy a secret with all her family.

"At our first interview, I expressed to the girl my dissatisfaction at her imprudent disclosures, and, as the only remedy, my willingness to send her away to some distant place, until vacation, when it would be easy for me to take her to France, and to leave her with my family, whom I should inform of what had taken place, but without saying a word about her having been my servant. Had such a plan been put into execution, everything could still be repaired, or at least the impending danger was indefinitely removed. There might be vague rumors about her absence, but nothing more. I should have left off drinking whiskey, in consequence of my mind being more at ease, and attended to my daily occupations with a new courage. Such is, at least, what I then intended to do. Unfortunately, my proposal was drily rejected; she would not go away; she was afraid I should leave her; she wanted to live in town, &c.; or she would make everything known.

"I submitted in despair to her haughty wishes, and gave her money for lodgings. She hired a room in a retired part of the town, and came to live there, not alone, but with her mother and a niece, the two latter saddling themselves on my shoulders, as if one incumbrance were not sufficiently heavy. Demands of money succeeded each other with a fearful rapidity, so that I found myself quite unable, for want of cash, to take my usual trip to France.

"At that period of the year (July), the harbor of Derry received a number of French vessels, which gave me a daily opportunity of acting as interpreter between the merchants and the captains; but at the same time I neglected my private lessons, a fault which had never occurred before. Being a constant prey to sinister presentiments about the future, I used to drink wine and brandy on board, without, however, being ever sick (this fact I cannot account for); only, every morning when I got up, there was a kind of tremulousness in my limbs. I could scarcely take up a glass to my mouth without spilling a part of its contents; my walk was unsteady, and my speech broken, more difficult than usual, unless I got animated. The mind seemed to preserve its soundness; I had several times to draw up reports, which scarcely took more time than that of writing them down.

"In this manner did I pass the month of July, be it said to my shame and deep regret. My visits to the girl were also frequent; it seemed as if an evil genius carried me there, though I well understood their danger and impropriety. I think that by that time I had lost a great deal of control over myself.

"In August, the reopening took place at Foyle College, and at three other schools which I used to attend. The Rev. Mr.

Henderson sent for me. I was not at home. Fortunately, a gentleman who also kept a school, and who was greatly attached to me, came on board an Italian ship, where he found me. He most justly said that he could not understand my way of living for the last month. There must be something wrong. That if I did not resume business immediately, he was afraid I should lose my pupils in town. He had been told something very painful to him, about my now taking to drink; but he did not believe that. He then carried me to his house for dinner. There he informed me that it was reported in town I had married my servant. This I denied.

"My friend's lecture seemed to shake off my torpor for some time; I left off visiting vessels, to resume business.

"Notwithstanding what had been rumored, every one received me well. New pupils came to me, so that I could number upwards of fifty of them. But if this increase was gratifying to me, there were repeated calls on my purse which produced a very different effect. I continued to drink, and drank the more, on thinking of the fast-approaching time when there would be a living proof of my guilt.

"This took place in November; as a rigorous consequence, I lost my situation at college and in another school. I did not repine. I acknowledged within myself that I deserved it. My remaining pupils were still in sufficient number to afford me the means of a livelihood. In order to avoid any further scandal, I earnestly advised and prevailed on the girl to leave town. I rented for her a house in the country, about four miles from town. Had I thought that marriage would not have made things worse, I would certainly have married her; but out of all the persons to whom I spoke on the subject, Mr. Henderson alone gave me to understand that it was the only means of atonement from an honest man. It is true, that when I asked him if my compliance with his advice would entitle me to a further attendance in his establishment, he answered that he could not employ me any longer, on account of the many respectable families whose children were at college, and who would object to the continuance of my tuition there.

"Matters remained in this state until December 28th, when I went out to the country (as if led by my evil spirit). Hard drinking there for several days, joined to quarrels arising from constant demands of money, brought on me sickness and such exhaustion that I could not leave my bed. From December 28th to January 13th, when I felt the real symptoms of the disease, I did not eat *one ounce of bread daily.* My only food was whiskey, which I am sorry to say they were always ready to minister to me.

"Until the 12th, I continued extremely weak, but felt so tired of the bed that I got up.

". Here, Monsieur le Docteur, I will endeavor to convey to you an exact idea of my disease in all its successive phases. I recollect everything so distinctly, that I can speak in the present tense, as if I were just *in the act of suffering.*

"My night, as many others before, has been altogether sleepless. Itchings, hitherto unknown, are felt all over the body, and render my skin sometimes painfully tender, sometimes quite benumbed, as if it were dead. Diarrhœa increases my sufferings; I am so dizzy, that I cannot walk in the room without groping along. It seems to me as if there were small flies before my eyes; I hear their humming. If I look out through the window, all the objects assume confused, but not yet fantastic shapes. The itchings do not leave me; they are very troublesome, and make me worse. Cannot taste any food, and this day abstain from taking whiskey. I retire to bed; no rest whatever; the itchings keep me in continual movement. Very early in the morning, and long before daybreak, I think I hear two or three peals of thunder, which frighten me very much. When I open my eyes, I see no more flies, but ignited small globules, like sparks. They are in myriads. I hear something like the ringing of many, many bells, and remark that if I rest my head on the pillow, the din is really frightful. At times I fancy that there are mice or rats running to and fro, with their usual cries, under my head, inside the pillow. The day breaks in; I want to get up. My bed has become a bed of torture for me. I try to walk a little in the room, but weakness compels me to sit down. My food consists only of a few cups of tea, without any bread, for which I feel no taste. Several times in the course of this day, I have *des envies de vomir,* but I cannot. I look at the fire; the burning peat has assumed strange fantastic forms, which seem to be animated. As I cannot sleep, I sit up very late, in the hope that I shall, from mere exhaustion, enjoy a little rest. Now and then, I take a cup of tea. I feel well nowhere. Sitting is often replaced by two or three turns about the room. Whatever position I may take, weariness, discouragement, anxiety, press on me. I attend to a conversation whispered between the mother and the daughter. They seem to talk about me and my affairs. I several times fancy they utter the word France, and my name, accompanied with curses. I think they are alluding to the possibility of my returning alone to my native country, but they will not let it be done; they will prevent my departure. The old woman says that her daughter had better have drowned herself. I then recollect that she for the last **few** days has been very moody, because my money (I imagined) **was** drawing to an end. Yesterday, I sent the son and brother of the two women for some money due to me, but he has brought back a cheque, which I alone can get cashed. I go on walking as if I did not listen. I am very far from being at ease, especially when I recall to mind that this is a lonely house, in a bleak, deserted part of the country, and that I should have to deal not only with the two women, but with the brother, a stout fellow, who has required no invitation to take up his abode with us, and who seems rather too much inclined to idleness. My apprehensions are, moreover, roused by the fact of my possessing the above mentioned cheque. They might believe that they too can get it cashed at the bank. At about twelve o'clock, I want to take another cup of tea with the two women, who are still up, and sitting near the fire. They prepare it; but I fancy I see the mother slip some black thing, like tobacco, to her daughter; I approach the fire, and again the mother tries to hand another lump of black stuff, but she drops it. I see the object of my suspicions lying on the ground; the mother tries to get it under her foot, which she stretches out in that direction; but she cannot succeed, and I suppose she is afraid I should notice her movements. The daughter looks uneasy. I am sitting between both of them, watching their motions in deep silence. At last, I avail myself of the first opportunity to pick up the obnoxious black lump, and I thrust it into my overcoat pocket. I am trembling from fear; I feel that I should hardly be able to speak. The sinister idea strikes me that they want to administer me poison, and the word vomica nux often presents itself to my mind. I get up from my seat, and resume my this time very unsteady walk, until the old woman presents me one of two bowls full of tea. I take it with a tremulous hand, and in a broken voice say to the daughter, ' Drink it; I wish you to drink it;' but she would not; she does not want it. I then see my suspicions confirmed. I seize the two full bowls, and run with them out of the house, crying out, 'You are two wretches, you wanted to poison me.' I take the direction of the nearest house, in order to show the contents of the two bowls; but before reaching it, I let them fall, and pursue my way. I knock at the house, entreating that the door should be opened to me. A woman (the only grown-up person I see in the house) asks me what I want. In a most agitated tone I say that I have been nearly poisoned, and that I shall make an application to the magistrates about that. As I am speaking, the brother comes up. He has been awakened by the two others. Assures me that I am mistaken. 'Well,' said I, 'come with me to any place where we may find a light, and I will show you that I am not mistaken. I have in my pocket an unquestionable proof of what your friends intended to do with me.' 'You are wrong, sir,' replies he; 'nobody wishes you harm; come you back to the house.'

"Fear prevents me from acceding to this request. I run off through boggy grounds in the direction of a public house on Derry road, about half a mile from the place. From the beginning of my flight I have lost my slippers, and have but a pair of stockings on. The night is very dark, and the rain is falling in torrents. I have to make my way through pools of water, dikes, rills, fences, and hedges. By day the task would be difficult, as there is but one very narrow and uneven path leading to the road—I do not keep the right direction for a long time; I hear close behind me the voices of the brother and sister; they are engaged in my pursuit. This idea increases my terrors. In the hope of escaping from that pursuit, which I ascribe to bad motives, I leave the path, and continue my run at random. I can assure you that I am not less than half an hour wandering about, often stumbling in the marshes, often finding myself back again at places I just left a few minutes before. I once keep myself hidden in a ditch with water up to my knees; the voices are but a few yards behind me. Here is the road at last, but I see no public house, and the darkness does not permit me to ascertain whether it is situated on my right or on my left. I take to the left, which is the wrong direction; I pursue my flight; the thought many times striking me that *God* has this time more obviously than ever saved me from an untimely grave. I pray along the road for the forgiveness of my past errors; I promise henceforth to behave like a true Christian, &c. . . . . I feel not only refreshed and encouraged by my prayers, but much stronger than I could have expected from the extreme weakness I felt on the preceding days. After half an hour at least of this run in the opposite direction to the pot-house, I begun to think that I must have found it if I had taken the right way. I therefore retrace my steps with unabated speed, determined to knock at every door, and to speak out concerning my escape from the lonely house. Strange to say, out of at least five or six houses where I stopped, knocking repeatedly for several minutes, and crying aloud for admission, I receive answer but from one. A man comes to the door without unbolting it, and rudely says the only words, *Cut away.* I am nowise disheartened.

"On my arrival at the pot-house I recommence rapping, and begging that they should be so kind as to open the door, for I am in great need of a shelter. A dog alone answers my knocks by his barking from inside. The fact is, that my pursuers got to the tavern before me, and there asking if anybody had called, said there was a man on the road who was out of his senses, and who perhaps would ask for admission; the landlord had better not let him in. Such is the account given since to me by the girl who went to the house along with her brother, and obtained admittance on pretence that they wanted candles. The landlord, being warned, does not move from his bed, and lets me stand out until I perceive that he has been prepared for my visit. I then make up my mind to return to Derry, where I should inform the police of what, in my fancy, has taken place. Indeed I have not the least doubt but a criminal attempt has been made against my life. Curiosity, however, soon altered my resolution. When I reach a place on the road where a lane branches off in the direction of the lonely house, an unconquerable desire bids me go and see from outside the window what is passing in there. As if I foresaw some bad encounter, I break from a hedge a short stick, which is to be my weapon in case of danger. I have not proceeded many yards in my new direction when I am stopped by two men carrying sticks. Who are they? The brother, and a fellow of his acquaintance, who is known under the name of the *dummy* (he was dumb). The former imperiously invites me to return to the house, where no harm is intended against me. I feel so frightened that, to show I do not wish to make any disclosures about the events of the night,

I throw the black stuff out of my pocket, and, though reluctantly, follow the two men.

"When I come in, I find there the woman to whom I first applied. She appears to be on good terms with the others, and I learn that the dummy is her son. This raises my suspicions about her. She endeavors to make me understand that I am quite mistaken about what I call *poison*, it was nothing but *soda*. How far this assertion is true, I cannot say; but cannot help thinking that *soda* is not black.

"They make me sit down and change my clothes, which are dripping wet. The brother goes out for some whiskey, which, they say, will do me good. On his return from the public house I take a small glass mixed with water, taking previously care that it should be tasted by the others. Contrary to my expectation I do not feel weary at all. I look at my feet and hands, which, to my great wonder, bear not one single mark of a scratch, although I have been running for two full hours shoeless, treading on sharp stones, and often obliged to jump over ditches, or to force my way through thick thorn-hedges.

"This I consider as the greatest proof that I was guided and protected by some supernatural Being. I say so to the people, but I am by no means reassured in mind. I reflect that I am in a sinful state, without any hope of forgiveness, were I to appear now before the Supreme Judge. My fears increase in proportion as the others endeavor to prevent my escape. I fancy they are all decided to make away with my life. I entreat them to let me go; I confess that I am afraid of them, &c. Strange visions throw my mind into great excitement; every object takes a hideous shape, and moves about. I look at the windows; diabolic faces are laughing at me. Their laughter makes me shudder. On whichever side I may turn, a chilling wind is hissing by my ears, with unearthly shadows passing before my eyes. If I look towards the door it is opening noiselessly, and I imagine I see somebody whose terrific head is peeping in. I start painfully at the least noise, and utter lamentable cries. This lasts for hours while I am sitting by the fire.

"I am prevailed upon to retire to bed. Do not feel any better. Vainly do I shut my eyes, in the hope of avoiding the sight of everything; horrid phantoms appear amidst the darkness. I feel as if I were pricked behind with a sharp instrument. The itchings are insupportable. I am a prey to a continual restlessness, mixed now and then with the cries produced by an unexpected noise, such as the fall of a chair, or by new visions.

" At the break of day the excitement subsides a little, and gives place to a fainting fit of short duration. For some time no new starts occur; but the confused ringing of bells continues; my sight grows very dim; I see nothing but monsters calculated to keep up my fright. Starts soon return more painful; even one of them throws me down on my knees, compelling me, as it were, to address a fervent prayer to our Lord for the pardon of my past life.

" From this day (13th) to the 27th no amelioration in my state. I look on the house as a cursed place, and remove to Derry, again followed, for my misfortune, by that family, whom I dread, in spite of all reasonings. As if their number were not sufficient, the sister had also made herself at home. I say repeatedly that I don't want their presence, that there is but one whom I ought to provide for; they stick to me like harpies, and take no notice of my remonstra- tions. They most likely will not go so long as there is anything to eat.

" Driven to desperation, if I take no food, I keep on drinking whiskey, not so copiously as before, but yet a great deal too much. I wonder how eagerly they give it to me, and advise me to take another drop whenever I complain of my extreme weakness. On my arrival in Derry, new fits of faintness : I sent for the priest, in order to receive his consolations; for I do not expect to live much longer. The reverend gentleman who has come to see me, perceives at once that medical assistance is to be had immediately. He therefore leaves me, and shortly after returns with a doctor, to whom I explain what I can about my complaint. The women are upbraided for having given me so much strong drink in my present state. The two gentlemen advise me to leave the place and the company, and to come *alone* with them. They take me to a respectable hotel, where they get a comfortable room for me ; a nurse is also engaged to sit up all night in case of need.

" Despite the excellent accommodation I have now obtained, I cannot enjoy one moment's rest. Besides many other sufferings, a new one came to complicate the symptoms of my disease. It is the fancy that I hear every one in the hotel speaking ill of me, and even the dreaded family is here too. They all proffer alarming threats; they want to have my life. It is wonderful how faithfully their voices are reproduced. I would swear that mother, daughters, niece, brother, and even the infant are below stairs in the kitchen. I cannot be undeceived by the kind words of the landlady. I am even so foolish as to believe that she has given them admittance, contrary to the orders of the doctor. The night-nurse does not escape my distrust either. In short, I see but the faces, I hear nothing but the voices of those which, from want of other words, I shall call my persecutors. They are here, now in the kitchen exciting their hearers against me, now outside the door, in the street. Cries distressing for me, such as, *Stop, stop the mad dog*, often fall on my ears, and cause me to spring out of the bed, and to look out either on the stairs or in the street. Such has been my daily state during the time that I stopped at the hotel. Meanwhile I received frequent visits from the priest and the doctor; my conversation with them was always sound, so far as the girl's family was not alluded to; for in the latter case I could not believe that I was the sport of a delirious imagination. Laudanum was several times administered to me in large doses, but to no purpose; on the contrary, I am of opinion that it did me more harm than good, for I then used to see everything more confusedly, and as if dancing before me. Unnecessary to say that appetite did not return; I had only some refreshing drinks prescribed by the medical gentleman.

" Reasons of economy, and the advice of the doctor, induce me to go to the infirmary. I am conducted there by the doctor himself, and I obtain a bed in a small quiet ward, generally used as a room for surgical operations. There are two other patients opposite myself, and the cook sleeps in a fourth bed on my left. Although restless, and unable to sleep, I have no starts, and make no noise whatever for many hours. It is two o'clock, A.M., I am wide awake. I look towards the bed on my left, and I have this painful vision :

" I am (in imagination) in the lonely house. Sleep has overcome me. The mother lies in the other bed, on which my eyes are fixed, with the little niece, who says: ' Grannie, where is Mr. D.?'

" *Grandmother*. ' He is away; let me alone.'

" *Child*. ' Grannie, where is Mr. D.?'

" *Grandmother*. ' Hold your tongue, he is killed, killed dead.'

6

"This lasts for several minutes, being repeated many times. All of a sudden I hear the mother ask the girl lying beside me: 'Does he sleep?'

"*Girl.* 'Yes.'

"*Mother.* 'Well, make haste off then, have done with him. It is two o'clock; we shall have time to run away.'

"*Girl.* 'I cannot find that cursed knife. Ah! here it is, I have got it.' . . . .

"Then I feel twice something like a pointed knife penetrating into my back. I utter a feeble cry, then all is silent. The mother again says: 'Well, have you done?'

"*Girl.* 'Yes; he has enough. Let us get off.'

"And it seems as if the mother were leaving her bed, and the girl slipping cautiously from mine. At the same time I hear from outside the voices of the sister and brother, who say: 'Quick, or we shall be caught.' . . . .

"They all escape, and immediately after two doctors come to examine my body, which I fancy is lying inanimate in an adjoining room. One of them says in French: '*Il est mort, il est bien mort.*' The other also, in French: '*Le pouls bat-il encore? Voyons. Oui. Alors il n'est pas mort. Non, non, il n'est pas mort.*'

"They carry me away, and another scene offers itself to my eyes.

"The mother and my ex-servant are gone; they are superseded on the tragic theatre by the sister and brother; the latter leading the little girl by the arm, and the former holding the infant. She is looking for the knife used against me. She finds it on the edge of a small well opposite the door. It was to be thrown into the water, but in the precipitation of her flight, my servant has missed her aim. I see (for you have not forgotten, Monsieur le Docteur, that my eyes are wide open) the sister stab the poor infant, and, to stifle his cries, she, with a curse, tears his tongue out and throws him into the well. The little girl is also got rid of, because she cries that they have killed Mr. D. and her cousin. I am so well awakened that I relate to the night-nurse particulars after particulars, as they are taking place. My sense of hearing acquires, on this night, such a degree of quickness, that I hear every quarter of an hour striking by the town-clock, and every time I say, 'It is half-past two, it is a quarter to three,' &c. . . . .

For me these are very audible sounds, which are hardly perceptible by others.

"A few minutes after, when I think they have all escaped, here comes the dummy's mother to fetch water; she discovers the infant's body, and cries out, *Murder!* The sister makes her appearance again. The woman accuses her of murder; a struggle ensues, the result of which is that the woman is strangled.

"Then I hear a confused noise produced by voices, and the sound of heavy steps. It is the police. They have arrested the murderers, and bring them back. I see every one of them. There is the mother, there are the three others, handcuffed, and closely watched by the officers, who are armed with carbines, and have received the order of firing, should the prisoners attempt to escape. Now, too, the body of the woman is discovered, and I hear several voices say : ' This is really a cursed place ; the house of murder.'

"Again the scene changes. I feel some one in my bed, who speaks to me. He says that he is my good genius ; he has come to protect me from the wicked ; but I must be truly repentant. I therefore pray for a long time in a low voice, until I fall asleep from exhaustion. My slumber is very short and agitated. I awake before daybreak. Now the scene of the night is continued. I hear criers in the street announce that the family ———, convicted of murder on the persons of ———, have been sentenced to death, and are to be executed on the same day. It seems to me that I am under a strange sky. The fog is very thick. I hear nothing but the cries of sinister animals, such as wolves, dogs, and the shrieks of geese, the croaking of frogs, mixed with the monotonous voice of the criers. I again fall into unconsciousness until it is light. I have been very restless, but not so noisy as to prevent the other patients from sleeping. The nurse alone knows what my imagination has seen.

"On awaking my eyes wander from one object to another, and remain fixed on many pieces of wood, used by the doctors in their surgical operations, and which lie topsy-turvy on a press in a corner of the room. I first shrink from the sight, for now the top of the press is occupied by living beings : here are the mother and my servant again ; then, on their rear, the sister and the brother. But in what state ? My good genius tells me that such is the visitation of God on great criminals. The mother has a cadaverous face ; her eyes are sightless and white ; her hair has assumed the color of flax; the rest of her body is concealed from me. The daughter is closer to me; she is dressed as for a fête, but her head is nearly bald; the hair has fallen off in the space of a few hours. There is a large stain of blood impressed on her brow, and a candle (like a sepulchral lamp) is burning beside her. They both stare at me now and then, like people who look but do not see. The two others, sitting exactly behind, present a disgusting aspect. The sister is as pale as a corpse; her hair, too, is white, and very thin on the forehead; the lips emit a kind of sanguinolent foam; the head performs the oscillations of a pendulum; she is an idiot. The brother's appearance is that of a hideous cripple; the head has decreased nearly to nothing, and would scarcely be visible, were it not for two green eyes obstinately fixed on me, but without any significance. He reminds me of what I have read about *cretinism.* I forgot to say that there is a fifth actor in this tragic tableau,—the young girl with curling hair, neatly clothed, leaning sometimes on her grandmother, sometimes on her aunt, and repeating at intervals : 'Grannie, or Auntie, where is Mr. D. ?' to which question the only answer given is : 'Hold your tongue; he is away, he is dead, killed dead.'

"This spectacle keeps my mind in excitement for the whole day. Visitors come in and look with wonder on those strange beings, from whom my eyes cannot be removed. Those visitors say : 'It is strange, very strange indeed !' In order to escape from the frightful sight, I once run out of the room. The doctor, who happens to be in the next ward, brings me back, but cannot persuade me that I am mistaken. At another time I fancy that an iron bar, placed to support a curtain above my feet, pours on me something whitish, like melted lead, which burns all my body. The same imaginary tube is sometimes turned against the family, and seems to produce on them the same effect as on myself. Again, I think I hear the voice of a gentleman, the head man of the committee, who visited the wards a few hours ago. He is upbraiding the doctor, in most unbecoming terms, for having given me admittance, while there are so many poor Irish dying out for want of medical cares and of bread. A quarrel and a fight ensue, the result of which is that the doctor is shot dead. I hear the report of the pistol, and the cries of many persons calling for the police, who, after much delay, arrive and capture the murderer. Before the arrival of the police, I once imagine that he is ascending the stairs to kill me; I jump from my bed, and conceal myself under another. I am dragged from under it by a day-nurse; then I run off again, at the risk of killing myself in rolling down the stairs. I am caught at the bottom. They carry me up again to the room, not without an obstinate struggle on my part; for I am afraid of new visions. The strait waistcoat is resorted to. They fasten me so tight that I can no longer move: my breathing is even greatly impeded, by a leather strap pressing on my chest. Night has come; I begin to utter cries of distress, because I see the unavoidable figures from the press quit their immobility, and join in infernal fits of laughter.

"Exhaustion again delivers me from consciousness. I am aroused from my torpor by the endeavors of the attendants to make me swallow some medicine. The idea immediately strikes me that the potion forced into my mouth is poison, and I spit it out. No more rest during the night. My eyes emit sparks of fire which fill the room. My persecutors are still there; no longer on the press, however, except the brother, who has resumed his natural form, and seems ready to spring on me. They are lying in the other beds; there seems to me as if an electric thread were carrying to them my inmost thoughts, which they repeat aloud. On the other hand, I can get through the same imaginary thread a knowledge of their designs against me.

"My good genius has not left me; he bids me look for strength in a sincere prayer, and pours on my enemies the same white fluid already mentioned. It is directed from my side to the places they occupy, and instantly reduces them to silence. From time to time, also, when I pray without fervor, or when I entertain any doubt about my good genius's power, the shower is turned against me from the iron bar, and especially directed to my head. This has the effect of fire; it burns my body all over so sorely, that I cannot help crying.

"The heat is oppressive; the room is full of a reddish smoke, at intervals chased out, through the door, by a blast of wind. I tell the nurse that, although the door is opened, I am afraid we will soon be blown up, if she does not put out the gas; she answers that there is no occasion for it, as we are in no danger, and I had better sleep, as if sleep were to come at my command. In my restlessness, I fancy that there is the head of a wolf, with glaring eyes, on the bolster; I pray for a long time; the head disappears. I am a little refreshed, but cannot sleep. My mind soon turns to other fantastic thoughts. I am no longer an inmate of the infirmary. I am kept a prisoner by my persecutors in a small house, where they endeavor to smother me by shutting the door, and lighting a fire of straw in the middle of the room. The mother and sister are more implacable than the others, and appear to enjoy my torments. Whilst I am a prey to great sufferings, and scarcely able to breathe, I hear from the street a voice, which I immediately know to be the voice of my brother-in-law. I wonder that he has come from Paris to Ireland. He answers that he has come with my sister, for the purpose of settling as a French teacher. I turn then his attention to my present miserable state. I implore his assistance; I entreat him, in the name of my sister and of our former friendship, to deliver me; but he laughs at my supplications, and even joins with my persecutors, whom he also excites to show no mercy and to take no heed of my cries, as there is nobody at hand to hear. I hear him walking up and down the street; he is with my sister; they both say, repeatedly, '*Il est perdu, il n'est pas perdu. Eh bien! Oui, il est perdu. Tant pis pour lui.*'

"At daybreak the visions disappear for a little time. My lips are parched from crying; my feet are now cold. I complain to the nurse. They give me a drink of milk, and place a jar of hot water at my feet. I remain thus quiet, and as if prostrated, until the doctor comes in on his round. He inquires of my state; feels my pulse; asks if I could sleep last night. He is told that I was noisy, speaking about dangers, praying aloud, &c., and that I would take no laudanum. He kindly remonstrates with me, saying that everything is prescribed for my good. (*That medical gentleman was well known to me, and he also knew me very well, as I used to give lessons in French to his family.*) Unfortunately, the subordinates have a rough way of discharging their duty. They, in my helplessness, ill-treat me, threaten me now with a stick, now with the red-hot poker, which they approach to my mouth. In these ill-treatments and menaces my delirious imagination sees nothing but a continuation of the tortures inflicted on me by my enemies. I look upon the night-nurse, the day-nurse, and especially on the *infirmier*, as people under the power of Satan, whom my prayers alone can drive away. Their drugs, too, I consider as being made by an evil hand, and only calculated to soil my soul. I have made up my mind to accept of nothing, except water or milk.

" In the course of the day, I come to think that my mother is dead, and that my eldest sister has arrived, and wants to see me. She stops with my brother-in-law and my other sister; but she cannot obtain any information about the place where I am kept. My persecutors reappear; I find myself in another house, quite unknown to me. Besides the family, there are strange faces, equally hostile. They want me to sign a promise of forty pounds, in return for my release. I consent to their request, but when the signature is given, they won't let me go; they now say that they must have their revenge. I am stretched on a mattress, tightly fastened with ropes and leather straps. I can hardly move my head. Presently my legs are stripped, and the toes of my feet covered over with a thick layer of fat meat. What do they intend to do? From their conversation I at last learn that my toes are to be devoured, along with the meat, by a huge dog of theirs, whom they have taken care to keep in good appetite for the *occasion*. The dog cannot be got for some time, during which I am a prey to frightful apprehensions. He is brought in by two men, and rushes, from the first, upon my feet, which he dreadfully mutilates. I hear the cracking of the bones under his teeth; I again cry and weep pitifully. There are many people—men and women—around me. They all seem to enjoy the spectacle, and take no notice whatever of my cries and tears. I have lost all remembrance of what followed; I suppose that I fainted. The fit, however, was short; for at night I have the following dream. (Let it be understood that all my dreams are nothing but visions; for they take place when I am wide awake, and when my eyes are open; my properly styled dreams have left no recollections in my mind.)

" I am dead. Like Seneca, I have been bled to death by my persecutors, who each had a cupful of my blood. I well remember that I have suffered death with resignation, and praying to God that he would forgive me my manifold sins. My voice has been heard; but I am not yet worthy of being numbered among the *Elus*. My good and bad actions during my lifetime are carefully weighed by our Supreme Judge; the latter are too numerous, but my repentance at the hour of death is taken into consideration. According to my belief, as a Roman Catholic, I am doomed to pass a certain lapse of time in purgatory. My murderers have already been overtaken and struck by the justice of men. They did not repent; they are damned for eternity.

"In atonement for my sins on earth, and before I may obtain the kingdom of heaven, I must be put to the test, and tempted by the infernal powers for several hours every night. I am, therefore, carried into the dominions of Satan, who endeavors, by a display of magic operations, to show me that his *puissance* is too great to be resisted successfully, and that sooner or later I shall give way. He also tries to persuade me that he can make me more happy than I am in purgatory. He points to a number of his subjects, among whom I recognize my persecutors, who seem to enjoy their present position.

"For the first time, I feel an invincible courage within myself. I firmly answer that I despise him, his threats, and his promises, and that, with my God's assistance, I fear nothing, and may defy all the monsters in his dark kingdom. The room then assumes a more gloomy appearance; it is vaulted like a cellar; a sulphuric smoke comes out of the fireplace, so thick as to conceal many objects from my sight, and to stifle me. The walls are covered over with grimacing, horrid monsters, at all of which I now laugh fearlessly, saying that this is nothing compared with what I saw many a time when I attended theatres. Now and then, if I perceive that the attacks made against me are too powerful, I am, as it were, inspired to have recourse to prayer. I therefore repeat uninterruptedly, aloud, and in any language I know, our Lord's Prayer, which I had nearly forgotten, together with *Glory be, &c.;* or I sign myself. I remark that no one of the Devil's attendants, or even himself, dare to touch me while I am praying. On the contrary, they seem to suffer a great deal inwardly, and slink away, in uttering curses; but they return to the charge as soon as I leave off praying. After a long, a very long struggle, I grow weaker and weaker; I can hardly speak for want of a drop of water, which I would not, however, accept from unholy hands. I am smothered; perspiration flows down my cheeks; my strength is exhausted; the evil spirits profit by my prostration; I feel crawling about me, and on me, repulsive reptiles or animals, such as serpents, toads, frogs, rats, mice, &c. There are myriads of them. Their size is so large that I must see them through a microscopic glass. Here my good angel comes to my deliverance. I am carried back to purgatory. Now I fall asleep.

"I have slept until eight o'clock—three or four hours, I should think. My head is clearer; I am not so restless; the noise in my ears is lighter. The two other patients tell me that I had a very bad night. My eyes were rolling in their sockets, like those of a madman. I was very noisy. I seemed to fight for a long time. I spoke sometimes in Latin, sometimes in English, but mostly in an unknown language. The night-nurse wanted to make me drink, but I could not, even with the assistance of the cook (man). It was fortunate that I could not stir.

"The doctor comes in, and finds that my pulse is less agitated. Notwithstanding the nurse's report about my excitement of last night, he orders that I should be free in my movements. The strait waistcoat and other *courroies* are taken off. No visions until night, when I fancy that Satan himself is lying by my side. I also imagine that my persecutors have resumed their places in the other beds. They say that it is a shame. I am sleeping with the Devil. They see his long flat feet hanging out of the bed, and from which I try in vain to disentangle mine. In my opinion, Satan has taken the shape of a wolf. His head is remarkable by two short horns. The whole of the body, with the exception of the two feet, which are as cold as ice, is covered with long yellow hairs, emitting a most nauseous smell. He again speaks to me in a threatening manner. I do not listen to him. My only answer is, that I no longer fear his power, because God is my protector. Then I commence to pray, sometimes in a low voice, sometimes aloud, but always composedly, as if I felt quite safe. I still hear the once dreaded voices; but reason seems to have returned—she tells me not to trust sounds.

"This was, Monsieur le Docteur, the third night I had visions since my admission into the infirmary; it was also the last one. From that time the visions completely vanished. It is true that I was still very far from being restored to health. My sight was greatly impaired for some more days. My appetite did not return all at once, but by degrees, and accompanied by a good sound sleep. I here must acknowledge that nothing was spared by the medical gentlemen which was likely to accelerate my complete *guérison*. They told me I had been very ill; and indeed I think they entertained very little hope of my recovery. I left the infirmary, when I asked for my dismissal, towards the 20th of February.

"On my return to town, I felt much more inclined to live as a Christian. I could not help believing that all the events, either real or imaginary, had taken place through God's will for my conversion. My first care was to consult the priest, and to take his advice about marrying the girl, notwithstanding my gloomy recollections concerning herself and her family. The reverend gentleman owned that the connection was altogether unsuitable, that it was a great pity, &c. But I had a great sin to expiate. Marriage had become a necessity. ·

"We were therefore married, although I had forgotten nothing. I first wanted to quiet my conscience, and was very much like a man who clings to any plank of safety, however rotten, to avoid drowning. In consequence of my new connection, now openly known, I lowered my usual charge, thus hoping that many pupils would avail themselves of it to learn French. My business was resumed without any loss of time. I abstained from any strong drink, and should have most likely been able to maintain my little family, had not my wife been badly advised by her friends, who did not dare to come to my house, but whom she visited.

"For reasons I cannot explain to myself, they, without any means of a livelihood, had taken up lodgings in Derry. I found her several times, when she returned from those visits, in a state bordering on intoxication. I then saw that the fruit of my labors was again going the wrong way. I got discouraged—disgusted with life. I drank again, lost my appetite, experienced new fits of faintness (no visions), accompanied by diarrhœa, and finally by want of sleep. My little money being gone, the pawn-office was resorted to; my watch and clothes were engaged, piece after piece, until there was nothing left. Then I saw that my only resource was to risk my return to France, after gathering up two or three pounds remaining due to me for tuition. My books, together with some furniture, were left to my wife, who, it was agreed, would try to live with her family until I should be able to get a situation, after my recovery, either in France or in England. She did not look much annoyed at my departure; but it is not the less my intention to discharge my duty as a husband as soon as Providence is pleased to give me the means. I would now work for her and the child much more than for myself. May this also be a lesson to her!

"Having described what I call the first period of my disease, I will now give an account of the second. When I left Derry, I had kept my room for two or three weeks, being unable to go on with my lessons, though the soundness of my mind was not once impaired again there, but from mere exhaustion. I resume my diary :—

 "Left Ireland on the 26th of June, with some cakes and a little bottle of whiskey. For saving expenses, took the steerage: could not eat; drank the whiskey; no sleep during the passage; very feverish; suffering much from diarrhœa. Arrived at Liverpool, 27th; no food, but one or two pints of porter. I feel very, very weak. For fear of being taken sick on my journey, and placed in the impossibility of proceeding, I take the mail-train, in order to get home sooner; there I have to pay 4s. 6d. more than I expected. In the carriage I endured great sufferings from vomitings. My stomach being empty, I expectorate nothing but bile. I can hardly sit up. No more sleep than on the preceding night. On the 28th, arrived in London, with about 10s. in my pocket. I am exceedingly depressed in mind, and wearied all over. I want to apply at a relation's temporary residence. I inquire of many persons about my way. Their information is very conflicting. At last I reach my destination, after a walk of more than three hours. The people of the house answer me, that my cousin returned to Paris three weeks ago.

"This sad announcement adds, if possible, to my despondency. There is my last hope gone, as to the possibility of getting home without a stoppage on my way. I can, however, through great economy in my expenses of the day, manage to save *eight* shillings for my passage to-morrow, on board the Bologne steamboat. Once in Boulogne, I shall at least be in France, and, as I carry about me my passport, my degree of A.B., with a great number of excellent testimonials, I may hope to interest the authorities in my favor, and to obtain from them the means of proceeding on my journey.

"I continue my walk for many hours, now and then stepping into a public-house to take a glass of ale or ginger-beer, when I feel too thirsty; but I do not taste any more substantial nourishment. It seems as if my stomach could not digest it. Though broken down with fatigue, and hardly able to stand up, I very seldom stop for a few minutes' rest. I feel that stopping is still worse than walking; because the absence of objects constantly

renewing deprives my mind of diversion, and makes it a more easy
prey to thoughts of despair. I therefore go on, unconscious and
unmindful of the direction I may take. In a narrow and dark-
looking passage through which I wander, a few French words fall
on my ears; I turn round and find that they come from a man in
a small stall, who sells cheap ices at one penny each. Being
anxious to get a modest bedroom for the night, and in the hope
that the man can give me some information about it, I enter the
stall and ask for an ice; then I beg the permission of sitting on a
chair; for, said I, I have been walking a great deal, and feel very
tired. The *ice-dealer* gives me a chair; he then inquires of me
if I am a foreigner; on my affirmative answer, he says that he
is a native of Switzerland, but knows France very well. He was
there for several years. I perceive that he does not speak English, or at least pretends not to know it. I see in the stall two
grown-up boys employed as assistants, and with whom the Swiss
converses in bad Italian. A great many customers, mostly of the
poorer class, and of little prepossessing appearance, come in and
ask for an ice. Some appear to be acquainted with the man,
although he has just told me that he commenced business this very
morning. No suspicions, however, strike my mind. I frankly
confess my distressing state; I should be very much obliged by
his taking me to a lodging-house where I may obtain a bed for the
night; I want to take the Boulogne steamer to-morrow, and I have
just enough for a bed, in a very modest lodging-house. The Swiss,
after much musing, takes me to a place where, he said, I shall be
well.

"Despite his assertions, however, I have no sooner set my foot
in the house, than I wish I had never come. This is a most mise-
rable-looking place, situated in a neighborhood which can have no
claim to respectability, from the number of rags and repulsive
individuals I have met on my way. I am conducted through a
dark alley up to a kitchen on the first story. The landlord and
landlady to whom I am handed by the Swiss, in a few Italian words,
are not likely to restore me to confidence. The former is a tall,
lean fellow, about fifty years, wearing moustaches, and smoking a
clay pipe by the fireplace. Were I in France, I would take him
for a *coupe-jarret*. His wife is an old woman whose face has been
greatly injured by the small-pox and the loss of one eye. I find
her very ugly. There are two young women in the kitchen, en-

gaged about I do not recollect what. They certainly have bold
looks. Several *orgues de barbarie* and *grosses caisses* let me guess
the kind of companions I shall have for the night, if I have
nothing worse.

"The old woman invites me to take a cup of tea. I decline
accepting of anything, and express my desire of retiring to rest
immediately, for I cannot sit up any longer from weariness. She
leads me up a very steep and dirty staircase to a room containing
three beds. One of them I may have. Before leaving, she wants
me to pay in advance the usual charge, sixpence. When I find
myself alone, I take a survey of the place. One table, the three
beds, and a few common chairs, make up the whole furniture. I
again observe a big drum on the floor, which affords me another
proof that showmen as well as strolling singers are the customary
lodgers of the house. No sinister suspicions, however, throw my
mind into distrust and fear. I address a sincere prayer to God ;
I think, when in bed, of those I have left behind. I cannot help
shedding tears ; but I hope in better days. So far as I can judge,
it may be six o'clock. I have therefore been walking many miles
since six in the morning. Sleep overcomes me. I have no
evil dreams; but a noise in the room puts an end to my rest.
I awake abruptly, and look about to see what the matter is. The
night has come. I see the old woman holding a candle. She is
with a man and a woman, whom she leaves an instant after. My
two companions take one of the vacant beds. The woman looks
very much like one of the two females I saw; but the man is not
at all the same as the tea-dealer, although the landlady told me,
when I was conducted to this room, that he sleeps there every
night. Both begin to talk in a low voice. From their conversation I perceive that they believe I am asleep. Imagination again
arouses my terrors. I fancy that they speak sometimes in French,
sometimes in English. I wonder how they have come to a knowledge of my language, especially the woman, who expresses herself with great correctness and a truly good accent. Then I imagine that she may be one of those Frenchwomen,`so numerous in
London, whose existence is derived from debauchery or theft. I
think that this one, after acting her part on the first stage, has
now fallen into the second. In short, I firmly believe that she is
connected with a gang of robbers. They, said I, intend to get rid
of me, in order to obtain possession of my few shillings. I sup-

trates into my heart. I cast stealthy looks about me. My companions do not sleep, for they are very restless. I suppose they have not yet given up their bad designs. I then examine carefully if there is no means of escape. Unfortunately, my *examen* confirms the worse suspicions in reference to the house. On my right, the window is secured by iron bars, and overlooks a small, dirty yard, surrounded by nothing but walls. My eyes turn to the other window, which is opposite a red tile roof, and so close to it, that I imagine I might jump out on that roof, were not the window exactly situated between the two beds occupied by the other lodgers.

"Being therefore convinced that all hope of escaping through the windows is to be abandoned as chimeric, I resolve to defend myself to the best of my power against the attack I expect every minute. There are in the small parcel that I brought with me two razors and a penknife, in the pocket of my trousers. I take out one of the razors and the penknife, which I open in silence, and which I place beside me on the bed. My companions have perceived these preparations. They seem to laugh in disdain at my means of defence. I think they say that the struggle will not be a long one. The idea of a longer weapon being in their possession, such as a dagger or a sword, again recurs to my mind. I then venture to speak. In a most trembling and scarcely audible voice, I say that I know their intentions against me, &c. I am determined to sell my life dearly. Perceiving that my words do not appear to produce any effect on my audience, I appeal to their humanity. I entreat them not to steep their hands in my blood, especially for such a trifling sum as *eight* or *nine* shillings. I am to return to my country this very morning. If they allow me to go, I promise to leave London without making any disclosures about them and this house. Let them take my money, if they like; I shall not complain.

"I go on for some time in the same strain; and at last, seeing that all my supplications seem to remain unsuccessful, and that the men will not alter their minds, I beg of them permission to grant me only a few minutes as a favor. No answer. I hastily slip out of my bed, fall on my knees by the bedside, and say a short prayer in a low voice. I feel a great deal more composed. There is now so much resignation in me, that I no longer fear death. I tell my companions that I am ready; they this time say that they wish me no harm. Though I do not believe in their friendly protestations, my terrors are gone. Let them strike me while asleep. This reflection does not prevent my taking two or three hours' rest, until seven o'clock strikes by the church clock. The other men are still in bed; one of them gets up at the same time as I do, because, says he, the doors below are not open. He leads me down the steep and narrow staircase. I find myself in the kitchen I saw yesterday. My guide is the tall man I remarked last night; he says he is the landlord's son. He takes me to the street door, and accedes to my request, when I express a desire to be put in my right way to London Bridge. He therefore accompanies me for some minutes, and leaves me in a wide street, saying that I have only to go straight on. I forgot to mention that he handed me two cards, to recommend the house to my friends, should any of them come to London. Those cards I took, but without any intention of ever using them as I was directed. They have been taken from me at the house where I was before my being brought here. The landlord's name is Cassanello (an Italian).

"I have been told by my guide that London Bridge is about a good mile off, and that the shortest way for me is to keep straight on. I therefore forget my state of exhaustion, and walk at a brisk pace, in order to be in time for the steamboat which is to sail at nine o'clock. I have already proceeded for not less than one hour, taking great care to follow the same endless street. There is, however, no London Bridge within sight yet. I venture to ask a policeman about it. He informs me that I am *three miles* at least from my destination, and points to another direction as the right one.

"On this day, Sunday, 29th of June, disappointments succeed disappointments. It seems as if London Bridge were moving and retiring before me as I advance towards it. Despite repeated inquiries, I think I should never have reached it, had I not at last, and in despair, given a little boy one sixpenny-piece to take me there. It was twelve o'clock when I arrived; the steamer was gone, and with her my last hope of leaving London on that day.

"I see everywhere people going to their places of worship. An interior voice tells me that it would be right on my part to do the same; for I stand in extreme need of our Lord's assistance. But on casting a look on myself, I feel ashamed of my wretched appearance, and content myself with praying to God that he may deign

7

not to abandon me. I go on at random until the divine service is over; then I enter a public house for the purpose of writing to my family, and apprising them of my being detained in London by illness, and unable, for want of pecuniary means, to proceed on my journey. When I have done, I recommence my wandering *marche* without interruption, without food, until night. I have been all day exposed to a scorching sun: I feel quite worn out; but I continue walking, like a machine, an automaton, without caring about any direction whatever. It is my intention to apply for lodgings to any police-officer I may meet on my way, when the streets are getting deserted. I thus hope to obtain a bed in a respectable house.

"At about ten o'clock, I find myself in a wide thoroughfare, where I see thousands of promenaders moving along the footpaths. From distance to distance, the landlords of several public houses have placed rows of chairs and forms, with tables, in the street. There sit many, many people, drinking beer and eating cakes. I am very thirsty, but I would not take any beer, because I am sure it does no good. I buy a cake, and draw a little water out of a pump.

"I then resume my walk for one hour perhaps; I perceive that the streets are not so thickly filled with people now, that it will soon be time for me to think of some accommodation for the night. Were it not that my step is more unsteady, my voice more trembling, my sight weaker, and my hearing subject to a constant humming, I feel nothing which may induce me to believe that I am worse than I was this morning.

"Presently, and all of a sudden, the real scene changes, so far as people are concerned. This is the same street, indeed, with the same buildings; but the promenaders, the women especially, are no longer strangers to me: they have assumed forms with which I am acquainted; I shudder on recognizing in two females the faces of my wife and her sister passing and repassing beside me; they are laughing a diabolical laughter; they cry out that I am *mad— yes, mad, and this time mad beyond recovery*. I shall die the death of a brute; I shall be damned for eternity.

"There is just enough *présence d'esprit* left in me to think that I am again the sport of a delirious imagination, and that I am destined to suffer under new trials. Notwithstanding the unceasing threats I distinctly hear about me, I won't believe, but at the same time I cannot help being more and more excited, and in spite of myself I answer those menaces as if they were real. It is time to apply to a policeman. After some minutes' walk, during which I get no relief, I find one whom I beg to conduct me to a decent lodging-house, in which I may find a bed for the night. I am a foreigner, quite a stranger in London; arrived yesterday, but would not like to return to the same house I slept in last night, because I think it is a bad one. I am ill, very tired, &c. The officer kindly takes me to a place where he is known. The people of the house, perceiving that I am unwell, desire me to take something before retiring to rest. I decline, and only drink a glass of ginger-beer. As soon as I am in bed I feel very much oppressed. I can hardly breathe. My eyes and mouth send forth sparks of fire. A stormy, hissing wind rages about my ears. All my body is in such a state of perspiration, that I put off my shirt. I fancy that a demon is on me, trying to smother me by pressing on my throat. I struggle with all my might, and pray repeatedly. My prayers drive Satan from me; but he is not far hence. I still see his hideous face in the room. The latter part of the night passes away in visions of a new kind. My memory has acquired a wonderful power of recollection. I see, in a succession of *tableaux*, as I should in a panorama, the faithful reproduction of what I have done wrong during my life. Many sinful deeds, never remembered before, and which I believed to be forever buried in oblivion, now spring up one after the other, and defile before my eyes.

"The day has long made its appearance, when I am able to snatch a little rest. At breakfast-time I am still in bed. The landlady has been informed, by two young men who slept in my room, that I was very restless, without, however, being noisy at all. She sends up to me a cup of tea and some toast. I take the tea, with very little bread. I cannot eat. I bought last night half a pound of meat, which remains untouched. When I have got up, I stop for some time in the parlor below-stairs with the landlady, to whom I sincerely confess my penury, and the reasons which compel me to tarry in London until I have received an answer from home. She happens to be a kind-hearted woman, and sympathizes with my sorrows. She accepts the money due for the bed, but refuses to receive anything for tea. I then tell her that, if she has no objection to it, I shall sleep in her house again, a proposal to which she readily consents. I take leave of her, with the intention of taking a short walk, and, in order to get rid of any incumbrance, I intrust her with the care of a small parcel, containing, among other things, my passport, my degree of A.B., and a number of testimonials. Although I have avoided strolling too far away from the place, I vainly endeavor to find it again. That the house is close to a railroad, and I was able to see the trains from my bed, is all I can say; for I have forgotten to ask the landlady for her name and the name of the street. At last I discover a railway which is quite, in its appearance, like the one I am looking for. Indeed, the aspect of the adjoining streets, cut, as it were, into two halves, makes me almost sure that I have come to the end of my anxious rambles. Unfortunately, appearances were never more deceiving. I walk over and over again through some twenty streets in the vicinity of the railroad, all to no purpose. I give up, for fear of being looked upon by the people as a suspicious character. I have thus been on foot for at least five or six hours, being sustained by nothing but ginger-beer, the only sort of drink I made a vow last night that I should taste again.

"In the hope that an application to the police may lead to the discovery of my papers, I hurry on to the nearest station, where I state the case to the best of my abilities; for I have very little strength even to speak. After hearing my statement, the chief officer tells me that it is very unfortunate; he can do nothing unless I let him know at least the name of the street where I met the policeman who took me to the lodging-house. I venture to express my opinion that it would be easy to find out the said policeman, by inquiring at all stations, which of the police conducted last night, about eleven o'clock, a Frenchman to a lodging-house; but all my reasons are not listened to. I therefore submit to try if I can find the street again. The officer tells me that I must come back as soon as it has been found, and assures me that he will spare nothing to have my parcel restored to me. I leave the police station, not at all despairing, in my ignorance, to be able, by dint of turnings and windings about the streets, to find at last the one I am instructed to look for, and of which I suppose I have kept a vivid recollection.

"Without wishing to weary the reader with a detailed narrative of my new perambulations, I shall only beg to say that, on that day, I did not even so much as sit down for more than twelve hours. I had no kind of food whatever; thirst alone compelled me to stand from time to time at a ginger-beer shop, *en plein air*, where I had a glass of the refreshing drink, and then on I went. I could not stop; it seemed to me as if somebody were again pricking me from behind, or whispering into my ears: *Walk on, walk on.* The objects grew confused. I heard imaginary conversations held in French. They related to me and my insanity. At times the prickings became so painful as to make me shed tears, and it was with the greatest effort that I could help uttering cries. Towards evening I was prompted, I cannot say by what invisible force, to go and give an answer at the police-station as to the issue of my errand. The difficulty was to get to it. It was very likely a good distance away. Frequent were my applications to policemen on duty in the streets, but either I gave them a wrong name, or they did not know the place. The fact is, that I never obtained the information I wanted. In fine, and, *en désespoir de cause*, I called at the first station-house on my way, and asked to be taken, if possible, to Finchbury station (so far as I can remember), where I desired to speak to the chief officer. They kept me waiting for a good while there, and it was dark when I was requested to follow a policeman who, they told me, was going to my destination.

"I purpose now to detail at some length the strange events, partly real, partly imaginary, that took place on the night of the 30th of June, from the moment when I left the station-house to accompany the policeman. I resume.

"This officer looks angry with me, as if I were a malefactor. I ask him if I have done anything wrong; he answers, *Nothing that I know of.* We have not proceeded many yards out when two ill-looking men come up and walk by my side. Their language is most abusive; they make threatening gestures at me. They say they are going to the station along with me, and there swear before the magistrate that I created a disturbance at their house. I call the policeman to witness that the accusation is quite false: I entreat him, with tears in my eyes, to disbelieve such a wicked report. The men I now take for two of those who slept in my room on Saturday night. They must be bad characters, said I, for they wanted to lay hands on me. The officer does not pay much attention to my supplications; on the contrary, he seems to be on very good terms with my accusers. He soon leaves me in a street, and, on going away, says that we shall meet again at the station, which is now within a few minutes' walk. I have, says he, only to go straight on. The two men are still by my side: they still abuse me; but, notwithstanding what they have just declared, about their intention of having me brought before the magistrate, they also leave me, and proceed on their way at a quicker pace. To my great dismay, I hear them crying aloud,— *Here is the madman coming. . . . Here is the madman.* This appears to be *un mot d'ordre* for every one. The two men are certainly new enemies. They try to set all London against me. Indeed, everybody is standing at his door, laughing at the madman; some speaking with compassion, others asserting that he ought to be locked up for the safety of all.

" The unavoidable cry is repeated from distance to distance, as if to invite the people who are in doors to make haste and look out, for there is the madman. I cannot understand how people may be so easily imposed upon by a set of slanderers, and thus rise up against one who does not remember having done any harm. I feel that resistance on my part would be great folly; my only resource is to suffer with new resignation. I, therefore, thinking it useless, throw the walking-stick which I carry over a wall I pass by.

"I now go on in a slow, quiet pace, with my hands in my pockets. I am entirely composed. Though I would swear to the reality of whatever I hear about me, there is in me an invisible adviser who commands me to bear up in silence against any kind of abuse. Sometimes, however, I cannot help exclaiming: *Je vous reconnais bien là, M. Diavolo ; encore un de vos tours contre moi ; mais je ne vous crains pas ; je vous défie ; car je suis sûr que le bon Dieu est pour moi,*—and many like sentences. Once, thirst obliges me to enter a tavern for a glass of ginger-beer. There are three men sitting on a bench in the bar-room; I imagine they speak of me, for I have caught the word *madman.* I complain of their behavior towards a helpless foreigner, who is only guilty of being poor. They politely answer, that I am under mistake. I am not at all the subject of their conversation. I then apologize for my blunder, and walk away with the conviction that every one has been roused against me. A little further on, I feel inclined to buy a penny loaf; but it seems as if all the bakers' shops were now closing on purpose, and that no one will sell me the food I am in need of. This universal bad feeling I ascribe to Satan's power; but I have full confidence in God,—I pray on fervently, being assured that I shall not be abandoned. How long did my walk last, through hundreds of streets, it is difficult to say exactly. Most of the shops had already been shut for a long time; the thorough-fares are no longer crowded with promenaders. It is very late. How is it that I am neither weary, nor cold, nor hungry? To these questions I know of no other answer than that I am under the care of Divine Providence.

"I meet many persons whom I take for acquaintances of mine. They have come to be present at what I call my *Passion*. There is a master whom I knew at Foyle College. He passes by with-out speaking. There is my brother-in-law, whom I have just passed. I know him well. He has a brown overcoat on, and smokes a cigar. There he is again. He won't leave me; he says he has come to have done with me at last. I presently hear his voice exciting every one to throw me into the river. I defy all in a loud tone; but at the same time, I wonder what interest my brother-in-law has in my death—what benefit he is likely to derive from it. I also feel much surprised at his uttering filthy words, mixed with oaths and blasphemies. This was not his habit. He is extremely excited. He says, that since Satan has got his soul, he must likewise get mine.

" On my side, the excitement becomes greater; I speak aloud to the crowd. The meaning of my speech being, that I fear no-body; that God is with me; that I am proud of having returned to better sentiments. I feel quite able to fight against Satan himself, because I am assured that I shall have an all-powerful as-sistant, already made manifest by the total absence of fatigue, fear, and want of food.

" Whilst I am talking in this strain, my eyes fall on a damp place in the street or lane. The said place is much darker than the rest. (Water had probably been spilt there.) I fancy that it has the shape of a large hide. It is the Devil's skin. I am told that my prayers and my faith have triumphed over Satan. I repeatedly trample on his remains, and only leave off to address the multitude around me. Fortunately my harangue is in French. They perhaps do not understand what I say; but they well enough perceive that I am not all right. A public house is hard by, in which I hear music and songs. The airs are French. They are interrupted only by the voice of my brother-in-law, who exclaims that they must have my life, because he is sure I am not yet in a proper state for salvation. A young man comes out of the tavern (I perfectly recollect this incident), and offers me a glass of porter, which I decline to accept, because, said I, I have promised to my God henceforth to abstain from *fermented* drinks.

"Some others among the crowd are not so kindly disposed in my favor. They would perhaps handle me somewhat rudely for my incomprehended discourse, were it not for the timely interference of a policeman, who has doubtless been enabled to perceive that if noisy, I am not a dangerous character. In answer to his questions, I inform him that I am the sport of the infernal *puissance*, who want to get possession of my soul, and who have caused me to be hunted down in this city like a malefactor, a madman. The officer shows me much kindness. He endeavors to prove that I have nothing to fear; he sees that I am a stranger, and would the less on that account let me be insulted. I then say that I am homeless, without one single acquaintance in London, but with money enough to pay for a bed. The policeman asks me if I should have no objection to sleep in a poor-house. On my reply that I have none whatever to any place in which I may pass the night, he takes me to the station, to communicate with the chief officer about what is to be done with me. Here, too, I receive a good *accueil;* but the chief officer cannot take upon himself to send me to the poor-house; I must sleep in a lodging-house. I am, therefore, conducted by the policeman, who has brought me to a decent place, where I am recommended to the landlord. Before proceeding any further, I shall here state that several times in the streets, and especially whilst in the police station, I most distinctly heard again the ringing of bells, as if coming down from above. The sound was sweet, harmonious, and seemed to be produced by silver bells. Another strange particular,—the sky appeared to be illuminated by immense and innumerable round lamps, while there was now and then something like the noise created by the fall of hailstones.

"I ask what o'clock it is. They inform me that it is nearly one. This is an eating-house, for many persons are at table, taking some food or a glass of beer. I should believe that they are carriers. I am told that the house keeps open all night, on account of the customers coming from the country. The room to which I am conducted is very spacious, and of neat appearance. It contains five beds, three of which are already occupied. I am scarcely in mine when I hear again from outside the voice of my brother-in-law more threatening than ever. He will not let me sleep. With Satan's assistance, he will get into the room : he will torment me to death. Then I fancy that he is in the yard, creating the same rattling noise as I heard once, by furiously driving an empty tumbril round a circus. He stops now and then; but it is to laugh a sarcastic laughter, to call me hypocrite, to defy God, or to indulge in an obscene discourse. This lasts until after daybreak. I am still wide awake, though I have not been in the least afraid; for there are two other voices close to my ears. They whisper to me that I have defensors, before whom Satan himself trembles. On my left I am addressed by my guardian angel, who informs me that I have been left to his care by our Lord. He says that I know him; that we were great friends; for he is the son of a neighbor of ours, with whom I used to play in my infancy. He died before he was ten years of age, more than twenty-five years ago, and became an angel in heaven. From that time he has been directed to watch over my actions. Had he been allowed to speak to me before, he would certainly have given me good counsels. For a number of years he has seen that I was running to eternal ruin, and he could do nothing but weep over my disorders, and pray that my eyes should be opened. I have many friends in heaven, many relations who also interceded for my salvation. But *what was written was written.* I was destined to rush headlong to the very brink of destruction.

"I then ask my guardian angel if he was not with me already, when I lay on a sick bed in Derry. He says he was; but he did not speak to me. I was then addressed by my full cousin, a young man of about twenty-seven years when he died, and who was a priest. To my question whether I shall be saved, my guardian angel gives no answer; but I hear, on my right, another voice, which says that I shall.

"This voice is clearer and more distinct than the first. It is the voice of God Almighty himself, who deigns to communicate with me. I listen in awe and silence to the revelations that are being made. They generally relate to the destiny of my family and friends in the world to come. Parents, brothers, sisters, uncles, aunts, &c., all have the secret of their respective fates unfolded before me. Every life is minutely reviewed one after the other; every action, good or bad, carefully weighed. It is incredible how there is nothing forgotten or overlooked; it seems as if an every moment account-book has been kept, not only concerning the deeds but the thoughts and intentions of each. Most of them are doomed to suffer forever ; some for a certain length of time, and *one*, only *one*, is to obtain the kingdom of heaven. Then do I recollect a passage of the Scripture, which I thought I had forgotten : '*Multi enim vocati, pauci verò electi.*'

"It is a long time since the men have got up. I am still listening. Sometimes I presume to venture a question as to my future line of conduct. Every time I receive kind instructions for my guidance. Lastly, my imagination carries me to a scene hitherto unknown. I behold a sea of fire, into which an invisible hand precipitates the sinners, who have all preserved their human forms. As they appear one by one before the Supreme tribunal, I hear these redoubtable words from the Almighty : '*Allez, fils de Satan, allez brûler dans le feu de l'enfer.*' Although free from fear, I cannot help exclaiming more than once : ' *Ô mon Dieu ! que votre justice est terrible !*' I feel that I should like to sleep now ; but I do not dare, for fear of displeasing God. The voice lets me know that I can rest myself after a short prayer. I therefore pray until I fall asleep. It must be at least five o'clock.

"My sleep has been quite refreshing, not at all troubled by bad, terrifying dreams. It is breakfast-time when I get up. The voice on my right is gone ; but my guardian angel is still here. He says he will not leave me. After dressing, I kneel down by the bedside and say my morning prayers. My mind is much at ease. I have more confidence in myself ; but no arguments could persuade me that the many events of last night are not real ; everything must be true.

"When I have done praying, I come down stairs. There are people engaged in breakfast. I ask for a cup of tea, with toast. They also bring me a little slice of ham, which I leave untouched, because I have no appetite to taste it. The rain has been falling a part of the night. It is not over yet. I wait in the room until it has abated. Then I resume my random strolls. I imagine that everybody knows what took place last night. Again the cries of '*there is a madman*' reach my ears. Whatever way I may go, they follow me ; I cannot get rid of them. After several hours passed in moving about, like a mere machine, I find myself out of town, in the open fields, with only a few scattered houses in sight. Here I hope that I shall be more quiet. Although I was very thirsty, I had not dared to step into any place for refreshment, because I feared to be recognized as the madman of yesterday. My guardian angel, whose advice I ask, tells me that I may take ginger-beer, but nothing else. The sky has cleared up; I sit down on the grass to rest myself a little. The place I have chosen is in the vicinity of a railroad. A train is coming, and, as it runs by, I distinctly and repeatedly hear the same annoying cry, '*there is the madman*,' as if all the passengers were acquainted with my history. I am extremely tired; I should like much to stop a little longer; but an invisible force bids me leave the spot and move on. I thus continue on my feet for some more hours, listening to the voice within me, and at times answering half aloud. I bend my steps back to town again, whither I am accompanied by the unceasing cry, to which I now submit with less reluctance. It must be late in the afternoon. The sky is overcast. I begin to be anxious about a place of rest. At last I find a chapel, and sit down at the door. I remain there for some time. The sudden idea strikes me that I am about to die; indeed, I feel something like two lobsters creeping up inside my chest. They are sucking my blood; and a voice tells me that I have but a few minutes more to live. This frightens me. My conscience is not in a right state yet; I am afraid to die. I go on in search of a chemist's shop, where I hope to obtain some relief. When I have found one, I complain of exhaustion, and ask for any strengthening medicine. The chemist gives me a cordial composed of—I don't know what,—which I swallow in the utmost confidence. I feel a little better, but not so well as to drive all fears of an imminent death away. My wishes are now to get to a Catholic chapel, and there to apply to a priest for confession. I therefore inquire about the nearest place of Catholic worship; I am directed to one about two miles off. Thither I direct my tottering steps: I find the door open, but no priest in. An old woman, whom I ask for him, says that she cannot tell me where he is. I leave this chapel to look for another; new wearisome stroll of nearly one hour. There is the object of my search, at last; but the entrance-door is locked: no possibility for me to get in. What to do? It is growing dark. The rain falls in large drops; I have no shelter, and I would not step into any public house for fear of being at once recognized as the madman, and, as such, exposed to the abuse, perhaps to the blows, of the people. I come to the conviction that there shall be no rest for me until I have found out the inn in which I slept last night. I imagine that I shall be able to find it, and it is only after much time has been spent in walking at random that I perceive my presumptuous mistake. During all the time, the harassing cry of '*there is the madman*' has not ceased to sound by my ears. I again see and hear my persecutors beside me ; now and then, too, the voice of my guardian angel keeps me up, as well as the silvery chime from above : this especially takes place when I have been praying fervently. Meanwhile, the rain has not abated ; I am wet through ; it is a late hour in the night, for I see lights nowhere except in very few public houses. I have made repeated applications for a bed—all in vain. There was no accommodation. My resolution is now to pass the night out, and, as the rain prevents me from sitting down, to walk on until day-light. I reach a sheltered place, where, for want of a seat, I have been standing up for some time, when a policeman passes by. He asks me how it is that I am there at such a late hour. I tell him that I could not find any lodgings, &c. . . . . . He can see by the gas-light that my clothes are very wet, and I appear to be ex-tremely fatigued. He wishes to afford me a shelter for the remainder of the night at the police-station. I follow him ; but the head officer cannot allow that I should stop in, because, says he, there is no charge against me. On the kind request of my guide, he, however, consents to send me to a workhouse, and writes a few words to that purpose, which he hands to the police-man. On our way to the poor-house, my imagination again works on my mind. I fancy that we are closely followed by an evil spirit, under the shape of a wolf, and with a human voice. I often complain to the officer that there is a demon behind us, who throws at me the same white-colored liquid from which I formerly suffered so much. The dreaded shower burns all my body like boiling lead; it is accompanied with imprecations and fits of laugh-ter from my pursuer. We arrive at the poor-house. They give me a bed, in which I soon fall asleep.

" This first night has been quiet. When I awake in the morn-ing, I expect that they are going to dismiss me ; but I must wait for the doctor's visit. The medical gentleman easily perceives that I am not so well as I think. He cannot grant my discharge, unless I have a place to go to. I feel quite surprised at the answer. I give way to despair, and reason leaves me altogether.

The sight and hearing, so much impaired already, may now be termed mere organs of delusions. Besides mine, there are five beds in the room. In one of them, I see a miserable victim, like myself. The four others are occupied by infernal spirits of the first order. They are the rebellious angels who presumed to revolt against God Almighty. Here, also, I shall meet with new attacks from my brother-in-law. I don't see him: I hear his voice and oaths as if he were in a room below. He said that it was himself who last night pursued me with the burning liquid, when on my way to the workhouse with the policeman. I shall not so easily escape now; for I am shut in, and he has powerful friends with him,—he means the evil spirits. He then discloses to me the secret and uncomprehended motives of his unceasing persecutions. I have done him no harm whatever; we ought, therefore, to be still on the same terms of good friendship as we were formerly. All this he cannot deny. However, he hates, he abhors me, and will only be happy when he sees me a corpse. My death must be the sinner's death. There must not be any time left for repentance; because, not content with selling his own soul to Satan, he has likewise disposed of mine. The condition imposed by the Prince of Darkness is, that I shall die in my present state of sin. It appears that Satan sets a great value upon my soul. My brother-in-law informs me that 15,000 francs are the terms of the agreement in which I am, unknown to myself, so seriously concerned. I wonder much how my soul may be so eagerly sought for by the *Evil One*. My brother-in-law's soul fetched only 80*l*. Is mine any better? I then learn that God has decreed, in his inscrutable wisdom, that I shall obtain a place in the kingdom of heaven. Satan is aware of it. He also knows that, after a life of sins, I am destined to endure great sufferings, and to show sincere repentance before departing this life. He therefore gives here another instance of his well-known presumption: though he is obliged to confess that his own power cannot prevent the accomplishment of my *destiny*, he wants once more to try if he will be able to surprise the Divine vigilance.

" During the first days my fears of a sudden death are extreme. Twice or three times I escape from my bed, because I fancy that one or two of the boards of the floor are lifted up to give passage to my brother-in-law, whose face I don't see, but whose threats I hear. He will shoot me with a pistol. He has received from

I see a window where I know that there is none.   There I behold
Almighty God, and our Lord Jesus Christ, such as they are represented in Catholic pictures.   Christ intercedes for me; I distinctly
notice a tear falling down his cheek, as if he were weeping over
my sins.   There also come two children, whom I take for the
Infant Jesus and John the Baptist.   Their mothers are with
them; they all want to implore God's forgiveness in my favor.
The sky outside is now bright, now it assumes a lurid appearance,
according as my prayers come from a contrite or a doubtful heart.
Towards the latter end of my confinement in the house, I am
informed that I shall be admitted into heaven.   My trials are
over; I need not fear or doubt any longer.   I am to be taken to
the celestial palaces in God's own chariot.   I feel very happy.
Shortly after, the voice tells me that my soul is gone.   My body
is now only animated by a *souffle*.   I cannot well understand, but
I believe.   Now, too, I fancy that God reveals to me the future
destinies of the world.   The kingdom of heaven is at hand:
mankind shall perish within a few days by a general conflagration.
The plague is raging in London and many cities on the Continent.
In France, the demon of murder and suicide exercises his sway
over the whole population.   Last revolution in Paris; the soldiers
are fighting against the people, then against each other, until
there is but one man surviving, who shoots himself.   Many times
I imagine that I hear a sinister voice in London: it says, '*Visited
such, such, and such streets; all dead:* may God forgive us!' &c.

"Such were the strange thoughts by which my mind was engrossed when I was removed from the poor-house.   The gentlemen
who came for me did not surprise me in the least on announcing
that I must get up, for they were to take me away.   I firmly believed that I was dead, and likely about to be admitted into heaven.
Nothing, in my imagination, could be expected.   On our way
hither, I saw houses, trees, carriages, passengers, all as it is on
earth; but I would have been averse to the idea that they did not
belong to another world, a kind of medium between earth and
heaven.

"When we alighted here, I came to think that I was to be shut
in for a limited space of time.   This was the last expiation for my
sinful life.   I kept in *sullen* silence, because it was my belief that
mutism was the condition, *sine quâ non*, for my speedy ascent to
heaven.   The attendants and patients with whom I was placed, I

considered as new temptators, whose attacks I should have to resist. Thus I fancied that my duty was to walk up and down the gallery with the least possible rest, and taking care always to tread on the same boards. I also considered it my duty to obey the attendants whenever they said, *I will*. In the yard the trial was of another kind. ' I must not,' said I, ' let any one make his way on the same path as I do; I must drive him away by constantly walking around him, and surrounding him with invisible lines, as the spider weaves his net around flies.'

" Once, I recollect, they retired to the shed. I took up my post right against them, and stood up for a long time there, moving three steps backward and forward. It seemed to me that I was ordered to do so some hundred times before allowing myself any rest. On the three or four first nights, I was in an excited state. A French book was kindly lent to me, which I did not dare to peruse, for fear it should be a snare set against my soul. In my room I used to pray and speak aloud, as I had done in the pauper-house, for I felt convinced this establishment (the purgatory) was swarming with invisible beings, some in need of my prayers, others of my exhortations. Any person approaching at that time and inviting me to be quiet, was sure to be taken for a temptator, at whom I threw the malediction, ' *Vade retrò, Satanas.*' Fortunately, I soon was enabled to see things in their proper light."

We append another interesting narrative, written by a lady after her recovery from an attack of insanity.[1] This patient possessed great accomplishments. Her imagination was active, and her character was most marked in its disposition to conceive projects and abandon them as soon as formed. Her insanity is said to have resulted from a misunderstanding that arose at a moment when she was already the victim of disappointed hopes. The conjunction of these circumstances became the exciting cause of her mental affliction. She had in Holland claims to a large sum of money, but the date of her right was at a remote period, while another family, and with all the appearance of justice, had made good their titles to the same possession. Advantageous offers, and the expectation of succeeding, by being present on the ground, urged her to proceed to Holland. After many useless plans, and

<hr>

[1] " Annales d'Hygiène."

after having seen all her efforts fail, she returned one day home with her feet very damp. The succeeding day she felt out of order, suffering much from cold feet, and pains of the head and throat. Instead of reposing in her bed, and promoting perspiration to recover her health, she sat at her desk to arrange a very long paper on her business, to which she devoted all her mind and means, so as to prove the justice of her claims. But notwithstanding the paper was written with great power, and she had presented the subject under every variety of aspect, it had no better success than the preceding memoirs. No answer was made to it; and when she called on the people to whom it had been transmitted, they always contrived to escape seeing her. Impatient, soured, and irritated at this cruel treatment, she had determined to return home, and had proposed leaving her lodgings, when she received a letter from her family, which induced her to protract her stay some time longer in Holland. The memorial which we have mentioned was the chief subject which engaged the disordered mind of this lady during the illness she had at that period. We now append the written detail which she gave of her feelings during her attack. Some few points in her history have been suppressed.

"During these transactions, I hired more retired appartments, and less dear. My landlord, a shoemaker, and all his family were worthy people, and obliging. I took them for Christians, though they were Portuguese Jews. When I was informed of that circumstance, I became painfully affected. I began to be under constant apprehension that they would rob me of my money. This fear increased to such an extent, as to deprive me of my rest. At last, I fancied that my host might some day make me swallow a narcotic draught, and assassinate me, along with my daughter, during the night, to get possession of my money. My suspicions received additional confirmation from the circumstance that these persons had prevailed on me to inscribe my name at the police-office as Madame H. A., and not Madame H. B. Tortured by fear, for the period of eight days, I scarce slept for a few instants. My food was composed of eggs, fruits, and tea, and one day, after having partaken of some bread which my landlady brought me, I was immediately attacked by a severe diarrhœa, and I had no more rest.

"My hostess explained the accident by a statement that the

police, in order to prevent an epidemic with which the country was threatened, had directed the bakers to introduce into the bread designed for the lower orders, medicines which would act as a general purge.

"My body and my head broke down, weakened by the low diet, and by the continual watching. Fear carried them away. I felt my judgment going apace along with the power of reflection; and at last I was unable to draw from any given fact conclusions in accordance with the relations of that fact. The persons around me became still more fully suspected by me; and the end was, the loss of my reason.

" Two dreams, one of my daughter, the other about myself, occurring in the same night, brought my disease fully out. My daughter told me, that she had witnessed me throwing myself into the street from the third flat of a house in the town, and that I remained stretched on the pavement broken in pieces, and dead. We went to try and discover the house which she had seen in her dream; it was the Court of Judicature. As for my dream, it was that a man, bearing a purse, had entered the house of the Portuguese Jew, and had cut my throat. The day after I was busy washing some clothes, when raising my eyes I saw (and I was wide awake) a long knife passing over the ceiling of my room. Struck with alarm, I bade my daughter to be silent. In great haste I placed all my money in my work-bag, I closed my trunk, and hurried my daughter into the street, taking with me all my most important papers. I cannot say whether some person, had not, by way of joke, passed a knife through a slit in the ceiling, or whether it was not altogether a vision, the creation of my excited imagination. This, however, is undoubted, that I was quite awake, and in full possession of all my wits, when I saw the instrument of death. I had met shortly before, in descending the staircase, a man with a large purse under his arm, probably a barber. The appearance of that man deprived me of my self-possession; and once out of the Jew's house, reason completely deserted me. I then went to one of the body-guard. I addressed a young officer, and begged him with fervor to carry immediately to the king the packet of letters on me; but as he hesitated, and left me under the pretext of calling a superior officer, I hastened away from him, and went to the German Chancery, where I compelled the worthy keeper of the records, M. Z——, to take my packet and preserve it for me. I also told him of my causes for alarm, and made him acquainted with the danger I dreaded. He took leave of me after having offered some commonplace consolations, and I found myself again in the street. Here, however, everything was changed as far as regarded me. The city, so tranquil but a moment ago, was in the height of an insurrection. The regiment quartered in the garrison was Jewish. The prince royal and the king had been made prisoners and condemned to death. The enemy had broken ground at Schevelingen. The Asiatic hordes were commanded by the Jews. Of what use could the gold be to me? I said to myself, and I returned to my landlord's door. I called his wife. I threw my money down on the work-table, advising her to begin a petty trade with it; and I concluded by a humble request for one louis, that I might return to Germany.

"The face of the poor Jewess must have actually been seen at the instant when she received so unexpectedly large a gift, to conceive the astonishing effect it had on her countenance—it actually became purple. She could not divine how to explain the matter; but she concluded in offering me a piece of gold, and would have allowed me to go away without any further remark, had not her husband come in. He took a handful of the louis, and slipped them, almost without my consciousness, into my bag. The louis, however, were restored too late, from which cause I was led to believe the family highly honorable. Having in this manner, as I supposed, got rid of my money, my dread of being assassinated vanished, and I reasoned with tolerable precision for an insane person. I said to myself, the people would have killed you on account of your money; let them have it; they will countermand the assassin, and you may return home without any fear. I made this all clear to my daughter, and I took the road to Delft. I wished to pass the night in that town, and travel by the boat to Rotterdam, whence I would have proceeded to Munster by Arnheim and Emerich. I was desirous to see Madame H. at Munster, and explain to her that it was a sacred duty she owed to her husband to recall him immediately from Holland, as he ran the hazard of being branded, as one individual had already experienced, who had put in his claims for a property.

"I had changed my louis at the banker L——'s, and I was already close by the gate of the city, when I saw a young Jewess following me; and though I had made different turns to avoid her, she nevertheless hung close on my footsteps. I then went up to her and exclaimed, in a menacing tone, 'Accursed pagans! you have already crucified Christ, and this day you vent your wrath on the prince royal!' The Jewess saved herself from this dreadful apostrophe, and from that moment I was fully satisfied that the prince, who was universally beloved, was in imminent danger. I then came in contact with an inclosed palisade. I asked what was the purpose of it? Being answered that it belonged to a Jew, I persuaded myself that it was the prison of the royal family. The absurd thought excited so much pain and sympathy in my heart, that I deserted my daughter, and desired with my nails, using all my force, to make an aperture in the inclosure, that I might save the prince and bring him out along with me. Nothing could withdraw that fixed idea from my mind, which led me to the belief of war.

" This idea was further substantiated by two new visions, which existed nowhere but in my disordered brain. I saw then on the canal a little boat, with black sails and colors. My eldest daughter, whom I had left at C——, had taken refuge there, and was miserably clad. The boat, however, could not move, as the king of the Jews, under the penalty of death, had forbid any of the boatmen weighing anchor. That I might not betray her, and let her understand that she was my daughter, I returned silently; and soon after I recognized the face of a young lady of H——, in full dress, coming out of a beautiful coach, and proceeding to an adjoining house. I followed this lady to address her, but those whom I spoke to said that they had seen no one. In all haste I then took the road to Delft, where I arrived at eight o'clock in the evening. I looked out for a respectable house for lodgings, but they would receive me nowhere. Finally, I was received into the house of Capt. B——, whose lady was sick and confined to bed. Nevertheless, the people of the house showed a great interest for me, and treated me with great kindness and humanity. A new accession of fever came on, and a host of visions, more or less fantastical, all relating to the imprisonment of the prince royal, excited a furious delirium of the most extravagant nature, in consequence of which the persons with whom I resided carried me, in the course of the night, to another house. On the subsequent day a letter was despatched to the keeper of the records, M. Z——: he came to me in a closed carriage, and took me to an establishment at a distance from the street, where I was put under the care of an old servant of M. H——. A physician was called in, and at the expiration of three weeks I was so far recovered, that my guardians could no longer trace my thoughts, though my ideas still clung to the same subject.

"After having left the house of M. B——, at Delft, I fell into a state of profound melancholy. I fancied myself to be in positions which only the extreme of madness can conceive. My recollections are by no means very clear of what occurred when we were at the hotel, where we had to pass three days; still, I have a floating idea of having conversed with different people, and that I answered different questions. I think, also, that when I went to bed, a great many people came to observe me, and they talked together about my condition, but all the rest was as a dream.

"The condition, however, in which I spent the first night, seems worthy of attention. I thought myself abed, perfectly conscious, but totally unable to make any movement, in an immense abyss, in which I believed I had been buried alive, and had now awakened in the tomb, in the condition I was to live for all eternity, with the perfect consciousness of my condition, to reflect on myself. My mind which, when awake a few hours previously, had been carried away by the most extravagant frenzy, still enjoyed all its perceptions clear. I discussed with myself whether I deserved so stern a fate, and as I was unconscious of any crime done with premeditation, I concluded by supposing that this severity of punishment had been awarded to me because, though I had fulfilled my duties as much as lay in my power, I had yet neglected to do any good beyond my line of duty, &c. In other respects, I was in the same condition as a person affected with tetanus.

"I recovered myself, however, though I was in a state of extreme debility, not having sufficient strength almost to support the weight of my body. Scarcely was I awake ere I relapsed into my illusions. I began to scrutinize my room, that I might discover whether I had not fallen into the house of a merchant of souls ('*Query*, Armi'). The burlesque motions with which I prosecuted this search would undoubtedly have provoked a smile in the most serious person, and at last I went into the chimney, reasoning thus with myself, that as it was made of stones, it could not be thrown down when the house was demolished. My fears were further augmented by the pictures which ornamented the walls.

In that posture I waited in trepidation the approach of the inmates of the house. A young girl appeared, who gave me some confidence, but when I saw my old landlady enter, my emotion could not be concealed; and lastly, when two keepers were brought into the room, who were not to leave me, my wrath was fired anew, and I broke a window that I might escape.

"After some time I was permitted to go to the garden; the open air soothed me, and yet everything around me was a source of illusion to me. The houses around the garden seemed to me to be prisons filled with prisoners. I fancied the kitchen of my landlady, in which a large pot was boiling, the place where the prisoners were put to the torture. The water of the pot in which they were going to throw me, I thought was boiling oil. Full of that notion, I tore the sleeve off my daughter's robe, desirous to retain it that she might not incur the hazard of being boiled alive.

"All this receives its explanation in the condition of a phrenetic lunatic, all whose actions are influenced by so many dreadful fancies; so it is always with me, that it is impossible to alleviate, even a little, those agonies, except I am completely enlarged from them. For if I had been shut up on that day, or even bound down by chains, either fright would have stopped the flow of the blood in my veins, or it would have circulated with such intense rapidity, that, with undoubted certainty, all the arteries would have burst in my brain. Most luckily I was left in the garden, though a violent storm was approaching. I felt myself very well when my keepers were forced to retire by the rain under the protection of the alley of the house, leaving me at full liberty to contemplate the rising storm. But how different was that storm from that I had seen before, and those I have witnessed since. The clouds which rolled up from the horizon appeared to me to be the billows of the deep, rising o'er the banks of the Schevelingen to the skies, fighting in the air together over my head; while a flotilla of the enemy, on the margin of the river, carried on a deadly combat against the inhabitants. The last hour had struck for the prosperity of Holland. I did not hear any thunder; I did not witness any lightning; but I perceived the explosion of a hundred blazes of fire; the cannonade, ceaseless, reverberated in my ears: from which we may infer, with all certainty, that the ear and the eye of the insane amplify and enlarge whatever is heard or seen.

"The same remark occurred to me afterwards. As my symp-

toms appeared better, my linen and my property were restored to
me. I took them out of my trunk, and arranged them on my
table. I was struck with their great number, and even with the
appearance of a cloth and towels, which, however, I had left behind
at C——. But this joy did not continue long; and when the
following day I again examined my linen, a great many objects
appeared to be wanting, which I had fancied to have had in my
hands the previous evening; so much so, that I supposed I had
been robbed. I did not, however, communicate my suspicions to
any one.

"These two circumstances justify me in affirming that the lunatic
fancies he sees and hears objects which have no real existence. But
what I am now going to mention proves the important influence of
an individual, opportunely seen, in giving a proper degree of
assurance to the sick person; for the earliest symptoms of my
recovery take their date from the day when I saw, amongst a great
many others, a form that particularly caught my attention.

"I cannot well say whether it was the second or third day
several persons came to talk with me in the garden, but I was
extremely insolent to every one, even to Captain B——, to whom
I owe my life. At the end two men opened the gate, and looked
on my side of the garden; one was dressed in a deep blue overcoat, and he almost immediately withdrew; the other was dressed
in very beautiful uniform; he also retired. After that a young
man of a very good expression entered, having all the outward
appearances of perfect health; he spoke to me in French, and I
answered him in the same language. I took this person for the
prince royal, and the bandage fell from my eyes. I felt myself
all of a sudden in great confusion for appearing before the prince
in a *costume* so unsuited for the occasion. I was surprised that
he was still alive, and as he appeared in perfect health, the anxieties I had experienced on his account, conceiving that the enemy,
which had beleagured the country, had made him suffer great
torment, all vanished in a moment. I felt myself as if inspired
with a new life, and from that hour the visions of horror were no
more.

"It will be easily understood that this young person was not the
prince, though he was a little like him. What an infinity of good
would be conferred on the lunatic could his thoughts be anticipated,
and scenes of a nature to affect him favorably be brought before

him. Had permission been given me to leave that day, I assuredly would have committed nothing either that was ridiculous or attended with injury to any one. But there were still more cruel trials in reserve for me, from which I was not to escape until I had gone through the ordeal of three additional days' illness.

"A coach was ordered, in which M. Z——, the keeper of the records, conveyed me to La Haye, where I was placed in a house near the castle. I then had a difference with M. Z——, as we did not leave the town by the same gate we had entered. I attempted to show him that he had mistaken the road, and I felt much offended in perceiving that he, with a smile on his lips, continued the same route, without paying any attention to my observations. When we stopped, this irritation was further increased on perceiving a child looking at us. I said to it that it deserved the rod, which caused it to run away. As I ascended the stairs I counted the steps; and I was again thrown into distress on getting to my room, when I saw that the door could not be locked from within.

"My alarm, however, became extreme, when I firmly believed that I thought I recognized in the person of my nurse an individual whom I had seen hanged some time before at La Haye, along with another criminal, and whom accordingly I took for a spirit. In the solitude of night, I perceive myself alone in company with this person, full of the most agonizing apprehensions. I would not allow the shutters to be closed at nightfall; and as, when I thought I had seen the prince, I had no longer any dread of war, I was fully persuaded that our soldiers had been victorious, so this idea stirred up in my breast the fears of being assassinated. When the pump was worked in the yard I fancied that they were going to throw the water up into my room, and I looked every moment to see it rushing in. Noticing three nails in my room, I supposed that they intended to hang us on them, myself, my daughter, and my nurse, because the latter had been condemned to death.

"Resting on my couch one evening, but quite awake, I watched every step of the nurse with my eyes, as I thought her a spirit; the candle ran, but I did not observe the tallow flow from *that* candle, but from a hole in the wall, whence it was discharged in an enormous quantity, resembling a furious torrent which has burst through its banks, so that I screamed aloud, and pretended that they were going to suffocate me. The incident made me suspect that they had the intention to poison the atmosphere, and ever from that moment I constantly experienced a disagreeable though sweet smell. All the viands offered to me had that taste. I thought that the meat they brought was human flesh, and insisted on the idea that they desired to poison me. Since my complete restoration to health I have discovered, in one of my walks, a poisonous plant, which had the disagreeable odor I allude to.

"The circumstance I have referred to, of the tallow running down the wall, is a convincing proof to me that persons laboring under disorder of the mental faculties, perceive objects which have no real existence, and that the sight of particular matters produces, spontaneously, images in the eye of the diseased person.

"Even at a later period, when I was improving, I still saw Dr. T——; then my brother-in-law; I heard the voice of my sister, as also another voice, which, speaking to me by my name, bade me 'lay down the petition.'

"I often requested of my keepers to have my clothes, my papers, and my money; but they answered me that they were to be kept till my husband appeared, who ought to come and inquire for me. On several occasions I objected to this arrangement (pleading the expense it would be attended with) to interest the persons who detained me to permit me to travel alone; this, however, they would not accede to, though I had become much more calm. Several dreadful dreams broke in on this state of tranquillity, tallying, however, very appositely with my condition. There I was, in the realms of Pluto below, which I examined with a remarkable degree of firmness and self-possession. I saw, moreover, the *aqua tolena* prepared. I had read an account of this horrible torture, the frightful details of which were all reproduced in the dream, and my children were the unhappy victims of this barbarity of the Italiani. I would rather suffer in reality every kind of imaginable torture, than again experience that horrible dream. On being awakened I found that I had been dreaming, but still one uneasy idea succeeded another, and the last of the kind was on my return, after having been in a *diligence*.

"We might be almost persuaded to conclude from these facts, that every visible object should be withdrawn from the eye of the lunatic; but if what I witnessed gave rise to misinterpretation on my part, those things which were concealed from me excited still more extraordinary conjectures.

"I converted the office in the house into a chamber where the torture was performed; every time I heard a packet sealed I thought it was the *coup-de-grace* of some unfortunate wretch. An old apartment, always closed, containing ancient records, and full of armories, was the charnel-house, and the armorer represented the coffins. I firmly believed that the story above me was a conservatory for the remains of those who had been assassinated, until one day, finding the door open, and all being still in the house, I went up quietly myself to ascertain how far my painful suspicions were well founded. Great, then, was my happiness, when, instead of bones, skeletons, and carcasses, I saw nothing but torn old waste paper. My curiosity was wound up to the highest pitch, and yet I had not courage to touch one of the leaves. I opened a window which looked into the royal garden; the windows of the apartment of the king also commanded a view of the garden. I noticed at one of the windows a tall lady in white robes; the moment I saw her she rose from her chair somewhat hastily, and I supposed she was the princess. From that moment all my fantastical notions were centred in that princess, as I thought she was detained as a prisoner in that room.

"I looked then by the windows in the front of the house where I was, and I noticed a range of buildings which surrounded the castle in the form of a circle. It would be interesting to ascertain whether, from the windows of that roof, the view which I describe here can be enjoyed in perfection, to determine whether my senses were not under the sway of an illusion, when I saw a crowd of magnificent mansions all around in that quarter. The front buildings could be perceived from my bedroom. I saw distinctly a small earthen pipe, which passed by the chimney of the house nearest the court of the castle; and it was not a long mental operation for me to conclude that the tube of that pipe was the only mode of the air having access to the house. So I likewise inferred that all the individuals who entered the house would be suffocated.

"On the day of my husband arriving, and in his presence, my whole system underwent a special change. Instead of feeling a satisfaction that I had in him a protector, I was harassed by the idea of being considered insane by him, and being placed under the control of a person whom I distrusted. Under the influence

of that fear I exercised all my self-control, that he might not suspect my insanity, though I was still far from being in full possession of my wits.   I also adopted the precaution to procure secretly
a strong dose of rhubarb.   I swallowed it all at once, and felt myself much better after.   I had done so formerly with benefit.

"Some days after the arrival of my husband, we began our
arrangements to return home.   We secured places in the diligence,
though we would have done better by hiring a carriage, as we had
to pay for three seats.   We were then fairly on our road, and the
shocks and jolts of the wretched vehicle in which we travelled,
were of no small service in restoring my addled brain.   I soon
found that my reason was restored.

"We arrived for the night at a town beyond A——, where we
were to stay till the morning.   We had a bedroom, but there was
no lock to it.   When my husband had undressed and gone to bed,
I noticed that he had left his pantaloons near the door, which was
ajar, and I was afraid lest he had left money in his pockets.   I
searched them, and found, to my great delight, thirty-two double
louis, of those which I had taken with me ; and in addition the sum
of two hundred *reichsthaler* in single louis.   I immediately concealed
the thirty-two double louis in my clothes, intending, if my husband
did not adopt better arrangements for our journey, to start alone
on foot, and manage the gold coins myself.   This money which I
had worked hard for in my early life, and which I had recovered,
imparted to me a new spirit, so that from that instant I felt that I
had entered on a new life.   My fears all vanished, and everything
about me appeared under a new light.   Desirous to give my husband some little annoyance, as a punishment for his want of prudence, I placed in his bed the money which belonged to him, retaining my own.   The following morning his alarm was great when he
found his pockets empty, though his pantaloons were on the chair
he had put them on the previous evening.   I comforted him,
restoring to him the money, and told him that his manner of
travelling, though it was highly extravagant, was not the more
pleasant on that account; that I would not contribute any more
to the general expenses, but pay only those of myself and my
daughter.   Notwithstanding my remonstrance, as he persisted in
travelling by diligence, I left him in a village, and proceeded alone
as far as the gates of Westphalia.   I should undoubtedly have

lost my way, had it not been for an incident which has much the appearance of the marvellous.

"Arriving at a place where three roads cross, I was going to follow that which would have brought me back to the point whence I had started, when I noticed the tracks of a man who had probably conveyed corn to the town of Minden : a sack had burst, and a considerable amount of the corn had escaped. My head was still feeble, and I had an explanation ready for this adventure : I conjectured then, and very luckily this time, that this corn had been spread on the road to enable me to escape from the labyrinth in which I was involved. I followed the marks with perfect confidence, and treading steadily on the corn, I passed over roads almost impracticable, and through several villages, getting finally into the highroad, where I met the diligence, which, taking that route, had made a long circuit : there I joined my husband and my daughter.

"At Minden, I took the arrangements for the continuance of our journey into my own hands, and hired a private carriage for ourselves. Notwithstanding this, the most trivial circumstance suggested erroneous fancies ; but as I was in a state of perfect liberty, I examined very attentively the subjects which had awakened surprise in my breast, and I gradually became conscious of my errors. I still recollect several of these very singular visions.

"At the period of which I now speak, I was in no way uneasy as to my own fate, or that of my family, but I was distressed by a feeling of sympathy for the Jews, discomfited, as I thought, in Holland, and scattered in the woods in the neighborhood of C——, where they were perishing of hunger and cold, along with their wives and children. I daily resorted to the woods and deposited bread and money, particularly near the cross-roads.

"Two regiments passing through the city at the same time, had a coffin in their escort : this circumstance affected me with alarm, for I thought that their king was in the coffin. To convince myself of the truth of the circumstance, I ran across the garden to meet the procession ; but the body had disappeared, and afterwards I understood that the coffin was tenantless. I called a young soldier, who was following the regiment at a distance ; I made several questions to him on the subject, but he did not answer me, but went away, without saying one word, to a hillock covered with verdure and thorns ; he there made a hole in the midst of the thorns with his cane. He still declined answering me, when I asked him whether a king had not been buried on one of the banks of the Rhine? I was soon, however, satisfied that the silent soldier was a spirit, which idea made me exceedingly uncomfortable.

"Fear, probably, and the stormy season to which I had been constantly exposed, again disturbed the harmony of my intellectual powers. From that day, as soon as I arrived in the country, I observed on the summit of all the mountains which circumscribe the horizon, machines which appeared to me to be telegraphs, and I fancied, at the conclusion, that the enemy, after having cut a canal, had beat back the Prussian army as far as the Rhine, driving it into the deep, and that they were anxious to preserve the vessels and the corpses of the parties so destroyed, as trophies of their victory. This idea excited in my mind a determined hatred against the barbarous men capable of so atrocious a deed: and to show that I could not be blamed for being a party to its execution, the strange notion came into my head to send some loaves and a bottle of brandy to several detachments of recruits on their route through the town: they took the brandy, and handed the loaves over to the poor."

Since this lady returned to her native city, her visions, though not exhibited by outward signs,—as she has now acquired sufficient self-control to conceal them from the world,—are still frequently renewed. She retained the notion for a long time, that the Jews had resolved to destroy the Christians. She also saluted with much courtesy and humility all the Jewesses; if they were clothed in rags, she addressed them in terms of extreme politeness, offered them her kind offices, and endeavored to comfort them. She sometimes gave the poor Jews a piece of money, in which she conceived there was some particular virtue.

At last, she gave up this notion, as she became daily convinced that her apprehensions were altogether chimerical; but she adopted a notion exactly the reverse. This contrast is often noticed in the dreams of the insane. She fancied that a great number of Jews were encamped in an immense forest behind a mountain in the vicinity of the town where she lived—that the government kept them prisoners there, and watched them, and that they were condemned to perish a wretched death by hunger. Actuated by sympathy for those unfortunate beings, and indignant at the cruel measures enforced against them, she ventured several times out near the forest, and placed at different parts by the wayside all kinds of food, such as loaves, fruits, eggs, &c., so that these unhappy creatures might pick them up, and that some of them at least might escape from the dreadful death to which they had been doomed.

The following is an account written by a physician, of his own case. When deranged, he imagined himself to be pursued by a demon. He had also other delusions. He fancied himself transported from street to street, and his imagination was active enough to exhibit to him every moment some different public place, in which his guards detained him on his bed. "I almost continually supplicated," says the author, "to be only carried to my house in *Holy Ghost Street.*" The persons about the patient, in endeavoring to pacify him, without complying with his wishes, only confirmed the delusion under which he labored. Their cry was: "It shall be done in a few hours, or early to-morrow, as it is now night." He lay pining in vain for the end of these few hours, and during the time his fancy created places not the most agreeable for his residence. Sometimes it pitched him between two walls, so close that he could not heave an arm; sometimes on a burial-ground; sometimes on the court before the hospital he attended. All the arguments of his friends availed nothing to prove to him that he was really in his own room. When they pointed out to him his own books, close beside which he lay, or the prints that hung opposite, he took it for a trick. Sometimes he did not recognize them for his own; and sometimes he conceived they had been removed to his present place of abode.

It was observed that the sound of a horn transported him in imagination to a public place for music and dancing; the neighing of a horse in the street to a stable; the bad odor of his own exhalations to a burying-ground.

He was under a delusion that he was hated and deserted by the whole world, that all his friends had forsaken and his patients renounced him. The foundation of fact on which this superstructure of despondency was raised, arose from his missing three of his most intimate friends, who were absent or incapable of attending upon him. With this must be considered a natural mistrust he entertained towards mankind, which his friends told him they had observed when he was in health. The number of unpleasant things he experienced from those about him, such as their refusal to let him quit his bed, forcing him to take medicines, applying blisters, must have added force to his morbid impressions.

"My other fancies were," he observes, "probably those most common in every form of delirium. The flowers on my curtains and tester, I took for men in continual movement. They all went towards the wall; and as there were none but my acquaintance, I often joined them. We found ourselves in large illuminated subterraneous chambers, where I learned such family secrets as every man in the world above keeps close locked up in the recesses of his bosom. Once I really called my wife to my bedside, and told her a shocking transaction, involving two of our friends, which I had learned in these subterraneous assemblies. I related the story with so much consistency, and gave it such an air of probability, as to make her take it for a real fact, which I must have known before my illness."

A patient, who had passed through a painful attack of insanity, was requested by the medical gentleman who had charge of the case to put in writing an account of the sensations he experienced at the commencement of his illness. I should premise that the patient imagined that among his friends and relations there existed a grand conspiracy against his life. He was also under the delusion that poison had been administered to him in his tea, and that he had escaped death only by drinking a small portion of the liquid. He thus describes the fancies he entertained in reference to a person under whose supervision he was temporarily placed. He says, "The attendant sometimes affected to smile at me with pity for my unhappy state of mind. Then he would lean back on the couch, close his eyes; open them a little, so that the eye could barely be seen through the lashes, and so as to prevent his being observed, as he thought. At those times he would cast the most infernal looks at *me*, and afterwards round the room for some weapon or other to finish what he had begun: the latter I could see not only from his looks, and the hardness his muscles used to assume, but also from the posture he would put himself into, ready to jump, if he discovered what would answer his purpose."

"From July, 1847, to November of the same year," says the Rev. Mr. Walford, when describing his attack of insanity, "I was highly nervous, and experienced a considerable loss of strength and flesh. I spoke sometimes so sharply to those around me as to startle them and make them fear me. About this time (the beginning of the attack) I felt great anxiety for the eternal salvation of my employer. His brother was lying ill, and I begged that I might visit him, but my offer was refused. I therefore prayed earnestly for his recovery, and had the satisfaction of hearing next day that he was better. Strong hope, mingled with fear, now took possession of me. When at prayer something would pull at my back, blow in my face, as if in derision, and, hovering round my mouth, try to snatch the words from my lips. At night, when in bed, I felt something press upon my chest, and awoke in great trepidation in the middle of the night, when I sometimes heard music at a distance. These impressions terrified me so much that I dreaded to lie down. Then, again, I was afraid of forfeiting God's confidence by committing some undefined sin that I could not resist. Therefore I felt a strong inclination to leave the house of my benefactor, which desire was increased by my imagining that the persons in it would fall into apostasy. Hence I had recourse to prayer with all my heart, and all my power; and while praying I nearly fainted. It next occurred to me that my employer had become rich by unjust gains, and that he and his wife would be trodden down in the streets and trampled to death. One evening, while at prayer, I saw a circle descend slowly on my head, and afterwards told my wife that I was the anointed of the Lord, but she did not appear to understand my meaning. Felt that I was very ignorant of the Scriptures, but expected every day that the power of God would instruct me, and that I should be commanded to leave the house on a sudden : so I put all things in order for my departure. On the 9th of March I left; but I was greatly agitated, and wept frequently, being unable to restrain my feelings. About this period I began to see objects, like gnats, floating before my eyes, and thought they were wicked spirits watching me; however I felt satisfied that I was anointed in a very high degree, and that my mission from the Holy Spirit was to walk incessantly about and convert the people I met with. As I passed near to them I believed the Holy Spirit transferred itself from me to them ; so I selected the most crowded thoroughfares in the metropolis for the work of conversion, and extended my walks daily, sometimes even into the adjoining counties; and I thought the people often turned round and looked at me as I passed with great satisfaction, as if conscious of the blessing I had conferred on them. To see the crowds I had converted greatly encouraged

9

me in my labors; and now, delighted with my office, I had special revelations. One night, while in bed, I saw the glory of the moon. It was like a horizontal pillar across the moon, which increased in size and radiance as it approached my bedroom window. I now believed that I was to be a prince, and the high prince of our Saviour. Upon the approach of the morning I felt a burning flame around me, and conceived that it was the glory of God sanctifying me for the work I had to perform. My sensations frequently alarmed me. More than once I was afraid I should go mad, and then I alternately laughed and wept. One day I heard my feet speaking to me, telling me that I should be a king, and reign at Jerusalem; and I also heard other voices telling me that I was Dan, the son of Jacob, and should have large possessions at Jerusalem. Thus, having left my home, I wandered over miles of ground, imagining that I was forbidden to sit down or stand still; and, after having walked the whole night, one morning I arrived in Sion lane, and was, by one of the cottagers, conducted to the house, where I expected to find food and rest. The proprietor, I supposed, was a high churchman; and I expected all the inhabitants would come while I was asleep and look at me, in order that they might be converted. During the first few weeks of my residence there many strange fancies came across my brain; with my new companions and the medical gentlemen I conversed freely, and gradually became quite conscious that I had been under delusions, which have happily passed away, and my mental health is now, I am grateful to believe, quite restored."

CHAPTER V.

How deeply interesting are the descriptions sometimes given
by the insane of their state of mind when passing *out* of a *deranged into* a *sane* condition of intellect. In some cases, the
reason is restored suddenly to its sovereignty; in many cases,
however, the mind appears gradually and almost imperceptibly to
awaken, as it were, out of a fantastic and fairy-like dream, into
a healthy state of consciousness. In one case, the patient described his mental condition during the period when it was considered to be *in transitu*, as follows : " I felt as I was recovering,
the delusions gradually losing their hold upon my fancy. I then
began to entertain doubts as to their reality. I felt disposed to
listen patiently to the judicious advice of my physician. I was
no longer irritated at being told that my perceptions were false,
and began to appreciate the absurdities of other patients. One
fellow-sufferer, who firmly believed that he was endowed with
supernatural power, and divine authority, and whom I had always
considered as *sane*, and improperly confined, and had invariably
treated with great awe and deep reverence, I now thought must
be mad!" The dark clouds that had so long obscured, enshrouded,
and embittered this patient's mind were gradually dissipated, and
the bright sun of reason shed its joyous and effulgent light upon
his hitherto darkened and bewildered understanding. As he progressed towards recovery, his mental perceptions became daily
more clear and intelligible. Whilst in this intermediate phase of
morbid thought he was forcibly reminded of Milton's majestically
poetical, and profoundly philosophical passage in which he makes
Adam relate to the angel what passed in his mind immediately
after awakening into life :—

" Whilst thus I call'd and stray'd I knew not whither,
From where I first drew air and first beheld
This happy light, when answer none return'd,
On a green shady bank, profuse of flowers,
Pensive I sat me down ; there gentle sleep
First found me, and with soft oppression seiz'd
My droused sense ; untroubled, though I thought
I then was passing to my former state
Insensible, and forthwith to dissolve." . . .

PARADISE LOST, b. 8, l. 283.

Another patient described his state of mind when recovering, as follows :—" During the whole of my illness, which lasted for eighteen months, I always fancied myself surrounded by a dark cloud. I never could appreciate that there was any difference between day and night. Even when the sun shone most brightly, it produced no alteration in my feelings. I fancied that I was doomed to live for the rest of my days in a state of perpetual gloom and never-ending darkness, as a punishment for sins I had committed in early youth. No bright object, alas! looked so to my mind. I found that I could gaze, without the least inconvenience, at the sun, even when at its height. It did not, in the slightest degree, dazzle me.

"I date the commencement of my recovery from the time when this mysterious darkness began gradually to fade away." "When I was getting well," the patient continues, "I fancied I saw objects more clearly and less through a haze. My mind appeared, during this distressing illness, as if it were covered, if I may so speak, by a dark veil. This is the only comparison that occurs to me. It was as if I were looking through a piece of green glass at every object. This cloudy condition of mind did not disappear altogether for some months, but as I began to see things with my natural vision, I felt that I was getting well. This state of progressive recovery continued until I saw everything through a clear and sunny atmosphere, and then my happiness and peace of mind were restored ; in other words, I was well."

A gentleman who imagined, without the slightest foundation for such an impression, that his wife had been unfaithful to him, persisted in entertaining this delusion for a whole year. He declined, during the greater part of his illness, having any communication with, and rarely speaking civilly to her when she called to see him. His general health was much shattered by a sedentary occupation and neglect of the ordinary rules of hygiene. His mind had also, for a long period, undergone much anxiety. At times he suffered from severe mental depression. His general health, in course of time, became greatly improved, but there were symptoms of local disturbance in the head that at first led to the suspicion of the existence of some form of organic disease of the brain.

A few months before his recovery, a large carbuncle made its appearance in the lumbar region. This caused great pain, and confined him to his bed for some weeks. Subsequently, numerous *furunculi* broke out in various parts of the body, attended with great general irritation and serious disorder of the assimilative functions. He was invalided for many months. He, however, entirely recovered, still, however, entertaining the delusion with regard to his wife, but in a somewhat modified and less acute form. At first he began to reason with himself as to the reality of this impression. He asked himself the following questions:— "Is my suspicion founded on fact? What proof have I of the infidelity of my wife? Could I establish an accusation of the kind against her, in a court of law? If I were to apply for a divorce on the ground of infidelity, who would be my witnesses?" Up to this time, he had resolutely maintained a firm belief in his wife's gross acts of immorality, and it was not until after his serious bodily illness that he began to waver on the subject of his delusion.

For nearly three weeks, a contest of this character took place in his mind. It was a struggle between healthy and disordered impressions. Occasionally, he appeared entirely to lose the delusion. It then recurred to his mind, but much less strongly than before. I advised a complete change of air and scene, and suggested a residence at Boulogne for a few weeks. He obeyed my instructions, went to this place, participated in the amusements it afforded, had a course of sea-bathing, and returned in a few weeks to England, in the full enjoyment of the "*mens sana in corpore sano.*" He informed me that one day when returning from a tepid salt-water bath, which had greatly exhilarated him, all idea of his wife having behaved even with indiscretion, vanished entirely from his mind. "I felt," he says, "a gush of joyous feeling take possession of my thoughts, that produced an indescribable state of happiness, which made me almost leap for joy."

A lady who had been for a period of nine months insane, believing that she was forsaken of God, appeared suddenly to recover. Her restoration to health of mind, however, was not so rapid as her friends were at first led to suppose. She gave her husband, after she returned home, a detailed and deeply interesting account of the gradual return of reason, and of the steady battle she had been carrying on for two months with the insane delusions. For more than eight weeks she had been struggling with the morbid impressions which had so poisoned her mind. The commencement of this contest occurred contemporaneously with a return of the uterine functions, which had been suspended for a considerable period. This improvement in her general health appeared to shake her belief in the existing delusion. At that period, she said, " I, for the first time during my long illness, asked myself seriously the question, ' Am I under a delusion ?' " For some days the morbid impressions caused her less mental distress; but having, owing to an attack of stomach disorder, passed two or three sleepless nights, the delusion returned in full force to her mind. After the lapse of a week, she again began quietly to reason with herself as to her insane religious notions. She then went regularly to church, without feeling, as she did previously, that "she was only mocking God by so doing." " I felt," she said, " a comfort in the prayers, and could listen with repose and satisfaction to the sermon." But even at this time, her mind was occasionally much distressed by some, but less acutely manifested, morbid and gloomy apprehensions as to the salvation of her soul. She continued, however, gradually to recover a sane state of thought. She no longer persisted in refusing to adopt the remedial measures suggested for her cure, and *pari passû*, with an improvement in the *physical*, did I witness the return of a healthy state of the *intellectual* functions. She informed me, after her recovery, that she was impelled by an internal voice to refuse compliance with everything that was proposed by myself in the way of treatment. She fancied that she was doing God service by resisting all the attempts that were made to improve her bodily and mental health.

I have, in a previous page, referred in detail to the deeply interesting history which has been published of the Rev. Mr. Walford's state of morbid religious despondency, as described by himself after his recovery. It will not be out of place here to put upon record Mr. Walford's account of his gradual restoration to mental health. He says :—

"The blissful recovery which I experienced was not to be ascribed to any medical process whatever. I had, indeed, much against my own inclination, been so importuned by my friends as to consent, three or four years before my recovery took place, to consult one or two medical advisers; but the effect proved, as I fully expected, that nothing was to be hoped for from this expedient, and I positively refused to see any other medical persons. About the same time, I was over-persuaded, on account of my general inability to sleep, to keep laudanum by my bedside, and to have recourse to it when sleep was found to be impracticable. I tried this measure two or three times, without any sensible effect, and firmly resolved to take no more. I adhered to my purpose, and no other experiments of the kind were ever adopted. A few months before any symptoms of improvement appeared, I now and then prevailed on myself to walk up and down a few hundred yards in the road adjacent to my house, when I was concealed by the darkness of the night from the notice of any who might pass me. Soon after, I went several evenings, when the light of day had departed, into my garden, and paced up and down for some time. On these occasions, I sometimes felt an impulse, during my walks, to pray, with deep fervency, that some measure of relief might be afforded to me. These prayers were short and broken, yet I trust they found acceptance in heaven.

"Some weeks or months after these occurrences, an old friend from Suffolk, a most worthy minister, came to see me, and stayed a day or two. I had formerly smoked many a pipe of tobacco in company with my friend, though for the preceding five years I could not bear the sight of a pipe. My wife, aware of his habits, had the materials for smoking set before him, which he employed, and earnestly pressed me to accompany him, which I passionately refused to do. On the evening of his departure, when, as usual, I was the only person sitting up, it occurred to me to try if I could smoke, which, for four or five years I had discontinued, on account of the manifest bad effects it produced on my pulse. I instantly procured for myself the smoking apparatus, and found I could perform the operation without the injurious results which had induced me to relinquish the practice. Soon after this experiment, I resolved to try if I could read, though I was under a great difficulty to select a book that did not seem likely to awaken painful associations, and I especially shunned all such as treated of religious subjects. Accident determined my choice. I had not relinquished a book society of which I was a member, though the books that came to my house were carefully concealed from my notice. At the time of which I am now writing, I found that a 'History of the Cotton Manufactory,' by Mr. Baines, was brought to my house, and as it seemed not very likely that anything in it would excite my feelings, I resolved, though with extreme apprehension, to try this book. In a day or two, I found nothing in it that much distressed me, and I perused it to its close. It amused me, and after reading it again, I wrote out a pretty extensive abridgment of it. I then attempted a work by Mr. Babbage, the title of which is, I think, 'The Economy of Manufactures.'

"After reading and epitomising these works, I was so much quieted as to regret that I had no others of similar character: and I then engaged in writing a translation of the history of Herodotus. Before I had completed my translation of the first book of that history, the spring brought the month of May. My son entreated his mother to take a ride in a carriage with him, and I joined in the entreaty, as I greatly wished she should enjoy some refreshment of this kind. The carriage was brought to the door, when my faithful wife positively refused to go, unless I would accompany them. This, I both thought and said, was impossible. She, however, persisted in her refusal; and for some time I warmly remonstrated with her, and urged her going. While I was thus engaged, a sudden inquiry offered itself to me: Why I could not go? I could discover no reason; and calling for my hat, I jumped into the carriage, when I directed the driver to take us to Epping Forest, through Wanstead and Woodford, a ride which, in former years, I had often taken with great pleasure. The verdure of the grass, trees, and country in general, with the fineness of the weather, so affected me, that all my fears, disquietudes, and sorrows vanished as if by a miracle, and I was well, entirely relieved, and filled with a transport of delight, such as I had never before experienced. My hope and confidence in God were restored, and all my dreary expectations of destroying myself or others were entirely forgotten. On my return home from this reviving excursion, every desire to shut myself up and exclude my friends was departed, and I could with difficulty restrain myself from being always abroad.

"This extraordinary change of feeling took place, as I have said, in May; and on the first day of the following August, I set out in company with my son and an active friend, who had before travelled on the continent, for France, Switzerland, and Germany. The delights of that journey were so enhanced by contrast with the events of the five preceding years, that I was in a species of rapture throughout the whole. I felt no apprehensions of danger in going so far from home; and the glorious scenes I witnessed so enchanted me, that my pleasure overflowed the limits of ordinary enjoyment. One only regret was occasioned by the unavoidable necessity, under which my companions in travel were placed, of returning at the end of the month to business; by which I was hurried from scenes of surpassing grandeur and interest, before I had half gratified myself with gazing upon them. Enchanted and fascinated as I was with this tour, I attribute no part of my recovery to it, as I had been entirely free from my sad condition, both of body and mind, before it took place; if this had not been the case, no wishes of my own, nor any entreaties of my friends, would have had power to persuade me to set out upon it, so deeply was I affected by the remembrance of former disappointments. Immediately after my return, I was seized with a most unexpected and severe diarrhœa, which I thought would terminate my joys and sorrows alike: it yielded, however, to skilful medical treatment, after some days; and one of my medical attendants, who had long been acquainted with my constitution, assured me when the vehemence of the paroxysms was abated, that the effects of it were far more beneficial than any medical treatment could have produced, and he anticipated a perfect freedom from the return of my distressing nervous disease. This anticipation has been verified by several successive years of established health: and though I am now occasionally in some measure disturbed by some of the minor symptoms of my disorder, for short periods, chiefly during the hours of night, my general health is remarkable for my years; and the condition of my feelings tranquil and cheerful, though seldom much elevated."[1]

[1] "Autobiography of the Rev. William Walford." Edited by the Rev. John Stoughton (of Kensington), 1854.

CHAPTER VI.

ANOMALOUS AND MASKED AFFECTIONS OF THE MIND.

BEFORE proceeding to the discussion of the various stages of incipient insanity, previously referred to, I propose to consider briefly, certain anomalous, generally unobserved, because *masked* conditions of brain and mind. I would, however, premise, that in the majority of cases of insanity, it is difficult to trace back to its origin, the first inroads and dawnings of morbid and insane perceptions, to demonstrate when the boundary-line between healthy and disordered idea has been traversed, at what precise periods certain normal states of eccentricity of *thought*, singularity and oddity of *conduct*, have passed into actual insanity. Unfortunately, there is no psychical test to which we can with safety and satisfaction, judicially and psychologically appeal, when difficult, doubtful, obscure, and subtle conditions of suspected mental disorder are submitted to us for medical, metaphysical, and legal analysis. Each case must be examined by, and *in relation to, itself*, and not in reference to any preconceived definition, or *à priori* hypothesis of insanity.[1] The vain attempt to frame a definition of this disease,

---

[1] When speaking of the degrees of departure from presupposed conditions of health, either of body or mind, perhaps the term *latitude* would be a more philosophically correct expression than the phrase *standard*, now commonly adopted. How imperceptible and shadowy are the gradual transitions from a state of health to one of disease! Who can accurately define their characteristics? We are able, however, to appreciate when there is any positive deviation on either side of the line. In the case of colors, it has been well remarked, "that we know blue and red perfectly well, but they may be blended together, in an infinite variety, in forming a purple color, and it may be impossible to say where the red and where the blue prevails. Yet this does not deprive us of the power of forming a very distinct conception of both colors, apart from each other." The experienced physician is able to appreciate when the boundary-line between reason and insanity has been traversed, although he is not competent to frame a definition that can be used as an unerring test in all doubtful cases of mental disorder.

will, in a measure, account for the great difference of opinion, as
well as unhappy conflict of testimony exhibited in courts of law by
medical men supposed to be conversant with the phenomena of disordered mind.

Before enumerating the symptoms characteristic of the commencement of insanity, I would premise that mental disorder often
first manifests itself in a marked and significant manner at a very
early period of life.   Decided paroxysms of insanity have occurred
in young children when at school, and in persons more advanced
in age whilst at college, all traces of the transient attack of mental disorder having passed, like a dark cloud, entirely away, there
being no recurrence of the disorder for many years.   Several remarkable cases of this kind have come under my observation.   In
one singular instance, a young gentleman whilst studying for university honors had an attack of insanity.   He was sitting up late
at night, busily occupied in reading, when he was suddenly seized
with an impulse to destroy everything within his reach.   He first
broke the lamp on the table, then a pier glass.   He subsequently
tore up and destroyed a number of books, and did great injury to
several articles of value in the room.   He left home about three
o'clock in the morning, and came back at eight, covered with filth,
apparently in full possession of his senses!   He refused to give
any explanation of his conduct, or to say where he had been.
When pressed upon the subject, he became irritable, sullen, and
morose.   This gentleman continued mentally well for *twelve* years,
when insanity again developed itself, and he has remained from
that period in a deranged state of mind.   A patient, now insane,
manifested, at the age of *ten*, decided symptoms of mental aberration, and to such an extent, that, occasionally, for days it was
deemed necessary to confine mechanically the hands, so mischievous were the child's tendencies.   At the age of fifteen, he, appearing like other boys, was sent to a public school, and it was not until
he was *thirty* that his insanity again manifested itself, and then it
was considered necessary to place him under restraint.

When referring to this class of case, and of the possibility of
insanity commencing at a very early age, then becoming arrested,
and even remaining dormant for *five, ten, twelve,* and *twenty* years,
Esquirol remarks, "I am more than ever convinced that the existing causes of insanity do not act abruptly, except when the
patients are strongly predisposed.   Almost all the insane exhibit,

before their disease, some alterations in their functions, alterations which commenced many years previously, and even in infancy. The greater part had had convulsions, cephalalgia, colics, or cramps, constipation, and menstrual irregularities. Several had been endowed with great activity in the mental faculties, and had been the sport of vehement, impetuous, and angry passions. Others had been fantastical in their ideas, their affections, and passions; some had had an extravagant imagination, and been incapable of continuous study; others, excessively obstinate, could not live, except in a very narrow circle of ideas and affections, whilst many, void of moral energy, had been timid, fearful, irresolute, indifferent to everything. With these dispositions, a mere accidental cause is sufficient to make the insanity break out."[1]

M. Pinel was acquainted with a case of insanity that had been going on unnoticed for a period of *fifteen* years. In several other cases, the maniacal and melancholy state had begun *four, six, ten, fifteen,* and *twenty* years previously. It is often easy to go back months or years in this way, and we finish by discovering that circumstances taken for causes by the friends, are frequently only the consequences of unobserved disease. In fact, it often happens at that period of the malady, that a slight contradiction, or fit of anger, or some cause equally insignificant to a person in good health, provokes the immediate and complete subversion of their reason, and gives rise to mistakes as to its true cause and duration. It does not, however, necessarily follow that when these symptoms of insanity appear in early life, that the disease will recur at a subsequent period. Children, as well as adults, are subject to sudden, transient, and paroxysmal attacks of temporary mental disorder, which pass entirely away, the mind retaining its healthy state for the remainder of life.

Dr. Brierre du Boismont has recently published some remarks upon the insanity of early life, in noticing the dissertation of Dr. Paulmier. This able and accomplished physician (Dr. Boismont) accounts for the comparative exemption of childhood from mental aberration, by the absence of many of the causes so potent in its production in adult life; not that children do not feel acutely, but their sensations are of a fleeting nature, and in this lies their protection. Nevertheless, children who inherit a disposition to mental

---

[1] "Dictionnaire des Sciences Médicales," T. 16, p. 195.

disease, or who possess a highly nervous temperament, and who are exposed to favoring circumstances, occasionally manifest undoubted symptoms of the malady. Haslam, Perfect, Franck, Burrows, and Spurzheim, have recorded cases of insanity occurring in children under eleven years of age. Greding gives an account of a child of eighteen months, who died of marasmus. She was brought into the asylum at Wuldham with her mother (who was insane). The child was then scarcely nine months old. She was subject to paroxysmal nervous attacks, which ended either in an indescribable laugh, or in a fit of mania, during which the little creature tore everything she could lay hands upon. Jacobi refers to several cases of insanity in children, then in the asylum of Siegburg. Esquirol treated two children, one of eight and another of nine years, and a girl of fourteen, all laboring under mania; he was also consulted about a child of eleven, in which the disease assumed the form of melancholia.

Marc gives an account of a little girl of eight, who freely admitted that she wished to kill her own mother, her grandmother, and her father. Her object was, to be possessed of their property, and to have an opportunity of indulging her passions. The child was morose, pale, and silent; when spoken to, her answers were very abrupt. Her health was improved by a residence in the country, but on being brought back to town, she became again pale and melancholy. For a long time the cause remained undiscovered; at length it was found that she was addicted to bad habits, which she openly avowed, regretting at the same time that she had not the opportunity of indulging her animal passions. Dr. Brierre du Boismont noted four cases, of children of six, seven, and ten years of age, in whom the symptoms of mental disease were manifest; and at present he has under his care a female child of three and a half years old, born of a paralytic father, which shows the strangest caprices; at one time sad and melancholy; again in the most violent fits of rage, without any cause, and not to be appeased. The intelligence of the child is far beyond its years. The cases of insanity brought under notice by Dr. Paulmier cannot be said to belong to childhood; his children are young people; ·for of thirteen examples, three are fourteen, two fifteen, three sixteen, and five seventeen years of age. Before, however, analyzing Dr. Paulmier's work, Dr. Brierre du Boismont turns to English, French, and American authors for information on the subject. In Dr. Thurnam's "Observations and Statistics of Insanity," there is a table of 21,333 cases. Under ten years, eight cases, and from ten to twenty, 1161 cases are noted. According to Dr. Thurnam, the greatest number of cases of insanity occurs between thirty and forty. In the United States, however, physicians have remarked the disposition to mental disease is stronger between twenty and thirty than between thirty and forty; and this is fairly ascribed to the earlier age at which young men enter the world and engage in business and politics. One of these beardless men of business said to his physician, "I am convinced this kind of life which I lead will drive me mad or kill me; but I must go on." In four American asylums, which contained 2790 patients, 33·73 per cent. were between twenty and thirty, and 24·41 per cent. between thirty and forty years of age. That the kind of education which the youth in the United States receive has a powerful influence on the development of insanity is proved by Evans and Worthington, in their reports of the Pennsylvania asylums. Dr. Wigan gives, in his unpublished writings, an account of crimes committed by young people without any object. The age of the youthful malefactors was between sixteen and seventeen for girls, and between seventeen and eighteen for boys. There was this in common, that there had not previously existed the slightest animosity towards the persons against whom they perpetrated outrages. According to Wigan, the great number of these young people had epistaxis, which, among the females, appeared with the regularity of menstruation. The crimes were generally committed after the temporary cessation of this habitual flux.[1]

Drs. Delasiauve and Schnepf have also published some particulars relative to the insanity of early life. The statistics of Dr. Boutteville exhibit insanity amongst children in no insignificant proportion. The maximum is presented between the ages of thirty and thirty-four. From five to nine, 0·9 per cent.; ten to fourteen, 3·5; from fifteen to nineteen, 20 per cent. Drs. Aubanel and Thorpe observed in the Bicêtre, in the year 1839, eight cases of mania in children, and one of melancholia, from the age of eleven to eighteen years. Mental disease is undoubtedly more frequent in childhood than is generally supposed. Hereditary tendency to disease, and ill-directed education, play an important part in its

[1] Dr. Winslow's "Psychological Journal," vol. xi, p. 497.

production. A writer in the *Revue des Deux Mondes*, for August, 1848, has with much ability accounted for the frequency of insanity in France. Dr. Paulmier recognizes three forms of mania,—maniacal excitement (*excitation maniaque*), mania, and incoherent mania. In the first grade of mania, the dissociation of ideas is not always recognizable—it nearly resembles the early stage of drunkenness; in the more advanced degree, the dissociation of ideas is remarkable; while in the highest it is such, that no longer two sentences, and sometimes not even two parts of one sentence, are connected. The diagnosis of the mania of children is at times difficult; meningitis may be confounded with it; but in general the headache, the dilatation of the pupils, and the nausea and repeated vomiting, afford means of fixing the line of demarcation. Mania with stupor (*d'une sorte de stupeur exaltique*) approaches closely certain forms of mental alienation which occur after epileptic seizures, and in which the excitement is associated with obtuseness and hallucinations (*obtusion hallucinatoire*). With respect to prognosis, the insanity of early life, according to the observations of Dr. Paulmier, ends in recovery; however, Dr. Delasiauve has made the remark, that a great susceptibility and disposition to a return of the mental disease often remains. Accordingly, many patients are found in the wards appropriated to adults, who had formerly been successfully treated as insane in the division assigned to children.

Dr. Brierre du Boismont concludes his notice of Dr. Paulmier's dissertation, by giving the results of his own experience. He says, that in a list of forty-two young people in whom the mental disease commenced between fourteen and sixteen years of age, eighteen times was it inherited from their parents. In by far the greater number of cases, the disease manifested itself under the influence of hereditary predisposition, and was connected with the age of puberty and menstruation. On inquiring of the parents the character of the children, the answer has almost always been, that they were, without any cause, sometimes sad, and at other times wild and ungovernable. They could never apply themselves steadily to work. They had no talent, or if it existed, it only flared up brilliantly for a moment. They would submit themselves to no rules. Some were apathetic, and were not to be excited by emulation. Others exhibited a volatility which could not be restrained. Many had been subject to spasmodic attacks. The incubation period was often protracted. In eighteen instances recovery took place, but the persons were liable to relapse. There also remained a remarkable strangeness of character, and an inability to assume any fixed position in life. Some afforded insecure evidence of the recovery being permanent. The conclusion is, that though, in a certain number of cases, recovery takes place, the mental alienation of children and young people is a most serious disease, partly from their antecedents, and partly on account of the imperfect development of the cerebral and other organs.[1]

At the commencement of insanity, the derangement of the intellect is so slight and transient in its manifestations, as to render its recognition, as a formidable malady impending over the patient, a task of grave doubt, and great difficulty. To the unskilled, untutored, and untrained eye, the disease is, in its early stages, occasionally altogether invisible. Even to the practised apprehension of the experienced physician, it is almost indiscernible, or, at least, of a dubious and uncertain character. In its incipient stage, mental disorder is characterized, generally, by acute morbid sensibility, physical and mental, accompanied by a difficulty of fixing the attention. In investigating this subject, it is necessary, as a preliminary inquiry, to endeavor to trace the disease back to its origin, and to examine accurately and minutely that degree or stage of the malady in which it is *not yet*, but from which it *may* become, insanity. At an early period of the incipient stage, the patient complains of being very ill, and exclaims that he is losing his senses, often pertinaciously asserting that his mind is not his own.

These symptoms will be considered more in detail, when I proceed to speak of the stage of consciousness. On investigating the history of those who have become insane, it will be ascertained, that long before any mental disease was apparent, they were subject to fits of apathy, had been in the habit of sitting for hours together in a state of moody abstraction, or brown study, and this, too, at a time when they had important domestic and other duties to occupy their attention.

Upon analyzing the patient's antecedents still more closely, it will be found that, for a long period, there has existed much irre-

[1] *Vide* Dr. Winslow's " Psychological Journal," No. XIII (New Series).

gularity and absurdity of thought, eccentricity and singularity of conduct. He has been considered as an oddity in his family, being rarely seen in the domestic circle. When his friends and relations are engaged in social union and converse, he retires quietly to his own room, where he is discovered musing, brooding, and muttering nonsense to himself. · At other times, he is forward and obstreperous, loud and vociferous, wild, ungovernable, and untrainable. On these occasions, the eyes exhibit a bright, brilliant aspect, and the physiognomy is lighted up by an unnatural degree of intelligence. At other times, the patient is restless, abstracted, and moody, during the day, and at night, slumbers and sleeps uneasily, often, when awaking, complaining of headache, mental confusion, or vertigo. During his sleep, he is occasionally subject to slight attacks of muscular convulsion, somnambulism, temporary illusions of the senses. He is liable to frightful and distressing dreams. All these symptoms are often indicative of the commencement of organic disease of the brain, as well as of alienation of mind.

In the early period of insanity, the most material elements of character undergo strange transformations. The man naturally remarkable for his caution and circumspection, becomes reckless, extravagant, and imprudent. If orderly and economical, he is confused and prodigal. If noted for his preciseness, he exhibits great carelessness and negligence. If gay and communicative, he is sullen and morose. If previously neat and particular in his dress, he becomes slovenly, dirty, and indifferent as to his attire. If timid, he is brave, resolute, overbearing, and presumptuous. If kind, gentle, and affectionate, he is rude, austere, irritable, and insulting in his intercourse and communications with others. If benevolent, he becomes parsimonious and miserly, hoarding up, with the greatest care, the smallest sums of money, sometimes under the insane apprehension that he will eventually be obliged to go into the workhouse. If, when in health the patient is known for his attention to his religious duties, he becomes, when insanity is casting its dark shadow over the mind, sadly neglectful of them, not paying even decent respect to the ordinances of religion. The man of business, who never, when well, was found absent from his counting-house, or known to neglect his vocation, now shows great indifference as to his affairs, and refuses to take any part in, or even to converse about them.

10

Insanity often first shows itself in a *morbid exaggeration*, a diseased *excess*, in the development of normal healthy mental conditions. The naturally timid and reserved man shuns society, isolating himself altogether from the companionship of his family and friends. The bold man is boisterous, noisy, presuming. The courageous, officious and talkative. The strictly conscientious person exhibits a morbid exaltation of conscience respecting his moral, social, and religious duties, and, when insane, or becoming so, will manifest the acutest misery at the notion of thinking or doing anything in the remotest degree at variance with his strict and literal interpretation of Holy Writ. In this condition of mind, the patient, suffering from *pseudo*-religious feelings, will refuse to comply with any instructions that are opposed to his own morbidly conscientious and sadly perverted notions of right and wrong, good and evil. The naturally cautious and suspicious man manifests an excess of these mental qualities, when in an abnormal state of mind. He will weigh with scrupulous exactness, cautious prudence, and watchful vigilance, everything that is said and done, surmised and hinted at, in his presence, hesitating and doubting as to the tendency, truth, and sincerity of all remarks addressed to him.

In a more advanced stage of this type of morbid thought, the patient (his insanity still consisting in a diseased perversion of a state of mind *normally* in an *excess* of development) often has delusions as to his food being poisoned, refusing for a time all sustenance, occasionally resisting (as I have heard patients confess after recovery) the efforts made to induce them to eat, at a time when they were tortured and agonized by the acute cravings of hunger! The naturally jealous man exhibits his insanity by suspecting his wife's affection, and even fidelity. The man of active poetic imagination manifests in his disease a disposition to indulge in the most wild and fantastic excursions into the regions of fancy, often, in his paroxysms of morbidly excited imagination, seeing

" More devils than vast hell can hold."

" In investigating," says an acute observer, " the nature of insanity, the first caution to be observed, is not to confound disorders of mental functions with natural qualities, which sometimes strongly resemble them. Many men, in the full enjoyment of health, are remarkable for peculiarities of character and idiosyncrasies of thought and feeling, which contrast strongly with the general tone and usages of society; but they are not on that account to be held as insane, because the singularity for which they are distinguished is with them a natural quality, and not the product of disease; and, from the very unlikeness of their manifestations to the modes of acting and of feeling of other men, such persons are, in common language, said to be eccentric. It is the prolonged departure, without an adequate external cause, from the state of feeling and modes of thinking usual to the individual when in health, that is the true feature of disorder in mind, and the degree at which this disorder ought to be held as constituting insanity, is a question of another kind, on which we can scarcely hope for unanimity of sentiment and opinion. Let the disorder, however, be ascertained to be morbid in its nature, and the chief point is secured, viz., a firm basis for an accurate diagnosis; because it is impossible that such derangement can occur, unless in consequence of, or in connection with, a morbid condition of the organ of mind; and thus the abstract mental states, which are justly held to indicate lunacy in one, may in another, speaking relatively to health, be the strongest proof of perfect soundness of mind. A brusque, rough manner, which is natural to one person, indicates nothing but mental health in him; but if another individual, who has always been remarkable for a deferential deportment and habitual politeness, lays these qualities aside, and, without provocation or other adequate cause, assumes the unpolished forwardness of the former, we may justly infer that his mind is either already deranged, or on the point of becoming so. Or if a person who has been noted all his life for prudence, steadiness, regularity, and sobriety, suddenly becomes, without any adequate change in his external situation, rash, unsettled, and dissipated in his habits, or *vice versa*, every one recognizes at once, in these changes, accompanied, as they then are, by bodily symptoms, evidences of the presence of disease affecting the mind, through the instrumentality of its organs. It is therefore, I repeat, not the abstract act or feeling which constitutes a symptom, it is the departure from the natural and healthy character, temper, and habits, that gives it this meaning; and in judging of a man's sanity, it is consequently as essential to know what his habitual manifestations were, as what his present symptoms are. Just as, in investigating stomachic affections, we do not compare the variations of appetite, or the strength of digestion, with any fixed or imaginary standard, but always judge of their value, as symptoms, in relation to their former state; because the moderate appetite, which is natural to one constitution, occurring in a person who had previously been remarkable for keenness and power of digestion, would justly be considered as an indication of loss of health, while the voracious appetite, natural to a third, would, in a different constitution, be as sure an index of stomachic disease."[1]

In the ordinary practice of medicine we occasionally meet with cases of *bodily* disease which are at variance with past experience and *à priori* notions, set at defiance preconceived views of morbid *physical* phenomena, resist every attempt to embody them within the *nosological* chart, and repudiate all reduction to any of the acknowledged orthodox pathological standards or tests. These affections are anomalous or *pseudo* in their character, are with difficulty defined, not easily diagnosed, occasionally altogether escape observation, and often resist, too successfully, the operation of the best directed remedial measures.

If among the diseases more particularly implicating the ordinary organic functions, we witness these pseudo or eccentric deviations from the recognized pathological character, *à fortiori*, are we not justified in anticipating that in the subtle, complicated, varied, and often obscure affections of the cerebral structure, deranging the operations of thought, we should have brought within the sphere of our observation extraordinary, anomalous, and eccentric deviations from certain predetermined, morbid, cerebral, and psychical conditions?

I presume it to be a generally admitted axiom that the mind may be *disordered* without being *insane*, using this phrase in its strictly legal acceptation. These conditions of morbid intellect may be considered by some as only degrees of *insanity;* but I would suggest that this term be restricted to those mental disorders, accompanied with positive loss of control, clearly justifying the exercise of moral restraint, and to those morbid conditions of the intellect which sanction an appeal to the protective influence of the law. In other words, I would confine my remarks to those cases in which the mind may be said to be *pathologically* disordered, but not invariably *legally* insane.

---

[1] Dr. Andrew Combe on "Mental Derangement;" 1831.

Have we in practice sufficiently appreciated this distinction? Fearful of committing ourselves to an opinion that might authorize an interference with the free agency of the patient, and justify the use of legal restraint, there has existed an indisposition to admit the presence of positive mental disorder, even in cases where it has been obviously and painfully apparent? This excessive caution—originating in motives that do honor to human nature—has often, I fear, been productive of serious, fatal, and irremediable mischief.

The subject under consideration is one, I readily admit, of extreme delicacy, but, nevertheless, of incalculable importance to all sections of the community. It is, I admit, beset with difficulties, and surrounded by dangers. In the hands of the inexperienced, the ignorant, indiscreet, and the wilfully designing, the facts that I have to record, and principles which I am about to enunciate, might be productive of much mischief; but, I ask, ought any apprehensions of this nature to deter the philosopher from entering upon so important an inquiry?

The subject of latent and unrecognized morbid mind is yet in its infancy. It may be said to occupy, at present, untrodden and almost untouched ground. What a vast field is here presented to the truth-seeking observer, who, to a practical knowledge of human nature, adds an acquaintance with the higher departments of mental and moral philosophy, as well as of cerebral pathology! How much of the bitterness, misery, and wretchedness, so often witnessed in the bosom of families, arises from concealed and undetected mental alienation! How often do we witness ruin, beggary, disgrace, and death result from such unrecognized morbid mental conditions! It is the canker-worm gnawing at the vitals, and undermining the happiness of many a domestic hearth. Can nothing be done to arrest the fearful progress of this moral avalanche, or arrest the course of the rapid current that is hurling so many to ruin and destruction?

This type of morbid mental disorder exists to a frightful extent in real life. It is unhappily on the increase, and it therefore behooves the members of the medical profession, as guardians of the public health, as philosophers engaged in the loftiest and most ennobling of human inquiries, as practical physicians called upon to unravel the mysterious and complicated phenomena of disease, and administer relief to human suffering, fearlessly to grapple with an evil which is sapping the happiness of families, and to exert their utmost ability to disseminate sound principles of pathology and therapeutics upon a matter so intimately associated and so closely interwoven with the mental and social well-being of the human race.

These unrecognized morbid conditions most frequently implicate the *affections, propensities, appetites,* and *moral sense.* In many instances it is difficult to distinguish between normal or healthy mental irregularities of thought, passion, appetite, and those deviations from natural conditions of the intellect, both in its intellectual and moral manifestations, clearly bringing those so affected within the legitimate domain of pathology. Are there any unfailing diagnostic symptoms by means of which we may detect these *pseudo-forms* of mental disorder with sufficient exactness, precision, and distinctness to justify the conclusion that they result from diseased cerebral conditions? This question it will be my duty to consider. The phases of mind of which I speak are necessarily obscure, and, unlike the ordinary cases of mental aberration of every-day occurrence, they frequently manifest themselves in either an exalted, depressed, or vitiated state of the moral faculties. The disorder frequently assumes the character of a mere exaggeration of some single predominant passion, appetite, or emotion, and so often resembles, in its prominent features, the natural and healthy actions of thought, either in excess of development or irregular in its operations, that the practised eye of the experienced physician can alone safely pronounce the state to be an abnormal one. I do not refer to ordinary instances of eccentricity, to idiosyncrasies of thought and feeling, or to cases in which the mind appears to be absorbed by some one idea, which exercises an influence over the conduct and thoughts quite disproportionate to its intrinsic value. Neither do I advert to examples of natural irritability, violence, or passion, coarseness and brutality, vicious inclinations, criminal propensities, excessive caprice, or extravagance of conduct, for these conditions of mind may, alas! be the natural and healthy operations of the intellect. These strange phases of the understanding, *bizarreries* of character, vagaries of the intellect, singularities, irregularities, and oddities of conduct, common to so many who mix in every-day life, and pass current in society as healthy-minded persons, present to the moralist and philosophical psychologist many points for grave contemplation and often suspicion. Such natural and normal, although eccentric states of the intellect, do not, however, legitimately come within the province of the *physician*, unless they can be clearly demonstrated to be *morbid results*, and positive and clearly established deviations from cerebral or mental *health*.

These forms of unrecognized mental disorder are not always accompanied by any well-marked disturbance of the bodily health demanding medical attention, or any obvious departure from a normal state of thought and conduct such as to justify legal interference; neither do these affections always incapacitate the party from engaging in the ordinary business of life. There may be no appreciable morbid alienation of affection. The wit continues to dazzle, and the repartee has lost none of its brilliancy. The fancy retains its playfulness, the memory its power, the conversation its perfect coherence and rationality. The afflicted person mixes as usual in society, sits at the head of his own table, entertains his guests, goes to the stock-exchange, the counting-house, or bank, and engages actively in his professional duties, without exhibiting evidence, very conclusive to others, of his actual morbid mental condition. The change may have progressed insidiously and stealthily, having slowly and almost imperceptibly induced important molecular modifications in the delicate vesicular neurine of the brain, ultimately resulting in some aberration of the ideas, alteration of the affections, or perversion of the propensities and instincts.

The party may be an unrecognized monomaniac, and, acting under the despotic influence of one predominant morbid idea, be bringing destruction upon his home and family. His feeling may be perverted, and affections alienated, thus engendering much concealed misery within the sacred circle of domestic life. His conduct may be brutal to those who have the strongest claims upon his love, kindness, and forbearance, and yet his mental malady be undetected. He may recklessly, and in opposition to the best counsels and most pathetic appeals, squander a fortune, which has been accumulated after many years of active industry and anxious toil. He may become vicious and brutal, a tyrant, a criminal, a drunkard, a spendthrift, and a suicide, as the result of an undoubtedly morbid state of the brain and mind, and yet pass unobserved through life as a sane, rational, and healthy man.

We witness in actual practice all the delicate shades and grada-

tions of such unrecognized and neglected mental alienation. It
often occurs that whilst those so affected are able to perform with
praiseworthy propriety, scrupulous probity, and singular exactness,
most of the important duties of life, they manifest extraordinary
and unreasonable antipathies, dislikes, and suspicions against their
dearest relations and kindest friends. So cleverly and successfully
is this mask of sanity and mental health sometimes worn ; so
effectually is all suspicion disarmed, that mental disorder of a dangerous character has been known for years to progress without
exciting the slightest notion of its presence, until some sad and
terrible catastrophe has painfully awakened attention to its existence. Persons suffering from latent insanity often affect singularity of dress, gait, conversation, and phraseology. The most
trifling circumstances stimulate their excitability. They are mar-
tyrs to ungovernable paroxysms of passion, are inflamed to a state
of demoniacal furor by insignificant causes, and occasionally lose
all sense of delicacy of feeling and sentiment, refinement of manners and conversation. Such manifestations of undetected mental
disorder are often seen associated with intellectual and moral
qualities of the highest order. Neither rank nor station is free
from these sad mental infirmities. Occasionally the malady shows
itself in an overbearing disposition. Persons so unhappily disordered, browbeat and bully those over whom they have the power
of exercising a little short-lived authority, and, forgetting what is
due to station, intelligence, reputation, and character, become
within their circumscribed sphere petty tyrants, aping the manners
of Eastern despots. They are impulsive in their thoughts, often
obstinately, unreasonably, and pertinaciously riveted to the most
absurd and outrageous opinions, dogmatic in conversation, and
litigious, exhibiting a controversial spirit, and opposing every endeavor made to bring them within the domain of common sense
and correct principles of ratiocination. All delicacy and decency
of thought are occasionally banished from the mind, so effectually
does the spiritual principle, in these attacks, succumb to the animal instincts and passions.

The naturally gentle, truthful, retiring, and self-denying, become quarrelsome, cunning, and selfish; the diffident bold, the
modest obscene. We frequently observe these *pseudo*-mental conditions giving undue prominence to a particular faculty, or seizing
hold of one passion or appetite. Occasionally it manifests itself

in a want of veracity, or in a disposition to exaggerate, and tell absurd and motiveless lies. It may show itself in a *disordered voli-tion*, in *morbid imitation*, in an inordinate vaulting ambition, an absorbing lust of praise, an insane craving for notoriety. The disorder occasionally manifests itself in a depressed, exalted, or vitiated state of the reproductive function; in morbid views of Christianity, and is often connected with a profound *anæsthesia* of the moral sense. Many of these sad afflictions are symptomatic of unobserved, and consequently neglected, cerebral conditions, either originating in the brain itself, or produced by sympathy with morbid affections existing in other tissues in close organic relationship with the great nervous centre.

The majority of these cases will generally be found associated with a constitutional predisposition to insanity and cerebral disease. These morbid conditions are occasionally the sequelæ of febrile attacks, more or less implicating the functions of the brain and nervous system; they also often succeed injuries of the head inflicted in early childhood. Modifications of the malady are unhappily seen allied with genius. The biographies of Cowper, Burns, Byron, Johnson, Pope, and Haydon, establish that the best, exalted, and most highly gifted conditions of mind do not escape unscathed. In early childhood this form of mental disturbance may, in many cases, be detected. To its existence may often be traced the motiveless crimes of the young, as well as much of the unnatural caprice, dulness, stupidity, and wickedness often wit-nessed in early life at our great schools and national institutions.

I cite a few illustrations of this *type* of undetected mental dis-order. A lady, who up to the age of forty-three was never known to manifest anything resembling a passionate disposition or a bad temper, became, after the birth of her last child, subject to paroxysms of overpowering and ungovernable passion, induced by the most trifling and apparently insignificant causes. This continued for several years, her state of mind never having been considered otherwise than sound. I had several opportunities, after her morbid condition was recognized, of observing her fits of rage, and certainly I never witnessed any demonstrations of anger off the stage so truly appalling. There was no aberration of idea in connection with the case, appreciable delusion, perver-sion of the affections, or hallucinations of the senses. Her mental affection manifested itself solely in sudden paroxysms of intense

passion. These attacks generally occurred once a week, sometimes
only once during the month ; but for a short period she had them
more frequently.   They were almost invariably preceded by vertigo, pain in the occipital region, and a dimness of vision.   It was
the presence of these physical symptoms that led to the supposition of the existence, in this case, of some undetected cerebral mischief.   I ordered leeches to the head a few days in advance of the
expected paroxysms, regulated the bowels and secretions, and thus
greatly diminished the intensity of the passionate excitement, but
failed in entirely curing the case.[1] Dr. Cheyne refers to a somewhat similar instance.   He says a friend of his was one day riding
with a clergyman of refined manners, who for many years had
been devoted to the service of God.   To his amazement his companion, without any adequate provocation, fell into a paroxysm of
ungovernable fury, swearing at a wood-ranger, and threatening
him with vengeance, because he had been dilatory in obeying an
order which he had received relative to a matter of little importance.   Had (observes Dr. Cheyne) this fact become public, all the
devotedness to his profession for which this excellent man was distinguished, would by many have been considered as assumed, and
his habitual humility of demeanor, arising from a sense of his own

---

[1] " *Ira furor brevis est*," is an admitted axiom. Such is certainly the fact, if a condition of violent, unjustifiable, ungovernable anger or passion arises from inadequate
causes, is prolonged to an unreasonable degree, is without intermissions, and refuses
to be controlled, kept in subjection, and governed by the reason or the will.

An old writer compared the course of man to that of a chariot on a wide but dangerous road.   Urged onwards by the passions, the feeble hand of *Reason* tries in vain
to restrain the fiery coursers.   Destruction threatening on the one side, she snatches
at the reins, and rushes into equal danger in the opposite direction.   Thus by a series
of gyrations is the course maintained—a steady undeviating transit never is attained.
In avoiding *Scylla* he runs into *Charybdis*.   The *modus in rebus* is disregarded, and he
loses sight altogether that there are—

" Certi denique fines,
Quos ultra citraque nequit consistere rectum."

PINEL observes, " That he who has identified anger with fury, or transient madness, has expressed a truth, the profundity of which I am more or less disposed to
acknowledge, in proportion as my experience on the subject of insanity has been
more or less extensive.   Paroxysms of insanity are generally no more than irascible
emotions prolonged beyond their ordinary limits : and the true character of such
paroxysms depends more frequently upon the various influences of the passions, than
upon any derangement of the ideas, or upon any whimsical singularities of the judging faculty."

unworthiness, as the result of hypocrisy. It appeared that this gentleman had a short time previously undertaken a duty which led to over-excitement of the brain. He was quite conscious of the incongruity of his conduct. It appears that his only brother had died in an asylum.

I had a young child, ætat. 12, under my care, whose only appreciable morbid condition was that of being subject to violent and uncontrollable fits of passion. These attacks frequently occurred during the night. The poor little creature was painfully conscious of her sad infirmity, and assured me that she struggled heroically against it.

We sometimes in practice see a modified form of this affection exhibiting itself in a bad, morose, and capricious disposition, called by the late Dr. Marshall Hall, who had seen several of these cases, " *temper disease.*"[1] This affection is not, however, confined to females. A member of the House of Commons, many years deceased, had periodical attacks of this nature, particularly after his brain had been overwrought. I was informed by a particular friend of the gentleman to whom I refer, that he once saw him in a terrible paroxysm of fury after making an electioneering speech, being perfectly conscious that at these periods he was temporarily deranged. He was in the habit of dashing cold water over the head during the fit, and occasionally, when suffering from much physical exhaustion, he has been known, with great benefit, to drink at a draught a pint of port wine. The celebrated Spanish General Galvez was subject to attacks of this nature. A

[1] " The most frequent, yet the most extraordinary, of these perversions of temper, are seen in young females. It is a species of aberration of the intellect, but short of insanity—real enough, but exaggerated, fictitious, factitious, and real at the same time. It frequently has its origin in dyspepsia, hysteria, or other maladies, and in emotion of various kinds—such as disappointment, vexation, &c. Its object is frequently to excite, and to maintain, a state of active sympathy and attention, for which there is, as it were, a perpetual, morbid, and jealous thirst. It was rather aptly designated, by the clever relative of one patient, an *ego mania.* I do not regard it as entirely a *feigned* disease. It is, originally at least, the result of malady, or of some mental or bodily affection. It is allied to hysteria; and hysteria—hysteric palpitation, for example—is a real disease. It is best illustrated by the effects of derangement of the stomach and bowels in infants,—and who would think of correcting a child for temper, which was the immediate, natural, and inseparable effect of bodily disorder? It is a perversity, an insaniola, originating in bodily disorder or mental affection, and perpetuated by a morbid indulgence of temper, and desire for sympathy and attention."—" *Observations in Medicine,*" by Dr. M. Hall. Series No. I, pp. 87–9.

bottle of claret generally cured him, probably, as Dr. Rush remarks, by overcoming a weak, morbid cerebral action, and producing agreeable and healthy excitement of brain. Would not, adds Dr. Rush, a dose of laudanum have been the appropriate remedy? A young gentleman was thrown from his horse, and fell upon his head. For ten minutes after the accident he continued in a state of coma. Since his recovery he has been subject to furious fits of passionate excitement. These attacks are generally preceded by severe headaches. His mental faculties do not appear much, if at all impaired, but he continues to suffer from these morbidly painful ebullitions of temper. Prior to the injury, he exhibited the most extraordinary degree of self-control and equanimity of temper. Dr. Beddoes refers to the case of a lady, who, after her recovery from an attack of brain fever, became extremely irascible. This was the reverse of her natural disposition. She made herself so offensively disagreeable to all her family, that her husband, a most amiable and self-denying man, was compelled to separate himself from her, and abandon his once happy fireside.

A somewhat similar case I visited in consultation with Dr. Webster. In this instance the lady was in the habit, during her paroxysms of passion, of seizing hold of her husband's hair, and tearing it out by the roots in large quantities. This poor fellow has often come to me in great distress, having a full assurance of his wife's insanity, beseeching me to protect him from her acts of insane violence. She was clearly disordered in her mind, but we could not detect, in our examination of her, evidence sufficiently conclusive to justify us in signing a medical certificate authorizing her being placed under control. We lamented that, owing to a defective state of the law, we could not grapple with the case. In this, as in numerous anomalous instances of disordered mind, it was felt that nothing could legally be done for the protection of the patient, and the disease must be allowed to take its course.

I have referred to a certain morbid mental condition, exhibitin_ itself exclusively in acts of *cruelty* and *brutality*. This form of unrecognized disorder may exist unassociated with delusion. There is much of this latent and undetected alienation of mind in existence, producing, within the sacred precincts of domestic life, great irregularities of conduct and a fearful amount of domestic misery. It often coexists with great talents and high attainments, and is compatible with the exercise of active philanthropy and benevolence.   The ordinary actions or conversation of those so affected, in many cases, would not convey to a stranger an idea of the existence of such a sad state of the intellect.   Howard, the celebrated philanthropist, affords an unhappy illustration of this type of disorder.   He is represented to have been a tyrant in his own house.   His cruel treatment caused the death of his wife.   He was in the habit, for many years after her death, of doing penance before her picture.   He had an only son, whom, for the slightest offence, he punished with terrible severity. He was in the habit of making this son stand for hours in a prescribed grotto in the garden.   The son became a lunatic as the result of this brutal treatment.   Several similar cases have been brought under my observation.   In one instance, temporary confinement was resorted to, but without positive advantage.

A lady, moving in good society, happily married, accomplished, well educated, of sweet temper, and with a mind under the benign influence of religious principles, manifested, at the age of forty-five, a sudden and extraordinary change of character and habits. She became irritable from trifling causes; was continually quarrelling with her husband and servants; discharged her tradesmen, accusing them of acts of dishonesty; and offended many of her most intimate friends and relations by her cold, and often repulsive manner.   This state of mind continued for two years, during which period she played the capricious tyrant within the sphere of the domestic circle.   Her husband became nearly broken-hearted; his friends and relations could not enter his house without being insulted; he neglected his business, and his health became seriously impaired from constant anxiety.   A new phase of the malady, however, exhibited itself.   She one day accused her husband of gross infidelity.   Proofs were demanded.   She immediately produced several anonymous letters which she had received, containing a minute, circumstantial, and apparently truthful account of her husband's misconduct.   These letters appeared to substantiate, as conclusively as such documentary evidence could do, her accusation.   No person doubted the genuineness of these letters.   Her friends, however, refused to recognize, even at this time, her actual morbid state of mind.   She subsequently had an epileptic seizure, followed by partial paralysis. I then saw the case.   Her cerebral condition being at this time apparent, she was removed from home. It was now discovered, beyond a doubt, that this lady had written the anonymous letters to herself, accusing her husband of infidelity, had addressed and posted them, and had eventually become impressed with the conviction that the letters were actually written by a stranger, and contained a true statement of facts. They had, as it afterwards appeared, been concealed about her person for nearly six months!

I was requested to visit a lady, who, after a painful and dangerous accouchement, exhibited, without any adequate exciting cause, an inveterate feeling of hatred towards one of her children. She treated this child with great and systematic brutality. To such an extent did she carry this morbid and unnatural feeling, that her husband was obliged to remove the child from the house, and place it under the care of a relative in a distant part of the country. I had no doubt at the time that this person's mind was disordered. Such was my written opinion. The idea was, however, repudiated by nearly all the members of the family, who obstinately closed their eyes to her sad and melancholy condition. The only evidence that existed, at that period, of mental disorder, was her unnatural alienation of affection, and her brutal conduct towards one of her children. This state of mind appeared unassociated with any appreciable delusive ideas. Three weeks had scarcely elapsed since my first consultation in this case, when I was informed this lady had made an unsuccessful attempt at suicide. It was then obvious that she was not in a sane state of mind, and her family no longer hesitated in placing her privately under close restraint. We occasionally observe evidences of this morbid state at a very early period of life, and it is indicative of an original organic defect in the constitution of the intellect.

Thomas Pepper, fourteen years of age, a pot-boy, a clever lad, but of sullen and morose disposition, committed suicide by hanging himself in an arbor in his master's bowling-green. It appeared from the evidence that the mind of the deceased was peculiarly formed, his conduct frequently evincing a predisposition to cruelty. He had been frequently known to hang up mice and other animals for the purpose of enjoying the pain which they appeared to suffer whilst in the agonies of death. He would often call boys to witness these sports, exclaiming—" Here's a lark; he is just having his last kick." He had often been known to catch flies and throw them into the fire, that he might observe them whilst burning.

He had also been observed, whilst passing along the street, to pull the ears of the children—lifting them off the ground by their ears; and when they cried out with pain, he would burst out into a fiendish paroxysm of delight at their sufferings. Witnesses deposed that about four years previously, when only ten years of age, he attempted to strangle himself in consequence of his mother having chastised him. He locked himself up in a room, and, when discovered, life was nearly extinct.[1] I refer to this as an illustration of a *type* of mental depravity, occurring in early life, arising from a congenital malorganization of the brain and intellect. This morbid disposition may be either connate, hereditary, or be the *sequelæ* of disease affecting the healthy condition of the brain. It occasionally supervenes upon injuries of the head.

I saw, some years ago, a youth whose whole moral character had become completely changed in consequence of a severe injury that he had sustained. This young gentleman, when of the age of eighteen or nineteen, was attacked by fever. In a paroxysm of delirium he sprung violently out of bed, and severely cut his ankle; considerable hemorrhage followed. After his recovery, his whole moral character was found to have undergone a complete metamorphosis. From being a well-conditioned boy, kind and affectionate to his parents, steady in his habits, sober, of unimpeachable veracity, he became a drunkard, liar, and thief, and was lost to all sense of decency and decorum! He was clever, intelligent, sharp-witted, but his every action was perfectly brutal. This boy, prior to his illness, was known to hang with endearing affection round the neck of his mother; but after this sad change, I have seen him attack her with brutal and savage ferocity. This patient was for some years in close confinement. He was subsequently sent abroad; but during a voyage to the East Indies he mysteriously disappeared one evening from the quarter deck of the ship, and is supposed to have committed suicide by throwing himself into the sea. We occasionally meet another *type* of unrecognized mental disorder. I refer to cases in which there appears to be a *paralysis of the moral sense*. Such cases are not inappropriately termed *moral idiots*.[2]

---

[1] From the *Times*.

[2] Grave exceptions have been taken to the term "*moral idiotcy*," by writers who have entirely misconceived the medico-psychological import of the phrase, as well as by others who have never had an opportunity of becoming practically acquainted

A young gentleman, who had been greatly indulged and petted at home, exhibited, shortly after going to school, a morose, cruel, and revengeful disposition. He quarrelled with the other boys, committed several petty acts of robbery, accusing others of being the culprits. He pursued his studies with intelligence, and was generally at the head of his class. His conduct became so systematically brutal, savage, and untruthful, that his father was requested peremptorily to remove him from the school. The gentleman under whose care the youth was placed, was induced, by the earnest persuasions of the father, to alter his determination and retain the boy. For several days he was noticed to be unusually morose and taciturn. He was perceived to be busily occupied one morning in writing. Being called suddenly out of the room, his letter was examined, and it was found to contain the details of a plan he had carefully concocted for the murder of one of the other boys, towards whom he entertained feelings of rancorous animosity. His letter was written to a boy who had left the school for misconduct, and who appeared to be in his confi-

---

with this singular type of congenitally defective intelligence. A modern author thus refers to the popular prejudices on this subject :—

"To some minds, the idea of a moral idiot involves painful notions of the Creator. I may be permitted to remark, that they rest on the false philosophy of the Eudaimonist. So long as we consider happiness as the great end of life, and virtue only its instrument, so long shall we find difficulties to solve in the mischiefs wrought by beings whom ignorance or fatuity renders irresponsible. To the Eudaimonist such mischief appears a final evil; and, as he is forbidden to attribute it to the irresponsible agent, he is driven to attribute it to God. But the difficulty ceases when we perceive that the end of creation is the perfecting of souls, and the production of happiness is altogether secondary thereto. Sin is now seen to be evil, not for the external mischief it produces, but for its own sake, as the most evil of all things. The outward act, be it ever so mischievous, is not *sin*—the Will constitutes the sin. Thus, when offences are committed by an irresponsible agent, God does not become the author of any sin; for sin is nothing but the conscious, wilful delinquency of a free creature, and there is no sin without it, any more than in the ravages of the storm and flood. The *mischief* done takes its place along with the suffering which is necessary to the end of creation; and, when the Great Drama is further advanced, we shall understand the reason of what seems unaccountable in the one short scene we now behold. To ask further, why moral idiots should have been created, is equivalent to asking why there should be intellectual idiots, children dying in infancy, &c. We must deem their existence on earth motived by reasons which (while ignorant of all life beyond us) we may not guess. The children at a school marvel why a parent withdraws his son soon after entrance, or does not suffer him to learn with them; but it is all understood *at home*."—"*Essay on Intuitive Morals, being an attempt to popularize Ethical Science.*" Part I. *Theory of Morals.* 1855. P. 113.

dence. He had procured a long, sharp-pointed bodkin, which he intended, whilst his victim was asleep, driving into his heart, by means of a hammer with which he had armed himself! In the letter, giving a minute description of the contemplated murder, he says: " *To-night I will do for the little devil.*" This boy was immediately placed under the care of his father, and on the advice of an eminent provincial physician, he was, without loss of time, subjected to close restraint. I am informed that there is now no doubt of his insanity. I did not see this case myself, but I obtained these particulars from the father of the young gentleman who had so providential an escape of his life. If this youth had committed murder, what would have been the plea urged in his defence, and the verdict of the jury ?

N. B——, ætat. sixteen, of singularly unruly and intractable character, selfish, wayward, violent, and without ground or motive, was liable, when under paroxysms of his moodiness, to do personal mischief to others. He was not, however, of a physically bold character. He was of fair understanding, and exhibited considerable acuteness in sophistical apologies for his wayward conduct. He made little or no progress in any kind of study. His fancy was vivid, supplying him profusely with sarcastic imagery. He was subjected at different times to a firmly mild and to a rigid discipline. Solitary confinement was tried, but to this he was impassive. He was sent to school, where he drew a knife upon one of the officers of the establishment, and produced a deep feeling of aversion in the minds of his companions by the undisguised pleasure which he showed at some bloodshed which took place in the town during a political disturbance. He manifested no sensual disposition, and was careful of property. His conduct became worse, and more savagely violent to his relatives. It is recorded that, at the early age of thirteen, he stripped himself naked, and exposed his person to his sisters. Dr. Mayo cites this interesting illustration as a type of what I term moral idiotcy or congenital depravity. When referring to this painfully anomalous class of affections, the late Dr. Woodward, Physician to the State Lunatic Asylum of Massachusetts, observes :—

"Besides a disease of the intellectual powers there seems to me to be cases of moral idiotcy, or such an imbecile state of the affective faculties from birth as to make the individual irresponsible for his actions. The persons to whom I refer have rarely much vigor

11

of mind, although they are by no means idiots in understanding."

A boy under Dr. Haslam's care, only thirteen years of age, appeared to possess no one of the moral faculties, and yet he was conscious of his lamentable state. He often asked, "why God had not made him like other men." Has not Shakspeare placed in Edgar's mouth a faithful portrait of this class of case? When delineating his own character, Edgar exclaims:—

> "I was a serving man, proud in heart and mind,
>   That served the lust of my mistress's heart,
>   And did the act of darkness with her;
>   Swore as many oaths as I spake words;
>   Wine I loved deeply, dice dearly:
>   I was false of heart, light of ears, and bloody of hand;
>   Hog in filth, fox in stealth, wolf in greediness,
>   Dog in madness, lion in prey."

A boy, in early life, was struck violently upon the head when at school by a brutal fellow employed as an usher in the institution. He was partially stunned, but recovered from the effects of the injury. When of sufficiently advanced age, he joined his father in business. He became subject to attacks of headache, particularly if exposed to much anxiety. For some months he continued sullen, was often absent from the counting-house, became the associate of the lowest class of society, and was detected in abstracting several large sums of money from his father's private desk. In this condition he remained for seven or eight months, no one suspecting a morbid state of the intellect. One morning whilst sitting in the counting-house, he suddenly seized one of the clerks by the throat, and attempted to throttle him. A severe scuffle ensued. Upon separating the combatants, it was discovered that the gentleman's mind was obviously affected. He became suddenly, as it were, demoniacally possessed. He poured forth a volley of filthy oaths, and an amount of obscenity terrifically appalling to those who witnessed his paroxysm of maniacal furor. There appeared no impairment of the reasoning powers, the memory, or reflective faculties. He suddenly lost all perception of truth, and all notion of decency and propriety. I saw this poor fellow in several of his attacks, and must confess, if I were disposed to believe in the possibility of demoniacal possession I should cite this case as one conclusively demonstrating the phenomenon. I have previously referred to instances of unrecognized monomania floating upon the surface of society. I am acquainted with two cases of this form of mental disorder where disease of the mind is not suspected. These latent and masked attacks of monomania frequently lead to overt acts of violence, crime, brutality, and suicide, and very often to alienation of property, no departure from health of mind being suspected.

A few years back I received a summons from a London police magistrate, to examine a case of alleged insanity. It appeared that a laboring man had committed several serious assaults, and was consequently arrested by the police. This man was examined by a medical gentleman, who said he had no doubt as to his insanity, without, however, being able to assign sufficient reasons for such an opinion. The magistrate had, on more than one occasion, himself investigated the case, and had taken the evidence of the surgeon referred to, but could detect no insanity in the prisoner's appearance or conversation. The medical gentleman asserted it to be his belief that the prisoner was insane, basing his conclusions upon the man's apparently unreasonable conduct, and mad acts of motiveless violence. I examined the prisoner publicly in court, and it was not until after the expiration of nearly three-quarters of an hour, that I obtained a key to the actual state of his mind. I then discovered that he was unequivocally insane. He was under the delusion that a stranger having evil designs upon his life, was in the habit of placing daily a small pill upon the mantel piece of his bed-room; that this pill (which he was compelled to swallow) contained an ingredient that greatly excited him, destroying all power of self-control, and leading him to commit the acts of violence of which he stood charged. His insanity then became obvious, and the magistrate signed a warrant for his committal to an asylum. It appeared that this insane man had been severely punished on previous occasions for different acts of unexplained violence, no one suspecting the existence of mental disorder. It was not until I had subjected him to a close and rigid examination for nearly three-quarters of an hour, during which the lunatic showed extraordinary ingenuity in concealing his delusion, and great cleverness in fencing with my questions, that I could establish, with satisfaction to myself, the presence of an insane idea.

Do we sufficiently estimate, in our appreciation of others, the effects of *physical* disease upon the character and actions of those upon whose conduct we are sometimes called to adjudicate and pronounce judgment ? How slight are the changes in the corporeal health, how subtle the variations in the delicate organization of the brain, that precede and accompany remarkable alterations in the *moral* and *intellectual* character ? The brave and heroic become as timid and bashful as coy maidens in particular states of ill-health. Mild, inoffensive, and humane men are driven to acts of desperation and cruelty, under the influence of certain physical diseases disturbing and deranging the operations of thought. " Men (it has been observed) have their ebbs and flows of bravery, and some distempers bring a mechanical terror upon the imagination."

The celebrated General CUSTINE, possessing at the dreadful battle of Mayence high health and vigor, could dauntlessly advance with heroic courage to the mouths of the Austrian cannon, yet after having suffered severely from bodily disease, and loss of nervous energy, he proved a dastardly poltroon and coward at the sight of the guillotine ![1]

A gentleman was, for many years, remarkable for great irascibility and violence of temper. He was constantly quarrelling with his relations, friends, and domestics ; in fact he became notorious for being an ill-conditioned man, with whom no person could for many days live, or associate on amicable terms. He suddenly became ill, complained of a feeling of great uneasiness in his head. This was followed by a violent attack of epilepsy. He recovered from the paroxysm, and, to the astonishment of all his relations and friends, his character had undergone a complete metamorphosis. He became a mild, good-tempered, and placid man, disposed to live on the most friendly understanding with everybody. This state of mind existed for eighteen months, when, in the act of getting out of a railway carriage, he had a second epileptic fit. This was succeeded by a return of his former violence of conduct. He again exhibited great irritability, with occasional paroxysms of ungovernable rage. This mental condition continued for six months, when he had a recurrence of the epileptic fits, followed, singular to relate, by a condition of mental composure, great self-control, and astonishing equanimity, when exposed

[1] Referred to by Dr. Thomas Beddoes, in his " Hygeia."

to extreme provocation. In a few weeks he had a succession of severe attacks of epilepsy, associated with maniacal symptoms. It was considered necessary to place this gentleman under restraint, and he is now in confinement.

In some conditions of nervous disorder, the slightest meteorological changes give rise to singular alternations of despondency, despair, hope, and joy, so completely does the mind succumb to physical influences. I have known a person subject to attacks of suicidal melancholia during the prevalence of a cold, blighting, depressing east wind, who appeared happy, contented, and free from all desire to injure himself, under other and more congenial conditions of the atmosphere![1] An Italian artist never could reside a winter in England, without the distressing idea of self-destruction repeatedly suggesting itself to his morbidly-depressed mind. I have known natives of France, accustomed from early life to the buoyant air and bright azure sky of that country, sink into profound states of mental despondency, if compelled to reside many weeks in London during the earlier portion of the winter season. A military man, suffering from severe mental dejection, was in the habit of promenading backward and forward in a certain track, towards evening, on the ramparts of the town in which he resided. When he walked forwards, his face fronted the east, where the sky was hung with black, as was, alas! his poor soul. Then his grief pressed doubly and heavily upon him; he was hopeless and in deep despair; but when he turned with his countenance towards the west, where the setting sun left behind a halo of glory and beautiful evening's red, his happiness again returned. Thus he walked backward and forward, with and without hope, alternating between joy and melancholy, ecstasy and grief, in obedience to the baneful and benign influence of the eastern and western sky! To this sad extent are the functions of the nervous system and operations of the mind under the dominion of ordinary physical laws.

A young man, of proverbial gentleness, one evening formed one

[1] "Could we penetrate into the secret foundation of human events, we should frequently find the *misfortunes of one man* caused by the *intestines of another*, whom the former endeavored to inspire with sympathy in his fate, at a moment when the frame of mind of the latter was affected by impeded secretion. An hour later, and his fortune would have been made."—Feuchtersleben's "Medical Psychology."

of a party (of young men of his own age) at billiards. Contrary
to his wont, he played badly, and he quarrelled and wrangled with,
and in the end offended, everybody in the room. Two hours after,
he was seized with nephritic pains, caused by the irritation of a
calculus, which was expelled, on the following day, from the kidney
and bladder. A very nervous man, suffering from stone, underwent, occasionally, the operation of *lithotrity*. To spare him the
pain and spasm inseparable from the introduction of the instrument into the bladder, he was placed under the influence of chloroform. Impressions were never completely extinguished, but they
were blunted. Thus, at the moment when the lithotrite was introduced, the patient manifested the struggles of anguish; he resisted
with energy, but when the pain reached its acme, he cried out:
"*You shall not conquer me! What means this violence? Peter!
Antony!* (said he, calling loudly to his domestics) *drive away these
men!*" and he added, "*You will have done well! You will obtain
nothing; I shall not consent to an unequal division. My children
are all equal in my affections!*" Thus a general sentiment of anguish, occasioned by *physical* pain, excited in him the idea of a
moral constraint.[1]

In what respect do these phenomena differ from the state of the
mind in insanity, except in their temporary and transient character? Suppose a continuance of the nephritic irritation, accompanied by the same psychical manifestation, and a loss of volitional
power over the actions, and we observe that irritability, tendency
to violent conduct, disposition to motiveless acts of violence, so
often witnessed in the early as well as advanced stages of mental
derangement. Again: if we could conceive the condition of mind
which followed the administration of chloroform to be in existence
for any length of time after the acute effect of the *anæsthetic* agent
had subsided, would not the state be one of insanity? These illustrations could be multiplied *ad libitum*.

There are many conditions of eccentric thought, transient states
of intellect, temporary manifestations of irregular and erratic
emotion, and evanescent phases of violent, ungovernable passion,
which would constitute insanity, and insanity, too, of a formidable
type, if such states of mind were of a *persistent*, and not of a *fugitive* and transient character.

---

[1] These two illustrations are taken from Dr. Gratiolet's work, referred to in p. 170.

Psychical phenomena, analogous to what has previously been referred to, are occasionally observed in patients suffering from temporary attacks of delirium, caused by the absorption into the blood of some form of poison.   There is upon record a remarkable and deeply interesting illustration of the kind, which I offer no apology for quoting in detail.   The case was one of *hydrophobia*, occurring in a female aged twenty-one.   A few days after the attack she commenced raving, imagining that she had been accused of some crime, for which she was in prison.   Under the influence of this delusion, she sprang up to make her escape, and tried to throw herself out of the window, saying, with great agitation, "I have done no harm."   It was then deemed necessary to confine her by means of a strait waistcoat.

About eight o'clock at night, upon Dr. Lister and Dr. Hamilton (the physicians of the hospital) entering the ward, they heard a female voice speaking thick and eagerly in the dark (for the other patients in the hospital had been removed).   A candle was brought to the bed, and the curtains were undrawn.   The young woman was lying on her back, exerting all her force to get up; terror in her countenance, eyes glistening, pupils much dilated, whole face and neck uniformly red, steaming with perspiration; pulse incredibly swift and small.   She became very restless.   Her tongue was clear, and saliva was running from the corners of her mouth.

She was in a state of great terror, with fear in her looks, and struggling to get away, calling out, "Let me go! let me go!" By transitions, too quick to be marked, she seemed to fancy herself at the entrance of some horrid place, exclaiming, "Now, do go in first; well, I will enter."   Quick as her own thoughts, and as if exposed to the violence of ruffians, with alarm still in her look, and in an earnest and imploring manner, she said, "As you are a gentleman, you will not leave a helpless girl to these . . . ." Her agony of terror increased, and she cried peremptorily and wildly, "Don't leave me, sir; don't leave me, I beseech you." Her mind was in a moment hurried from this idea to an imaginary place, where she fancied she was going to be used cruelly by a woman.   "She will tie me up! break my bones!" she cried, with terrified looks, exerting all her force to escape.   She then sunk into a state of calmness for a minute, but soon her frightened looks and averted head and neck expressed a renewed conflict with danger.   Her mind became a little more tranquillized, but still unhappy from fancying herself detained by force from obeying some order of her mistress. "Let me go," she cried; "my mistress wants me." The apprehension of her mistress's anger increased, and she vociferated, "I beseech you, let me go;" then, with imploring looks, added, "I pray, as if at heaven's gates, let me go, but for five minutes; I will return to you; indeed I will. My mistress calls me."

While she was thus occupied with the thoughts of her mistress's anger, a piece of orange was offered to her to eat. She said, "I will; do let me go to my mistress." She then received the orange into her own hand, muttering, "It will choke me." Then struggling hard, as with an idea to get home, she, as if designedly, dropped it under a fold of the blanket, exclaiming, in accents of wild despair, "As you are a gentleman, do not hinder me; I must go." In a moment she fancied herself again exposed to acts of cruelty, for with sudden terror she cried out, "They are breaking my legs!" After this emotion, she appeared, in her excited fancy, to have reached a place of safety, where she lay quiet a minute or two, as if breathing from the toils and dangers she had escaped.

The opportunity of her being calmer was seized to engage her attention to a present object. A teaspoonful of gruel was offered her to drink, and she was urged to take it. She said, as if returned to the knowledge of her real situation, she was not dry, and then began to rave again about her mistress. It was said it would do her good. Upon which she seemed by her manner as if she wanted to have the spoon in her own hand. It was given to her; but she only kept the spoon in her hand, requesting to be allowed to go to her mistress, until she spilled the contents, by little and little, on the bedclothes. Her attention having been thus called to present objects, she seemed to return to the knowledge of herself.

Another teaspoonful was offered to her, upon which she signified that she was prevented from properly taking it by her hands being confined. The cords of the sleeves of the waistcoat were slackened, and she was requested to swallow the gruel. She held it in her hand, beginning to be intent again to get to her mistress; and it was remarkable, that without knowing what she was doing, or at least without giving attention to the act, she put the teaspoon into her mouth, and swallowed the contents. As she was miserably restless, and sometimes violently struggling, it was said, if she would be still, her hands and arms should be set at liberty. She seemed to assent to this proposal, and the cords were untied; but the moment she felt her arms and body at liberty she began to turn down the bedclothes. Her looks kindling afresh, and expressing that she was bent on escaping, or doing something dreadful, the cords were drawn tight again, and her body confined.

The medical gentlemen remained about twenty minutes at her bedside, and in that short time she underwent the sufferings previously enumerated, and many more not described. It was deeply distressing to witness her appearance and agitations. It was painful to leave her in such poignant misery without being able to give the smallest relief. As the physicians went out of the long ward they heard her exclaiming, as if in a fresh conflict with some new overpowering danger; and when the door was shut after them, her eager, interesting voice, was still heard at a distance, complaining, beseeching, shrieking, in darkness, despair, and solitude! She died about one o'clock that morning.[1]

Is it not possible that, in this case, the mechanical restraint which was resorted to, with the view of preventing her doing serious mischief to herself during her violent paroxysms of excitement, may, to some extent, have suggested to her morbidly agitated thoughts the idea of parties physically overpowering her? Dr. Gratiolet, after relating several cases illustrative of the influence of temporary physical irritation on the intellectual ideas and moral emotions, remarks : " What ferocious duellists, what assassins have, perhaps, owed their cruelty to similar causes! How great the interest to physiology will be attentive *autopsies* of those who have been executed, and who have been urged to crime by inexplicable impulsions! There, also, is doubtlessly found the reason of those suicides which nothing explains, if it be not this profound and indefinite inquietude, which gives to every incident of life, to conditions of perfect happiness, a sombre color, and repulsive aspect. In reality let us conceive an inquietude pushed to its acme. An unfortunate individual feels vaguely the presence of an enemy. This inquietude, of which the object is not defined, demands explanation; the anger that it excites requires to be satisfied. Who has not, in certain hours of indefinable anguish, desired an adversary to combat, and sought an object for his blind fury? In these

---

[1] " Morbid Anatomy of the Brain," by A. Marshall, M.D. London, 1815.

terrible moments anything serves.   One tears his vestments; another kills the dog that caresses him; while a third cuts the throat of a passer-by, of whom the dress displeases him, and who by chance has regarded him.   Here is, without doubt, the point of departure of a great number of fixed ideas and delirious impulses.   These ideas, when they do not incite immediately to a fatal result, are transformed, and very often change their object, so that we can consider them as the result of a general tendency which seeks an end, and often attains it by chance."[1]   Dr. Darwin relates the case of a clergyman who, under the influence of *pseudo* and morbid religious opinions, was in the habit of bruising and wounding himself for the sake, as he said, of "*mortifying the flesh.*"   This patient occupied much time at his devotions, and continued whole nights alone in the church.   As he had a wife, and a family dependent upon him, an unfavorable prognosis was formed of the case, it being supposed that the sympathizing affection and devotedness manifested towards him, as well as the preoccupation of mind so afforded, might have checked the insanity in its early stage.   This gentleman was removed to an asylum. He subsequently returned home, and died in consequence of self-inflicted injuries, combined with the continued abstinence from food, which he practised in obedience to his insane religious hallucinations.   Dr. Darwin endeavored to reason him out of his delusions.   He once told him that "God was a merciful Being, and could not delight in cruelty; but that he (Dr. Darwin) supposed that he (the patient) worshipped the devil."   The clergyman was struck with this idea, and promised Dr. Darwin that he would not beat himself for *three* days.   He, however, only abstained from so doing for four-and-twenty hours.   Dr. Darwin adds: "When these works of supererogation have been of a *public* nature, what cruelties, murders, and massacres, has not this insanity introduced into the world!"   A person who had been very active in leading and encouraging the bloody deeds of St. Bartholomew's day at Paris, on confessing on his death-bed his sins to a worthy ecclesiastic, was asked, "Have you nothing to say about St. Bartholomew's day?"   He replied, "*On that occasion God Almighty was obliged to me!*" •

[1] "Anatomie Comparée du Système Nerveux, considéré dans ses Rapports avec l'Intelligence." Par Fr. Leuret et P. Gratiolet. Tome II. Par M. P. Gratiolet. Paris, 1839, 1857.

Can any person acquainted with the confession of Ravaillac entertain a doubt as to his insanity and moral irresponsibility at the time he assassinated Henry IV of France, for which he suffered the prolonged and agonizing tortures of the rack, followed by being torn to pieces by four horses drawing in opposite directions?

A young gentleman, aged twenty-nine, died of consumption. A *post-mortem* examination of the body was made. The brain itself showed no marked deviation from health, but the *dura* and *pia mater* presented evidences of organic change. The former membrane was found to be three times its healthy consistence. In appearance it was like a piece of *tanned leather!* There were also tubercular depositions on the *pia mater*. The alterations discovered in the *meninges* immediately investing the brain must have existed many years; and these, no doubt, disordered his mind. This person had for some time been a cause of much unhappiness to his family without their suspecting him to be insane. He drank to a frightful excess, indulged in the society of the most degraded, depraved, vicious men and women, and squandered in a few years a splendid patrimony. He married a respectable girl, much below him in social rank and station, whom he, in a short time, brutally ill-treated. He then deserted her and an infant child, leaving them both to the charity of friends and distant relatives. Towards his own immediate family he manifested no kind of interest or affection. His father, who was a man very advanced in years, was subjected to a murderous assault on one occasion, because he refused to attach his signature to one of his son's reckless acceptances. This wretched man was eventually accused of various acts of gross bestiality, as well as of theft. There never was known such an instance of accomplished vice and cold-blooded depravity. Without declaring him to have been actually *insane,* I would ask, whether there can be any doubt as to the *pathological* relation between his *cerebral* condition and the extraordinary *psychical* manifestations referred to?

A young lady, who had been subject for many years to violent hysteria, accompanied with occasional flightiness of manner, alternating with depression of spirits, suggestive of the possibility of insanity one day supervening, conceived an intense passion for a married clergyman whom she had never seen but on *one* occasion, and then only for a short period, in the pulpit! Her family knew nothing of this circumstance until they received a visit from the clerical gentleman, who had in his possession a number of epistles from the lady, couched in very high-flown and amatory language. Upon investigating the matter, a question at once arose as to the *sanity* of the lady, and her condition of mind was immediately made the subject of careful consideration. It was then discovered that her intellect was (unknown to any member of the family) disordered upon other subjects, but that the prominent and salient feature of her mental malady was a vague, unintelligible, morbid erotic feeling for the gentleman to whom she had so indiscreetly addressed the letters. Twelve months elapsed before the mind was restored to health. The cure was, apparently, a perfect one. After her recovery, she often adverted to her insane passion for the clergyman, and said that she now fully realized that her ridiculous *penchant* for him was only a *symptom* of insanity! Her mind, she said, during the time of her illness, appeared to have been enveloped in a dark thick mist.

A maid-servant exhibited, by her wild looks, singular conversation, strange manner, &c., decided symptoms of disordered mind. She was placed under treatment, and was restored to health. A short period after her recovery she met the medical man who had attended her. Upon being questioned as to the state of her health, prior to being placed in an asylum, she hung down her head, and said, "If you will not betray me, sir, I'll tell you a secret." Upon his assuring her that he would not, she said, "Why, sir, that physic that you give those mad folk is very comical sort of stuff, for when I was first sent to you, nothing in the world was the matter with me, but I was most desperately in love as ever poor wench was, and your physic has quite entirely cured me. I am now as happy as the day is long, and I mind the man no more than I do you or any one else." The medicine so effectual in the removal of the love-madness was an emetic, and two or three active calomel purges! The fact was, the girl's love affair was the first manifestation of her insanity, which the medicine was successful in arresting and curing![1]

A merchant, fifty-five years of age, father of a large family, of a strong constitution, although of a lymphatic temperament, mild and gentle in his disposition, who had acquired a considerable

[1] Bingham on "Mental Diseases," p. 137-8.

fortune in business, experienced some domestic troubles, not sufficiently serious, however, to affect any one possessing a vigorous
mind, and healthily organized brain. About a year previously he
formed a large establishment for one of his sons, and shortly afterwards became very active, and expressed, contrary to his usual
habits, the delight which he felt at his increasing prosperity. He
was also more frequently absent from his warehouse and business
than usual : but notwithstanding these trifling changes, neither his
family, friends, or neighbors, suspected the existence of mental
disorder. One day, whilst he was from home, a travelling merchant brought to his house two pictures, and asked fifty louis for
them, which he said was the price agreed upon by a very respectable gentleman, who had given his name and address. His sons
sent away both the pictures and the seller. On his return, the
father did not mention his purchase, but the children began the
conversation, alluding to the roguery of the merchant, and their
refusal to pay him. The father became very angry, asserting that
the pictures were very beautiful, were not dear, and that he was
determined to purchase them. In the evening the dispute became
warmer, the patient flew into a passion, uttered threats, and at last
became *delirious*. On the next day he was confided to Esquirol's
care. His children, frightened at their father's illness, and
alarmed at the purchase which he had made, looked through their
accounts, and great was their astonishment at seeing the bad state
of his books, the numerous blanks which they presented, and the
immense deficiency there was of cash ! This morbid irregularity
had existed for more than six months. Had this discussion respecting the pictures not taken place, and his actual state of mind
been detected, one of the most honorable mercantile houses in
France would, in a few days, have been seriously and fatally com-
promised; for a bill of exchange of a considerable amount had
become due, and no means had been taken to provide for its payment.[1]

The conduct and conversation of a gentleman holding a high
position in the commercial world, excited in the minds of his relatives a grave suspicion as to his sanity. I was consulted about the
case by the family, and gave an opinion that the symptoms were
of such a character as to justify their apprehensions as to his

[1] Esquirol on the " Illusions of the Insane," p. 34.

mental condition.   I advised that the gentleman's conduct should
be closely observed, but that no measures of actual personal restraint should be resorted to until the disease of the mind was
more obviously demonstrated.   The patient was, contrary to my
advice, permitted to be at large, under no kind of supervision,
and previously to any step being taken to exercise control over
him, he had, unknown to his friends and family (without being
able to assign a sane motive for so doing), disposed, for an amount
considerably less than its value, of a small but beautiful estate in
the country that had belonged to the family for nearly a century.
An attempt was made to set aside the sale on the ground of insanity, but it was argued, that the gentleman in question being
permitted to be at large, allowed to go to his counting-house, to
draw cheques, and execute, unrestrained, other important matters
of business, the transaction relative to the sale of his property
must be considered as one made by a person fully competent to
understand the nature of what he was doing, and was therefore
void in point of law.

In another case, a gentleman was allowed, in a very doubtful
state of mind, to continue to transact business of an important
character for some period after the family had been advised as to
his mental incapacity.   In this state of mind, he embarked in a
wild and mad railway speculation, by which he lost *fifty thousand
pounds*.

A gentleman whom I saw last year, in consultation with Mr.
John Propert, made purchases of stock to the extent of *one hundred thousand pounds*, when clearly not in a condition of mind to
manage his own affairs, but not yet sufficiently insane to justify
the family in interfering with his free agency by preventing him
from going regularly to his counting-house.   Fortunately, a near
relative was informed of the nature of the monetary transaction
alluded to, soon after its being completed, and was enabled, after
representing to the parties the true state of the gentleman's mind,
to cancel the investment, but not without the sacrifice of a considerable sum of money.

I was requested to visit a clergyman residing in the north of
England, whose condition of mind had caused his family great
anxiety.   I found him unquestionably insane.   His derangement
was marked by clearly manifested delusions.   His conduct for
many years previously to any symptom of mental aberration

being noticed, had been characterized by actions quite irreconcilable with the supposition of the existence of perfect soundness of intellect. He had, for four or five years, before his state of disordered intellect became obvious to those constantly associated with him, ordered a number of valuable trees to be cut down on the estate, without his being able to offer a sane justification for such an outrageous proceeding. He had also sold a quantity of valuable land adjoining his glebe, to a neighboring squire, that had belonged to the family for many generations (unfortunately not entailed), and which he never would have parted with had he been in a state of mind to enable him to form a sane judgment of the character of the proceedings. At this time, and for many years subsequently, his conduct was marked by great eccentricity and caprice. Nevertheless, he did not exhibit in his conversation any symptom of mental derangement or impairment, mixed as usual with society, attended the annual visitations of his diocesan, wrote and preached capital sermons; attended faithfully and zealously to all his parish duties, at a time when many of his actions were clearly the offspring of a mind decidedly off its balance, if not closely verging upon actual insanity.

I saw a gentleman, some years back, who belonged to the Southern States of America; he was then suffering from general paralysis, associated with ideas of high rank and great wealth. I ascertained, whilst investigating the case, that the gentleman had, for nearly *eight* years previously to his insanity being recognized, been guilty of conduct incompatible with the hypothesis of sanity and moral responsibility. He had in a most reckless manner, involved himself in a number of law proceedings against numerous members of his family upon the most frivolous and ridiculous grounds. He had unjustly accused his servant of having robbed him, and had initiated legal proceedings, with a view of prosecuting in a court of law one of his oldest and most valued friends for libel, without any kind of justification for such a proceeding. On another occasion he assaulted a stranger whom he accidentally met on board an American steamer, alleging that he had grossly insulted him by his looks and gestures. A quarrel soon arose between the parties, which nearly ended in a fatal *rencontre*. At one time he became niggardly, and, in fact, miserly in his habits. Although he was a man of considerable property, he refused to supply his family with the common neces-

saries of life. When asked for money, he was in the habit of
flying into a furious passion, cursing and blaspheming those near
him in a most dreadful manner. This symptom of insanity continued for several months, when he suddenly lapsed into the opposite extreme. He became recklessly improvident, and extravagant.
He squandered, in an unaccountable manner, nearly *fifteen thousand dollars* in the course of six months, utterly regardless of all
counsel, expostulation, and protest. During the whole of this time
(strange to relate), no one even *suspected* his mental sanity. His
conversation, on general topics, was not only coherent and rational,
but it was marked by vigorous intelligence, and great sagacity.
His letters also were free from all symptoms of aberration of intellect, and occasionally he attended public meetings, and spoke
with great eloquence and effect. His state of mind did not excite
suspicion, until one day, whilst attending a railway meeting as
one of the directors, he arose, and addressing the chairman,
offered to purchase, on his own account, all the disposable shares
in the possession of the company, and this, too, at a time when it
was believed to be, and literally was, on the verge of *bankruptcy!*

Let us charitably hope that many extraordinary and apparently
unreasonable and motiveless acts of brutality, violence, cruelty,
passion, and crime, that result from trifling and inadequate exciting causes acting upon congenitally weak and badly organized
intellects, may have their origin in some form of latent disease of
the brain, concealed, or unrecognized disorder of the mind. Is not
the sad history of crime fraught with illustrations of this kind?

Let it not, for one moment, be conceived, that I have the least
desire to screen the criminal from the just and *legal* punishment
awarded for flagrant violations of the law, or that I am disposed
to raise a false issue, or encourage a morbid sentimentality, or
maudlin sympathy in his favor. Such are not my views. Whilst
desiring to urge everything that can *scientifically* be said in defence of the culprit, I am not unmindful of what is necessary for
the safety of society, as well as what is righteously due to those
whom the criminal has so grievously injured.

But is there nothing, I ask, to be advanced in the way of apology, for the poor, wretched, heart-broken lunatic, irresistibly
driven by a diseased brain, and a perverted imagination, to an act
of murderous violence, whilst under the overwhelming dominion of
a fearful illusion of the senses, or crushing hallucination of the

intellect, destroying the power of healthy reason, and paralysing all freedom of the will? Poor Cowper, himself the subject of a severe form of *hypochondriasis*, when writing a congratulatory letter to a friend who had recently recovered from an attack of severe bodily disease, says, "Your illness has indeed been a sad one, causing, no doubt, great distress to yourself, and considerable anxiety to your relations and friends; but, oh! what are your *bodily* sufferings, acute as they undoubtedly were, to the unceasing *mental* torture I suffer from *a fever of the mind?*" I am afraid, in our sympathy (natural though it be) for the murdered victim, and in our feelings of deep compassion for those who survive to bitterly bemoan his loss, we are occasionally disposed to ignore the extent of acutely agonizing suffering the lunatic often experiences before he yields to the delirious impulse, and commits a crime so opposed to the strongest instincts of his nature.

In homicidal insanity, the victim is, alas! frequently related to the lunatic by the closest, the fondest, and dearest ties. A morbid desire to shed human blood (caused by particular affections of the brain), from a conviction that something dreadful *must be done* to relieve the mind of its terrible pressure, occasionally overpowers all feeling of fraternity and love. "It *must* be done—it *shall* be done—blood must be shed—my dear wife—my darling infant must perish by my own hand, before this mental anguish can pass away." Such was the sad description given of the morbid feelings of the most loving and affectionate of husbands and fathers.

The lunatic, driven to destroy human life, by a fearful delusion, which has obtained a complete ascendency over his reason, imagines that he hears a voice authoritatively commanding him to murder himself, and, occasionally others. He struggles, for a time, with these dreadful suggestions, but, alas! (the *cerebral* disorder extending), they eventually master him, and, when in a state of brain and mind, utterly extinguishing his knowledge of right and wrong, effectually paralysing the natural affections, and entirely destroying all power of self-control, he rushes blindly and unconsciously, in the frenzy of wild and delirious despair, on himself or his unhappy victim. In this condition of intellect, he is no more responsible for the crime he commits, than if he were a ferocious bull in the arena, goaded on to deeds of blood and

12

violence, by the ingeniously practised irritation, of the courageous, well-trained, and accomplished *torreador*.[1]

Far be it from me in any sentiments of compassion I may express for the unhappy lunatic doomed to an ignominious death, to be otherwise than keenly alive to the wailings of distress proceeding from the once happy dwelling made desolate by the ruthless hand of the murderer; sorry should I be, if I could ever ignore the terrible sufferings so often entailed by crime, on the widow's hearth and the orphan's home.   The fearful results—the sad con-

---

[1] The following is an extract of a beautiful poem published some years ago in the "Examiner" newspaper, from the pen of Mr. Edmund Ollier, descriptive of the *wail of the maniac* after realizing the fact of his having murdered his wife, in a temporary paroxysm of drunken homicidal insanity :—

" No, no !   I did not kill her !   No !
I say I will not have it so—
I will not hear it !   'Twas a dream
From which I woke with sudden scream,
And found the sweat upon my brow,
And that dull pain which even now
Is heavy on my heart and brain :—
*   *   *   *   *
" I have a wife—a dear one.—Nay,
Start not !   I have one *still*, I say,—
Or shall, when from this dream I wake.
We were heart wedded : we did slake
Our miseries in each other's tears,
And grew, through all the strange, sad years,
Quiet in grief's own quietness.
*   *   *   *   *
" Beware !   You'd tell me she is dead !
But I will dash my desperate head
Against these walls, before you speak
That cruel word !—Oh foul !   You seek
To crush me, seeing I am weak.
You have no touch of human ruth ;
You shake me with mere shows of truth
Which *must* be false, or heaven would pass
In shudderings to one formless mass.
Why, look in one another's eyes—
How calm they are !   You tell me lies,
Or your own tears would fleck the ground !—
I dreamt it, if this brain be sound.
*   *   *   *   *
" I wail and wander like a ghost,
Houseless, about a glimmering coast,
Where one lost face makes red the night.
—Oh, lingering dawn !   Oh, day !   Oh, light !"

sequences of crime—should never be lost sight of, whilst endeavoring by carefully considered scientific principles of medical psychology to shield the criminal, under the plea of insanity, from the legal penalties attached to his act, but no amount of public odium to which the medical witness may be exposed,—no extent of scurrilous abuse which may be levelled against him, should influence or deter him, when called upon to give evidence in cases of alleged criminal insanity, even to the weight of a hair, in the steady, fearless, and unflinching discharge of one of the most important, sacred, and solemn functions that can be delegated to a responsible being.

> ———— " Ambiguæ si quando citabere testis
> Incertæque rei; Phalaris licet imperet, ut sis
> Falsus, et admoto dictet perjuria tauro,
> Summum crede nefas animam præferre pudori,
> Et propter vitam vivendi perdere causas."
>
> "Juven." Sat. 8, v. 80.

The position of a psychological "*expert*," is one not to be ambitiously coveted. In cases of alleged insanity, he is occasionally compelled, when elucidating, in courts of law, the phenomena of mental derangement, to enunciate principles, as a pioneer of truth, *in advance* of the knowledge possessed by those who sometimes examine, and often severely, unjustly, criticise and calumniate him. When giving evidence on scientific points, he is occasionally and unavoidably obliged, in the expression of his opinions, to go counter to what is termed the "generally received" notions on the subject of insanity.[1] If it be his desire, in imitation of certain *dilettanti* psychologists, to sail with the popular breeze, and to pander to the opinions of the vulgar, by making his views of insanity square with those ordinarily entertained by the non-professional, psychologically uneducated, and, medically inexperienced, part of the community, his task is a facile and an easy one, but if he forms a just estimate of his position, as a lover and

[1] Dr. Whewell ("History of the Inductive Sciences") remarks, "that the general voice of mankind, which may often serve as a guide, because it rarely errs widely or permanently in its estimate of those who are prominent in public life, is of little value when it speaks of things belonging to the region of exact science." The opinion of the majority upon questions, within the comprehension and grasp of men of ordinary intelligence, and natural sagacity, is entitled to profound deference and respect. It may be, and often is, right. But does not history satisfactorily establish, that what in common parlance is designated as the "generally received opinion," is, occasionally, very remote from the truth?

"Interdum vulgus rectum videt, est ubi peccat."—Hor.

cultivator of science, and possesses a philosophic appreciation of his responsible vocation as a citizen of the state, physician, and medical jurist, and is resolved not to yield one inch of ground, in his honest exposition of scientific truth, in deference to popular fallacy, or in slavish obedience to ignorant abuse and noisy clamor, he must expect to pay the penalties attaching to his exhibition of moral courage, and firm and unflinching adherence to the path of public and professional duty. He may be maligned, misrepresented, and traduced for adopting this honorable principle of conduct, but the cause he has espoused must eventually triumph over all difficulties, temporarily obstructing its steady, onward, and advancing progress.

"Experts in madness! mad doctors!" indignantly, and offensively, exclaimed Mr. Baron Bramwell, in his charge to the jury at York, in the celebrated case of William Dove, the insane necromancer. "Experts in madness!" Why not? We have recourse to able, skilled, and scientific witnesses to elucidate difficult and disputed points in engineering, architecture, mechanics, navigation, feigned writing, chemistry, and many of the exact, as well as speculative sciences, and upon what ground should we repudiate the testimony of learned and experienced men, practically acquainted with the phenomena of insanity? What man of judgment would think of publicly throwing discredit upon the well and deliberately considered opinions of a Faraday, Brande, or a Graham, when called upon to unravel vexed and subtle questions of analytical chemistry? Who are better fitted than these eminent and learned men to decide such doubtful matters? Should we be justified in repudiating a Stephenson or a Brunel (if still among us) if selected to throw light in a court of law, upon an obscure, and litigated point connected with the science they so successfully cultivated and adorned? Why then speak contemptuously and disparagingly of the opinions of an educated and experienced class of *specialists*, when requested to solve knotty, and recondite questions, connected with alleged states of mental alienation? Is insanity so obviously apparent, so glaringly self-evident, and so palpably on the surface, that medically uneducated and inexperienced persons are competent, immediately to detect its existence without being assisted in their judgment by the testimony of men whose lives have been devoted to its careful study? Does a knowledge of the morbid phenomena of mind (the most profound and abstruse of all subjects) come by intuition, and is it dependent upon the *minimum* amount of time that has been applied to their investigation? Is the competency to pronounce a sound, scientific, and trustworthy opinion, on subtle forms of disordered thought, in exact correspondence with the smallest extent of opportunity afforded of becoming practically acquainted with their phenomena? Such, I fear, is the too commonly received view of the matter. Agreeably to vulgar and popular notions, a person alleged to be insane, is expected to exhibit all the usual stereotyped, artistic, poetic, and melodramatic characteristics of madness. If a genuine lunatic, she must resemble poor Ophelia, and have pieces of straw permeating various parts of her hair, and tied round the waist, and show her insanity by singing plaintively and incoherently snatches of melody. No one would be considered as *bona fide* insane, that did not foam at the mouth, gnash the teeth, tear the hair, clench the fist, roll the eyes in a "fine frenzy," talk gibberish, rave, and converse of being possessed by the "foul fiend," as Poor Tom in "King Lear," is heard to do, when acting the part of the madman on the stage. If such were the ordinary characteristic manifestations of the forms of insanity, with which juries and judges have generally to deal (in civil as well as in criminal courts) I quite concur in the opinion, inferentially expressed by Mr. Baron Bramwell, that the evidence of experts is quite superfluous, and may safely be dispensed with. But this is not the type of cases usually submitted to legal adjudication. The annals of our courts of law establish, beyond a doubt, that the criminal and homicidal lunatic almost invariably belong to the class of' quiet, cunning, subtle, clever, and what Esquirol terms, "*reasoning*" madmen. How rare it is to see a person laboring under *acute* insanity tried for a capital crime? In the majority of criminal cases, the lunatic, although suffering from a dangerous and homicidal form of mental derangement, has sufficient self-possession and control over his disordered thoughts, to converse and comport himself like a person in healthy possession of his reasoning powers. This is a type of case that so often deceives the most conscientious judge, puzzles and perplexes the most painstaking body of men impanelled (as a jury) to try the issue of sanity or insanity, life or death. Subtle cases like these present but few difficulties to the *practical* physician, thoroughly conversant with the phenomena of insanity, and well acquainted with the physiognomy and idiosyncrasies of the insane.

He, alone, is competent to scientifically and accurately test the more obscure forms of mental derangement; he, above all others, is best able to discover, unmask, and bring to light the latent disease. It is, therefore, likely to be most fatal to the administration of justice, to deliberately ignore, when analyzing judicially such recondite conditions of mental alienation, the valuable co-operation of men of admitted science, great observation, and of enlarged experience. The coarser and more demonstrative symptoms of insanity are obviously patent to men of common intelligence, and ordinary knowledge, but the less manifested, more obscure and *hidden* types of mental disease, require for their satisfactory elucidation, an intimate and profound acquaintance with the physiology, as well as pathology, of the human mind. Without the aid of the testimony of experienced witnesses, juries are much more likely to arrive at a wrong, than a right conclusion. It is irrational to expect any other result, when we consider the great and peculiar difficulties with which they have generally to combat, when subtle, and disputed forms of criminal insanity, are submitted to their consideration and decision.[1]

[1] If an expert propounds in a court of law an opinion in relation to an alleged case of criminal insanity, in strict conformity with the experience of the great bulk of men practically engaged in the study and treatment of the disease, and gives expression to views in harmony with the principles of enlightened psychological science, he is exposed to the imputation of entertaining, and inculcating, dangerous, and, forsooth! "crotchetty" theories. This insinuation is often made by ignorant, presumptuous, and conceited men, just as competent to appreciate the more obscure, recondite, and subtle forms of deranged thought, as the common house, sign painter, or scene dauber, would be, to estimate, to their full artistic extent, the delicate and beautiful coloring, shading, and tints of a *Raphael, Claude, Correggio, Titian, Carlo Dolce, Guido*, &c.

Whilst considering this subject, perhaps it would not be deemed irrelevant, if I were to correct a gross misrepresentation of an opinion I expressed when attempting to rescue from the gallows, a poor idiot of the name of Atkinson, who was tried for murder at the York Assizes, in 1858. It was reported, and generally credited, that I was guilty of the imbecility of declaring, when in the witness-box, that I made it a rule never to give testimony in support of the sanity of any man who had committed, and was tried for murder! If I had given expression, at the time, to such a "monstrous" absurdity, I certainly should be disposed to believe that I was much farther advanced in idiotcy, than the poor demented criminal, whose life I was then endeavoring, by my evidence, to save.

The statement I made on the occasion referred to, and which gave rise to so false an interpretation, was in substance as follows: I remarked, that if a man were accused and tried for a murder, committed some time previously, and the plea of insanity were urged in his defence, upon what was conceived to be the strong, and *bonâ fide* evidence of *competent eye-witnesses, practically acquainted with the prisoner's*

I do not venture to reconcile with known and admitted facts, the singular inconsistencies pervading the public mind, on the subject of insanity. A man commits suicide. At the coroner's inquest it is established, that previously to the catastrophe, the self-murderer was observed to have been odd in his manner and depressed in spirits. These symptoms are sufficient to satisfy the jury as to his irresponsible state of mind, and a verdict of " temporary insanity" is without hesitation, in many instances, properly returned. It is notorious, that in these cases, juries eagerly avail themselves of the slightest evidence of mental derangement, and appear pleased to find, that they have a fair and reasonable excuse for a verdict of lunacy. The same jury, however, impanelled to try a similar issue before another tribunal, the question raised not being the insanity of the self-murderer, but the soundness of mind and capacity of a person to manage himself and his property, will perseveringly refuse to recognize the existence of insanity, and incapacity, even if established by the clearest, and most conclusive medical and general testimony. The faintest, and *minimum* amount of proof, in the former case, immediately determines the verdict of the jury; the *maximum* degree of evidence, adduced before a different court, is generally required, and often set aside, as totally unworthy of regard. The jury, in the one case, is most anxious (influenced, no doubt, by right and charitable motives) to protect the memory of the *suicide* from the imputation of *sanity;* and in the second instance (totally ignorant of the extent of desolation and misery that are, alas! so often entailed upon families by an obstinate determination not to recognize the existence of insanity), they stretch a point to shield the subject of inquiry from what is unphilosophically termed, the *stigma* of mental derangement. If the evidence in the former case, so demonstratively conclusive to the mind of the coroner's jury of the presence of insanity were adduced, to establish unsoundness of mind at a commission " *De Lunatico Inquirendo,*"

state of mind, at the time he committed the crime, I should consider it a duty to hesitate in pronouncing in a court of law (the life of the prisoner being dependent upon *my* evidence) a *speculative* opinion of his perfect sanity of mind, and moral responsibility, in direct opposition to the *positive* testimony of others, basing my conclusions on the examination I had made of the prisoner's state of intellect, some time after the perpetration of the imputed crime, and immediately previous to his trial.

it would bring severe censure and reproach upon those who attempted to obtain a verdict upon such inadequate testimony.

It may be argued, that these two illustrations are essentially
different in their principal features. In the former case, no possible harm can accrue to the unhappy man (whatever may be the
effect of the suicide upon his family) by a verdict of temporary
insanity, even if the jury were to come to a wrong conclusion;
but in the latter case a person, it is alleged, may be seriously
injured, by being deprived of the control of his person and property, if wrongly accused of being insane, and pronounced mentally unsound, and thereby deemed incapacitated for the management of his own affairs. The point at issue is undoubtedly open
to this grave objection. But, on the other hand (whilst advising
the exercise of extreme caution before recording a verdict of
insanity), we are bound to consider the serious and fatal mischief
that might follow an inconsiderate and hasty repudiation, on the
part of the jury, of *un*soundness of mind. If a lunatic be discharged from supervision through the ignorance or mistaken kindness of the jury, the most disastrous consequences are likely to
ensue from his being permitted, when in a state of mental derangement, to deal with his property. How often have families
been brought to beggary and ruin by the insane proceedings of
persons thus prematurely and improperly liberated from all control, whilst in a state of mind utterly unfitting them either to
understand or to transact important matters of business. Wills,
and other important deeds, have been executed under such conditions of disordered and enfeebled mind, and large possessions have
been cruelly alienated from the heir-at-law and bequeathed to un-
principled and designing men, by persons obviously incompetent
to exercise testamentary capacity. Juries impanelled to try the
question of mental soundness at a Commission of Lunacy are
generally disposed to ignore all evidence of insanity and incapacity, unless it be of such a character as to clearly render the person, alleged to be insane, positively dangerous to himself as well
as to others. A jury, as ordinarily constituted, is incompetent to
estimate the delicate coloring, tint, and shades of the ever-varying
phases and degrees of disordered and unsound mind. It often requires the well-trained and exquisitely-educated eye of the accomplished medical artist to appreciate the subtle manifestations of
the more obscure and latent forms of mental alienation. A per-

son whose derangement of intellect is not prominently manifested, has therefore a reasonable chance of obtaining a verdict in his favor, and this probability is very much enhanced, if he has been fortunate enough to retain for his defence the services of an astute solicitor, and an eloquent and sagacious advocate, fully competent to deal skilfully and successfully with the facts of the case, presenting them in a most convincing light to the jury. It is not my province to censure the lawyer for doing his best to establish the sanity of his client, even in the teeth of evidence clearly proving him to be insane.[1] My object is simply to direct professional attention to the serious and irremediable injury that is likely to accrue, unconsciously to the lunatic himself, as well as to the interests of those nearly related to, and dependent upon him, by an erroneous decision as to the state of his mind. A man having at command, and under his exclusive control, a large amount of property is, upon clear and undoubted evidence, alleged to be insane. It may be the wife, the son, or the daughter, who, recognizing in the head of the family a state of mental unsoundness, has, with a view of saving him, as well as his family, from the workhouse, mooted the question of his mental capacity. The alleged lunatic, unless acutely deranged and demented, indignantly denies the imputation (a common occurrence in such cases), exhibiting, at the time, much natural irritation and anger against those with whom the allegation has originated. The case eventually becomes a matter of judicial inquiry. The jury, sworn to try

---

[1] Much vulgar abuse has been directed against the members of the legal profession, for the assumed readiness they are alleged to exhibit in accepting any brief that may be presented to them, irrespectively of the actual and *bonâ fide* merits of the case they are retained to advocate. The counsel is presumed to know nothing of the matter to be litigated except what is embodied in his instructions. With these alone he has to deal. It is his duty to act upon such instructions, and to do his best to conduct the case intrusted to him, in strict conformity with the recognized rules of evidence. It is not a part of his vocation to sit in judgment upon the facts of the case placed before him; neither is he called upon to throw up his brief, should he perceive, in the course of the trial, that (as far as the justice of the case is concerned) he is unfortunately on the wrong side, and that the evidence is telling against the interests of the party he is engaged to defend. Dr. Johnson has placed this matter in a correct light. In answer to a question put to him by Boswell, in relation to the point mooted, he remarked, that "a lawyer has no business with the justice or injustice of the cause he undertakes, unless his client asks his opinion, and then he is bound to give it honestly. The justice or injustice of the cause is to be decided by the judge."

the issue, confounded by the eloquent and impassioned appeals of counsel, confused by the frequently conflicting character of the medical evidence, puzzled by the apparent rationality of the party affirmed to be afflicted with mental alienation, are unable to come to a unanimous decision as to the sanity or insanity of the person whose state of mind is the subject of their investigation. Nevertheless, if there be a majority of the jury in his favor, the person alleged to be insane is fully entitled to their verdict, and being declared of sound mind, is consequently discharged from all supervision and control, and placed, *legally*, in a position to deal as he pleases with his person and property.[1] It is not difficult to conceive the course which a person who has been able, thus cunningly and cleverly, to mask, from the eyes of a section of the jury, all evidence of his mental derangement, might be induced to take after being so liberated, and to what extent the interests of his family would be fatally imperilled and involved by his testamentary, as well as other acts, executed under the combined influence of *legally undetected* insanity, and natural anger, directed towards those who, influenced by the kindest and most honorable motives, have incurred his severe displeasure by initiating proceedings in the Court of Chancery, with a view of enforcing (for the man's own advantage), a statute of lunacy against him. It would be useless, if the claims of relationship were to be ignored in a will, made soon after the execution of the commission, by a person smarting under what he conceives to be an unjust imputation of insanity, to dispute its validity upon the death of the testator. If such an attempt were made, by raising the plea of testamentary incapacity, the verdict of sanity recorded by the jury at the Commission of Lunacy would, except in extreme and exceptional cases, be viewed as valid and conclusive evidence in favor of the will. Thus, misery and destitution of the acutest kind, would be entailed on the surviving relatives of the unhappy man, by their inability to upset a disposition of property clearly made

---

[1] According to the present state of the law, there must be at a Commission *De Lunatico* a majority of twelve of the jury before a verdict, either way, can be received by the Master. It often happens that the jury in number amounts to fifteen, twenty, and five-and-twenty. In many cases, there are often twelve jurymen for the sanity, and eight or ten entertaining strong opinions adverse to a verdict of mental soundness. Under these circumstances, the reader will be able to appreciate the facilities that exist for persons, obviously insane, escaping through such an ordeal.

when the testator was manifestly incapable of exercising a sane memory, judgment, and reflection.'

I would point out another anomaly in reference to the state of the law as well as to the condition of public opinion in relation to this interesting subject. A man commits a murder. He is tried for the crime. The plea of insanity is raised in his defence, upon what is conceived to be *bonâ fide* evidence of the existence of mental derangement at the time of the murder. The attempt thus made to protect the criminal, immediately rouses the public indignation. Such an excuse is not in many instances listened to, and the unfortunate medical witnesses who have been called upon to exercise an important, and often thankless duty in support of the plea, are exposed, for giving an honest expression of opinion, to the most unmeasured ridicule and vituperation. In defending the memory of the suicide from the disgrace that would accompany a verdict of *felo de se*, the evidence of the medical man *proving insanity* is regarded with great respect and treated with profound deference ; but in the effort to rescue a poor lunatic from the agonies of a painful death upon the scaffold, on evidence much stronger than was adduced before the previously mentioned court, the expert is exposed to unmitigated abuse. Instead of being considered as an angel of mercy, engaged in the exercise of a holy and righteous mission, he is viewed with suspicion, and often treated with contumely, as if he were attempting to *sacrifice*, instead of to *save* human life. Again, the attempt to prove sanity of mind and mental capacity at a *Commission of Lunacy*, with the object of preserving intact the liberty of the subject and establishing his right to an unfettered management of his own property, is applauded to the very echo ; but the endeavor to excuse, on the plea of insanity, an act of crime consigning the unhappy wretch, alleged to be an irresponsible lunatic, to penal servitude for life, or, alas ! to the hands of the public executioner, is denounced in unqualified language, as a most monstrous, unjustifiable, and iniquitous interference with the course of justice. The excuse of insanity will not, in many cases, under these circumstances, be tolerated by a portion of the press, in the slightest degree countenanced by the judge who tries the criminal, or deferred to by the jury, whose duty it is to decide the fate of the prisoner. The public mind is violently shocked at the commission of a horrible and brutal murder. The act is viewed in the abstract as one of

great and barbarous atrocity, apart altogether from all its concomitant extenuating medico-psychological considerations.   The cry is
raised for " vengeance !"   The shout is,—"an eye for an eye !"
—"a tooth for a tooth !"—" blood for blood !" forgetting, in the
paroxysm of indignant emotion, and frenzy of excited feeling, engendered by the contemplation of a dreadful violation of the
majesty of the law, that JUSTICE must ever be tempered with that
DIVINE MERCY which sanctifies and enshrines

> " The throned monarch better than his crown,
> *   *   *   *   *
> And is the Attribute of God Himself."

CHAPTER VII.

THE STAGE OF CONSCIOUSNESS.

IF we were to closely scrutinize into the fathomless mysteries of the inner mental life, and fearlessly analyze the nature of the terrible conceptions that occasionally throw their dark phantasmal shade across the anxious and troubled breast, what a melancholy, degrading, and profoundly humiliating revelation most men would have to make, of the dark corners, secret recesses, and hidden crevices of the human heart! If this self-examination were faithfully and honestly executed, it would cause the best and fairest of God's creatures to shudder with terror at the possibility of such ideas ever intruding into the soul's solemn sanctuary.[1]

---

[1] A neglect of the practice of self-inspection and self-interrogation, is said to be one of the most serious imperfections, moral and intellectual, of the present system of mental discipline and education. The defect is not confined, it is alleged, to listless, vacant persons, who permit life to glide over them amidst frivolities, and waking dreams, but is perceived among those who intensely and actively employ themselves with objects external to themselves. An able moral philosopher observes, when alluding to this subject: "that after a certain period of life, few have the hardihood sternly to look within. For a high degree of moral courage is required to face the disclosure which awaits the mind, when it is thus turned inwards upon itself; a disclosure, it may be, of the result of years and years that have passed over it in listless inactivity, which yields nothing to reflection but an empty void; or in the eager pursuit of objects which are seen to be worthless; or in the acquirement of habits which are felt to be destructive of the health of the mind; the disclosure, it may be, of important duties neglected and important pursuits overlooked, and the conviction that life is drawing to a close, while its great business is yet to begin. Few have moral courage to meet this disclosure; and when it is met with an attention in some degree adequate to its supreme interest, the impressions which it yields are encountered by the force of confirmed moral habits, which seem to claim every faculty and feeling of the mind as theirs by hopeless bondage. Hence the supreme importance of cultivating in early life the habit of looking within; the practice of rigidly questioning ourselves as to what we are, and what we are doing; what are our leading pursuits, and what our mental habits; what are our plans and prospects for life, and what influence over the whole of our moral discipline have the solemn realities of a life which is to come."—*Dr. Abercrombie on the " Culture and Discipline of the Mind."*

Moral philosophers, intimately acquainted with the anatomy of the human heart, have often asked, who has not occasionally had a demon pursuing with remorseless impetuosity his every footstep, suggesting to his ever-active, and often morbidly-disturbed and perverted imagination, the commission of some dark deed of crime, from the contemplation of which he has, at the time, shrunk back aghast with horror? What mind is alleged to be so pure and untainted, that has not been disposed to yield, when the reason and moral sense have, alas, been transiently paralyzed, and God's grace ceases to influence the heart, to the seduction of impure thought, lingered with apparent pleasure on the contemplation of physically unchaste images, or delighted in a fascinating dalliance with criminal thoughts? Who has not conceived how easily he might, with his own hand, "shuffle off this mortal coil," and penetrate into the dark and mysterious secrets of futurity? What heart has been, at all times, free from malevolent passion, revengeful emotion, lustful feeling, unnatural, and, alas, devilish impulses? Is not every bosom polluted by a dark, leprous spot, corroding ulcer, or portion of moral gangrene? Does there not cling to every mind some melancholy reminiscence of the past, which throws at times a sombre tinge over the checkered path of life? We may flatter our pharisaical vanity and human pride, by affirming that we are exempt from these melancholy conditions of moral suffering, and sad states of mental infirmity, but, alas, we should be belying human nature, if we were to ignore the existence of such, thank God, only temporary, paroxysmal, and evanescent conditions of unhealthy thought, and abnormal phases of passion, which occasionally have been known to cast their withering influence and deathlike shadow over the mind, blighting, saddening, and often crushing the best, kindest, and noblest of human hearts.

"Who can tell," says a learned divine, "all the windings, turnings, depths, hollowness, and dark corners of the mind of man? He who enters upon this scrutiny, enters into a labyrinth or a wilderness, where he has no guide but chance or industry to direct his inquiries, or to put an end to his search. It is a wilderness in which a man may wander more than forty years, and through which few have passed to the promised land."[1]

Among the obscure, and, as yet, inexplicable phenomena of dis-

[1] Dr. South.

ordered intellect, stands prominently forward a condition, incipient phase, or pre-existing abnormal state, in which the patient (long before he becomes, or is considered actually insane) is fully sensible, painfully, keenly, and exquisitely conscious of the predominance of certain morbid and unnatural states of emotion, idea, and impulse.

For a considerable period before the mind has lost its equilibrium, or is appreciably disordered, the patient admits that he is under the influence of certain vague apprehensions, undefinable misgivings, and anxious suspicions, as to the *sane* character of his emotions, healthy condition of his ideas, and normal state of his instincts. He detects himself, when unobserved, occasionally asking, can my impressions be healthy ? Is there any good reason for my entertaining these strange and singular feelings ? Why am I adverse to *this* person's presence, and why do I feel a repugnance to and shun the society of *that* individual ? Am I in a sound state of mind ? Are unnatural ideas and strange impulses like those suggesting themselves to and influencing my mind, consistent with a healthy condition of thought, and a sane state of the intellect ? Am I in possession of my senses ? Is this state of feeling, this condition of weakened volition, these strange inclinations that appear blindly and irresistibly to drive me to the commission of overt acts, so adverse to my natural character, so antagonistic to my sense and knowledge of what is right and wrong ;—are these flittings of sombre melancholy, these scintillations of perverted thought, so contrary to my nature, and opposed to every principle of my being, the dawnings—obscure, faint tints, shadowy outlines —of approaching insanity ? Am I mad or becoming so ? emphatically and frantically interrogates the unhappy person subject to this incipient manifestation of disordered and disturbed thought.[1]

---

[1] In a conversation between the stoic *Damasippus* and *Horace* (Sat. iii, lib. ii), the poet asks the former, " in what kind of folly do you think my madness consists ?"

" Qua me stultitiâ (quoniam non est genus unum),
  Insanire putas ?"

and adds,
          "Ego nam videor mihi sanus."

" Quid ?" responds the Stoic,

          "Caput abscissum demens cum portat Agave
          Gnati infelicis,"

(and then immediately asks),

Such sad doubts, fearful apprehensions, mysterious inexplicable forebodings, and distressing misgivings as to the healthy condition of the mind, often induce the heart-broken sufferer, convulsed with pain, and choking with anguish, prayerfully, and in accents of wild and phrenzied despair, to ejaculate with King Lear,

> "O, let me not be mad, not mad, sweet Heaven!
> Keep me in temper, I would not be mad!"

This agonizing consciousness of the presence of morbid and insane ideas, painful recognition of the first approaches and foreshadowings of insanity, are occasionally so acute, and the mental misery induced so crushing and overwhelming, that relief from the terrible sufferings they occasion is occasionally sought for in self-immolation.

In the incipient stage of insanity, I repeat, the patient is fully sensible of entertaining exaggerated and unnatural impressions; is acutely conscious of the mind dwelling morbidly, and sometimes irresistibly, upon certain trains of absurd, unhealthy, and it may be, alas! very unholy and *impure* thought. He painfully recognizes the fact, that insane conceptions are struggling to master his reason, obtain an ascendency over his judgment, an abnormal influence and control over his passions, and the subjugation of his instincts. In some cases (and this is a distressing and dangerous type of insanity), he is impelled (why and wherefore he knows not) to commit suicide, and even to sacrifice the lives of those related to him by the closest ties of relationship, as well as to give utterance to blasphemous, revolting, and impure expressions! He finds it, occasionally, extremely difficult, and almost impossible, to dismiss from the mind, and keep in subjection, these morbid impulses to acts of homicidal and suicidal violence, or to conquer the insane desire to clothe in grossly obscene language conceptions, from the contemplation of which his delicate and sensitive nature would, when unclouded by disease, have instinctively shrunk with horror, loathing, and disgust.

A gentleman of great accomplishments, of high order of intel-

"Sibi tum furiosa videtur?"

It would thus appear that this illustrious poet had a clear conception of the phase of conscious insanity of which I am now speaking.

lect, of known literary reputation, and of admitted personal worth, had his mind for years tortured with morbid suggestions to utter obscene and blasphemous expressions. He eventually destroyed himself; and in a letter which he wrote to me a few days before committing suicide, and which did not reach me until after his death, he said his life was embittered and made wretched by these terrible suggestions; but he thanked God that he had never once yielded to them, and that, although he was a Christian in principle, he felt he was not sinning against God by committing self-destruction, with the object of effectually destroying all chance of his giving utterance to thoughts that might contaminate the minds and morals of others!

In the incipient, as well as in the fully-developed conditions of insanity, the instincts,—the coarser parts of animal nature,—make, occasionally, a bold, determined, and vigorous effort to forcibly seize the sceptre, and exercise supreme authority and despotic dominion over man's "sovereign reason." An awful, terrible, deadly, "hand to hand" struggle sometimes ensues between these antagonistic elements. "The reason *may* resist," says Coleridge (when referring to this appalling contest), "it *does* resist for a long time, but too often, alas! at length it yields, and the man is mad forever!"

BISHOP BUTLER records that he was, all his life, struggling against the horrible morbid suggestions (he termed them "devilish") which, he says, would have maddened him, if he had relaxed the stern wakefulness of his reason for a single moment.

A lady writes: "Can I obtain no relief for my acute and horrible sufferings? Hell, with all its torments, cannot be equal to the tortures I endure! I feel all the misery of a lost soul, all the agony of the damned! With this heart-breaking misery, I know I cannot be in my right senses! Would that I could have administered to me some opiate to deaden the sensibility of my poor brain, or to make me mad, and thus destroy all consciousness of suffering! Dr. —— has given me a powerful medicine, but it is of no service. Night and day is my mind bewildered by this intense feeling of being or going mad! Do tell me frankly what your opinion is as to my state. Is this insanity, or am I becoming deranged?[1] Have you known any case similar to mine? and if

---

[1] Sir James Mackintosh alludes to this form of unhealthy and distempered mind in his celebrated letter to Robert Hall, addressed to this distinguished minister of the

so, did they recover or die in a madhouse? I am advised to separate myself, for a time, from my family. It breaks my heart to think of so cruel a severance. If I went abroad, could not Col. —— and my precious children go with me? If foreign travel is decided upon, where would you advise me to go? Paris never did agree with me. I spent, a few years ago, a miserable winter there when I lost my poor H——. I am sure the associations of the place would aggravate all my mental symptoms. Last night I never closed my eyes for five minutes in sleep. Would that I could cease to think of the horrible suggestions of my exquisitely sensitive nature and terribly diseased imagination. I cannot sustain this state of mind long. I have a nervous horror of death, and yet I sigh for destruction. I often wish I had never been born. Should I be committing a sin if I were to commit suicide in my present condition of intellect? Would I be held responsible for what I did whilst tortured and driven to despair by these dreadful thoughts?"

A lady prayed passionately that she might be relieved from the horror of the fearful delusions that tortured her imagination by a complete deprivation of reason and loss of consciousness, exclaiming, with intense emotion,

> "Come, madness! come unto me, senseless death!
> I cannot suffer this! Here, rocky wall,
> Scatter these brains, or dull them."—JOANNA BAILLIE.

Another patient confessed that she had resolved upon committing suicide on *six* different occasions, and once had a dose of deadly poison to her lips; but her courage failed when she thought of her dear children, the youngest being only a year and a half

---

Gospel, after his recovery from his first attack of insanity. Sir James Mackintosh writes:—

"We are all accustomed to contemplate with pleasure the suspension of the ordinary operations of the understanding in sleep, and even to be amused by its nightly wanderings from its course in dreams. From the commanding eminence which you have gained, you will gradually familiarize your mind to consider its other aberrations as only more rare than sleep or dreams; and in process of time they will cease to appear to you much more horrible. You will thus be delivered from *the constant dread which so often brings on the very evil dreaded;* and which, as it clouds the whole of human life, is itself a greater calamity than any temporary disease. Some dread of this sort darkened the days of Johnson; and the fears of Rousseau seem to have constantly realized themselves."

old. This lady was apparently in possession of her reasoning faculties, and was perfectly capable of managing, and did superintend with great skill, a large domestic household; but she was occasionally subject to paroxysms of intense mental depression, associated with horribly impure suspicions respecting her husband, which she knew and confessed to be morbid and entirely visionary. These attacks were generally of some days' duration, and on one occasion she was in this state of mind for four continuous weeks. Whilst the paroxysm existed, she talked to those about her, describing with painful minuteness and extraordinary exactness, her acutely agonizing feelings. Her husband informed me, that he never could detect the slightest defect in her powers of reflection, or in the reasoning faculty, judgment, or memory. At one time, whilst suffering great mental distress, wringing her hands in wild despair, and praying passionately for instant annihilation, it was necessary for him to persuade her to concentrate her attention to some important matter of business, involving a retrospect of minute circumstances that had occurred nearly five years previously. He was struck with the remarkable accuracy of her memory, clearness of perception, and soundness of her judgment. Yet conjoined with this state of intellect did this poor lady entertain impressions (too disgusting to detail) about her husband, which she knew and readily admitted were creations of her distempered imagination.

A gentleman, after recovering from an unquestionable state of lunacy, confessed that for two years previously to his believing and acting in conformity with his conceptions, he was perfectly conscious of their being morbid. Occasionally his mind wavered on the subject; but, on a little reflection, he was in the habit of saying to himself, " Nonsense !" " Pooh, pooh !" and then laughing at the absurdity of his own disordered thoughts. On one occasion he attended a political meeting where there was much speaking, and great accompanying noise and excitement. He, like those about him, took an active part in the proceedings, and participated in the agitation that so generally prevailed. This brought matters to a crisis. It was after returning home from the meeting referred to, with his mind in a state of great exaltation, that he imagined he saw the heavens open, and special revelations made to him. Then a firm belief in the reality of his impressions commenced; he, in fact, at that time emerging out of a morbid, but not yet deranged state, into one of positive insanity! "I am," said a man subject to attacks of alienation of mind, "fully conscious of the operation of thought, and of the gradual, insidious advances of absurd, unreasonable, and morbid thought, up to a certain period, when I am no longer conscious of anything," the mind then passing out of an *unhealthy* into a *disordered* condition.   •

"Such a state as mine," writes a patient, "you are probably unacquainted with, notwithstanding all your experience. I am not conscious of the suspension or decay of any of the powers of my mind. I am as well able as ever I was to attend to my business; my family suppose me in health, yet the horrors of a madhouse are staring me in the face. I am a martyr to a species of persecution from within, which is becoming intolerable. I am urged to say the most shocking things. Blasphemous and obscene words are ever on the tip of my tongue. Hitherto, thank God! I have been able to resist; but I often think I must yield at last, and then I shall be disgraced forever and ruined. I solemnly assure you that I hear a voice which seems to be within me, prompting me to utter what I would turn from with disgust if uttered by another. If I were not afraid that you would smile, I should say there is no way of accounting for these extraordinary articulate whisperings but by supposing that an evil spirit has obtained possession of me for the time. My state is so wretched that, compared with what I suffer, pain or sickness would appear but trifling evils."[1]

"I have met," says a distinguished authority, "with more than one patient in private practice who confessed that his life had for many years been rendered completely miserable by the constant effort required to suppress morbid impulses, even when their manifestation tended only to acts of folly and not crime."

A very active and meritorious clergyman, who expended a large portion of his small income in works of charity, told Dr. Wigan in confidence, that after hard study, or want of rest, this state of mind made him greatly apprehensive of insanity; and that often, when preaching, there would seem to be placed before his eyes some profane book, which the devil tempted him to read in lieu

---

[1] "Essays on Partial Derangement of the Mind in supposed connection with Religion." By the late John Cheyne, M.D.   Pp. 64, 65.

of his sermon! That the more he prayed for aid against the temptation, the more he found himself oppressed by it; and that at last he discovered that violent efforts for an hour with the dumb bells, or fencing, immediately before service, would entirely re-move it. His great difficulty was to use the necessary exercise without attracting notice. A good gallop would have been the proper course, but the money which should have kept his horse he gave to the poor. A similar modification of diseased action in one brain controlled by the other is found, says Dr. Wigan, in the propensity which some persons with a tendency to insanity possess, to blaspheme at church, and interrupt the most solemn part of the service by violent or obscene language. Such impulses are not known to others till they become ungovernable, but they exist in a slighter degree in some who are called *sane*.

A young gentleman of ancient family and historical name, of good general disposition, and fair though neglected education, had an ungovernable propensity to run up into an organ-loft in the middle of divine service, and play some well-known jocular tune, attached, perhaps, to profane or indecent words. This he would do so suddenly that it was impossible to prevent it before he had thrown the congregation into confusion. He was always sorry for it, and declared that he tried with all his might to prevent it; and he always abstained from going near a church in service time, though he would read the prayers at home with apparently sin-cere and tranquil devotion. If he accidentally passed an open church door the temptation was irresistible, and he often got him-self into serious embarrassment by indulging these freaks. He conversed coherently and rationally, and in all other respects was perfectly sane; but he was subject to periodical epileptic fits, and the propensity was at last traced to this malady.

Many years elapsed in this very mild and equivocal form of mental disturbance; he went abroad, and I lost sight of him, but was informed that he entered into great sensual indulgences, his fits became more and more aggravated, and he at last died of what his friends called brain fever. The persons who attended him at the last moments knew nothing of his previous history, and the brain was not examined.[1]

A gentleman, after recovering from a protracted attack of men-

1 Wigan's "Duality of the Mind," pp. 237, 238, 239.

tal derangement, assured me that for more than *nine* months prior to his losing all *voluntary* power over his thoughts and actions, he was conscious of his approaching insanity, and of the presence of certain morbid trains of thought! He was frequently in the habit of acting in a most singularly eccentric manner when walking in the public streets, grinning at strangers, putting his tongue out, and laughing hysterically at persons whom he accidentally met. He involved himself on one occasion in a serious altercation, having hustled violently against some ladies coming out of a place of public amusement, which led to an explanation and apology. The patient informed me that at the moment *he knew* what he was about, and had not altogether lost the power of self-government. At another time, when it must be *presumed* he was on the brink of an attack of actual insanity, he began repeating, with extraordinary rapidity and accompanying energy of muscular action, a string of unmeaning and unintelligible words. He continued for nearly an hour uttering this jargon as he was walking towards the city. He was fully conscious of the nonsense he was talking, and recognized the folly of his conduct, but the disposition to so indulge, he says, was fascinating and quite irresistible, defying all power of control! At other times he was quite free from these oddities, and comported himself with singular propriety and decorum.

On another occasion he saw, printed in large characters, a ridiculous and unusual name on a placard. For an hour and a half he kept repeating this word until he was obliged to stop from feelings of muscular fatigue! This gentleman became, at the expiration of nine months, quite insane, imagining that he was pursued by the police for the commission of an offence he had committed against public morals. This was a complete delusion, which was, after a few months of treatment, entirely dissipated.

A gentleman who, when insane, attempted to murder three different persons, assured me that during the height of his paroxysm, he felt as if his mind were enveloped in a dark cloud. In another case of homicidal insanity, the patient, whilst being impelled to sacrifice life under the incontrollable desire to commit some act that might divert his attention from his own harrowing thoughts, confessed that for some days before the murder everything he saw was tinted with blood. He believes that this perversion of the perceptive faculties first suggested to his mind the dreadful crime which he subsequently perpetrated.

In this stage of insanity, the patient occasionally suffers most acutely from *phantasms*. He is quite conscious of the spectral illusions being dependent upon a disordered state of the visual and perceptive faculties (often caused by gastric and hepatic derangement), and is able to reason with himself, and talk to others respecting their nature and origin. I have often been consulted by patients suffering from this type of hallucination. These cases are not difficult to cure. One gentleman, for three months was constantly followed by a terrible spectral image, resembling, to a remarkable degree, in figure and countenance, a brother who had destroyed himself twelve years previously whilst at sea! In this case, the patient had, previously to the appearance of the hallucination, complained of headache, great nervous depression, and lowness of spirits. He confessed, that he never for one moment believed in the reality of the image. When he sat down to dinner, the spectre took his seat opposite! If he walked in the street, the phantom was by his side! When travelling by rail, the apparition was seated in the same carriage! The patient was fortunately a man of good strong sense, possessing a vigorous, well-cultivated, and severely disciplined understanding. He was, therefore, competent to reason with himself philosophically in relation to the illusion, and to keep in check any disposition that might occasionally exist to believe in the reality of the spectral image. He eventually parted company with his mysterious phantom, but not until he had a severe attack of confluent smallpox, which nearly proved fatal. After recovery, he never complained of the hallucination. In a second case, a lady said, that her life was made wretched by a similar illusion of the senses. She was constantly tortured by a number of singularly grotesque figures, dressed in most fantastic costumes. These phantoms danced round her during the day, and at night, appeared about, and sometimes *in* her bed. It was with great difficulty she could obtain continuous and refreshing sleep. This patient never for one moment believed in the *material* character of these spectral illusions. She was in the habit, occasionally, of taking sketches of these curious phantasmal figures, many of which I was permitted to see.

A worthy clergyman, now under my treatment, is subject to the most singular aural illusions. Several years back, he had a severe attack of carbuncle at the nape of the neck. After recovering from this affection, he began to hear voices audibly speak to him.

They often addressed him in the Welsh language, occasionally using particular phrases, idioms, and endearing epithets, that he had been in the habit of indulging in *forty* years previously when paying court to his wife. He is rarely free from the influence of this conscious illusion.[1]

The particulars of the following interesting case of hallucinations were communicated in writing by the young lady who was their subject, to the physician who attended her, a gentleman of great experience in mental affections :—

"I was born April 9th, 1840, and am just 19. My health is good, and constitution strong, I think, though as a child I was delicate, owing to over study. My temperament is melancholy, though not gloomy. I seldom, if ever, suffer from what people call the 'blues.' My mother's uncle drove himself mad trying to solve the problem of perpetual motion. My father never exhibited any peculiarities of mind, or saw visions, until his last illness. He always had a presentiment that he should die when about 43 or 44 years of age. He was not superstitious, but always laughed at my visions as fancies.

"The first time I was alarmed by an apparition was, I think, in 1855, when I was on a visit to Ireland. One day I was preparing to attend a party, and had gone to my room early in the afternoon to lay out my clothes ready for the evening; also to sew some rosettes on my shoes, in which I was engaged just in front of the looking-glass, where, glancing up, I saw reflected a face with gray hair, looking over my shoulder. I was not afraid, but thought, 'How foolish I am!' worked on a little, and looked up again. It was still there. Trying to believe I had been deceived, I worked

---

[1] On one occasion he was seated by my side whilst I was occupied in writing a prescription. Appearing somewhat abstracted, I asked, " whether he then heard the voices speaking to him?" He replied, " Yes, quite distinctly." I said, " What are they saying?" He rejoined, " I would rather not repeat the words, as they are not very complimentary to yourself." After begging him to inform me what observations these unseen spirits hovering about us were making, he replied that they were ejaculating, " Don't leave your living; don't go abroad; remain in England; don't do what he recommends, don't take the medicine he prescribes." I had endeavored to impress upon this patient's mind the importance of his relieving himself for a time from all anxious and responsible clerical and parochial duty. I advised a continental tour, with a view of trying the effect of a thorough change of air and scene, having found, in cases similar to his, much benefit from this mode of treatment. Whatever I suggested for the re-establishment of this clergyman's health, these imaginary persons did their best, most uncourteously, to oppose!

on for a few seconds, and then looked again—and there it was! Thoroughly frightened, I ran from the room, not to re-enter it alone. Next day I wrote home to ask if anything was the matter. They answered me that all were well but my uncle, who had been very ill, *but was better then.* When a month later I returned, I learnt that he had died just about the time I had seen the face in the glass; but that they did not like to tell me, for fear of spoiling my pleasure. When I returned to England, the brother of the young lady whom I went to visit came to stay at our house for a time. He was a fine youth of twenty, with very large and peculiarly earnest hazel eyes, very curly hair, and altogether of very unmistakable appearance. He remained with us for about two months, when, having an appointment in India, he left us. Arrived there, he wrote home regularly, saying that he liked the place *so* much, that it agreed with him *so* well, and that he was never better in his life.

"One morning, either two or three days after what we call 'Guy Fawkes' day' (5th of November), I woke suddenly—with all my senses perfectly clear, which was the more strange as I had ever been most difficult to arouse. The moment I opened my eyes, I saw my friend, George B——, bending over me, his face within a few inches of mine, his eyes so fixed into mine that I could not withdraw my gaze. It was broad daylight, being about eight or after, and I saw he was in his usual dress, and, even to the curls of his hair, looking as distinct in form and color as a living figure. Much surprised, though not in the least frightened, but on the contrary, experiencing a most unearthly calmness (as I always do when I see these visions), I arose to a sitting posture. He also arose till he stood upright, and still looking earnestly at me, he receded a few steps, then disappeared. I did not feel alarmed, but got up and dressed at once, for fear that when I told my friends they should say it was all a dream. All that day, wherever I went, a ceaseless knocking followed me; and though our house was very large, I heard it in every part. If I went into my dressing-room, I heard it there on the toilet-table, and in the drawing and dining-rooms, though each on different stories. Going through the halls and passages it rapped along the walls. In fact, I heard it everywhere, except in the streets. My friends laughed at me, when I said I was sure I should hear some evil of George.

"A day or so after, I went from my own room to sleep in that of a young lady who was staying with us at the time. It was a large double-bedded room, and the night was bright and moonlight. The candle had been out some little time, and my friend was asleep, as I could hear by her heavy, regular breathing. Suddenly I saw a tall, white figure near the door at the foot of the bed. It walked right up on it, and came close to me. Thinking it was Miss B—— walking in her sleep, I sprang up, saying, ' Miss B——! oh, Miss B——! where are you going?' at the same time trying to clasp her. My arms went through the figure, and then I knew it was no mortal. Somewhat frightened now, I cowered down, and ere long fell asleep, more than ever convinced that my friend George was either dead or dying. Very soon afterwards we heard that he had died of fever on the 8th of November, the date of the first appearance.

" This happened in November, 1855, and the following May we came to Canada, and settled in G——. One evening, papa, mamma, sister, and myself were invited to the house of an acquaintance to spend a social evening, with cards, music, &c. Not feeling inclined to join the card-players, I sat down at the piano, feeling unaccountably sad. The door was just, or rather nearly opposite to me, being on the left of the piano. Of a sudden I looked up, and was astonished to see poor George B—— standing in the doorway, the lights shining full on him, and he looking earnestly at me. Thinking I had deceived myself, I played a little, and looked up. Yes, there he was, without doubt. I turned away, played on, then looked again; still he was there. Calling my sister, I asked her to go into the hall with me. We went. Not a soul—or rather nobody—had been near the place. I told mamma of the occurrence; and when we looked to see the day of the month, we found that it was the 8th of November.

" The next time that I saw anything of the kind, was just before we left G——, to come to T——. I had gone into the kitchen for something. The girl was in the garden, and I distinctly saw a woman standing in the doorway. A few evenings afterwards, we were all sitting around the supper-table, on which burned two large spirit-lamps, when I saw a woman, dressed in black, standing behind papa's chair. Leaning on it, the light fell full on her. She was a stranger to me, and bore no resemblance to any one I knew. I did not at the time, but do now think it was a warning of my papa's death. I told him, and, as usual, he laughed at me.

I saw nothing more till just before my papa's and sister's illness. My health was delicate at the time, owing perhaps to change of climate. We were at this time in T——, and residing in Ann Street. One evening, feeling tired, I left the rest of the family at supper, and came to bed by myself. In passing my dressing-room, on my way to my bed-room, I saw a head looking out on me from behind the door. I called out to them to come quickly up, as I was lonely or ill, or some such excuse, I forget what, but I did not say a word of what I had seen, not liking to make the rest nervous. A few days after this, I was in my dressing-room. It was in the afternoon, about two o'clock, perhaps. I stood in front of the looking-glass arranging my hair, when I saw reflected a bright, fresh, rosy-looking face, just such a face as my poor sister's. I turned round, and heard at the same time, and for a quarter of a minute and more after, a sound resembling the dropping of a number of pieces of tin or silver coins all over the floor of the room. Greatly surprised, I told papa at once; also what I had seen a few nights previously.

"Not long after this, and on the very night-week before that on which papa was taken ill, we were all invited to spend the evening at the house of a friend. Mamma was too ill to go; and partly because I was fatigued, and partly to keep her company, I determined, though nearly dressed, to stay at home. So papa and my sisters went. I took a book, and sat down at the table to read, as mamma soon fell asleep. Our girl went to bed about nine, and I was the only one in the house awake. I was so deeply interested in my book that I did not notice how time passed. Presently I heard some one with, judging from the sound, very long nails beating on the table. Looking up, I saw seated opposite me, so close that by stretching out my hand I could have touched him, a man in ordinary black clothes. He was on the chair at the foot of mamma's couch. Directly I looked up the nails ceased tapping the table. As I looked at him he vanished. I saw him for about four seconds, I should think. You may fancy I was neither nervous nor excited, when I tell you I did not disturb mamma, but sat there for three or four hours longer, till papa came in. I own I was shocked, but not nervous or excited. Papa was surprised and grieved to see me looking so ill when he came, and attributed it to being up too late. Not wishing to frighten mamma, I said nothing about the vision till next day; when papa, anxious to dispel my fears, said: ' Why, you silly child, what nonsense! Here am I, strong and well, and yet a night or two since, when I went to bed, I saw opposite me a bed, myself lying dead on it; and every time I opened my eyes, I saw the same.' Within a week from this he was taken ill, and died in a few weeks. During the last week of his illness scarcely a night passed but I saw some apparition. The first time I was disturbed was just about a week before his death. I was lying awake, not at all nervous, for I had not the least idea that I should lose my papa. My face was turned to the wall, when I felt the pressure as of a heavy hand on the pillow behind me. Ice-cold fingers touched me, and a cold hand encircled my neck. Such horror seized me that I must have become insensible, for sense and recollection left me. Next morning I mentioned this to mamma. All that week, to the time of papa's death, I saw women in white, and sometimes in black, at my bedside. What was very strange, too, all the night that poor papa was dying, I saw two women in the room besides mamma and the nurse. When I entered, or looked up from papa, who required our unceasing care, I saw a strange woman in black standing behind nurse, and another at the door. After his death I saw no more of them, at least not till my sister was seriously ill. She, at the time of papa's death, was poorly with influenza; nothing serious. She had taken a powder to induce perspiration the previous night; but hearing about seven next morning, from our cries, that papa was going, she rushed from her bed without throwing anything round her, and kissed him just as he breathed his last sigh. Then she refused to go to bed again, threw herself down on the rug in the parlor, with her head to the fire, where she persisted in lying, and kept calling for brandy-and-water, which was foolishly brought her by the servant and nurse, we being too distracted to notice anything. The consequence was she became feverish, and was obliged to take to her bed. In the meantime I bore up as well as I could, feeling that as eldest child I should not give way, but endeavor to comfort the others and poor mamma; so till night I never shed a tear, but went in with every one who called, to where papa lay. But in the evening I could not restrain myself any longer, and had hysterics. On one of these occasions a gentleman friend carried me fainting into the street for air. It was very quiet, when suddenly we both heard a loud voice, coming from we could not tell where, and saying, in distressed and agonized tones, ' Fanny, Fanny, Fanny!' as much as to say, ' Oh, do not, I entreat you, distress yourself so !' In a moment I was calm and strong. We neither of us said a word about the voice, but entered the house at once. Next day he asked me if I had heard it. I told him I had ; and seeing that the thought greatly agitated me, he added, ' Oh, I dare say it was some one calling Harry !' but I knew better, for nothing could be more distinct than the voice and words. A day or two afterwards I went to my sister's room to sit with her, as she was lonely. It was about seven in the evening. As I ascended the stairs with a lamp in my hand, I saw two women robed in black at the top, one each side of the stairway. I was suffering too deeply to feel fear, so went on. The figures disappeared as I neared them. As I entered the room where my sister lay, I saw papa behind the door, looking very pale. I looked several times to make sure I had not been deceived, and each time saw him there. I sat down on the bed, with my back towards the figure, until I could bear it no longer, when I called some one else to take my place, for I knew no one else in the house could see the spectre. I think it was the next day the doctors said we must all leave the house at once, or we, too, should have the fever ; so we went to the house of a friend.

"One evening, a few days after my arrival, a loud ring at the door-bell woke me. I started up, and saw, as I imagined, one of the ladies of the house by my side. I spoke to the figure, and it vanished ; and at the same time I heard my friends saying something about ' poor Sophia,' my sister's name. Greatly alarmed, I called to them to bring a light, as I was sure I had seen some one in my room. I then asked who it was that rang at that early hour (about four or five o'clock). They told me it was one sent out to say that there was a change in my sister. I thought they meant a favorable change, so fell asleep, feeling happier and more hopeful than I had felt since papa's death. The same day my friends broke the tidings of my sister's death to me as gently as possible. It had taken place about three o'clock in the morning, and mamma had at once sent to acquaint us with the melancholy intelligence.

"From that time till last May I saw nothing. Last Queen's birthday I had been out, walking about with a gentleman friend. Towards evening we came in, and I went to my room to change my walking-dress. I had nearly finished dressing, and had only to get on my slippers, when, turning round, I saw papa standing near the door. So distinct was it that I felt frightened, and, snatching up the lamp, I rushed from the room. When I reached the parlor, where they were all sitting, I felt reassured and somewhat ashamed; and as in my hurry I had forgotten my slippers, I determined to return for them. So, taking the lamp, I opened the folding-doors between the front and back parlors, and ran up against the figure. I met no resisting power; had I done so, I should have hurt myself severely, no doubt. I was greatly agitated when I saw it, and rushed back to mamma, who inquired what was the matter with me, I looked so ill. I told her what I had seen.

"One night, some months after this, a gentleman friend called. He had not been long present before I had occasion to go up-stairs for something. I did not take a lamp, not being afraid, but went in the dark. Coming down, just as I reached the bottom of the stairs, I saw papa standing within a foot or two of me. A soft phosphoric radiance seemed to surround him. He was very pale, as I saw distinctly by the strange light, though all was dark around me. I was very much frightened, as I should have to pass close to him to re-enter the parlor. My brain seemed to reel as I ran desperately past and gained the room where they were all sitting. When I told them how I had been alarmed, some one went into the passage, but saw nothing.

"The last, and by far the most horrible vision I ever had, was on the 8th of December last (1858). I woke up one morning before dawn, but, as mamma burns a lamp every night, it was quite light in our room. I had been awake about ten minutes or a quarter of an hour, and could not go to sleep, do what I would. However, as my mind was very pleasantly occupied, I did not mind much. Of a sudden I heard a heavy stamp, as if some one were trying to attract my attention by stamping with the foot. I raised my head, and to my horror saw an old person, who might have been a man or a woman; for the figure had on a white dressing-gown, and a kind of black skull or Glengariff cap. I could not see any hair, or should have been better able to judge of the sex. The face was that of a corpse, pinched and drawn by long illness and old age. The profile was turned towards me, and was delicate and regular, and clearly defined against the wall at the side of it. One hand was across the chest or waist, and the other

hanging straight down. I rose on my elbow the better to make
my observations.   There were no clothes hanging in that part of
the room, so that I could not have been deceived by anything of
that kind.   It stood by mamma's side, and as I gazed took three
steps, each accompanied by a heavy stamp, and stopping at every
step.   I was perfectly calm while taking in all these particulars,
but after the third step I was overcome by terror, as the figure
was coming round my side; and clasping my little sister, as if
even her tiny form would yield me protection, I prayed that the
Almighty would remove the vision, and cause mamma to wake.   I
only heard one step after that. After a few minutes I determined
to tie a knot in my handkerchief, under the pillow, as I knew
mamma would say in the morning it was all a dream.   Just as I
was about to do this she woke. I spoke to her, and taking courage
looked at my watch, and found that it was about twenty minutes
to six.   I did not mention what I had seen till next day, or rather
until it was light.   I feel convinced that it was a forewarning of
either my grandfather's or grandmother's death, as they have both
been failing rapidly of late.

"I forgot to mention one case that happened before the last,
and which should have had the precedence.   One morning in
March, 1858, I was giving a lesson at Miss M——'s school here,
and, looking up, I saw a thin man in blue cloth coat, with turn-
down velvet collar, standing by the side of my pupil.   His figure
was just like poor Mr. G——, the violinist.   His face I could not
see, as my pupil's head came between us.   I was startled, and
screamed, thinking it was one of the masters at the first glance.
I just had time to notice it when it vanished. I told mamma when
I got home.   Next day we heard that poor G—— had died at just
about the time I saw his figure.   I had not even heard that he
was ill, and knew nothing of it till I was told he was dead.

"Another case, I forgot to mention, occurred, I think, some
time in last November. I was aroused from my sleep by a loud
knocking at my bed-head.   After I woke I listened, and in a few
minutes heard it again.   I said to mamma, 'Do you hear that?'
'Hear what, child?' 'Why, that loud knocking.'   She said,
'Why, I have been awake for more than a quarter of an hour,
and there has not been a sound that I could hear.'   Afterwards, I
heard it again at the window.   It was daylight, and I could see if
there had been any one there; but I saw nothing.   I told mamma

I was sure we should hear of the death of some one we knew; and sure enough, a few weeks after we heard that my aunt's father had been found dead in his room, just about the time I heard the knocking. I was a favorite of his when he was living.

"I cannot remember anything more now; I think I have mentioned every apparition that I have ever seen."[1]

Accompanying the other symptoms characteristic of the stage of consciousness are the following: The mind is harassed and bewildered by odd notions, unusual feelings, unnatural trains of thought, strange inclinations, intense irritability, unequal powers of attention, confused, irregular, painful, disturbed, and sometimes ludicrous association of ideas. As these unhealthy feelings are *forcing* an entrance, and trying to obtain a *settlement* in the mind, the patient is vexed, and irritated with himself for permitting them to intrude upon the sanctity of his thoughts. An heroic effort is often made to dissipate and dislodge these morbid scintillations of insanity, or, when this cannot be accomplished, to studiously, artfully, and ingeniously conceal their existence from others.

A morbid aversion of a parent to his children entwining itself into the secret recesses of thought;—a growing, unreasonable, and unaccountable dislike to the companionship of old friends (often to those formerly dearly and tenderly loved), creeping insidiously and stealthily into the mind;—strange, inexplicable misgivings;—motiveless, unaccountable, and unreasonable suspicions as to the affection of a loved son, a favorite and tenderly attached daughter;—apprehensions as to the chastity of the wife;—doubts as to the constancy and fidelity of the husband, flit sometimes, like a thick mist, dark shadow, and a troubled dream, across the morbidly disturbed and anxious mind, years before insanity is imagined to have commenced its ravages.[2] These symptoms (long

---

[1] "American Journal of Insanity." Oct. 1859.

[2] There are no delusions so sad and fatal in their consequences as those relating to the fidelity of the wife. Many valuable lives have been sacrificed to this frightfully dangerous hallucination. A man was confined in an asylum while suffering from this delusion. For many months this idea was uppermost in his mind, and appeared to absorb all his thoughts. At the expiration of eight or nine months he appeared to be much improved in bodily and mental health, and the delusion had apparently less hold of his imagination. Eventually, he cunningly declared that his mind was quite at ease respecting his wife, and that he no longer believed that she had or *could* have been unfaithful to him. Under a mistaken impression that he had recovered, the patient was discharged from the asylum, and permitted to return home. In about a

before they are recognized to be morbid) cause much acute and bitter anguish, masked and concealed suffering, great and unobserved misery in the bosom of families, often sapping the foundation of domestic happiness. A contest of this character in an *unhealthy*, but not yet *insane* mind, has continued for a long period unknown, except to the wretched sufferer, before the intellect has entirely succumbed to its baneful and destructive influence. In this state of disordered health, the patient endeavors, whilst pursuing regularly his ordinary occupations, frequenting places of amusement, and mixing daily with his family and friends, to *appear* to those about him in good mental health, and to act like a rational man. In many cases he is able, for a period, effectually to simulate perfect sanity of mind, and to effectually mask from others his disordered condition of intellect.

When influenced by physical stimulants, a person in the incipient stage of intoxication will make a determined effort to comport himself like a sober man, being fully conscious of the lamentably degrading and brutalized condition to which he is reduced. Under these circumstances, he endeavors to conceal from observation his actual state, will make a great effort to control his ideas, talk rationally, and walk steadily, and, although much under the potent influence of intoxicating drink, he is able, by a resolute and determined effort of the will, for a time to play well his part, and thus disarm all suspicion as to his actual condition of inebriation.

Such is often the state of a person in the incipient stage of insanity, battling courageously, and it may be successfully, with eccentric, unnatural, odd, singular, impure, and unhealthy mental impressions, clearly the first beginnings and early manifestations of derangement of mind.

A clergyman of the Church of England, who had led a life of

---

week or ten days afterwards, he murdered his wife and child, believing that the former had committed adultery, and that the child was not his own! For several days after joining his family he appeared quite well, so cleverly and effectually did he mask his lunacy from those immediately about him.

A baker suspected the fidelity of his wife. He was clearly deranged on the point. He eventually, whilst under the influence of this delusion, emasculated himself, and when spoken to on the subject, insanely argued that as his wife was with child, the fact of his mutilation would clearly establish to the world the truth of his accusation as to her unfaithfulness, as no one would, for a moment, *then* believe that he could be the father of the child with which she was pregnant!

14

Christian purity and active benevolence, became (as a consequence of over-study) the subject of this type of mental disorder.   He was in the habit frequently of knocking his head violently against the mantelpiece, until the skin was covered with contusions, in the fruitless struggle to dissipate the physically impure images and blasphemous thoughts that originated involuntarily in his mind. This patient entirely recovered his reason after the lapse of nine months.[1]

In some women the insanity (particularly if it be of the puerperal type) is characterized by a singularly distressing perversion of thought, connected with a morbidly exalted state of the reproductive instincts.   The conversation is, in these cases, occasionally tinctured with expressions, from the contemplation of which the unhappy sufferer would, like a sensitive plant, have recoiled when in health.   The gentlest of the sex, the purest and most delicate of feminine minds, pious, refined, and cultivated of moral natures, are often, alas ! the first to exhibit, when suffering from particular

[1] With what consummate knowledge of the human mind has Dr. Johnson portrayed the incipient stage of insanity, when the intellect, still to a certain degree conscious of the dawnings of morbid thought, endeavors to struggle, and for a time does so successfully, against the suggestions of a disordered and rampant imagination. I refer to his account in " Rasselas" of the astronomer's recognition of, and conflict with, delusive impressions, as well as his description of their eventual and melancholy triumph over his reason. Addressing himself to Imlac, the astronomer says : " I have possessed for five years the regulation of the weather and the distribution of the seasons; the sun has listened to my dictates, and passed from tropic to tropic by my direction; the clouds, at my call, have poured their waters, and the Nile has overflowed at my command; I have restrained the rage of the Dog-star, and mitigated the fervors of the Crab. The winds alone, of all the elemental powers, have hitherto refused my authority, and multitudes have perished by equinoctial tempests, which I found myself unable to prohibit or restrain."

" Might not some other cause," said Imlac, " produce this concurrence ? The Nile does not always rise on the same day."

" Do not believe," said he, with impatience, " that such objections could escape me. *I reasoned long against my own conviction, and labored against truth with the utmost obstinacy. I sometimes suspected myself of madness,* and should not have dared to impart this secret but to a man like you, capable of distinguishing the wonderful from the impossible, and the incredible from the false."

" Why, sir," said I, " do you call that incredible which you know, or think you know, to be true ?"

" Because," said he, " I cannot prove it by any external evidence, and I know too well the laws of demonstration to think that my conviction ought to influence another, who cannot, like me, be conscious of its force. I therefore shall not attempt to gain credit by disputation. It is sufficient that I feel this power, that I have long possessed, and every day exerted it."

types of mental derangement, this painful moral and psychical degeneration. Such melancholy manifestations of poor human nature, fallen, crushed, perverted, and often destroyed by disease, suggest to the man of the world, medico-psychologist, theologian, and moralist, sources of deep and profound thought, and subjects for grave philosophical meditation. It is, however, consolatory to reflect, that the mind may pass through this terrible and mysterious phase of alienation intact, emerging from the fiery furnace without the slightest remnant of moral taint, injury, or contamination! How true it is that,

> " Thoughts impure
> May pass through minds of angels and of man
> And leave no stain."

When analyzing these sad states of morbid idea, distressing forms of disordered emotion, and painful types of excited passion, we are obliged, alas! to confess, that there is very little in connection with them to elevate, expand, and purify the taste, or to charm, captivate, and enchain the poet's fancy. In this malady, the emotions, sensations, and appetites are unhappily in a melancholy state of degradation, perversion, and alienation; and, as a general rule, the conversation and conduct of those so afflicted reflect and are in unison with this derangement of the intellect, and disordered state of the instincts. The reason is dethroned and taken forcibly captive by the animal impulses; and these, when in a state of supremacy, exercise an undisputed and tyrannical sovereignty over the judgment, conscience, and the will. Hence, the sad and distressing *tone* of thought (as indicated in the conversation), previously referred to as occasionally observed in attacks of mental derangement, caused by, or complicated with, ovarian irritation, uterine irregularities, and disorders, among very young women, possessing naturally the most refined, innocent, and sensitively organized minds.

Shakspeare, in one of the most touchingly affecting creations of his transcendent genius, threw a poetic charm, a brilliant flood of fancy, around the character of Ophelia,

> " Sweet as spring-time flowers,"

so redolent of feminine gentleness, purity, and grace; but ever true to nature, this great magician, and all but inspired poet, could not sacrifice truth to fiction, fancy to fact, and he therefore makes this love-sick girl, during her insane warblings, give utterance to conceptions that never could have suggested themselves to her exquisitely chaste and delicate mind, before it was prostrated and perverted by disease.[1]

When addressing herself, almost unconsciously, to the king, in reply to his question, "How do you do, pretty lady?" Ophelia, after plaintively exclaiming, "Lord, we know what we are, but know not what we may be," utters the following rhapsody:—

> "To-morrow is Saint Valentine's day,
> All in the morning betime,
> And I a maid at your window,
> To be your Valentine:
> Then up he rose and don'd his clothes,
> And dupt the chamber door,
> Let in the maid, that out a maid
> Never departed more."

"I have been most careful in the education of my child," said a gentleman, in deep distress, to me one day, whilst listening to the incoherent ravings of his poor daughter (scarcely nineteen

---

[1] A young woman was seduced in early life and carried off to London. The man with whom she eloped, finding that she had no children, cruelly abandoned her. She became dreadfully depressed in spirits, and ultimately losing her reason, was confined in an asylum. The narrator of the following particulars says, that when he first saw this poor girl she was apparently about eighteen years of age. She had a pretty bouquet of flowers in her hand, and whilst arranging them, like poor Ophelia, she sung very sweetly, snatches of various favorite melodies. On being asked why she left her late habitation, she answered, "Because I was obliged to do so." She was asked, how she employed her time last night? "I walked all about Dover." "What! did you not go to bed?" "No! no! I could not close my eyes. Give me a strong stick and a nice lantern, and I will be your watchman. Oh, I shall make a very good watchman. You must let me sleep in the day, you know." She had some slips of paper in her hand, and these she called "fairings:" she distributed them among the poultry in the yard, whom she emphatically styled her children. She then commenced singing, "The ocean wide," &c., and then burst out instantaneously into "Push about the joram." Finding at length her little heedless charge of fowls basking in the morning sun, she tenderly exclaimed, but in a wild accent, "My pretty children are all gone to sleep; they have no hard-hearted lovers; but I can't sleep. Macbeth has murdered sleep. Ah! he was a naughty man; was he not?" A young man approached her, when somebody observed, "Look, here's your lover come!" "Oh, now! do not give me too many lovers; they will break my heart! My fate, you know, is very hard, is it not?"

years of age!) "She has," he continued, "seldom been out of the house, and has only been allowed to associate with our own limited and select circle of friends and relations, all of whom are morally, if not religiously, disposed. I never knew a more pure, delicate, and unsophisticated mind, than she possessed previously to her illness; and now, when deranged, she manifests an accurate acquaintance, not only with the most corrupt ideas, but with the improper *phrases* ordinarily used by the most depraved street-walkers!"

These sad manifestations of perverted and disordered instinct are susceptible of the subjoined explanations: In the first place, we are bound to consider the orthodox scriptural doctrine of the *innate* corruption and *natural* depravity of the human heart. The prophet Jeremiah says, that " *the heart is deceitful above all things, and desperately wicked: who can know it ?*"[1] Again, our Saviour himself declares, " *that out of the heart proceed evil thoughts, murders, adulteries, fornications, thefts, false witness, blasphemies.*"[2]

As long as reason reigns supreme, and is unclouded by disease, and whilst the will retains its normal and healthy sovereignty over the higher faculties of the mind, and its control of the instincts, the natural tendency that exists towards evil thoughts and vicious actions is kept, by man's own efforts, aided, if not happily by Divine grace, by exalted moral considerations, in a state of subjugation; but contemporaneously with a paralysis of the co-ordinating principle (the *executive* element of mind), and a perversion of the reasoning faculty, caused by some type of physical, it may be, *cerebral* disease, does the effect of early training, educational discipline, carefully cultivated habits of thought, strictly considered social companionship, and zealously directed moral and religious influences, cease, alas! (in many cases) to restrain the passions, and curb the animal instincts and appetites. Hence, the painful character of the *expressions* almost unconsciously used by some young women when insane.[3]

I am now only addressing myself to the results of *diseased* brain, and *disordered* mind. There are, of course, often witnessed many

---

[1] Jeremiah, chap. xvii, v. 9.   [2] St. Matthew, chap. xv, v. 9.

[3] "Why need we talk of a fiery hell? If the will, which is the law of our nature, were withdrawn from our memory, fancy, understanding, and reason, no other hell could equal, for a spiritual being, what we should then feel, from the anarchy of our powers."—*Coleridge's "Table Talk."*

sad exhibitions of depraved thought, and vitiated taste, the effect
of a voluntary and sinful abandonment of the reason and passions
to gross habits of sensuality, vice, and even crime.   These melancholy manifestations of perverted intellect have no *necessary*
relation to the conditions of *diseased* mind, of which I am now
particularly speaking.

There are, however, other sources of moral contamination and
mental deterioration in operation, which the most vigilant parents
are not always able to detect or guard their children from.   I refer
to the pernicious example, and wicked suggestions of depraved,
irreligious, and profligate servants (a frightful cause of moral
pollution, as well as of mental idiocy in early life), occasionally,
unhappily, admitted into the bosom of families by false characters
(alas! too easily procured), to a perusal of vicious books, surrep-
titiously smuggled into the nursery, as well as of the details of
gross acts of impropriety and indecency, made matters of judicial
investigation, so minutely and faithfully reported in some of the
ordinary channels of communication.   These frightful records of
vice and crime, so palpably exposed, elaborately and artistically
developed, in all their naked depravity and deformity, are fearfully
and fatally suggestive to the minds of the young.

Apart altogether, however, from this view of the question, we
are bound to consider the effect of a morbid exaltation (as the effect
of diseased *brain*, as well as of other organs) of natural instincts,
inciting prematurely into activity feelings and inclinations normally
(until a certain period of life) in a torpid, and latent state.   We
may hence account, pathologically, for the development of natural
physical tendencies, usually manifested at, and after the age of
puberty, but it does not explain the actual knowledge and use of
particular prurient phrases and obscene modes of expression.   This
phenomenon can only proceed, either from the parties having
heard the identical words used by persons with whom they have
unfortunately associated, or from having seen them in print, or
heard them uttered in the public streets.

Let me not be misunderstood.   In many cases of sad mental
alienation, the unhappy patient, although a prey of distressing
delusions, often exhibits great elevation of sentiment, exquisite
taste, profound elevation, and purity of thought.   The insane are
frequently heard giving utterance to expressions that would reflect
the highest honor upon healthy and cultivated understandings.

The light of reason is occasionally seen permeating with undiminished lustre, the dark cloud that has threatened, for a time, altogether to overshadow, if not to eclipse, its effulgence. Natural sweetness, unaffected gentleness, and marked amiability of disposition, are often witnessed triumphing over fearful types of mental disease, struggling to crush the lofty inspirations of the mind, obliterate kindly sympathies, and to pervert and paralyze the noble aspirations of the heart.

The unselfish consideration which the insane so frequently manifest towards persons temporarily deprived, like themselves, of unrestrained freedom of action;—the affectionate and assiduous attention they pay to their companions in affliction and sorrow;—their endeavors to assuage their bitter anguish, by repeated assurances that their removal from home, although apparently an act of unnecessary harshness, and unkindness, on the part of their relatives) could not, under the circumstances of their illness, be avoided, and would ultimately tend to their advantage, conclusively establish, that insanity often leaves intact some of the best principles that ennoble and dignify human nature. I have known men and women decidedly insane, although not conscious of the fact, thus administer comfort and consolation to the wounded spirits of those recently admitted as patients within an institution in which they themselves were most unwillingly confined. I have heard the insane, with a view of soothing and mitigating the sorrows of those about them, freely admit that they had, like others, been mentally afflicted, but had recovered, or were convalescent from the symptoms of the malady, and although, at the commencement of their illness, they were firmly persuaded that they were perfectly sane, and ought never to have been removed from home to an asylum, they were *now* fully satisfied of having been deranged, and felt grateful to their friends for recognizing the fact, and placing them under moral control and medical treatment. I have had the pleasure of hearing the insane pray by the bedside of other patients when afflicted with severe and dangerous bodily illness, and do so, too, with pious fervor, and great propriety of language, never once making the slightest allusion to their own unhappy and disordered thoughts.[1]

[1] I had a patient under my care who suffered from great dejection of mind, associated with a delusion, that he had committed the unpardonable sin, and was, in consequence, forsaken of God. This gentleman had always been remarkable, previously

The state of unhealthy feeling, previously described as often symptomatic of incipient insanity, is occasionally observed in certain anomalous conditions of the nervous system allied to hysteria, and may exist apart altogether from any actual disorder, or even a tendency to derangement of mind. These distressing nervous symptoms sometimes are seen in young girls, when passing at the age of puberty into womanhood, and occur to females of a mature age at the critical period of life. This morbid exaltation of the nervous and mental functions, is generally found associated with visceral complications, easily curable, however, in many cases, by remedial measures. In some patients these symptoms are the effect of long-continued and neglected stomach and hepatic derangement. In other instances the uterine system is the seat of the mischief; and in some types of the malady which have come under my observation, the condition of mind could be traced to irritation and congestion established in the brain itself. In one remarkable case the patient was tortured by an intense fear of losing his

to his illness, for his orthodox views, and strict attention to religious duties. Before I was consulted, he had made an ineffectual attempt at suicide. This patient took an affectionate interest in another invalid confined like himself in the institution. They were generally engaged several hours during the day in close companionship and conversation. In fact, they were almost inseparable. This gentleman was seized with an attack of dangerous bodily illness, threatening life. His friend took a deep and kind interest in his case, and was rarely absent from the sick chamber. On one occasion I asked him to offer up a prayer at the bedside of his friend. The request appeared somewhat to stagger him. He was evidently most anxious to comply with my wishes, but was afraid of committing himself. After a little hesitation he fell upon his knees, and prayed with great force of expression, and with touching tenderness. There was not the slightest indication in the prayer (which was extemporary), of his own morbid religious hallucinations. He told me some time after his recovery, when referring to this circumstance, that he experienced considerable difficulty in avoiding (whilst praying on this occasion), alluding to his own unhappy state of mind. The case of Simon Brown, as recorded in "The Gentleman's Magazine" for 1762, illustrates the point referred to.

Simon Brown was a dissenting minister of great intellectual powers. He became insane. His delusion was that he had fallen under the sensible displeasure of God, who had caused his rational soul gradually to perish, and left him only, in common with brutes, an animal life; that it was therefore profane in him to pray, and incongruous to be present at the prayers of others. In this opinion he was inflexible. Being once importuned to say grace at the table of a friend, he repeatedly excused himself, but the request being still repeated, and the company kept standing, he discovered evident tokens of distress, and after some irresolute gestures and hesitation, expressed with great fervor this ejaculation: "*Most merciful and Almighty God! let thy spirit which moved upon the face of the waters when there was no light, descend upon me, that from this darkness there may rise up a man to praise thee !*"

senses, combined with confusion of ideas, strange dislikes to his
relatives, and a disposition to conceal himself from his family.
He had for some time suffered from headache and a general feeling
of *malaise*. This gentleman soon recovered after a few ounces of
blood were taken from his head, and two or three active calomel
purges administered. In less than three weeks from the time he
placed himself under treatment, he was able to resume his ordinary
occupations. In the case of a lady, presenting the same symptoms, great congestion was discovered in the neighborhood of the
cervix uteri. This morbid state of the vessels was removed by the
local application of leeches. The blood so abstracted, conjoined
with other treatment, entirely relieved the mind of all fear and
apprehension of insanity. In another case the mental disturbance
could be clearly traced to engorgement of the liver, consequent
upon a long residence in a tropical climate. Calomel, taraxacum,
nitro-muriatic acid, internally, combined with a persevering use of
the "nitro-muriatic bath," as recommended and described by Mr.
Ranald Martin, in his able treatise,[1] very speedily dissipated all
mental despondency, and morbid anxiety as to the existence or
approach of mental derangement.

Closely allied to the state of conscious insanity of which I have
been speaking, or, to use the language of Coleridge, "*the mind's
own anticipation of madness*," is, what may be designated a morbid
presentiment of threatening and approaching alienation of mind.
This condition of disordered thought is occasionally recognized in
cerebral, as well as in *mental* diseases. The patient has, in a few
instances that have come under my observation, exhibited in the
early stage of brain disease, a mysterious prophetic power, a
singular presentiment or warning of his cerebral and insane attacks. In one case, the patient assured his friends, for some weeks
prior to an apoplectic seizure, that he should soon be the subject
of the malady, and that it would be fatal! Alas! he proved to
be a true prophet! In another case, a patient said that he had
received a warning of the advent of insanity, and was positive
that he should be attacked. I knew *three* instances of patients
who for several *years*, predicted the accession of mental derangement, and who ultimately became insane!

"We cannot," says Portal, "hear without astonishment, the

---

[1] "Diseases of Tropical Climates," by J. Ranald Martin, F.R.S., 1859.

remarks sometimes made by those who are threatened with attacks
of apoplexy.   All their senses appear perfect and entire, but their
minds appear to have acquired an inspired and prophetic power.
Their first impression is, that they are about to quit the world.
Then they predict the future by the present; and the event justifying the prediction, they are regarded as true prophets.   I saw
a patient who foretold his death six days previously to its actual
occurrence, there being at the time no symptom in connection with
the case that at all justified so unfavorable a prognosis.''

Sir Walter 'Scott had sad forebodings as to the final close of
his active, eventful, and anxious life!. He appears to have had a
melancholy presentiment of the attack of brain disease of which
he died.

His son-in-law and biographer, Mr. Lockhart, says, when referring to the final scene of the great magician's life, " A more difficult and delicate task never devolved upon any man's friend, than
he had about this time to encounter.   He could not watch Scott
from hour to hour—above all, he could not write to his dictation
—without gradually, slowly, most reluctantly, taking home to his
bosom the conviction that the mighty mind, which he had worshipped through more than thirty years of intimacy, had lost
something, and was daily losing something more of its energy.
The faculties were. there, and each of them was every now and
then displaying itself in its full vigor; but the sagacious judgment, the brilliant fancy, the unrivalled memory, were all subject
to occasional eclipse.

> ' Along the chords the finger strayed,
> And an uncertain warbling made.'

Ever and anon he paused and looked round him, like one half-
waking from a dream, mocked with shadows.   The sad bewilder-
ment of his gaze showed a momentary consciousness that, like
Samson in the lap of the Philistine, 'his strength was passing
from him, and he was becoming weak like unto other men.'   Then
came the strong effort of aroused will—the clouds dispersed as if
before an irresistible current of purer air—all was bright and
serene as of old, and then it closed again in yet deeper darkness.
Under these circumstances, it was no wonder that his medical advisers assured him repeatedly and emphatically that, if he persisted
in working his brain, nothing could prevent his malady from recur-

ring with redoubled severity. His answer was, ' As for bidding
me not work, Molly might as well put the kettle on the fire, and
say, *Now, don't boil.*   .   .   .   I foresee distinctly, that if I were
to be idle, I should go mad !' The fate of Swift and Marlborough
was also before his eyes ; and in his journal there is an entry
expressive of his fear lest the anticipated blow should not destroy
life, and that he might linger on, a driveller and a show. ' I do
not think my head is weakened—(this was a subsequent entry)—
yet a strange vacillation makes me suspect. *Is it not thus that
men begin to fail—becoming, as it were, infirm of purpose ?*

> ' That way madness lies—let me shun that.
> No more of that.' "

And when at the Court-house of Jedburgh he faced the rabble
populace, and braved their hootings, the same idea of impending
calamity was still present to his mind, as he greeted them on
turning away, in the words of the doomed gladiator, " *Moriturus
vos saluto !*" " As the plough neared the end of the furrow," to
use Scott's own expressive phrase, he was still urged on by his
fixed habits of labor. " Under the full consciousness that he had
sustained three or four strokes of apoplexy or palsy, or both combined, and tortured by various attendant ailments, cramp, rheumatism in half his joints, daily increasing lameness, and now of
late gravel (which was, though last, not least), he retained all the
energy of his will, and struggled manfully against this sea of
troubles."

Dean Swift had a singular presentiment of his imbecility. Dr.
Young, walking one day with Dean Swift some short distance
from Dublin, suddenly missed the Dean, who had lagged behind.
He found him at a distance, gazing in a solemn state of abstraction at the top of a lofty elm, whose head had been blasted by a
hurricane. He directed Dr. Young's attention to the summit of
the tree, and heaving a heavy sigh, exclaimed, " I shall be like
that tree, I shall die at the TOP first."

It is not difficult to account physiologically as well as pathologically for the singular phenomena previously referred to. I
had under my care a lady who informed me, that for *six* years
previously to her becoming insane, she was perfectly convinced,
from her mental and bodily sensations, that the seeds of the

malady had taken root, and that insanity had, even at that time, commenced to germinate.

Another patient said, that in early life, when at college, he was convinced that the mind had received, as he termed it, a " *twist*," in consequence of his having passed many sleepless nights, caused by several weeks of continuous, and unremitting laborious mental work. So conscious was he, at the time, of the mischief that had been done to his brain, that he exclaimed, whilst 'anxiously pacing the room, " I shall die a lunatic !" He subsequently repeated the same expression to a college friend. At the age of forty-eight he became insane, and tried on several occasions to commit suicide. I have known several patients who have had, for a long period prior to the manifestation of insanity, these singular warnings of approaching brain and mental disorder.

If damage is done to the delicate cerebral structure in early life by moral or physical causes, and the material lesion, whatever be its nature, is (as is usually the case) of slow and progressive growth, we can easily understand the existence of abnormal *physical* sensations within the head, as well as of morbid *mental* impressions (engendered by changes in the nervous tissue of the brain), which would, in many cases, necessarily give rise to the anticipation of insanity, or to the dread of some type of disease of the brain developing itself at an after period of life.

CHAPTER VIII.

STAGE OF EXALTATION.

THIS stage will be considered in its twofold relation, viz. :—

1. *Psychical Exaltation.*
2. *Somatic Exaltation.*

1. PSYCHICAL EXALTATION.—For some period before the more active symptoms of cerebral and mental exaltation are manifested, the patient is observed to be wayward, capricious, passionate, and impulsive. He is irritable and fractious, peevish and pettish, exhibiting, what would (under less suspicious states of mind, and more favorable conditions of bodily health) be termed, an "unhappy infirmity of temper." These symptoms of psychical exaltation are occasionally associated with alternate fits of vital depression and mental confusion. The patient is subsequently morbidly anxious about trifles, slight ruffles on the surface, and trivial annoyances, occurring in the family circle or during the course of business, worry, flurry, tease, and fret him, nothing satisfying or soothing his mind, and everything, to his distempered fancy, going wrong within the sacred precincts of domestic life. He is quick at fancying affronts, and greatly exaggerates the slightest and most trifling acts of supposed inattention. The least irregularity on the part of the domestics excites, angers, and vexes him. He is suspicious of, and quarrels with his nearest relatives, and mistrusts his best, kindest, and most faithful friends, often harboring the most absurd and unfounded misgivings in regard to the purity and fidelity of his wife, attachment and affection of his children.

When in this premonitory stage of mental derangement, bordering closely on an attack of acute insanity, he twists, distorts, misconceives, misconstrues, and perverts in a most singular man-

ner every look, gesture, action, and word of those closely associated
and nearly related to him. The expressions of love, affection,
kindness, endearing sympathy, and friendship which greet him,
without reservation, on all sides, are viewed as evidences of enmity
and ill-will, or as well-contrived, cunningly devised, carefully and
adroitly arranged masks, to hide some latent design and artfully
veiled conspiracy against his life, liberty, and property!

All objects within the range of his perverted senses are tinctured and distorted by a disordered vision, jaundiced eye, and
morbidly exalted and excited fancy. In this incipient phase of
mental derangement, he shakes with fear at the reflection of his
image—crouches with apprehension at the reverberating sound of
his own footsteps—trembles at the melancholy sighing of the wind
through a neighboring copse—turns pale at the echo of his voice—
falls back aghast with horror at the recognition of his shadow,
mistaking it for a frightful phantom, or grim spectral image,

> " Fierce as ten furies; terrible as hell,"[1]

following, with a determined energy and malignant aspect, closely
in his wake, and with resistless impetuosity dogging his every
footstep !

> " Black Melancholy sits, and round her throws
> A deathlike silence; and a dread repose:
> Her gloomy presence saddens all the scene,
> Shades every flower, and darkens every green,
> Deepens the murmur of the falling flood,
> And breathes a browner horror on the wood."[2]

The patient often exhibits, at the commencement of an attack
of insanity, what, to a superficial observer, would be considered
only an unnatural elevation of spirits. He is at other times
loquacious, and talks loudly and dogmatically. He subsequently
becomes querulous, peevish, irresolute, and undecisive, not being,
for two consecutive minutes, in the same frame of mind. He
quarrels with his best friends, argues with great warmth, pertina-
city, and vehemence, the most trifling matters, is excessive and
extravagant in his expressions of friendship, bitter and rancorous
in his feelings of dislike, hatred, and aversion.

In this state of morbidly active brain, and unhealthily excited

[1] Milton.   [2] Pope.

mind, the fancy runs rampant, taking discursive and airy flights, every circumstance being viewed by the patient *couleur de rose.*

There is associated with this exaltation of the imagination great exaggeration of expression, forming a striking contrast with the patient's usual modesty and sobriety of conversation, strict urbanity, repose, and propriety of conduct. He talks ostentatiously of his vast wealth, boasts of his elevated social position, speaks exultingly of the profound respect he can command, appears vain of the high rank which has been conferred upon him, and is proud of the still greater distinction he is destined to acquire!

As the insanity advances, the patient, in direct opposition to his usual habits and tastes, delights in low society, is neglectful of his personal appearance, drinks stimulants to excess, is extravagant in pecuniary matters, and often squanders his property in visionary and absurd speculations. He subsequently exhibits some form of mental obtuseness, or moral obliquity. He is lost to all sense of truth, respect for decency of thought, regard for good breeding, and all notion of decorous conduct. He magnifies, exaggerates, twists, distorts, and falsifies everything connected with himself, being the hero of every incident accidentally mentioned in his hearing.

These mental characteristics are often in direct opposition to his natural or healthy modes of thinking and acting. Occasionally, for some months before any positive morbid *alienation* of mind is recognized, the intellect is clearly off its balance. The patient has violent paroxysms of extreme irritability and passion, produced by the most insignificant causes.

Contrary to his ordinary practice, he swears, deals in loose inuendoes, talks obscenely, and acts indecently, breaking out in loud fits of sobbing, or in wild paroxysms of laughter, being alternately under the influence of agony and hope, joy and despair,

> " Moody madness,
> Laughing loud, amidst severest woe."

The attack of insanity is, occasionally, ushered in by excessive and boisterous paroxysms of animal spirits, kindled into activity by the most trifling causes. A gentleman, naturally quiet, of grave habits of thought, and of reserved manner (who had never been known to indulge in any demonstrative act of merriment) was suddenly seized with an apparently uncontrollable disposition to indulge in *loud and immoderate fits of laughter*. The most trifling observation, the most insignificant circumstance, such as a look or gesture, excited his mirth to an intense and inordinate degree. For several days previously to this remarkable change of disposition, he had been sitting up late at night perusing and analyzing a lengthened correspondence relating to some property, respecting which there had been a disagreeable and vexatious family dispute. He had complained to his valet of want of sleep, as well as of headache. These were the only *observable* symptoms that preceded this unnatural overflow of spirits, and, in fact, outbreak of insanity. For nearly a week none of his relations could perceive anything in connection with the case approaching to false perception, aberration of idea, or illusion of the senses. He laughed, like an hysterical girl, indiscriminately at every occurrence.

On the tenth day from the seizure, he (after a violent and uncontrollable paroxysm of laughter) solemnly proclaimed himself, whilst in church, to be the saviour of the world! It required this palpable demonstration of insanity to bring conviction home to this patient's friends as to his actual state of mental disorder. I have seen several cases of insanity occurring in women developing itself in a similar manner.[1]

---

[1] Mrs. Trollope, when speaking of Strasburg Cathedral, says: "I entered the church with the intention of climbing to the top of its spire: but gave it up on hearing the sacristan's account of the ascent. It is on record, that three females have been, at different times, so overpowered by the giddy eminence which they had reached, that they have thrown themselves off *in a momentary fit of delirium*, and been dashed to atoms. The latest of these awful accidents occurred within the last ten years (she wrote in 1833); and the man who recounted the tale to Henry (Mrs. Trollope's son), while he was standing on the self-same pinnacle, told him that he had himself witnessed it. He said that the unfortunate creature was quite a young girl; and the first symptoms she gave of the suicidal delirium *was excessive mirth*. She *laughed and shouted as if in ecstasy*, and having reached a point where nothing intercepted her view of the abyss below, she sprang off, screaming wildly as she fell."

"Exuberant gaiety," says Dr. Mayo, "bursting forth in one whose ordinary state is extreme depression, constitutes an ominous symptom, when the tendency to suicide is suspected. The patient has often, at that moment, achieved just that state of orgasm which will enable him to commit the act, and he exults fearfully in the consciousness of this."

"Furor est, agnoscere solis
Quem liceat quos jam tangit vicinia fati."

—("*Elements of the Pathology of the Human Mind*," p. 79.)

In the stage of morbid exaltation previously referred to, the patient frequently exhibits a talent for poetry, mechanics, oratory, and elocution, quite unusual and inconsistent with his education and opposed to his normal habits of thought. His witty sallies, bursts of fervid and impassioned eloquence, readiness at repartee, power of extemporaneous versification, and mechanical skill and ingenuity, amaze those who were acquainted with his ordinary mental capacity and educational attainments. There is an unusual display of vigor of mind;—an ability to converse fluently on subjects not previously familiar to the mind, and an aptitude to discuss matters wholly unconnected with the patient's particular situation in life. A quickness of perception, a facility and propriety of utterance quite unusual, become, in some cases, as the disease progresses, daily more manifested.

" The records of wit and cunning of madmen," says Dr. Rush, " are numerous in every country. Talents for eloquence, poetry, music, painting, and uncommon ingenuity in several of the mechanical arts, are often evolved in this state of madness.[1] A gentleman whom I attended in an hospital in 1810, often delighted as well as astonished the patients and officers of our hospital by his displays of oratory in preaching from a table in the hospital yard every Sunday. A female patient of mine who became insane after parturition in the year 1807, sang hymns and songs of her own composition during the latter stage of her illness, with a tone and

---

[1] The most exquisite poetry, replete with splendid imagery, genuine feeling, and touching pathos, has been composed by the inmates of asylums, and by those, too, unquestionably insane. The following simple verses were written by a lady confined as a lunatic in the Ohio Asylum, U. S. America. They were addressed to a rose just budding into life, in the lattice window of her sitting-room.

> " I have often seen the flower spring,
>   From out the mould'ring wall—
> I have seen the clust'ring blossoms cling
>   And grace the ruin'd hall.
>
> " But here, 'mid scenes of human woe,
>   This little rose intends to blow.
> So in life's shades, however drear,
>   Some ray of mercy will appear.
>
> " Bloom, tiny flower, a gracious hand
>   Invisible, unfolds thy leaves
> O'er scenes of grief, by his command,
>   Joy still with sorrow interweaves."

15

voice so soft and pleasant that I hung upon it with delight every
time I visited her. She had never discovered a talent for poetry
or music in any previous part of her life. Two instances of a
talent for drawing evolved by madness have occurred within my
knowledge. And where is the hospital for mad people in which
elegant and completely-rigged ships and curious pieces of machinery have not been exhibited by persons who never discovered
the least turn for a mechanical art previously to their derangement ? Sometimes we observe in mad people a resuscitation of
knowledge; hence we hear them describe past events, and speak
in ancient or modern languages, or repeat long and interesting
passages from books, none of which, we are sure, they were
capable of recollecting in the natural and healthy state of their
mind.''[1]

A gentleman, whilst insane, and confined in an asylum, wrote an
able philosophical and critical essay on *"Original Sin."* It was
found among his MS. papers after death. He was, when he
penned the dissertation, under a delusion that there was a family
conspiracy to poison him. Occasionally, he admitted that he
struggled resolutely against this delusion, but never thoroughly
succeeded in mastering it. After his decease, the valves of the
heart were found to be ossified. As asphyxial sensations are
known to give rise to erroneous mental impressions, it was presumed that the idea of poisoning was suggested by the uneasiness
which he felt whenever the stomach was overloaded and distended
with food. Everything he ate disagreed with him; the heart
labored to propel the blood through its ossified and constricted
passages, the lungs became engorged and congested, and the
breathing spasmodic and difficult. When in this state of physical
suffering, he was wont to exclaim, "The villains have been poisoning me again !" Nevertheless, in his happier and more lucid moments, a more charming companion was never met with. No one
ever sat down in his society without being amused and interested,
or having derived some information from his vast erudition, and
great literary and scientific accomplishments. But while he could
reason clearly and ably on philosophical subjects, his moral apprehensions and affections were still perverted. If the name of one
particular member of his family were alluded to, he would utter

[1] "On the Diseases of the Mind." By Benjamin Rush, M.D. 1835.

violent imprecations against him, and accompany them with the most bitter homicidal threats. Among his manuscripts was found another document, which contrasts somewhat strangely with the theological essay alluded to. It was entitled "My Last Will and Testament," and clearly indicated the morbid state of his feelings at the time it was penned.[1]

I have known men naturally most dull of apprehension, in fact nearly half-witted, exhibit, both in the early as well as advanced stages of insanity, considerable intellectual acuteness and capacity.[2]

"I was troubled sometimes," says Pinel, "to follow the incorrigible garrulity, and a sort of flow of unconnected and incoherent words of an old scholar, who at other times fell into a stern and savage silence. When any piece of poetry in which he had formerly delighted suggested itself to his memory, he became capable of continuous attention, his judgment seemed to regain its rights, and he composed verses in which there reigned not only a spirit of order and of justness in the ideas, but also a regular supply of fancy, and some very happy sallies." In another place the same author observes :—

"Certain facts appear so extraordinary, that they have need of being borne up by the most authentic testimony, in order not to be called in question. I speak of the poetical enthusiasm which is said to have characterized certain paroxysms of mania, even when the verses recited could nowise be regarded as an act of reminiscence. I have myself heard a maniac declaim, with grace and exquisite discernment, a longer or shorter succession of the verses of Virgil or Horace, which had been a long time effaced

---

[1] The will was as follows: "In the name of God. Amen! This is the last Will and Testament of me, ———. I bequeath all my property, consisting of * * * in the Three Per Cents., and about * * * in Messrs. ——— Bank, and a security upon the Estate of ———, in the county of ———, which security is in my brother's desk, to Mr. ———, artist. To all my own family I bequeath my curse for having administered, and bribed other persons to administer, poison to me, by which I am reduced to a very weak state, and for having bribed two doctors to certify me insane, when I was not so, by which I have been confined for two years and six months without having been insane. May Jehovah visit these wrongs upon them is the last prayer of ———."

[2] This interesting subject is considered at length, with great philosophical acumen, elegance of taste, and literary ability, by M. Octave Delepierre, in two essays (privately published) entitled : 1. "*Études Biobibliographes sur les Fous Littéraires ;*" 2. "*Essai Biographique sur l'Histoire Littéraire des Fous.*" An analysis of these brochures will be found in Nos. XIII and XIV (New Series) of my "*Psychological Journal.*"

from his memory, inasmuch as, after his education was terminated, he had been twenty years absent in the American colonies, given up to the pursuit of wealth ; and the reverses occasioned by the Revolution, had alone thrown him into this distraction of mind. An English author, whom I have already cited, attests that a young girl, of a feeble constitution, and subject to nervous affections, had become insane, and that during her delirium she expressed herself in very harmonious English verses, though she had before shown no disposition for poetry." Van Swieten relates the case of a woman who, during her paroxysms of mania, showed a rare facility for versification, though she had before been occupied with manual labor, and her understanding had never been enriched by culture.

Tasso composed his most eloquent and impassioned verses during paroxysms of insanity. Lucretius wrote his immortal poem, "*De Rerum Naturâ*," when suffering from an attack of mental aberration.[1] Alexander Cruden compiled his celebrated "Concordance" whilst insane.[2] Some of the ablest articles in Aikins' Biography were written by a patient in a lunatic asylum. Cibber says in his life of Lee—"I have seen a ship of straw finely fabricated by a mad ship-builder, and the most lovely attitudes have been represented by a lunatic statuary in his cell."[3]

---

[1] It has been maintained by some writers, arrogating to themselves great critical penetration, that they were competent, from internal evidence, to point out in this celebrated poem, those passages that were evidently composed during Lucretius's attack of insanity. They refer particularly to portions of book iii, in which the poet speaks of death and the state of the soul.

[2] Alexander Cruden, during his first attack of insanity, was asked whether he ever was mad? He replied, "I *am* as mad *now* as I was *formerly*, and as mad *then* as I am *now ;* that is to say, *not mad at any time*."

[3] Nathaniel Lee was known by the name of the "mad poet." He was confined for some time in Bethlem Hospital. Langbaine observes, "It is to be regretted that his madness exceeded that divine fury described by Ovid as characterizing all true poets."

"Est Deus in nobis agitante calescimus illo."

In a satire on the poets, Nathaniel Lee's state of mind while in the asylum is thus described :—

"There in a den removed from human eyes,
Possest with muse, the brain-sick poet lies,
Too miserably wretched to be named ;
For plays, for heroes, and for passion famed ;

I attended, a few years ago, a young gentleman whose attack of insanity was supposed to have been caused by rough and ill-usage whilst at school.   I was informed that this youth had never exhibited any particular talent for arithmetic or mathematical inquiries ; in fact, it was alleged that he was incapable of doing even a simple sum of addition or multiplication.   After recovering from the acute symptoms of his maniacal attack, and when able to employ his mind in reading and conversation, it was found that an extraordinary arithmetical power had been evolved during his illness.   He was able, with wonderful facility, to solve several rather complex problems.   This talent continued for several months, but after his complete restoration to health, he relapsed into his former natural state of arithmetical dulness, ignorance, and general mental incapacity !

Last year I attended the wife of a clergyman who exhibited, during her paroxysms of maniacal excitement, a wonderful talent for rapid and clever versification.   The nurse, who was in constant attendance upon the patient, was so struck with the phenomenon, that she had transcribed, before calling my attention to the fact, a number of verses evidencing poetical powers of no ordinary character.   The disposition to improvise was manifested mostly at night.   After her recovery, all capacity for rhyming appeared to subside.   I understand that, previously to her mental illness, she had not exhibited the slightest poetical inclination or ability.   Insanity in young women of a certain temperament often commences and progresses as follows: (Dr. Haslam has called our attention to this type of mental disease, and has graphically delineated its insidious approaches).   "It usually manifests itself in persons distinguished by prompt capacity and lively disposition, who, in general, have been the favorites of parents and tutors, by their facility in acquiring knowledge, and by a precocity of attainment they have manifested.   This disorder commences about or shortly after the period of menstruation, and, in many instances, has been unconnected, as far as could be ascertained, with hereditary taint.   The attack is almost imperceptible.   Some months usually elapse before it becomes the subject of particular notice ;

Thoughtless he raves his sleepless hours away,
In chains all night, in darkness all the day.
And if he gets some intervals from pain,
The fit returns," &c.

and fond relatives are frequently deceived by the hope that it is only an abatement of excessive vivacity, conducing to a prudent reserve and steadiness of character. A degree of apparent thoughtfulness and inactivity precede, together with a diminution of the ordinary curiosity concerning that which is passing before them; and they therefore neglect those objects and pursuits which formerly proved sources of delight and instruction. The sensibility appears to be considerably blunted; they do not bear the same affection towards their parents and relations; they become unfeeling to kindness, and careless of reproof. To their companions they show a cold civility, but take no interest whatever in their concerns. If they read a book, they are unable to give any account of its contents. Sometimes, with steadfast eyes, they will dwell for an hour on one page, and then turn over a number in a few minutes. It is very difficult to persuade them to write, which most readily developes their state of mind; if they do so, much time is consumed and little produced. The letter is repeatedly begun, but they seldom advance beyond a sentence or two. The orthography becomes puzzling, and by endeavoring to adjust the spelling, the subject vanishes altogether from the mind. As their apathy increases they are negligent of their dress, and inattentive to personal cleanliness. Frequently they experience transient impulses of passion, but these have no source in sentiment; the tears which trickle down at one time, are as unmeaning as the loud laugh which succeeds them; and it often happens that a momentary gust of anger, with its attendant invectives, ceases before the threat can be concluded."

Whilst analyzing the incipient symptoms of insanity, as manifested during the stage of exaltation and excitement, it will not be irrelevant for me to consider an important subject closely connected with the matter under consideration, but perhaps more immediately bearing upon a medico-legal point of great interest to the jurist, as well as to the practical psychologist. I refer to the subtlety, quickness of apprehension, ready wit, biting sarcasm, great power of self-control, extreme cunning, and extraordinary shrewdness of the insane, as well as the wonderful mastery they have occasionally been seen to exercise over their acknowledged delusions, whilst under the searching analysis of the ablest and most accomplished advocates of the day. In many cases it has been proved to be useless to possess the "key note" to the insanity of the person under examination, or "to touch the chord," supposed to be in unison with, and likely to awaken into activity the latent insane delusion and cunningly concealed hallucination. The lunatic, if he be carefully trained and skilfully tutored, having an important purpose to accomplish, by effectually *masking* his mental disorder, will, under, these circumstances, act with wonderful ability and singular ingenuity, on the *defensive*, and, in the teeth of the most stringent examination, make "no sign." How often have I seen the insane (*who have been previously well prepared*) thus baffle the acumen of the most experienced and sagacious members of the bar.

It is a commonly accepted notion, that the delusive idea will immediately develope itself, provided its character be known, and special reference made to it by those engaged in testing the sanity of persons alleged to be of deranged mind. Nathaniel Lee, who acquired no inconsiderable degree of practical knowledge of the phenomena of insanity, during his long incarceration in Bethlem, and prolonged association with the inmates of that hospital, appears to have been inoculated with this fallacy, for he says, in his description of the madness of Cæsar Borgia,

> "Like a poor lunatic that makes his moan,
> And for a while beguiles his lookers on,
> He reasons well. His eyes their wildness lose.
> He vows the keeper his wronged sense abuse ;
> *But if you hit the cause that hurts his brain,*
> *Then his teeth gnash, he foams, he shakes his chain,*
> *His eyeballs roll, and he is mad again.*"

It requires no ordinary amount of tact and skill, as well as practical acquaintance with the subtle psychology of insanity, to fully qualify a person to examine and unravel successfully a complex case of lunacy. I have often found it necessary to pay two or three protracted visits to a patient, conversing with him on general subjects, before I have considered it prudent to make any reference to the alleged delusions. By this process the confidence of the patient is effectually secured, his suspicions disarmed, and the expert able gradually to direct the attention to the points upon which the mind is thought to be disordered. If the lunatic clearly perceives the object of the physician's visit, the drift of the questions addressed to him, and fully realizes the importance of concealing impressions that are represented to be creations of a diseased imagination, it will require much persevering ingenuity to extract from him anything like an admission of his actual state of insane mind.

Feigned insanity is often unmasked by placing the patient under the influence of chloroform. Might not the same anæsthetic agent be found serviceable in analyzing a case of cunningly concealed lunacy? There can be no doubt as to the effect of chloroform in giving, in a particular type of case, great temporary prominence to insane delusions. I have occasionally observed, that when it has been found necessary to administer this anæsthetic agent by inhalation to persons mentally deranged, its immediate effect has been to develope and drag from their hiding-place, hallucinations that were previously if not in a latent, but faintly and feebly manifested state.[1]

Dr. Haslam remarks, that " a successful examination of an insane person is not to be effected by directly selecting the subject of his delusion, for he will immediately perceive the object of such inquiries, and endeavor to evade or pretend to discover them; the purpose is more effectually answered by leading him to the origin of his distemper, and tracing the consecutive series of his actions and the association of ideas; in going over the road where he has stumbled he will infallibly trip again."

The power of concealing delusions which confessed and even dangerous lunatics have been known to possess when under the strictest and most searching examination, has often astonished persons unaccustomed to deal with them, and not fully conversant with the subtle phenomena of insanity. The illustrious LORD ERSKINE observes, in one of his most able and eloquent speeches, " that in all the cases which have filled Westminster Hall with the most complicated considerations, the lunatics and other insane persons who have been the subjects of them have not only had the most perfect knowledge and recollection of all the relations they stood in towards others, and of the acts and circumstances of their lives, but have, in general, been remarkable for subtlety and acuteness. These are the cases which frequently mock the wisdom of the wisest in judicial trials; because such persons often reason with a subtlety which puts in the shade the ordinary conceptions of man-

---

[1] It will be important not to confound the hallucinations and illusions occasionally induced, in persons of healthy minds, by the administration of chloroform, with those that are clearly symptomatic of a state of mental derangement.

kind; their conclusions are just, and frequently profound; but the premises from which they reason, when within the range of the malady, are uniformly false;—not false from any defect of knowledge or judgment, because a delusive image, the inseparable companion of real insanity, is thrust upon the subjugated understanding, incapable of resistance, because unconscious of attack."

A repudiation (for a short period) of the existence of insane thought, admitted by the patient, and known by others to have previously existed; the ability to converse continuously and rationally, with great shrewdness and sagacity, on matters requiring for their comprehension a vigorous and well-balanced intellect, are no conclusive and demonstrative tests, *per se*, of legal soundness of mind, or of recovery from an attack of insanity. In the great majority of cases, evidence of this character should, however, be viewed as establishing a *bona fide* restoration to health of mind.

Some years ago, I had under my care a young gentleman who had tried, on more than one occasion, to murder his sister when under the delusion that she had prevented, by her unjustifiable interference, his marrying a lady of large property and of high rank. The idea was altogether an insane one. For nearly a year this notion was never absent from his mind. He, however, manifested other symptoms of mental derangement. Eventually, the delusion with regard to the sister appeared to have been removed from his imagination. I spoke frequently to him on the subject, and he declared that his impressions with regard to his sister no longer existed. He once observed, "I wish to see my dear sister for the purpose of craving her forgiveness for permitting such bad thoughts to enter my mind." To all appearance he seemed to be restored to mental health, or at least to be convalescent, yet I had (from a variety of trifling circumstances, when viewed by themselves) my doubts and misgivings as to the *bona fide* character of his apparent recovery. For more than a week his mind, he alleged, was free from all delusion. I called one day to see him, and placed myself in such a position that I could closely observe his conduct, and hear his conversation, without his being aware of my presence. When I first saw him he was reading. In about ten minutes he left the sofa where he was sitting, and approached towards the looking-glass. He gazed fixedly at himself for a few minutes. He then began, whilst in this position, to indulge in the most malignant grins. At last he clenched his fists, and walked about the room in an agitated manner, exclaiming, "The villain," "the miscreant," "the viper," "the snake in the grass," "I'll do for her on the first opportunity." I was now satisfied that the lunatic had been playing an artful part for a purpose, and that he was still in a dangerous state of insanity. I did not converse with him on this occasion, but did so on the following day, when, strange to say, he persisted in declaring that he had no delusions with regard to his sister, or any member of the family. I made no reference to what I had observed on the previous day, and being convinced, in the course of a week, that it was not my intention to allow him to be at large, he threw off his disguise, and his insanity then became evident to every person who approached him.

"I remember," says the late Sir Henry Halford, "hearing Lord Ellenborough express, in the strongest terms, his conviction that an insane person had completely recovered, after having observed him to sustain a lengthened conversation upon an important subject with great good sense and sobriety. Nevertheless, this patient was detected, a few days afterwards, under the full influence of his delusion, using Latin, however, to express his thoughts, that he might effectually elude, if possible, the watchful observation of his attendants."[1]

"The insane," says Esquirol, "group and arrange their ideas, carry on a reasonable conversation, defend their opinions with subtlety, and even with a rigid severity of logic, give very rational explanations, and justify their actions by highly plausible motives. When they have a great object to effect, they will combine all their means, seize every opportunity, remove all obstacles, have recourse to threats, force, cunning, dissimulation, prayers, promises, and tears; they deceive the most experienced, their perseverance is indomitable; convinced that what they think is true, that what they wish is just and reasonable, they cannot be convinced of their error. Their conviction is occasionally stronger than their judgment. 'You are right,' said a lunatic to Esquirol, 'but you cannot *convince* ME that you are so.'"[2]

[1] Essays and Orations read and delivered at the Royal College of Physicians by Sir H. Halford, Bart., M.D., p. 142.

[2] A patient, who was confined in a public asylum, stoutly and ingeniously maintained that he was considered and incarcerated as insane because nature had blessed him with acuter powers of discernment, judgment, reason, and fancy, than his less fortunate neighbors. Unfortunately, however, he had not the good sense and prudence to conceal these superior gifts and endowments of mind from the observation,

Are phenomena like these susceptible of a psychological solution? There can be no doubt that, in certain types of insanity, unconnected with much, if any, cerebral disorganization, the intellectual and perceptive faculties are, although influenced by the prevailing delusions, in a state of unnatural exaltation. In ordinary cases of disease implicating the brain, producing a state of vascular congestion on its surface, or a great rapidity in the circulation of the blood through its vessels, the psychical functions are, generally, in an active state of manifestation.

In attacks of fever, accelerating the cerebral circulation, and in the incipient stage of the brain affections of early life, the patient often exhibits an unnatural acuteness, occasionally amounting to a brilliancy of intelligence. There is also great sensorial activity. Analogous phenomena are observed in some forms of ordinary cerebral disorder affecting the operations of thought; and on this principle we may, in a measure, physiologically and philosophically account for the subtlety and cunning of the insane. But does not the fact admit of another solution?

The *instinctive* appetites, as contradistinguished from the *intellectual* faculties, are, as a general rule, in a state of activity, exaltation, and ascendency, in many types of deranged, as well as originally defective and impaired mind. In the various gradations of imbecility, and in some cases of profound idiocy, we often observe a high manifestation of the instincts. In the lower grades of stupidity and congenital idiocy we occasionally see exhibited that extraordinary sagacity and cunning which is so characteristic of the higher class of animals. Mechanical ingenuity, acute sense of hearing, seeing, and smelling, as well as wonderful powers of adaptation to all possible physical conditions, are often observed among a certain class of the insane utterly incapable of appreciating a rational idea. Hence, we may, to a certain extent, explain the *subtle instinctive sagacity and acuteness* so frequently seen associated with the various forms of deranged mind. It would appear that in proportion as the reasoning and reflective powers are in an arrested, latent, and dormant state, do the instinctive propensities (as a compensating balance) ascend the scale, occupy the seat of reason, and arrogate and exercise the right of undisputed and often unbridled sovereignty.[1]

jealousy, and envy of his contemporaries; hence he was declared to be a lunatic, and sent to and detained in a madhouse.

[1] "Madness," says Coleridge, "is not simply a bodily disease. It is the sleep of

Mr. Dugald Stewart thus attempts, metaphysically, to account for the acumen and subtlety of the insane. He maintains that the phenomena may, to some extent, be attributed to the physical influence of the disorder in occasioning, together with an increased propensity to controversy, a preternatural and morbid excitation of the power of attention, and of some other intellectual faculties; but much more in his opinion to its effect in removing the check of those collateral circumstances by which, in more sober understandings, the reasoning powers are perpetually retarded and controlled in their operation. Among these circumstances, it is sufficient, says this able writer, to specify, for the sake of illustration, 1. "That distrust, which experience gradually teaches, of the accuracy and precision of the phraseology in which our reasonings are expressed: accompanied with a corresponding apprehension of involuntary mistakes from the ambiguity and vagueness of language; 2. A latent suspicion that we may not be fully in possession of all the elements on which the solution of the problem depends; and 3. The habitual influence of those first principles of propriety, of morality, and of common sense, which, as long as reason maintains her ascendant, exercise a paramount authority over all those speculative conclusions which have any connection with the business of life. Of these checks or restraints on our reasoning process, none are cultivated and strengthened, either by the rules of the logician, or by the habits of *vivâ voce* disputation. On the contrary, in proportion as their regulating power is confirmed, that hesitation and suspense of judgment are encouraged which are so congenial to the spirit of true philosophy, but such fatal incumbrances in contending with an antagonist whose object is not truth, but victory. In madmen, where their control is entirely thrown off, the merely logical process (which never stops to analyze the meaning of words) is likely to go on more rapidly and fearlessly than before, producing a volubility of speech, and an apparent quickness of conception, which present to common observers all the characteristics of intellectual superiority. It is scarcely necessary to add, that the same appearances, which in this extreme case of mental aberration are displayed on so great a scale, may

the spirit, with certain conditions of wakefulness; that is to say, lucid intervals. During this sleep, or recession of the spirit, *the lower, or bestial states of life, rise up into action and prominence.* It is an awful thing to be eternally tempted by the perverted senses."

be expected to show themselves, more or less, wherever there is any deficiency in those qualities which constitute depth and sagacity of judgment."[1]

2. SOMATIC EXALTATION.—In the incipient stage of insanity there is great disturbance of the *motor* power. This is often, in the first instance, only indicated by a general muscular agitation, producing a *brusquerie* of manner, forming a striking contrast to the patient's natural state of quietness and repose.

As the mental disorder progresses, he comports himself like a person in a state of incipient intoxication. It is difficult to remove the impression of his being under the influence of vinous stimulants, from those who observe his erratic conduct, and listen to his wild conversation. His singularities of deportment, excited physiognomy, incoherence and extravagance of language, his unnatural elevation of spirits, paroxysmal attacks of exaltation, irregular muscular movements, indicated by his eccentric, odd, rolling, and unsteady gait, naturally suggest the question, is he *drunk* or *mad ?*

During the stage of physical agitation, previously referred to, the patient resembles a ferocious animal removed from his wild native forest, and confined in a cage. He paces and repaces the room, night and day, in a condition of extreme perturbation, rarely sitting or standing in a state of repose for many consecutive minutes. He suddenly starts from home, being tormented by a peevish, irresistible restlessness,—a constant, unwearied, never-satisfied desire for change,—walking, unfatigued, long distances with great apparent fixedness of purpose and accompanying vehemence of gesture, without having in view a sane or rational object. These rapid strides, forced and violent movements, appear to originate in an instinctive desire to throw off a morbid accumulation of muscular power, disperse an unhealthy excess of irritability, dissipate an abnormal redundancy of nervous energy, and keep in a state of subjugation corroding, anxious, and perverted thoughts, thus relieving the mind of

" A whirling gulf of phantasy and flame."

In vain the unhappy man so struggles to obtain peace of mind by yielding to an irresistible and uncontrollable desire to rush, al-

[1] " Philosophy of the Human Mind" (1848), p. 431, 2.

most unconsciously, from place to place ;—fruitless are his endeavors to arrest the creation of the morbid and gloomy imagery
desolating and bewildering his thoughts,—perverting his reason,—
deadening his sensibility,—searing his conscience,—benumbing his
moral sense,—distorting his judgment,—deluding his senses,—and
paralyzing his volition ;—abortive are his efforts to escape from
the "horrible shadows" and "unreal mockeries" that torture and
disorder his imagination.   Alas ! he cannot fly from himself.

> " Quid terras alio calentes
> Sole mutamus ?—Patriæ quis exul
> ———Se quoque fugit ?"1—Hor.

A convict in Van Diemen's Land, after quarrelling with one of
the overseers, brutally murdered him.   He immediately escaped,
with a few clothes and a gun, to the wild solitude of the bush.   The
murderer lived, for some time, like a savage, occasionally making
his appearance, armed to the teeth, at various huts, where he peremptorily demanded food.   The convict's mind ultimately succumbed to the severe mental agony and physical distress to which
it was exposed, and he became a dangerous lunatic.   He was eventually perceived to be under the dominion of a terrible hallucination.   He imagined that he was constantly being pursued by the
ghastly phantom of his murdered victim.   He was observed to
rush frantically from tree to tree, bush to bush, house to house,
from one part of the district to another, endeavoring to fly (like
an animal hunted to death by ferocious bloodhounds) from the
clutches of some person constantly in his wake, and steadily track-
ing his path.   The maniac eventually surrendered himself into the
hands of the police, alleging that annihilation was preferable to

---

1 A friend observed to Socrates, alluding to a mutual acquaintance afflicted with
melancholy, that " he had derived no benefit from his travels."   " I am not surprised
at that," replied the philosopher, " *for he travelled along with himself.*"

Sterne says : " The learned *Smelfungus* travelled from Boulogne to Paris, from Paris
to Rome, and so on ; but he *set out with the spleen and jaundice, and every object he
passed by was discolored or distorted*.   He wrote an account of them, but 'twas nothing
but the account of *his own miserable feelings*.   I met Smelfungus in the grand portico
of the Pantheon.   ' 'Tis nothing but a large cock-pit,' said he. . . . . I popped upon
Smelfungus again at Turin, on his return home, and a sad tale of sorrowful adventures
he had to tell. . . . . He had been flayed alive, and bedevilled, and used worse than
St. Bartholomew, at every stage he had come to.   ' I'll tell it,' cried Smelfungus, ' to
the *world*.'   ' *You had better tell it,*' said I, ' TO YOUR PHYSICIAN.' "

the agony of mind which he suffered.   In fact, although insane, he prayed earnestly for death at the hands of the public executioner, in order to extricate himself from the spectral image that was never absent from his mind!

Who can escape from the never-dying agony and unceasing tortures of a wicked and perturbed conscience?   What means are there of effectually obliterating that "damned spot" that must ever appear in terrible judgment against inexpiated and unrepented crimes, unforgiven by Heaven, and "unwhipt of justice" upon earth?

> " Exemplo quodcumque malo committitur, ipsi
> Displicet auctofi.   Prima est hæc ultio, quod se
> Judice nemo nocens absolvitur; improba quamvis
> Gratia fallaci Prætoris vicerit urna."
>   JUVEN. SAT. 13, v. 1.

I had an opportunity of seeing, some years ago, a singularly distressing case of confirmed insanity consequent upon a long, sad, and eventful career of vice and immorality.   The patient had lived, for fifteen years, a most extraordinary life.   He had been accused (but not *legally* convicted) of almost every description of crime.   He eventually went to Australia, and resided for a long time in an unfrequented part of that country.   He subsequently returned to England, discarded by his family in consequence of his gross and inexplicable acts of impropriety, and abandoned himself, without restriction, to all kinds of debauchery, vice, and profligacy.   He was supposed (upon what was at the time conceived to be valid evidence) to have been guilty of a barbarous murder; was accused of having committed an unnatural offence; and was publicly charged with acts of forgery, perjury, and theft!   In early life he squandered, in a most reckless manner, a fortune which he had obtained with his wife, and then cruelly deserted her and a family of three children, after forming a connection with a depraved woman of a most hideous and forbidding aspect, whom he met accidentally in the public streets!   During the whole of this period, he exhibited none of the ordinary symptoms of mental alienation.   At the age of fifty he became clearly insane, if he had not been so for many years previously.   His insanity was of a most painful type.   There evidently existed, associated with his mental derangement, occasional lucid and apparently sane reminiscences of his former vices and crimes.

He had a perfect horror of seeing any one enter the room in which he was confined; and if a stranger were introduced, he immediately rushed into a corner, where he would crouch like a wild and untamed animal, in an agony of frenzied despair. He then held up his hands in the attitude of wild distress, and with an expression of perfect terror depicted on his countenance, literally screamed, "Away, away!—don't come near me!—I don't know you!—why do you stare so at me?—I am not the man!—I am innocent!—falsely accused!—turn him out!—I won't speak to him!—I will confess nothing!" When contemplating this unhappy man's condition, I was forcibly reminded of the scene in Macbeth, where the gory spectral image of Banquo is conjured into existence by the guilty conscience of the king.

"No disease of the imagination," says Dr. Johnson, "is so difficult of cure as that which is complicated with the dread of *guilt*. Fancy and conscience then act interchangeably upon the mind, and so often shift their places that the illusions of the one are not distinguished from the dictates of the other. If fancy presents images not moral or religious, the mind drives them away when they give it pain; but when melancholy notions take the form of duty, they lay hold on the faculties without opposition, because we are afraid to exclude or banish them. For this reason, the superstitious are often melancholy, and the melancholy almost always superstitious."[1]

The Abbé de Rancé became insane from the effects of remorse. His insanity was manifested by a state of frantic grief. To this succeeded profound melancholy. He sent away all his friends, and shut himself up in his mansion at Veret, where he refused to see a single creature. His whole soul was absorbed in a deep and settled gloom. Hermetically sealed in a small room, he even forgot to eat and drink; and when the servant reminded him that it was bedtime, he started, as from a deep reverie, and seemed unconscious that it was not still morning. A faithful servant who sometimes followed him by stealth, often watched him standing for hours in one place, like a statue, the snow, rain, and pitiless storm mercilessly beating on his poor head, whilst he, unconscious of the wild fury of the elements, was wholly absorbed in the gloomy silence of black and hopeless despair.

[1] Rasselas.

Happily, there are many cases of insanity, even in the incipient stage, where the mind is intensely abstracted and pre-occupied in the contemplation of the most glowing, richly poetical, fanciful, and joyous imagery. The morbid imagination exalts its possessor into the purest and most elevated ethereal regions. The patient revels in the luxury of vast hoards of wealth; is elevated to positions that confer upon him the highest amount of physical enjoyment, and the maximum degree of intellectual gratification that the body and mind are susceptible of. He is in fancy a monarch, ruling over the destinies of a great nation. He is "every inch a king," having at command undisputed and despotic sovereignty. Occasionally, the lunatic is in imagination not only the emperor of a great and powerful nation, a happy, contented, and prosperous people, but sole arbiter and monarch of the universe, ruling, governing, and having under his exclusive control and subjection every kingdom, civilized and uncivilized, on the face of the globe! At other times he is an angelic being, enjoying all the rapturous pleasures and ecstatic bliss of the redeemed, in a brighter and a purer state of existence. I have occasionally seen such patients return to the dull, and often humble realities of *sane* life; in other words, restored to the possession of reason, and (comparing their normal with their abnormal condition of mind) have been disposed to ask the question, which was the happier state of the two?[1]

"In this stage of exaltation," says Pinel, "the patient overwhelms those about him with his extraordinary loquacity. If he

---

[1] Horace describes the feelings of a lunatic, brought down, by a restoration of reason, from the happy Elysium into which his morbid fancy had transported him, to the regions of poor common humanity :—

> "Pol! me occidistis, amici,
> Non servastis, ait, cui sic extorta voluptas
> Et demptus per vim mentis gratissimus error!"

"I always expected," said a patient to Dr. Willis, "with impatience, the accession of the paroxysms of insanity, since I enjoyed, during their presence, a high degree of pleasure. They lasted ten or twelve hours. Everything appeared easy to me. No obstacles presented themselves in theory or in practice. My memory, all of a sudden, acquired a singular degree of perfection. Long passages of Latin authors occurred to my mind. In general, I have great difficulty in finding rhythmical terminations, but *then* I could write in verse with as much facility as prose. I was cunning, malicious, and fertile in all kinds of expedient."—"*A Treatise on Mental Derangement*," by Francis Willis, M.D. 1843.

16

comes into a room he turns everything upside down, he displaces and shakes the chairs and tables, without seeming to have any particular motive for so doing. Scarcely have you taken the eye off him, when you perceive him on the promenade, and there, as aimlessly busy as in the room, he chatters, throws stones, and walks up and down the same way over and over again. Another speaks alternately of his horses, dogs, garden, and his wig, without waiting for an answer, or giving the hearer time to follow his rodomontade. He rambles about his grounds like an *ignis fatuus*, cries out, gabbles, torments his servants with trifling orders, his relations with absurdities; and the next moment no longer knows what he has said or done."

The preceding *resumé* conveys a general idea of the precursory symptoms of insanity, as far as they relate to morbid cerebral, or mental excitement. This state of mind, however, is also premonitory of other affections of the great nervous centre, not associated with aberration of the ideas.

It frequently precedes ordinary attacks of *meningitis* and *cerebritis*. It is observed in the affections of the encephalon that occur in childhood, and the symptom is characteristic of those conditions of the brain so commonly associated with attacks of acute, as well as of low typhoid fever, producing great rapidity of the cerebral circulation, depression of the vital, and exhaustion of the nerve force.

A state of *mental excitement* is frequently precursory of apoplexy. For some days prior to an attack of this disease, the patient has been known to exhibit symptoms of unusual irritability and irascibility.

A gentleman, whose mind had been severely harassed by anxious business, complained for some period prior to an attack of apoplexy of odd sensations in his head. He said he felt as if his brain were a "lump of lead," and as if "thousands of insects were creeping over it." He had no headache. A week before being seized with serious cerebral symptoms he became extremely irritable, spoke angrily to his wife (the first occurrence of the kind in a long and happy wedded life), quarrelled with, and appeared disinclined to have the children about him. It was thought that some matter of business, unknown to his family, had worried him, or that he had experienced a serious pecuniary loss. On the day before his attack of cerebral hemorrhage, he showed symptoms of

acute mental excitement, which greatly alarmed his wife and
family.   On the following day, after a disturbed night, he rose
very early in the morning and entered his bath-room, and, about
half an hour afterwards, was found by his valet in a state of profound insensibility!   The pulse being scarcely perceptible, and
the action of the heart feeble, stimulants and restoratives were
immediately administered.   After the lapse of an hour, consciousness partially returned; he, however, died in the course of the
evening.   On the examination of the brain after death, a clot of
blood was found on the *corpus striatum*, with slight evidences of
softening in the right cerebral hemisphere.

A tradesman, ætat. forty-seven, fell from the top of an omnibus
in Oxford Street, injuring his head.   Symptoms of concussion
followed.   He continued in a state of semi-consciousness until
late in the evening, when he opened his eyes, gazed listlessly
about him, and, in a faint tone of voice, asked, " Where am I ?—
What has happened?"   In the course of a fortnight he was able to
resume his business.   About *twelve months* after this attack, a
marked difference was observed in his mind.   He became peevish,
quarrelsome, discharging his principal managing clerk for some
trifling inaccuracies.   A short time subsequently to this change
being observed, he had, whilst in his counting-house, an attack of
epilepsy.   His mind appeared clearer and more composed, after
recovering from the acute effects of this seizure, than it was previously.   He exhibited great self-command and acuteness in matters of business, and appeared to be less irritated by family affairs.
In about six weeks he showed symptoms of mental depression,
which were soon followed by *uncontrollable paroxysms of violent
and furious passion!*   His wife was much alarmed at his altered
mental state, considering that he was on the eve of an attack of
insanity.   In the course of the night he had a second epileptic
seizure.   He recovered from this fit, and the mind appeared once
more from under a dark cloud, and his natural kindliness of disposition and warm-heartedness again showed itself.   The change
in the state of his intellect, and altered condition of his affections
after each attack of epilepsy, was remarkable.   He had, during
the succeeding six months, *eleven* similar epileptic seizures, and in
one of these attacks, which was more of an apoplectic than of an
epileptic character, he died.   The epilepsy was always preceded
by great irritability and excitement, but without any appreciable

delusions. After death, the right hemisphere of the brain was found to be considerably indurated, and in the left hemisphere, near the seat of the injury, was found a small scirrhous tumor of the size of a pigeon's egg.

In one peculiar and often fatal type of insanity, known by the name of progressive, or "*General Paralysis of the Insane*," the premonitory stage is marked (in many, but not in all instances) by exalted, grand, and ambitious ideas, referring principally to wealth, social position, worldly honors, mental and physical capacity. For a long period, before any mental disorder is generally suspected, the ideas are observed to be only of an absurd and extravagant character. The patient talks of the amount of money he has made; of the success of his commercial speculations, his good fortune, extraordinary luck, and of the bright future in store for himself and family. He magnifies the amount of his daily or weekly receipts, whether realized in the practice of a profession, in trade, or in commerce. I have known this tendency simply to distort facts and look extravagantly at the bright side of everything, through an intensely magnified and highly colored, because *morbid* medium (when the actual circumstances of the party did not in the slightest degree justify such sanguine ideas), to exist for *five* or even *ten* years, before the mind presented any decided and recognized symptoms of alienation!

A gentleman, who died at the age of sixty-two, of general paralysis, for *seven* years previously to his being considered as insane, manifested a most extraordinary disposition to falsify and exaggerate everything with which he had to do. His want of a right appreciation of existing facts, his constant and singular untruthfulness, gave rise, among his relations, to much anxiety and distress of mind. Some of his most intimate friends became estranged from him in consequence of his gross want of veracity. As the disease of the brain progressed, his mind became perceptibly more disposed to indulge in wild, visionary, and illusory notions. He eventually imagined that he had discovered the philosopher's stone, the art of making gold, was possessed of great wealth, and had the coffers of the Bank of England at his disposal. A few months before his death, he was busily engaged in a scheme, exhibiting great arithmetical cleverness and ingenuity, for paying off the national debt, out of his own vast, but, alas! imaginary hoard of wealth!

In another case, the disease could be traced back for *ten* years, when the patient's habits, thoughts, and disposition were observed to undergo remarkable alterations, following, what was at that time thought to be, a severe *fainting* fit, but which, undoubtedly, was an *epileptic* seizure.   Previously to the attack of epilepsy, this gentleman was noted for being a prudent, cautious, careful, and unimaginative man.

A few days after the attack referred to, a marked change was observed in the patient's deportment and conversation.   He exhibited an unnatural flow of animal spirits, unusual buoyancy and elasticity of mind, and subsequently indulged in the most absurd, but still not irrational, or insane notions of grandeur and wealth. This condition of mind continued *for nearly a year*, without exciting any suspicion as to his real state of mental or bodily health. He then visited the United States of America.   During the voyage out he suffered greatly from sea-sickness, and his ideas (perhaps as a consequence) were more subdued, toned down, manner less restless, and his general conversation in a condition of healthy repose.   He remained in America for several years, indulging in many innocent oddities, vagaries, and eccentricities, but continuing, *apparently*, in healthy possession of his intellectual powers. He amused and busied himself, whilst there, in ascertaining the value of property that was offered for sale, talked of his wish to make investments in land and houses, and made himself, in a business manner, well acquainted with the particulars respecting several large tracts of waste land that were advertised to be sold. He returned to England (singular to relate) without committing *one act* of what might be termed insanity or even of extravagance. His wife could not be otherwise than diverted at the absurdly exaggerated and sometimes ludicrous tone of her husband's strangely wild and often flighty conversation, but never for one moment suspected that his mind was suffering from a phase of incipient alienation, or that he was afflicted with obscure disease of the brain !

A few months after his arrival in England, he had a second epileptic fit.   It was, however, transient in its character, and accompanied with but little muscular agitation or convulsion.   On his recovery from this attack, his mind manifested decided symptoms of aberration.   Under the influence of medical treatment, all signs of mental disorder rapidly disappeared, and to the astonishment of every one, he appeared to entirely recover ! A few months subsequently, the extravagant ideas again took possession of his mind. He proposed to abandon the pursuits of commerce in which he was engaged, and to study for the bar. He expressed a desire to enter one of the English universities, and selected Oxford for his *alma mater*. He talked wildly of what he should accomplish in his new profession ; of his capabilities of adroitly examining witnesses ; of his extraordinary knowledge of the law of evidence (never having read a law work !), of his magical powers of oratory, and marvellous gifts of elocution ! From this period the disease rapidly progressed, and he became paralytic and demented ! The brain revealed, after death, evidences of long-existing disorganization, particularly in its investing membranes. There was also considerable softening of one of the hemispheres, conjoined with atrophy of the convolutions.

CHAPTER IX.

STAGE OF MENTAL DEPRESSION.

In the early stage of insanity, the patient is at first seen to mope, he is then heard to complain of extreme *ennui*, and, subsequently, he becomes abstracted, moody, and sullen. Acute morbid melancholy afterwards manifests itself. This condition of mind often exists for some time before derangement of the perceptive faculties or mental delusions are recognized.

It is occasionally difficult to draw the line of demarcation between ordinary attacks of *ennui*, the more severe types of hypochondriasis, and the mental depression symptomatic of the commencement of insanity.

In these cases, so insidious is the advent, so imperceptible the stealthy march of this form of mental disorder, that it is often difficult to diagnose its existence, and to trace it to its origin.

With what poetic and psychological truth has our great dramatist delineated, in the character of Hamlet, the incipient symptoms, slow gradations, and almost inappreciable advances of the *æsthenic* type of insanity!

This state of mind often leads to suicide. There is, alas! in existence a frightful amount of unrecognized and untreated mental depression associated with suicidal impulses. The daily channels of communication convey to us this sad intelligence in language that does not admit of misconstruction. The melancholy history of one case recorded is but a faithful record of hundreds of others that are occurring within the range of our own vision. If the evidence generally adduced at the coroner's inquest is to be credited, in nearly *every case of suicide, cerebral disorder has exhibited itself, and the mind has been clearly and palpably deranged.* In many cases, the mental disorder had clearly existed for weeks, and, occasionally, for months, without giving rise to the suspicion of the presence of any dangerous degree of brain or psychical disturbance likely to lead to so disastrous an issue. There are few morbid mental conditions so fatal in their results as these apparently trifling, evanescent, and occasionally fugitive attacks of depression. They almost invariably (in certain temperaments) are associated with a disposition to self-destruction. I am never consulted in this type of case, without fully impressing upon the relatives and friends the importance of the most careful and uninterrupted vigilance. These slight ruffles on the surface, apparently unimportant attacks of mental despondency, and trifling paroxysms of morbid *ennui*, accompanied, as they frequently are, with intense weariness of life, a desire for seclusion, love of solitude, and longing for death, *are indicative of acute states of brain, and mind disorder*, and are fraught with fatal mischief to reason and to life! How much of this character of disordered mind not only escapes observation, but is subjected to no kind of medical treatment or supervision! Occasionally it may happen (but how rare is the occurrence!) that the unhappy suicide may have exhibited no appreciable symptoms of mental derangement; but even in these cases we should be cautious in concluding that perfect sanity existed at the time of the suicide.

It often occurs that a person is impelled to self-destruction by the overpowering and crushing influence of some *latent and concealed delusion*, that has for weeks, and perhaps months, been sitting like an incubus upon the imagination. Patients confess that they have been under the influence of monomaniacal ideas and terrible hallucinations for a long period without their existence being suspected even by their most intimate associates. "For six months," writes a patient, "I have never had the idea of suicide, night or day, out of mind. Wherever I go, an unseen demon pursues me, impelling me to self-destruction! My wife, friends, and children observe my listlessness and perceive my despondency, but they know nothing of the worm that is gnawing within." Is this not a type of case more generally prevalent than we imagine? May we not say of this unhappy man, with a mind tortured and driven to despair by a concealed hallucination, or unobserved delusion, urging him to the commission of suicide, as the only escape from the acuteness of his misery,

> " HE hears a voice WE cannot hear,
>   Which says, HE must not stay,
> HE sees a hand WE cannot see,
>   Which beckons HIM away?"

This morbid condition of the intelligence is commonly observed as one of the precursory signs of *organic* disease of the brain unallied with insanity. Acute softening, cerebral hemorrhage, general paralysis, and cerebral tumors, are occasionally seen in the early stage, associated with severe mental depression.

I have observed several cases of inflammatory, as well as white softening of the brain, preceded by great lowness of spirits, occasionally amounting to acute melancholia. In one case a gentleman who had lived, what is termed a hard life, showed symptoms of hypochondriasis, preceded at first by ordinary attacks of profound *ennui*. This was so opposed to his usual temperament that the alteration in his natural character was made the subject of observation. He suddenly became quite hipped, refused to go into society, and always appeared unhappy if any of his former associates called upon him. He became soon afterwards quite a recluse. This gentleman, after the lapse of some years, during which period his condition of physical and mental health underwent many changes and modifications, died of white softening of the brain. His state of mental depression, however, existed for some time before the sensor or motor powers gave evidence of disease. I have known cases of apoplexy preceded by great depression of spirits.

CHAPTER X.

STAGE OF ABERRATION.

INCIPIENT aberration may manifest itself in,

1. *The Intellectual Faculties.*
2. *The Perceptive Faculties.*
8. *The Moral Faculties.*

I have already alluded to the contests which so frequently take place in the mind (some extent off its balance) with impressions clearly of a morbid character, but not actually fixed and insane ideas. This is clearly an incipient stage of aberration.

THE INTELLECTUAL FACULTIES.—How obscure, gradually progressive, subtle, and insidious are the inappreciable approaches of insane thought! At what period does the exaggerated, false, and eccentric conception traverse the fatal boundary line separating the *sane* from the *deranged* mind, and become, instead of an erroneous notion, illogical conclusion, error of judgment, mistaken conviction, absurd and extravagant thought, a *bona fide* insane *delusion*, a morbid *creation* of the distempered and diseased imagination?

"An attentive observer, tracing the first period of the evolution of a fixed idea, witnesses one of the most curious spectacles imaginable. He sees a man, the prey of a disposition imposed by this malady, striving from time to time to rid himself of it, but ever falling back under its tyrannical influence, and constrained by the laws of his mind to seek for some form under which to give it a body and a definite existence. He will be seen successively to adopt, and to repel, the divers ideas which present themselves to him, and laboriously striving to deliver himself of a delirium which shall be the expression, the exact image, of an internal condition of which he himself, after all, suspects not the existence! This first phase in the evolution of the fixed idea, this gradual and progressive creation of delirium, constitutes the period of incubation of insanity."[1]

A man has received an offence, perhaps a series of offences, trifling in their character. His mind at first dwells slightly upon the fact: he then allows the impression to absorb the attention to a degree quite incommensurate with their importance, other trains of healthy thought being rigidly excluded from his mind. Eventually, these notions become extravagant and exaggerated. The injury which was, in the first instance, considered a trivial and insignificant one, assumes, however (as the mental disease progresses), grave and significant character in the estimation of the person whose mind is almost exclusively occupied in its morbid contemplation. The intellect at last yields to the pressure, and the general health becoming deranged, the idea which was, originally, only an extravagant conception, becomes a clearly manifested delusion; in other words, *a fixed and settled insane idea*, the insanity consisting, not in a creation of the fancy *de novo*, but in a morbid *exaggeration*, and insane *perversion*, of actually existing circumstances.

"It is the character of insanity not only to call up impressions which are entirely visionary, but also to *distort* and *exaggerate* those which are true, and *to carry them to consequences which they do not warrant in the estimation of a sound mind.*"[2]

Dr. Johnson has traced with the hand of a master, the insidious advances of deranged thought :—

"Some particular train of ideas fixed upon the mind, all other intellectual gratifications are rejected: the mind, in weariness or leisure, recurs constantly to the favorite conception, and feasts on the luscious falsehood, whenever it is offended with the bitterness of truth. By degrees, the reign of fancy is confirmed. She grows first imperious, and in time despotic. These fictions begin to operate as realities, false opinions fasten upon the mind, and life passes in dreams of rapture or of anguish."[3]

THE PERCEPTIVE FACULTIES.—The perceptive powers are often the first to yield to the influence of disease. A gentleman, who eventually became insane, and died, alas! by his own hand, for

[1] Falret.   [2] Abercrombie.   [3] Rasselas.

months before he yielded to the delusion that led to his confinement, and self-destruction, battled strongly and heroically with an illusion of the senses, which he was conscious had no existence apart from himself.

He often conversed with his wife upon the subject of his horrible phantasy, and "unreal mockery," she trying, by soothing expressions of devoted affection, and arguments addressed to his reason, to dissipate the terrible image that pursued him, like an evil eye, night and day. This gentleman's state of brain was not made a matter of investigation until his insanity was obviously declared. His reason and life would, in all probability, have been saved, had timely medical aid been obtained for his relief!

A lady, ætat. fifty, wife of a merchant, well educated, head large, temperament bilio-lymphatic, experienced several family misfortunes, which gave rise to much bodily ill-health, and to a restless and irritable state of mind. The first indication of actual delusion and insanity, was the appearance of a transient halo around whatever she was engaged in reading, and ultimately encircling every object she steadfastly regarded. Her false perceptions became subsequently more numerous. She walked with difficulty, in consequence of the impression which she had, that a smooth surface was an irregular one; that deep chasms constantly occurred in the floor, over which it was necessary for her to stride, that the height of one step of the stair was greater than that of another, or that she tottered on the brink of a precipice. Noises, which were scarcely perceptible to others, annoyed her very much, both from their supposed loudness and harshness, as well as from their resembling voices addressed to her in conversation. Her language was likewise affected. She had a difficulty in recalling expressions, and misapplied or misplaced such as she used. Her memory of facts was much impaired. She was not cleanly in her habits, or careful as to the arrangement of dress, &c. These symptoms were occasionally entirely absent, when she regained her original acuteness and intelligence, but even when they were present, and inspired her with fear and anxiety, she doubted the reality of the sensations she received, and appealed to those around her for confirmation and assistance. While in bed, or resting recumbent, she was rarely annoyed by these delusions, but upon getting up, or upon any sudden change of position, she was surrounded by luminous spots, vacillating in her gait, and was for an interval, incapable of attending to any external object, or of disabusing her mind of those perceptions, or of the fear and agitation which they created. This circumstance led her former medical attendant to suspect organic disease of the brain. She complained of exquisite pain across the lower part of the forehead and temples ; and so intense were her sufferings that she was unable to bear the weight, or even the touch of glasses which she was accustomed to wear.[1]

The mind occasionally exhibits evidence of aberration in the precursory stage of *cerebral*, as well as *mental* disease, particularly in congestive and inflammatory conditions of the brain and its meninges. Illusions of the senses, as well as delusions of the mind, are sometimes noticed among the incipient symptoms of acute affections of the encephalon.

A state of mental terror and alarm, vague, shadowy, and undefined notions of approaching evil, very frequently precede actual aberration of intellect, the patient imagining that some dreadful, inexplicable, and mysterious doom is impending, or that some serious catastrophe is about to occur.

A gentleman, a few days previously to an attack of apoplexy, could not dispossess his mind of the idea, that he had committed a grave *moral* offence, for which he was to be tried in a court of law. He could not be reasoned out of this delusion.

In another case, the patient was subject to distressing phantasms. These symptoms have been observed as precursory of acute softening of the brain, as well as of cerebral hemorrhage. A patient conceived, for many weeks prior to an apoplectic seizure, that he was pursued by a spectre.

Inflammation of the brain is often preceded by a perversion of the sense of smell, and illusions of sight and touch. Bouillard, Parent Duchatelet, and Martinet, relate several interesting cases illustrative of these phenomena.

An eminent artist died of softening of the brain. The cerebral symptoms exhibited themselves several years previously to the attack in the form of flashes of light before the eyes,—and to these were afterwards added, pains in the head, and diminished distinctness of vision. This last symptom gradually increased till his sight was totally destroyed. The morbid phenomena, however, which chiefly annoyed this unfortunate gentleman consisted in a

---

[1] " Phrenological Journal," vol. xiv, pp. 77–8.

series of the most dazzling images, perpetually playing upon the optical apparatus, by day and by night. Their brightness was unspeakably distressing. Sometimes they would assume the forms of angels with flaming swords, every motion of which seemed, like an electric flash, to blind the eye and sear the brain by the intensity of their light. The forms and shades, however, of these spectral images were perpetually changing, but without any mitigation of the sufferings which they produced. With the exception of some irritability of temper, there was not the slightest affection of the intellectual powers. The memory, imagination, and the judgment were unimpaired. He was led about the streets by one of his servants; and he attended to all matters where his sight was not engaged, with the greatest punctuality. The eyes themselves presented no physical appearance of disease.

The symptoms above-mentioned were mitigated, from time to time, by counter-irritation to the nape of the neck, leeches to the temples, and aperient and diuretic medicines. In the spring of 1835, however, he was seized with all the usual symptoms of apoplexy. He lay in bed in a motionless and insensible state. The pupils were dilated, and the power of speech paralyzed. To the astonishment of his medical attendants, he rallied from this condition of severe cerebral disorder; and, after a few weeks, he was able to walk to the city, and transact business as usual! But the spectral images, of dazzling and exquisitely painful brightness, returned, with, if possible, increased intensity.

In the month of August, he was suddenly seized again with the apoplectic symptoms above-mentioned, and, notwithstanding the same means were employed as on the former occasion, he died at the end of three or four days from the commencement of the apoplectic invasion.

The body was examined on the day after his death. There was nothing unusual in the membranes of the brain. The right lateral ventricle contained nearly two ounces of clear fluid. The left ventricle was occupied by a series of hydatid-like cysts of various sizes, and filled with fluids of various consistencies and colors. This cluster sprung from the floor of the ventricle, by a kind of peduncle, and penetrated into every sinuosity of the cavity, pushing its branches anteriorly, so as to pass over and before the thalamus nervi optici of that side, and even into the opposite hemisphere of the brain, destroying those portions interfering with its march.

Both thalami were reduced to a pulp, as was, indeed, the whole of the anterior lobes of the brain, which would scarcely bear the slightest handling without falling into a state of deliquescence. The optic nerves were pressed upon by the cystic or hydatid mass, and reduced to little more than the size of threads, and these of very soft consistence. There was no change in the coats or humors of the eye.

The most remarkable phenomenon in the above melancholy case, was the intensity of brightness which always accompanied the spectral images. Whatever were their shapes, the dazzling and painful splendor never forsook them. These symptoms rendered his life, for some years, a scene of dreadful suffering.

It was considered remarkable that the intellectual faculties should have remained entire, while the anterior lobes of the brain were undergoing the process of softening which they displayed on dissection! "Did this *ramollissement* take place," asks the narrator of the case, "during the three or four days of apoplexy prior to death? If it existed long before the fatal event, there will be some difficulty in accounting for the integrity of the intellectual faculties up to the time of the apoplectic seizure. Was the serous effusion into the right ventricle the cause of the apoplexy? or the consequence of it? or was it a gradual accumulation, and not mainly instrumental in the final catastrophe? What was the cause of the first attack of apoplexy, and why did he recover from it?"[1]

A farmer in the neighborhood of Edinburgh, accustomed to drink freely, was invited to the funeral of a friend. He took a dram before he left home, and another at the house of his deceased friend. He had some of his acquaintances at dinner, with whom he continued to carouse until late at night. On the following morning, he imagined he heard five hundred people talking at once. He compared what he heard to the confusion of tongues at Babel. Portending the utmost danger from this sensation, he hurried across the farm-yard, and desired the surgeon who attended his family to be sent for without delay, and soon afterwards he became insensible. When the surgeon came, he bled him freely, and sent to Edinburgh for a physician. When that gentleman arrived, the patient was a little relieved, but still he labored under considerable

[1] Recorded by Dr. James Johnson, in the "Medico-Chirurgical Review."

stupor; he was again bled, and a third time next morning; and in a day or two, he felt himself restored to good health.[1]

A lady, a few days previously to an attack of paralysis, was thrown into a state of great terror by an apparition that she had fancied appeared to her in the night.

A young child, a short period before being seized with acute meningitis, imagined that a brother who had been dead for several years reappeared to him. In a case of fatal hydrocephalus, the first symptom that directed attention to the state of the child's brain, was a sudden expression of intense alarm which he exhibited, occurring during the evening, arising from an impression that an apparition was in the room, and near the bed. In another case an attack of meningitis was ushered in by an illusion of the senses, the patient fancying that the ghost of a deceased relative was gliding about the room!

Morgagni mentions the case of a man who, working at night in a cesspool attached to a hospital, suffered from an hallucination. He fancied he saw a spectre clothed in white. On his death, which quickly supervened, it was discovered that he was laboring under venous congestion, and cerebral softening.

"Some months ago," says Dr. Alderson, "I attended a patient who had been attacked during a voyage from America, with violent headache. He was relieved by the formation of an abscess beneath the integuments of the skull; his breathing was somewhat affected by other tumors which had formed in the throat. He complained of having fatiguing dreams, and even of dreaming when awake. A short time afterwards he told me that for the space of an hour or two he thought he saw his wife and family, although convinced by his reason that they were in America. The impression on his mind was so strong, and the conversation he had held with his son so circumstantial and important, that he could not resist telling it in all its details to his friends on the following day. He also desired to be informed if his wife and family had not arrived from America, and whether they were not in the same house. I was sent for a second time; he quickly perceived that he was considered deranged, when, turning towards me, he inquired if his disease could induce a belief in spectres, apparitions, and figures? 'Until now,' said he, 'I had no faith

---

[1] "Cases of Apoplexy and Lethargy." By J. Cheyne, M.D. p. 83.

in all the stories of this character.' He knew that he was perfectly sane, and that his friends also acknowledged him to be so, with a mind as strong as it had ever been.

" Having explained to him the nature and cause of his visions, and told him that they would cease with his bodily sufferings, both he and his friends grew composed. But the phantoms became more and more importunate, until he could not make up his mind to retire to rest, because he was immediately harassed by the souls of the dead, or visited by persons disagreeable to him. Having changed his room, the visions ceased for some time; but he soon perceived his friends of the New World pictured as on a piece of polished metal.

" Designedly occupying myself with a book, I detected him mentally conversing with them, and at times evidently imagining that I also saw and heard them. When he looked away from the polished bar, he talked sensibly on religion, medicine, and politics. At length he changed his residence, when the purulent matter being discharged, his condition was ameliorated. He is now convalescent, and entirely relieved of his phantoms."[1]

Dr. Hibbert relates the particulars of the following interesting case, which he says the learned and accomplished Dr. Gregory, of Edinburgh, used to refer to in his lectures :—

" A patient of some rank having requested the doctor's advice, made the following extraordinary statement of his complaint: ' I am in the habit,' he said, ' of dining at five, and exactly as the hour arrives I am subjected to the following painful visitation. The door of the room, even when I have been weak enough to bolt it, which I have sometimes done, flies wide open; an old hag, like one of those who haunt the heath of Forres, enters with a frowning and incensed countenance, comes straight up to me with every demonstration of spite and indignation which could characterize her who haunted the merchant Abudah in the oriental tale; she rushes upon me, says something, but so hastily that I cannot discover the purport, and then strikes me a severe blow with her staff. I fall from my chair in a swoon, which is of longer or shorter endurance. To the recurrence of this apparition I am daily subjected, and such is my new and singular complaint.' Doctor Gregory immediately asked whether his patient had invited

[1] "Edinburgh Medical and Surgical Journal," vol. vi, p. 291.

17

any one to sit with him when he expected such a visitation? He was answered in the negative. The nature of the complaint, he said, was so singular, it was so likely to be imputed to fancy, or even to mental derangement, that he had shrunk from communicating the circumstance to any one. 'Then,' said the Doctor, 'with your permission I will dine with you to-day *tête-à-tête*, and we will see if your malignant old woman will venture to join our company.' The patient accepted the proposal with hope and gratitude, for he had expected ridicule rather than sympathy. They met at dinner, and Dr. Gregory, who suspected some nervous disorder, exerted his powers of conversation, well known to be of the most varied and brilliant character, to keep the attention of his host engaged, and prevent him from thinking of the approach of the fated hour to which he was accustomed to look forward with so much terror. He succeeded in his purpose better than he had hoped. The hour of six came almost unnoticed, and it was hóped might pass away without any evil consequence; but it was scarce a moment struck, when the owner of the house exclaimed, in an alarmed voice, 'The hag comes again!' and dropped back in his chair in a swoon, in the way he had himself described. These periodical shocks were clearly established to arise from a tendency to apoplexy, and after the brain was relieved by the abstraction of a small quantity of blood, the patient entirely recovered."

A gentleman, immediately previous to being seized with epilepsy, imagined he saw a little old woman, in a red cloak, run up to him and give him a severe blow on the head.

A gentleman who was subject for nine years to epilepsy, previous to his attack was, as he expressed it, suddenly seized with a peculiar train of thought, which was not intelligible to him, but caused him intense anxiety. The ideas were always of the same character, and whilst he was in the act of making an effort to disembarrass himself of them, the paroxysm of epilepsy took place.

The following cases, as recorded by Dr. Devay (of Lyons) constitute good illustrations of those psychical states which so frequently precede and accompany brain affections :—

"I have known a man, aged fifty-seven, who having up to that time led a grave and even austere life, abandoned himself to the pursuit of amusements unsuited to his age, and was a few months after seized with sudden and complete apoplexy (*apoplexie fou-*

droyante). A man, most estimable for mental endowments, and for the qualities of his heart, called one day to converse with me on subjects not relating to his health. His conversation was clear, nothing morbid was indicated in his gait, but he had for a long time complained of inaptitude for work. Whilst I was occupied in writing a letter, I saw him rise, rummage a drawer in my room, and open a note. This act, on the part of a person of the most polite and discreet habits, struck me forcibly. I connected it with two other circumstances which were known to me. During the revolution of February, this gentleman, holding an important post in the administration, had engaged, from the most disinterested and praiseworthy views, in public agitation, from which his mind had received a strong impression. Three months afterwards the patient lost his sight, after attacks of violent headache, and subsequently died with all the symptoms of cerebral softening.

" A complete change in the character of the ideas (when not the result of advanced age), if manifested suddenly, and when it cannot be traced to the action of moral influences, is suspicious *quoad* the state of the mind and brain. I knew a young physician who exhibited this phenomenon in a very marked manner, and who, a short time after, was seized with general paralysis. At the time of my acquaintance with him, three years previously, he was very free in his assertions, and inclined to exaggerate, but he had become subsequently discreet and wary in his speech. His former condition, and the medium in which he had lived, showed sufficiently that this change could not be the effect of a progressive amendment. I therefore considered that there was some latent disease of the brain, and my opinion was ultimately fully confirmed."[1]

PERVERSIONS OF THE MORAL SENSE.—Insanity, and other forms of cerebral disease, often manifest themselves in the early stage by aberrations and perversions of the moral sense. For some time prior to the development of derangement of mind, or disease of the brain, patients have been known (contrary to their usual habits), to indulge in gross sensual excesses, to exhibit states of moral decadence, weakened and paralyzed volition; to be guilty of acts of private and public indecency, dishonesty, debauchery, and beastly intemperance. These symptoms occasionally exist for years, before insanity has clearly declared itself.

[1] " Gazette Médicale de Paris," January, 1851.

A lady, of good family and of affluent circumstances, accompanied by her maid, entered the shop of a fashionable jeweller at the west-end of London. The lady, as well as other members of her family, were in the habit, for years, of dealing with the tradesman referred to. After examining many articles of jewelry, she left the shop without purchasing anything. Soon after her arrival home, the master of the shop called at the house, and requested an interview with the husband of the lady. This was at once complied with. He then informed him that his wife had been to his shop, and had, as he suspected, abstracted a valuable diamond bracelet. The matter was immediately investigated, and the suspicion of the tradesman proved to be correct. The bracelet was found and returned to its owner; he, in the true spirit of a liberal and humane man, affirming to the distressed husband, that it was his firm belief that the circumstance had arisen either in a mistake, or was the result of a temporary fit of alienation of mind. No one acquainted with the character of the lady could, for one moment, believe that she had (whilst in full and unclouded possession of her senses) committed a deliberate act of felony! Such an idea was too preposterous to be, for a moment, entertained. This unhappy episode suggested an investigation, and, to the great astonishment of her husband and all the members of her family, a number of diamond rings, valuable bracelets, gold chains, &c., were found in her possession, of which no account could be given. About nine months after this affair, this lady's conduct became so remarkably and patently singular, that, for the first time, her husband began to suspect the existence of aberration of mind. Her mental disorder exhibited itself in a disposition to pilfer everything she could lay her hands upon. The articles so stolen were most cleverly concealed in various parts of her dress, in beds, and in parts of the house not generally frequented by the family.

Such was the state of the patient's mind when I was first consulted. I had no doubt as to the character of the case. It was my opinion that other and more decided symptoms of insanity would, in a short time, be observed. In three months from my first seeing this patient, her mind exhibited decided indications of aberration, rendering it necessary for her to be removed from home. Her mental health was re-established in about eighteen months.

The wife of a respectable tradesman, for twelve months before her mind was imagined to be disordered, was repeatedly in the habit of entering her husband's shop and stealing small sums of money from the till. With this she purchased a number of useless articles of dress, with which her wardrobe was crammed. She had shoes, gloves, petticoats, silk and satin dresses, for which she had no use; in fact, which she never wore, or intended to wear. She had a mania for stealing, secreting, and purchasing useless articles of dress quite unsuitable for a person in her station of life. This patient eventually exhibited religious hallucinations, and, under a delusion that she had committed the unpardonable sin, made an attempt upon her life.

A lady, well known in fashionable life, was repeatedly detected in the act of purloining articles of value from her friends. When she returned home from a dinner party or a ball, her maid invariably found several pocket-handkerchiefs and fans concealed about her person. She could not resist the temptation of picking and stealing. Her family sometimes suspected that there was some disorder of the intellect, but no medical advice was obtained until she exhibited decided symptoms of morbid mental excitement, accompanied with clearly manifested delusions.

A young gentleman, connected with the army, committed numerous petty acts of theft, which for some time he cunningly contrived to conceal from those about him. He was eventually detected in stealing a bottle of champagne at a time when he had a superabundance of this wine in his possession. His conduct was made the subject of formal inquiry. Many of his friends were of opinion that the young gentleman was not altogether of sane mind, and, in his defence, this plea was raised. It was proved by his servant that he had for some time been in the habit of walking about his room at night, frequently talking to himself, and laughing loudly at his own thoughts. He was occasionally found in a moody and abstracted state. He would sit for several hours staring at vacancy. At times he was unreasonably irritable, particularly on occasions when great command of temper and freedom from all passion were essentially important. On these, and other grounds, he was honorably acquitted of the criminal charge, but, considering his mental condition, his family were advised to remove him from the army. This gentleman died six years afterwards of disease of the brain, supposed to be softening, but the fact could not be positively ascertained, as no *post-mortem* examination was permitted.

A clerk, holding a confidential position in a provincial bank, was accused of repeated acts of theft. The evidence against him was conclusive. On searching his lodgings, nearly all the missing money was found, carefully concealed in the lining of some old clothes, apparently worn out and useless. He did not deny the accusation. He treated the matter with a nonchalance of so peculiar a character, that those occupied in the inquiry (which was strictly of a private character, as the party in question was connected by marriage with one of the firm) were disposed to question the soundness of his intellect. He was not in necessitous circumstances, his salary being a liberal one. Independently of this fact, his wife had a fair income, which she placed at his disposal. His habits of life were of a simple character. He was believed to be a most conscientious man, being scrupulously exact in all his dealings with his tradesmen. On one occasion he found an inaccuracy in an account that had been rendered to him by his wine merchant, and he at once pointed out the mistake, and immediately sent a check in payment of the extra amount due. The gentleman was obliged to resign his appointment in the bank. The private jury selected to investigate the matter affirmed that they *suspected* mental alienation, but declined expressing any authoritative opinion on the subject. Two years subsequently, the case came formally and professionally under my observation. At this time, the mind was manifestly disordered. He believed himself to be a person of rank, and destined by the Almighty to establish a state of religious equality throughout the whole world. The treatment I advised to be adopted in this case, after the lapse of a few months, appeared to be promoting his cure. He suddenly, however, manifested great mental confusion and excitement, and ultimately suddenly died in an apoplectic fit. There was found, after death, great thickening as well as adhesions of the *dura mater* to the skull, with opacity of the arachnoid. There was a slight patch of softening in the left hemisphere, which contained a clot of extravasated blood of the size of a small bird's egg.

I have had under my care a lady who invariably stole whatever she could lay her hands upon during certain uterine changes, and another patient always manifests the same propensity at the period of utero-gestation.

"A person high in office," says Dr. Brierre de Boismont, "had performed the duties of his station up to the time when I was consulted, and yet the details which were furnished to me by his wife left no doubt that his moral and affective faculties had been for some time impaired. From having been generous and honest, he had for more than six years exhibited great sordid avarice and unbridled licentiousness. With the progress of the disease, his avarice was manifested in mean actions; he refused to pay his debts, maintaining that he had already done so, and even purloined objects from the houses of his acquaintances. Until the last-named acts were committed, no one had suspected that his mind was disordered. Some time after, I was called in consultation to see a retired public officer, whose thefts had made much noise some years previously. The particulars with which I was furnished regarding this patient inclined me to believe that he was laboring under the premonitory symptoms of general paralysis. I felt certain that such was the fact. On my introduction to the patient, the first words that he uttered fully established the correctness of my anticipations. His delinquencies had been observed eight years previously. His mental alienation was only recognized a few months ago."[1]

A gentleman, whilst on a voyage from the West Indies to England, attempted to commit a criminal assault upon one of the female passengers! Up to the period of the sailing of the vessel he had shown no observable symptoms of mental derangement. His friends in the West Indies had never in this case *suspected* insanity. For some weeks, however, prior to his sailing for England, he had been exposed to great mental labor and anxiety, having to settle and arrange a complicated matter of business.

At the time of the commission of the assault, his conduct was singularly inexplicable and irrational. The offence was perpetrated in the broad light of day, at a time and under circumstances rendering detection, exposure, and punishment, prompt, certain, and inevitable! For the rest of the voyage he was closely confined to his cabin, under strict surveillance. On his arrival in London, *he was pronounced to be clearly in an insane state!* I subsequently saw the case, and as far as I was enabled to unravel its history, was satisfied that the act of immorality of which he had been guilty during the voyage was the *first* demonstration of his insanity.

[1] "Gazette Médicale de Paris," 1847, p. 393.

A young gentleman, holding a responsible situation in a banking establishment of repute, was walking in the neighborhood of Regent Street on a Sunday afternoon, when he suddenly committed an act of gross indecency. He was taken into custody. When asked for an explanation of his singular conduct, he appeared like a man in a state of delirium, and could offer no satisfactory excuse for his outrageous act. His previous character was unimpeachable, he never having been known to be guilty of any palpable immorality ; in fact, he was universally admitted, by those who were most intimately acquainted with him, to be a person of great purity of thought, and strict propriety of conduct. He was, however, accused by the police of the offence, but before the matter came under the cognizance of a court of law, his mind exhibited decided symptoms of disorder, and he was consequently released from the hands of the civil authorities, and properly placed under medical treatment and restraint. Was the immoral offence the *first* OVERT *act of insanity*, or did the mind become deranged in consequence of the dread of exposure, disgrace, and punishment ? I am inclined to the former hypothesis. It appeared that there was insanity, to a considerable extent, in the family, and that this gentleman had received, when a boy, a severe injury to the head, from the effects of which he was supposed never to have recovered. It was discovered that for some days previously to the commission of the indecent offence, he had been observed to have been singular in his manner, and was heard to complain of headache, restless and disturbed nights.

A young lady, up to the age of nineteen, comported herself with the greatest decorum and propriety, evidencing in her conversation a high moral tone. Between the age of nineteen and twenty, she had several attacks of acute hysteria, but was soon, apparently, restored to health. She then became pensive and sad, retiring often to her own room, where she was often found bathed in tears. She exhibited a great indisposition to associate with the family, or to converse with those about her. Apart from these symptoms she manifested no positive sign of mental aberration.

With a view of rousing her from a state of recognized mental torpor, she was taken by a member of the family to a public ball, and it was whilst there, and in the act of dancing with a comparative stranger, that she first exhibited, by a marked and painfully loose character of action and conversation, unequivocal symptoms either of grave moral depravity, or of serious mental disorder. The gentleman with whom she was dancing observing something peculiarly wild in her physiognomy, had his suspicions awakened as to her condition, and had no difficulty in arriving at a right solution of the character of the case. He lost no time in delicately mentioning the matter to the relative who accompanied the young lady to the ball, and she was immediately taken home. On the following day she became *acutely insane*, all her delusions and conversations having reference to a morbidly exalted state of the uterine functions.

"A woman, aged forty-two, for a year and a half gradually fell into a state denoting general softening of the brain, manifesting almost entire blindness, inability to walk, and semi-imbecility of intellect. Two years ago she felt severe and almost constant pain in the head: her general health was in other respects perfectly good and her intellect clear. *Three* years previously, this woman, though possessed of an ample competency, *committed a petty theft at a fair*. This was the first symptom of her approaching cerebral disease.[1]

[1] Related by Dr. Brierre de Boismont.

CHAPTER XI.

IMPAIRMENT OF MIND.

I PROPOSE to consider this subject in the following order :—

1. *General Weakness of Mind.*
2. *Morbid Phenomena of Attention.*
3. *Morbid Phenomena of Memory.*

GENERAL WEAKNESS OF MIND.—The intellect often presents evidences of general prostration and debility, long anteriorly to any serious disorder of the brain being diagnosed, or even suspected. This condition of cerebral lassitude, mental sluggishness, psychical weakness and impairment, is, in many of its features, analogous to the torpor of mind that so frequently supervenes upon certain acute forms of bodily disease, particularly those of a febrile character implicating the nervous functions.

In this state of mental ill-health, the patient is conscious of a want of brain tone, sluggish action of mind, and of a deviation from his normal condition of intellectual acuteness, activity, and vigor. He is painfully sensible of feeling mentally *below par*, and recognizes his inability to use efficiently his powers of mind. He suffers from a torpid state of the intellect, a psychical *malaise* unfitting him for any kind or degree of cerebral work. The effort to think is irksome and painful, causing, if persevered in, vertigo, headache, painful confusion of thought, and acute mental depression.

In this condition of nervous exhaustion, the patient is incapable of exercising, for any lengthened period, continuity of thought, and is at times quite unable to think at all. This mental listlessness, prostration, and apathy, disqualify him from any occupation requiring the active operation of the intellectual powers. He throws aside his favorite books, and even the newspapers, formerly the source of so much pleasure, become devoid of interest, and even distasteful to him.   He then neglects his ordinary vocation, feeling in mind *blasé*, and only able to sit quietly in a state of gloomy abstraction in his room, or saunter about the house or streets in a condition of dreamy reverie.   I have often witnessed these symptoms consequent upon an overtaxed and unduly exercised mind.

Men, naturally of the most active understandings, of a high order of intelligence, and capable, when in health, of a considerable degree of sustained and vigorous intellectual labor, have been reduced to this sad state of pyschical impairment, and "precocious senility," as the result of anxiety, or as the effect of an excessive and severe cerebral and mental strain.

Under these circumstances the mind is easily fatigued.   This condition of failing intellect is recognized by the difficulty which the person experiences in preserving intact the sequence of ideas and chain of thought.   The memory either wanders, or is vague and incoherent in its associations.   All power of healthy psychical combination is either lost, or greatly impaired.   The mind has no fixed hold upon its conceptions, and in consequence of an enfeeblement of the will, and weakened power of attention, the ideas are influenced by the most casual and accidental circumstances.   In general terms, all balancing or co-ordinating psychical power appears to be gone.[1]

---

[1] Among the incipient symptoms of softening of the brain, and apoplexy, are occasionally observed a torpor, and prostration of intellect, exhibited in an inability to undertake any kind and degree of mental work. The patient complains of a deficiency of psychical power, an exhausted state of the nervous energy, and of a want of *vis*, the brain appearing to have lost its healthy tone, and stamina.

M. Gendrin says, " Apoplectic attacks are often preceded for some days by a difficulty in executing intellectual work, by an incapacity for unusual attention, by an extraordinary irascibility, by a morbid weakness which exaggerates impressions, and produces terrors without a cause, or by unreasonable anxiety concerning ourselves or those related to us.ᵃ

These premonitory symptoms are not demonstrable in every case of cerebral hemorrhage, for many patients appear capable of severe brain or mind work up to the moment immediately preceding the apoplectic or paralytic fit, but in many cases this conscious diminution of vigor of brain and impairment of mind are important premonitory signs of approaching acute paralytic and apoplectic seizures.   The symp-

---

ᵃ " Traité Philos. de Méd. Prac."   Tom. I, p. 487.

This morbid condition of intellect is generally associated with, and, in a great measure, dependent upon, a depressed, debilitated, and exhausted state of the vital and nerve force. The blood is impoverished in consequence of being deprived of some of its important organic elements, and the whole system suffers from *anæmia*. The countenance assumes a pallid, haggard, lifeless, and exsanguine aspect. The assimilative functions are disordered, and the patient sometimes becomes seriously emaciated. Such is often the physical state of those whose minds have been prematurely exhausted. This phase of mental and bodily ill-health, in the majority of cases, speedily yields to the judicious administration of stimulants and blood tonics associated with appropriate moral treatment, provided no serious *structural* mischief has commenced in the brain.

The symptoms, however, previously detailed, are occasionally precursory of formidable attacks of organic disease of the brain, and are to be viewed, in some cases, as pathognomonic of the existence of cerebral tumors, softening, abscess, induration, and other formidable types of encephalic disorganization.

A gentleman, aged fifty-four, who died of softening of the brain, associated with hemiplegia, had for nearly twelve months previously to his loss of motor power, complained of no other symptom than painful prostration of mind. He had the greater portion of his life been actively engaged as the principal of a large academy, having under his scholastic supervision nearly sixty boys. Being a strictly conscientious man, and of an anxious temperament, he was always in a state of feverish excitement and painful apprehension lest he should fail in the discharge of the serious and responsible duties devolving upon him. His mind was thus kept in an unceasing condition of mental inquietude and perturbation. Under this severe amount of cerebral pressure and mental anxiety, he was conscious, as he admitted at the time to his medical attendant, of *his mind gradually fading away from him*. He eventually became quite incapable of personally superintending his establishment. On one occasion, fancying that his intellect had in a great mea-

tom, however, is present in other states of disease of the brain. Should this condition of mind be associated with giddiness, headache, depressed spirits, aberration or impairment of vision, or a slight sensation of numbness (even if circumscribed) in any part of the body, the patient may well be anxious as to the state of his cerebral health.

sure recovered its original strength, he entered the school, and occupied himself with his usual duties. He, however, soon found that he was quite incapable of directing his attention for five minutes continuously to any one subject connected with the business of tuition, and he immediately retired to his own private room, and seating himself in a chair, burst into a flood of tears, exclaiming, in wild despair, " *My mind is gone! altogether gone !*" In this case no symptom of *physical* disease of the brain was detected until *twelve* months anteriorly to death! The condition of mental impairment existed uninterruptedly for a period of four years prior to the attack of hemiplegia, which occurred shortly before death. In another case a solicitor was obliged to retire for a period of five years altogether from professional business, in consequence of an enfeebled state of mind, unassociated with aberration of intellect, or lesion of the sensor or motor power. This gentleman acknowledged that for *thirty* years he had not been for seven continuous . days absent from the anxious and responsible duties of his office! Two years prior to his decease, symptoms of cerebral amaurosis were recognized, and he nearly lost all visual power. During this time, he was subject to acute attacks of headache, accompanied with great depression of spirits, and distressing paroxysms of extreme nausea, and sometimes of vomiting. He suddenly, one day after dinner, became hemiplegic, and in a few weeks died. A tumor was found in close proximity to the optic thalamus, undoubtedly interfering with the special functions of this ganglion. In a third case, an officer who had gone successfully through several East India campaigns, became gradually imbecile. All the faculties of the mind simultaneously were debilitated and deteriorated. This did not manifest itself at first in a loss of any particular mental function, such as the memory or attention, but the whole powers of the mind appeared to gradually fade away, and succumb to a mysterious, inexplicable, and destructive influence. This patient continued in a chronic condition of imbecility for many years. After death, the brain was found in a state of sad disorganization. The *dura mater* and *tunica arachnoidea* were much thickened, and on the former was discovered a considerable extent of tubercular deposition. The *calvarium* was indurated (the *diploe* being entirely obliterated), the brain much atrophied, and in some portions, in a softened state. In this instance, there were no delusions or other symptoms of aberration until *a year and a half* before death.[1]

In the early stage of cerebral or general paralysis, the patient often *acts* as if he had (mentally) lost all confidence in himself. He rarely acknowledges that such is the fact, but exhibits in his conversation and deportment evidences of a state of enfeebled mind, paralyzed or vacillating will. These symptoms I have known to exist for years antecedently to the development of any clearly manifested sign of disease of the brain or disorder of the mind. A gentleman, who eventually died of cerebral paralysis, *two years* before there was any recognition of disease of the brain, was reduced to a state of complete childish and slavish dependence upon those about him. It was an unusual occurrence for him to write a letter, or reply to one. His wife or eldest son generally discharged these duties for him. Letters addressed to him on important matters of business remained sometimes unopened for several days. In consequence of this neglect, his wife was in the habit, occasionally, of searching his pockets, and when letters with unbroken seals were put into his hand, he merely exclaimed, with apparent surprise, "Oh dear me, how careless I have been!"

There was no obvious want of capacity, neither were there marked symptons of imbecility in this case, until the expiration of the period previously specified. Strangers never observed in this patient any diminution of mental vigor, but those in constant and loving association with him, and well acquainted with his previous condition of mind, were painfully observant of the gradual and insidious advances of his brain disorder and mental decrepitude. They could not but notice his singular and unnatural want of interest in his professional affairs, shown by his absenting himself from chambers and neglecting other important duties. His marked indifference to his children, and apparent loss of affection for his wife, without exhibiting any insane *alienation* of feeling,

[1] When speaking of the lesions of intelligence that precede or accompany diseases of the brain of an apoplectic type, Andral remarks (when recapitulating the morbid psychical phenomena observable in cerebral affections): " Many patients preserve all the clearness and strength of their intelligence up to the moment of the apoplectic attack. In others, there are observed, a shorter or longer time before this period, some changes in the intellectual faculties; sometimes they are, as it were, benumbed. Many, on the contrary, manifest an extraordinary degree of excitement. Some lose their memory; there are moments when they know neither where they are, what they do, or what they say."—*Andral's Clinique Médicale.*

was also a significant symptom, *quoad* his state of mind, caressed his wife and children with his usual warmth of aff(*when his attention was directed specially to them by others, and he was twitted for his coolness and neglect.* He was in the habit of sitting for hours, turning listlessly over the pages of a number of favorite books, and looking through portfolios of engravings and drawings, without apparently knowing what was occupying his attention. During the whole of this time he was fully capable of discussing, when the subject was suggested to him by others, the merits of any particular book or painting (for he was a man of great taste, and had a large and valuable library, and many first-class works of art in his house), but associated with this apparent but factitious power of concentrating his mind to, and considering any given subject, his intellectual brightness and vigor were gradually fading into the dark regions of imbecility.[1]

I cite the preceding cases with a view of establishing that serious fatal structural disease of brain may occasionally be preceded *by no other symptom than loss of mental power.* Undoubtedly many instances occur of great impairment of mind resulting from exhaustion of the psychical and nerve force, quite unconnected with apparent organic change in the structure of the brain.

It is occasionally the duty of the physician to see and prescribe for such cases. They often, alas! baffle his best and most assiduous attempts at cure. Occasionally, however, it is his pleasure to realize the beneficial effect of continuity of remedial treatment in restoring the mind to its original vigor, and that, too, in cases often justifying the most unfavorable termination.

In the preceding illustrations of that form of mental weakness, clearly arising from an abnormal exercise of the mind, and preternatural exhaustion of the vital energies, the *nutrition* of the brain is, in many instances, manifestly and often seriously impaired.

---

[1] After death, the relations found secreted in the pockets of the gentleman's clothes and in the house, a number of letters relating to important matters of business, unopened, and of course unreplied to. Many of these letters were of old date, and some contained remittances of money. One envelope contained a Bank of England note for 100*l.*, which had been transmitted fourteen months previously, and which was supposed to have been stolen or lost. At this time none of the family suspected anything wrong with his brain or mind.

CHAPTER XII.

MORBID PHENOMENA OF ATTENTION.

THIS subject will be analyzed as follows :—

1. *Impairment of Attention.*
2. *Heightened or Exalted Attention.*
3. *Concentration of the Attention.*

The faculty of attention is one of the most important of the varied powers of the mind. Without its possession, the understanding would be a blank. If we had no voluntary capacity to direct the thoughts to objects of consciousness, how abortive would be the attempt to expand, discipline, and improve the intellect!

"The difference," says Sir W. Hamilton, "between an ordinary mind and the mind of Newton, consists principally in this, that the one is capable of the application of a more continuous attention than the other; that a Newton is able, without fatigue, to connect inference with inference in one long series towards a determinate end; while the man of inferior capacity is soon obliged to break or let fall the thread which he had begun to spin. This is, in fact, what Sir Isaac Newton, with equal modesty and shrewdness, himself admitted. To one who complimented him on his genius, he replied, 'that if he had made any discoveries, it was owing more to patient attention than to any other talent.' "[1]

No sound knowledge of objects exterior to ourselves, no right appreciation of normal conditions of consciousness, or accurate insight into the morbid phenomena of thought, can be obtained, without the power of concentrating by an act of volition, the attention to subjects under the immediate contemplation of the understanding. Observation and reflection (two of the most important

---

[1] "Lectures on Metaphysics."

of the mental faculties) would have no existence apart from the possession of the power of directing and controlling the attention. The able, intelligent, learned, and sagacious man has this faculty of the mind fully matured and developed. It is essential that such should be the case.

The dull, vapid, and uninformed understanding exhibits this intellectual power in a very feeble state of manifestation. The absence of this faculty causes great intellectual weakness. The mind so organized has no power of concentrated thought. Objects of sense are *seen*, but not *observed* ; and all power of reflection appears to be destroyed. The man who has this faculty in the greatest activity and subjection, is best fitted to acquire and mentally retain the knowledge which, if properly applied, elevates him to political, professional, and social positions of influence, usefulness, and authority. Without the power of continuity of thought, and ability to direct the attention, by an effort of the will, to subjects of contemplation, no effectual intellectual progress in knowledge can be made.

" Genius," says Helvetius, " is nothing but a continued attention (*une attention suivie*)." " It is," says Buffon, " only protracted patience (*une longue patience*)." " In the exact sciences, at least," says Cuvier, " it is the patience of a sound intellect when invincible, which truly constitutes genius." Lord Chesterfield says, " that the power of applying the attention steadily and undissipatedly to a single object is the sure mark of a superior genius."

How desirable then it is, that this faculty should be perseveringly cultivated, and when fully developed, carefully and zealously preserved from injury !¹

" Attention forms the great link between the intellectual and moral departments of our nature, or between the percipient and what has been named the pathemic departments. It is the control which the will has over this faculty that makes man responsible

¹ Sufficient importance is not attached in the education of women to the cultivation and discipline of the faculty of attention. Great injury is undoubtedly done to the mind by the hurry and rapidity with which everything is required to be accomplished .n this express railroad era. Until the science of mathematics form an integral part of female education, no really efficient plan of mental training can be said to be adopted. Men in this respect have an advantage over women, by being obliged to go steadily through a course of mathematical study, the mind being thus early in life well-developed, disciplined, and trained by the severest of intellectual studies.

for the objects which he chooses to entertain, and so responsible for the emotions which pathologically result from them.

"The mind can be weaned from the influence of evil affections, by the withdrawment of its thoughts from those objects which both excite and supply the means of their gratification, and wooing the attention to other objects by which good emotions are awakened to occupy the whole man, and displace those hurtful sensibilities which war against the soul. It is thus that attention becomes the great instrument of moral discipline; and it is because of the command which the will possesses over this faculty, that man becomes responsible for the government and regulation of his thoughts.

"The faculty of attention, when employed on external things, is just as mighty an instrument of moral discipline as it is of mental discovery. It fetches that influence from without, which bears with efficacy on the springs of feeling and of action.

"It is by the attention shifting its objects, that the heart shifteth its emotions. The mechanism there is operating rightly, but it is in virtue of a touch from without. It is by looking outwardly and not inwardly, in fact, that the mind hath been set as it were to the right object, whose moving influence it is that brings the mind into its right state of emotion: and thus the cultivation of the dispositions is manifested to be a more simple and intelligible process than many are in the habit of conceiving it.

"The wayward tendencies of the heart are conquered, not so much by an operation at home, as by an operation abroad. The most effectual refuge is, in the contemplation of that ethereal and unclouded purity, by which the throne of Heaven is encircled—a lifting of the thoughts to the august and unpolluted sacredness which dwelleth there—the daily and diligent consideration of that awful sanctuary which is above, where nought that is unholy can enter—and a solemn invocation to Him, before the rebuke of whose countenance all the vanities of a distempered imagination will at once flee away."[1]

IMPAIRMENT OF ATTENTION.—In the incipient stage of disease of the brain, the patient complains of an incapacity to control and direct the faculty of attention. He finds that he cannot, without an obvious and painful effort, accomplish his usual mental work, read, or master the contents of a letter, newspaper, or even a page

---

[1] Dr. Chalmers's "Sketches of Moral and Mental Philosophy."

or two of a favorite book. The ideas become restive, and the mind
lapses into a flighty condition, exhibiting no capacity for continuity
of thought.

Fully recognizing his impaired and failing energies, he repeatedly tries to conquer the defect, and seizing hold of a book, is resolved not to succumb to his sensations of intellectual incapacity,
psychical languor, and cerebral weakness; but, alas! he often
discovers (when it is too late to grapple with the mischief) that he
has lost all power of healthy mental steadiness, and normal concentration of thought. In his attempt to comprehend the meaning
of the immediate subject under contemplation, he reads and re-
reads with a determined resolution, and an apparently unflagging
energy, certain striking passages and pages of a particular book,
but without being able to grasp or understand the simplest chain
of thought, to follow successfully an elementary process of reasoning; neither is he in a condition of mind fitting him to comprehend or retain, for many consecutive seconds, the outline of an
interesting story, understand a simple calculation of figures, or
narrative of facts.   The attempt, particularly if it be a *sustained*
one, to master and converge the attention to the subject which he
is trying to seize, very frequently increases the pre-existing confusion of mind, producing, eventually, *physical* sensations of brain
lassitude, and headache. " Going through a train of close reasoning," says an acute observer, when speaking of this condition, "is
an undertaking absolutely impracticable.   Indeed, to dwell upon
any one thought steadily is a task, and a task, too, that can only
be gone through at long intervals.   Some acute observer has remarked of a former King of Prussia, that his conceptions were
quick, but that on contemplating a subject he grew confused.
Whether it be true in this particular instance or not, the observation holds good of many individuals predisposed to epilepsy.
They are, generally, those who have tampered with their sensibility.   They seize a question dexterously, but their strength is
exhausted in the first assault. If you try to make them grapple
with a difficulty, they immediately flinch. To any proposition
requiring them to contemplate a number of ideas steadfastly, they
will yield a flat, unintelligible assent, or, to mask their want of
bottom, as the jockeys term it, they will endeavor to fly off to another topic. To conceive the condition of the head in such cases
more distinctly, we may recollect how it fares with the eye when

weakened in such a manner that the instant it is cast upon an in-
scription, the characters are perfectly plain, but that in a little
time they seem to run into each other, they become undistinguish-
able, and at last vanish altogether.   From misconduct of the
understanding, all frivolous people must be troubled with some
flightiness of attention.   We need no other reason to enable us to
understand why it becomes requisite in polite circles to change the
topic of·conversation every second minute.''[1]

How often these symptoms are premonitory of softening of the
brain, paralysis, epilepsy, and even apoplexy!   This weakened
power of attention often precedes, and is associated with, impairment and loss of memory.

States of brown study, distraction, and reverie, are often precursory of more demonstrative symptoms of impaired attention.
They are but shades, degrees, and varieties of that morbidly torpid
manifestation of the faculty which so often accompanies unhealthy
conditions of the intelligence, and abnormal states of the cerebral
tissue.

These irregularities of thought are frequently *self-created*, often
owing their existence to an obstinate determination on the part of
the patient to succumb to their fascinating and seductive influence.[2]

A medical gentleman, who exhibited symptoms of mental derangement, informed his medical adviser that his ill-success in his
profession filled him, as may well be supposed, with anxiety for his
own subsistence and that of his family.   He would sit at home for
hours ruminating, and in a state of profound abstraction; and
when he found, day after day, no summons arrive, he would saunter
abroad and occupy himself with a reverie of wishes.   These wishes
he would sometimes arrange into a climax of events, worthy of the
glass man in the "Spectator."   At length he would direct his
footsteps homeward, under a kind of persuasion that some person
of consequence had actually sent, during his absence, to call him
in.[3]

This indulgence in a state of *morbid reverie*, or disposition to

---

[1] Dr. Beddoes' "Hygëia."

[2] "Reverie," says Locke, "is when ideas float in our minds without any reflection
or regard of the understanding."   What are termed "waking dreams," are distinct
from that state of the mind previously described by Locke, viz., as "thoughts wandering without connection."

[3] "Hygëia," by Thomas Beddoes, M.D.   1803.

"build castles in the air," is fraught with serious mischief to the mind. Excessive, continuous, and prolonged reverie is often precursory of softening of the brain, and is also a symptom commonly observed in the incipient stages of some types of mental disorder. Hence the great value, in early education, of carefully regulating, directing, disciplining, and mastering the attention, thus fitting and training the mind to combat successfully with those mental influences and physical states of ill health which, when uncontrolled and unsubdued, so often sap and undermine its energies, prostrate and destroy its powers.[1]

"Reverie and castle-building is a kind of waking dream, and does not differ from dreaming, except by the consciousness which accompanies it. In this state, the mind abandons itself without a choice of subjects, without control over the mental train, to the involuntary associations of the imagination. The mind is thus occupied without being properly active; it is active, at least, without effort. Young persons, women, the old and unemployed, and the idle, are all disposed to reverie. There is a pleasure attached to its illusions which render it seductive and dangerous. The mind, by indulgence in this disposition, becomes enervated; it acquires the habit of a pleasing idleness, loses its activity, and at length even the power and the desire of action."[2]

"I have sometimes," says a distinguished living authority, "half believed, although the suspicion is mortifying, that there is only a step between his state who deeply indulges in imaginative meditation, and insanity; for I well remember when I indulged in medi-

---

[1] "There is hardly a person," says the Abbé de Condillac, "who in his idle hours has not had some reverie, in which he has imagined himself the hero of the romance. These fictions, which are called castles in the air, generally produce only a slight impression on the brain, because we seldom give way to them, so that they are soon dispersed by some real objects, with which we are obliged to occupy our thoughts. But suppose some sudden fit of melancholy seizes our mind, so as to make us avoid the company of our best friends, and dislike everything that pleased us before, we shall then find, in the transport of our grief, that our favorite romance will be the only idea that can divert us from it. The animal spirits, by degrees, will dig such a strong foundation to his castle, that nothing will be able to demolish it; we shall fall asleep in the building of it; we shall dream that we reside in it; and in fine, when the impression of the spirits shall insensibly arrive at that pitch, as if we really were what we have fancied ourselves to be, upon returning to ourselves we shall take our chimeras for a reality. Perhaps the madness of that Athenian, who imagined all the ships which entered the Piræum to belong to him, was owing to no other cause."

[2] Anchillon "Essais Philosoph." By Pascal.

tation to an extreme degree, that my senses appeared sometimes to be wandering. I cannot describe the peculiar feeling I then experienced; for I have failed in so doing to several eminent surgeons and men of science, with whom I have conversed respecting it, and who were curious to become acquainted with its nature. But I think it was, that I was not always assured of my identity, or even existence; for I found it necessary to shout aloud to be sure that I lived; and I was in the habit very often, at night, of taking down a volume, and looking into it for my name, to be convinced that I had not been dreaming of myself. At these times there was an incredible acuteness or intenseness in my sensations. Every object seemed animated, and, as it were, acting upon me. The only way that I can devise, to express my general feeling, is, that I seemed to be sensible of the rapid whirl of the globe."[1]

HEIGHTENED AND CONCENTRATED ATTENTION.—The attention is occasionally heightened, or in a condition of unhealthy exaltation, as well as of concentration. This is observed when the mind has been continuously, abnormally, and sometimes involuntarily directed to certain vivid impressions, trains of thought, classes of ideas, conditions of emotion, or states of physical sensation. That psycho-somatic disease termed hypochondriasis, which manifests itself principally in a morbid anxiety as to the health, is, in its primitive nature, essentially a diseased concentration to, and consequent exaggeration of, organic conditions of physical sensibility, resulting often from slight bodily ailments, which eventually assume, in the distempered and deluded imagination of the hypochondriac, a grave and significant character.[2] Much of the disturbed thought, predominance of insane ideas, consisting in wretched illusions as to the state of the health, may unequivocally be traced to an undue convergence and misdirection of the attention to unimportant mental impressions and trifling nervous sensations. The mind often dwells uninterruptedly upon particular emotions, fixedly upon certain states of thought, continuously upon specific classes of ideas, to the rigid exclusion of matters of healthy consciousness, and sane contemplation, *until it loses all right, or*

---

[1] " *Contarini Fleming*," by the Right Hon. B. Disraeli, M.P., D.C.L.

[2] *Dubois* divides hypochondriasis into three stages: 1. *Strained attention.* 2. *Disturbed psychical conditions induced by innervation.* 3. *Disorganization of tissue caused by functional disorder of the mind.*

sound appreciation of subjective and objective phenomena. The
condition of intellect, previously referred to, often exists, to a
certain extent, as a normal state, and as such only indicates the
presence of health. It is, however, often a sign of *cerebral* and
psychical disease.

It is a well-established fact that alterations of tissue have been
the result of a morbid concentration of the attention to particular
organic structures. Certain feelings of uneasiness, or even pain,
originate in the mind a suspicion of disease existing in particular
parts of the body, it may be the lungs, stomach, heart, brain, liver,
or kidneys. Some slight irregularities and functional disturbances
in the action of these organs being noticed, are at once suggestive
(to the hypochondriac) of serious and fatal disease being established
in the part to which the attention is directed. This deviation from
a normal state of certain functions, frequently lapses into actual
structural disease, as the effect of the faculty of attention being,
for a lengthened period, morbidly concentrated to their action.
The continuous direction of the mind to vital tissues, *imagined* to
be in an unhealthy state, undoubtedly causes an exaltation of their
special functions, and an increase of sensibility, by (it may be presumed) concentrating to them an abnormal quantity of blood, this
being followed, successively by 1, undue vascular action; 2, capillary congestion; 3, an excess in the evolution of nerve force, and
4, appreciable *structural* alterations.

Thus, the mischievous influence of *moral* agencies is exercised
upon the *physical* as well as *psychical* organism, laying the foundation of lesions of structure and perversions of thought originating
in the mind itself. Morbid anatomy painfully attests the visible
and tangible results of mental influences on the various physical
tissues.

How much of self-created bodily suffering, voluntarily courted
physical pain, carefully, and alas! zealously trained, distressing,
and incurable disease of the mind, arise from a lengthened anxiety,
and continuous fret and worry as to the state of the corporeal and
mental health! The unceasing dread of the presence and constant
morbid anticipation of approaching disease (whether of body or
mind) very frequently creates the mischief so much anticipated,
and so greatly apprehended. "*Non raro ægrum ab hoc sensu, et
medicum ab ægro falli, cum æger ex sensu communi, hausisse hinc*

*inde adfirmat quod imaginatio et præcepta etiam opinio illi sug-
gessit*,"[1] is advice that should not be incautiously neglected.

"Health,'' says an able divine, "is an important blessing of
which we should be careful, and for which we ought to be most
thankful to the generous God who bestows it, but in the care sometimes taken of health, even at the expense of more serious duties,
I have sometimes thought I saw exemplified the words of the
satirist,—

> ' Et propter vitam, vivendi perdere causas.'—JUV.

For the sake of life, neglecting the very causes for which life is
granted."

It is not difficult to explain satisfactorily the *modus operandi* of
heightened and concentrated attention upon certain trains of
healthy as well as of incipient morbid thought, exalted emotions,
disordered conditions of the instincts, and perverted states of the
appetites and passions.   Impressions that were originally false or
erroneous;—conclusions that could only be termed absurd, and
illogical;—judgments that might, consistently with fact, be designated merely as defective, and impaired, *become evidences of actual
disease of the brain and disorder of the mind, consequent upon an
unhealthy and unbroken direction of the attention to these mental
operations*.   Insane delusions often thus originate.   Hence the
extreme danger of not exercising, like trustworthy sentinels, a
watchful supervision, and active controlling influence over every
thought, and the evil that arises from not keeping in a state of
strict subordination the mental emotions.   The fearful mischief
that ensues from neglecting, by resolute mental efforts, to battle
with the erratic suggestions of an unduly excited and flighty
imagination, to keep in abeyance, and even to strangle in their
birth, unhealthy impressions struggling to fix and engraft themselves upon the easily moulded, plastic, and yielding fancy, cannot
be over-estimated, or exaggerated.   " *Vide ne funiculum nimis
intendendo aliquando abrumpas*," says Lucian, when referring to
the danger that arises from an excessive and prolonged concentration of the mind to any one subject of contemplation.

Whenever there exists a consciousness that a decided effort is
required in order to master, converge, and rivet the attention to

---

[1] Hartman's "Pathology," p. 261, as quoted by Feuchtersleben in his "Medical
Psychology," p. 215.

any particular subject, train of thought, and class of emotions, the patient may, *cæteris paribus*, be assured that the psychical functions of the brain have been overwrought, or that they are not (for a time) in a healthy or normal working condition. This symptom often accompanies slight irregularities of the arterial and venous cerebral circulation. It is also the effect of transient states of capillary congestion on the hemispherical surface of the brain, dependent, occasionally, upon functional disorder of the stomach, heart, kidneys, and liver, and need excite no alarm unless the mental paralysis be of some duration, is clearly encephalic in its origin, and associated with vertigo, headache, loss of memory, lesions of sensibility, and other well-marked signs of brain disorder. Nevertheless, it is a symptom entitled to serious consideration, when analyzing the incipient manifestations of cerebral and mental disease.

I am anxious not to attach undue importance to this evidence of morbid intelligence, but I cannot close my eyes to a fact, so often noticed by myself as well as by others whose observations have been directed to the subject, that *a debilitated power of attention is a prominent symptom in the early stage of cerebral disorder.* I have known cases of incipient brain disease in which patients have, previously to the manifestation of other symptoms, lost all ability to read, continuously, twenty lines of a printed book without a strong and painful effort of thought. This state of mind has continued for months, necessitating the abandonment of all intellectual work, and has been succeeded by obvious symptoms of organic cerebral disease, loss of memory, and even has passed eventually into mental imbecility. If an impairment of attention and debility of memory exist, it is illusory for the patient to imagine that he is able (until his *physical* condition of ill-health is attended to) by repeated and persevering efforts to resuscitate the lost powers. In his attempt to do so, he still further taxes the morbidly impaired state of these faculties, and, instead of invigorating, prostrates, debilitates, and often, alas! entirely extinguishes the intelligence.

A patient, when describing this condition of intellect, says, "I cannot read as I used to do, I am obliged to repeatedly go through a page of a book, and re-read a sentence, without having any idea of its purport. The attempt to fix and concentrate the thoughts requires a continuous, painful, and vigorous effort of the will."

In this state of ill-health, serious irreparable injury is done to the delicate organization of the brain and mind, by an attempt to exercise, stimulate, and *force* into activity, this morbidly flagging and sluggish mental power. The existence of symptoms like those previously detailed, conclusively establishes that the brain is quite unfit for any degree of *sustained* labor, and that conditions of perfect REPOSE, and states of prolonged and uninterrupted REST, are essential to a restoration of its enfeebled energies. The danger so often incurred by overtaxing the power of attention in enfeebled states of the bodily health, is well illustrated in the following case, drawn up by the patient himself.   The history is as follows: "I was this morning (says the patient) engaged with a great number of people who followed each other quickly, and to each of whom I was obliged to give my attention.   I was also under the necessity of writing much, but the subjects were various, and of a trivial and uninteresting nature, and had no connection the one with the other; my attention therefore was constantly kept on the stretch, and it was continually shifting from one subject to another.   At last it became necessary that I should write a receipt for some money I had received on account of the poor. I seated myself and wrote the two first words, but in a moment found that I was incapable of proceeding, for I could not recollect the words which belonged to the ideas that were present in my mind.   I strained my attention as much as possible, and tried to write one letter slowly after the other, always having an eye in order to observe whether they had the usual relationship to each other; but I remarked and said to myself at the time, that the characters I was writing were not those which I wished to write, and yet I could not discover where the fault lay.   I therefore desisted, and partly by broken words and syllables, and partly by gesture, I made the person who waited for the receipt understand that he should leave me.   For about half an hour there reigned a kind of tumultuous disorder of my senses, in which I was incapable of remarking anything very particular, except that one series of ideas forced themselves involuntarily into my mind. The trifling nature of these thoughts I was perfectly aware of, and was also conscious that I made several efforts to get rid of them, and supply their place by better ones which lay at the bottom of my soul.   I endeavored as much as lay in my power, considering the great crowd of confused images which presented themselves to my mind, to recall my principles of religion, of conscience, and of future expectations; these I found equally correct and fixed as before. There was no deception in my external senses, for I saw and knew everything around me, but I could not free myself from the strange ideas which existed in my head. I endeavored to speak, in order to discover whether I was capable of saying anything that was connected, but although I made the greatest efforts of attention and proceeded with the utmost caution, I perceived that I uniformly spoke other words than those I intended. My soul was at present as little master of the organs of speech as it had been before of my hand in writing. Thank God, this state did not continue very long, for in about half an hour my head began to grow clearer, the strange and tiresome ideas became less vivid and turbulent, and I could command my own thoughts with less interruption. I now wished to ring for my servant, and desire him to inform my wife to come to me; but I found it still necessary to wait a little longer, to exercise myself in the right pronunciation of the few words I had to say, and the first half hour's conversation I had with her was, on my part, preserved with a slow and anxious circumspection, until at last I gradually found myself as clear and serene as in the beginning of the day. All that now remained was a slight headache. I recollected the receipt I had begun to write, and in which I knew I had blundered, and upon examining it I observed, to my great astonishment, that instead of the words, '*fifty dollars, being one-half year's rate*,' which I ought to have written, the words were, '*fifty dollars, through the salvation of Bra*——' with a break after it, for the word '*Bra*' was at the end of the line. I cannot recollect any business I had to transact that could by means of an obscure influence have produced this phenomenon."[1]

This impairment of the faculty of attention occasionally supervenes upon febrile attacks. Dr. Abercrombie accurately describes this weakened state of the intelligence. "The patient," he says, "in the early or milder stages, is incapable of fixing his mind upon anything that requires much attention, of following out an argument, or of transacting business which calls for much thought or consideration. He is acute and intelligent as to all common occurrences, and shows no want of recollection, or of the power of

[1] " Mental Derangement," by Alexander Crichton, M.D. 1798.

reasoning, when his attention is excited, but he feels it an exertion that is painful to him. In a higher degree of this condition he is still intelligent as to what is said, or done at the time, or in recognizing persons, but in a short time forgets everything in regard to the person, or the occurrence. He is incapable of that degree of attention which is necessary for memory, though the powers of perception are entire. In the next stage he becomes incapable of receiving the full impression from external things, and in consequence of this he mistakes the objects of his own thoughts for realities. This is delirium, and there are various degrees of it. In some cases the attention of the patient can be roused for a time, and directed to the true relations of external things, though he relapses into his delirious impressions when he is left undisturbed; in others the false impression is constant, and cannot be corrected by any effort which is made to direct the attention; and in a third modification of this remarkable condition, he mixes up his hallucinations with external impressions in a most singular manner. He is still capable, however, of describing his impressions, that is, of talking so as to be understood, though what he speaks of relates only to his erroneous conceptions, or mere bodily feelings. In the next stage, he either does not attempt to express himself at all, or is entirely unintelligible. He is now cut off from communication with external things, and with other sentient beings; and the highest degree of this is what we call coma, or stupor, which resembles profound sleep.

" This description refers chiefly to the gradations in the state of the mental functions which we observe in continued fever. It is particularly interesting to trace them in this disease, because we see the various grades passing into one another, and thus showing in a connected series the leading peculiarities which in other affections we have to contemplate separately."

I have previously referred to the morbid phenomena of distraction (être distrait). This is an important and significant incipient symptom of disease of the brain. The patient, whilst engaged in conversation, suddenly pauses, is puzzled, confused, and appears to have lost the connecting media in the chain of thought. This condition of mind is occasionally precursory of epilepsy and apoplexy. It is also known to manifest itself in the early stage of softening of the brain, and in cases of ordinary as well as of general paralysis. This symptom has often, although existing, been unobserved, until the cerebral disease has made considerable progress.

A professional gentleman, who had for fifteen years led a most active life, encountering, during that period, many vicissitudes of fortune, occasionally prosperous, and at times reduced to great extremities in consequence of heavy pecuniary losses sustained by becoming security for a near relative, exhibited symptoms of declining general health, necessitating his going abroad for a few months to one of the German spas. At this time there was nothing special in connection with the case that justified any serious apprehensions as to his ultimate recovery. He appeared to be much benefited by change of air and scene, as well as from his exemption from all anxieties of business. On his return home, however, he manifested symptoms that betokened the commencement of disease of the brain. Although generally showing great activity of intellect, unenfeebled powers of attention, unimpaired capacity for continuous thought, and considerable capability of application to the minute and complicated details of subjects requiring, for their right comprehension, much concentration of mind, he, at times, gave indication of cerebral disturbance that could not fail to attract the anxious observation of the acute practitioner who then had charge of the case. He complained of headache, transient fits of mental confusion, paroxysms of vertigo, loss of self-command, irritability of temper, and occasional interruptions in the consecutive operations of thought. Whilst engaged in conversation, he would for a minute or two appear much distracted, then suddenly stop as if he had lost the link in the chain of ideas passing through his mind. This patient, under the judicious treatment adopted, appeared to recover his cerebral health, for he, during several subsequent years, conducted a complicated business without manifesting any indication of brain disease or impaired intellect. Six years, however, did not elapse before his health again showed serious signs of decadence, and his state of brain was once more made a matter of professional observation. It was at this period that I had an opportunity of seeing the case. The patient exhibited many symptoms of serious and fatal disorganization of the brain. There was loss of memory, occasionally much irritability at the merest trifles, slight thickness of the speech, defective articulation, a singular misplacement of words, and loss and want of co-ordination in the muscular power. His gait was rolling and unsteady. All these symptoms gradually increased, until he became generally paralytic in mind and body, and died, ten months afterwards, in a state of imbecility. His brain was found much diseased. There was softening both of the *cerebrum* (the left hemisphere) and *cerebellum*, with considerable thickening and opacity of the meninges, evidently of some duration. It was supposed that the disease of the brain, of which this patient died, had commenced *ten years* previously to his decease. The relaxation from the anxieties of a business, involving complicated calculations and grave responsibilities, for a short time appeared to arrest the cerebral disorder. His subsequent relapse was owing to .his premature return to active mental work. However, the disease was, evidently, a second time suspended by the local abstraction of blood (for the purpose of relieving evident congestion of the brain), mild mercurials, and afterwards mineral tonics. The mental distraction, hesitation in the speech, and occasional want of sequence of thought, were clearly among the earlier symptoms of the disease of the brain which ultimately destroyed reason and life.

The preceding case very closely resembles in its main features that of Oscar, the late King of Sweden, the particulars of which are detailed with great minuteness by Dr. P. O. Liljewalch, first physician in ordinary to his late Majesty.

It appears that the King (I abridge the subjoined account from Dr. W. D. Moore's translation of the official report of the King's last illness, as well as the *post-mortem* examination) had enjoyed the greater part of his life tolerably good health. He had, early in life, a severe attack of typhus, and, subsequently, of rheumatic fever. He rallied, however, completely from these seizures. His Majesty exhibited great activity and cleverness in the discharge of his regal duties. His general health was excellent, with the exception of a slight irregularity in the heart's action, observed generally in the spring of the year. His Majesty was in the habit of making yearly excursions to remote parts of his kingdom, and returning to the capital late in the autumn. From these journeys he derived great benefit. In 1851, his Majesty's health again showed symptoms of failure. The heart became very irregular in its movement, and the digestive functions were impaired. The liver also increased in size, and the brain manifested signs of disorder. His Majesty, on the advice of his physician, took to the baths of Kissengen, and, subsequently, made a tour through Switzerland. He again returned home much improved in health. He soon afterwards lost a beloved son. The shock caused by this heavy bereavement induced another attack of typhus fever, which nearly proved fatal. The King, however, recovered from this severe illness, and would, it was thought, have continued well, had he not, zealously but indiscreetly, devoted his mind to anxious political matters, omitting his annual summer excursion. In 1857, his Majesty's health again gave way, causing great uneasiness to his family. The symptoms, at this time, were those of congestion of the brain. Dr. Liljewalch says :—

" The lower extremities, the muscles of which were always weak, began to totter under the weight of the body, and at the same time that the power of combination for the motions of these parts was impaired, his Majesty was troubled with vertigo, particularly accompanying the movements of the head, and with vomiting, which symptoms, in combination with diminution of strength, and the occurrence of involuntary muscular spasms, indicated the existence of a more deeply-seated affection, probably a softening in the central nervous system. Incapacity to discharge his royal functions now brought on a deep melancholy, and his Majesty, even in the commencement of his illness, expressed his conviction of its incurability. Although this conviction could not, unfortunately, but be participated in by those who were privileged to be his Majesty's physicians, we did not at that time consider it our duty publicly to express it. The means employed to combat the disease were, moreover, without any essential efficacy ; the paralysis, which commenced in the lower extremities, gradually increased; and after the King, feeling his inability any longer to fill the high position to which Providence had called him, transferred into the hands of his then Royal Highness, the Crown Prince, the Government of the United Kingdoms, his deep melancholy gave way to a progressive indifference, even for those things which in his health he had regarded with the most lively interest. The disease, henceforward, progressed slowly towards its end, and the paralysis began so steadily to extend to the other voluntary muscles, that towards the end of last June both lower and upper extremities, and the sphincters of the excretory passages were almost entirely paralyzed, while involuntary spasms from time to time agitated the right leg. The appetite, too, had now disappeared, and, although digestion continued undisturbed, the body had greatly emaciated, while the hitherto superficial bed-sores, which had often been nearly healed, and had already existed more than six months without causing any great pain, began to extend and to assume a gangrenous appearance.   Under all this the patient's strength gradually sank ; the power of speech, previously very limited, latterly was altogether lost; the lungs filled with mucus, which, in consequence of incipient paralysis of the muscles of respiration, could only, with increased difficulty, be expectorated ; and, on the 8th of July, at eight o'clock in the morning, his Majesty quietly expired, supported in the arms of his royal consort, who, during his more than two years' illness, never left his side, and surrounded by all the other members of the royal family, kneeling with her and weeping bitterly around the death-bed of the never-to-be-forgotten and long-tried head of their illustrious house.

"The first trace of the nervous disease, the development of which I have now described, and which brought the late King to the grave, manifested itself long since, although it was not until within the last six or eight years of his Majesty's life that, as we have seen, it occurred with more definite, and at last with such threatening symptoms.   No one, who had the good fortune to approach his Majesty's person, and who had an opportunity of observing him during a long period in his daily intercourse, could avoid being amazed at the very extraordinary power his Majesty always exhibited of retaining in his memory the most varied details, or could cease admiring the rapid apprehension, the unerring judgment, and the singular clearness of statement which were exhibited whenever he spoke. *But at the same time he would not fail to recollect how his Majesty sometimes, in the middle of a conversation to which he was directing all his attention, would of a sudden appear to be abstracted, and would really transfer his thoughts to some other subject on which, unless he might be disturbed, he would allow them to rest, usually only for a few moments, but sometimes for many minutes ; after which the conversation would be resumed, as if it had not been interrupted.*   The peculiar expression of his Majesty's features, particularly his look, assumed on such occasions, and the spasmodic state, or the involuntary movements which at the same time took place in one or other part of the muscular system, render it probable that this distraction, which at times was of frequent recurrence, was due to an incipient affection of the central organ of thought. This symptom, referrible to the most important organ of the nervous system, was of late years accompanied, as has been already mentioned, with increasing weakness in the muscles of the lower extremities, and with uncertainty in the combination of movement, probably depending on a commencing organic change, either in the organ alone, on which the power of motion depends, or else in that by which the co-ordination of movements is effected."[1]

I was consulted in the spring of 1857 in the case of a gentleman, connected with the Stock Exchange, who was suspected to have disease of the brain. His symptoms, at the time of my first seeing the case, were as follow: General muscular weakness, occasional paroxysms of severe headache, slight paralysis of the superior palpebræ of the left eye, occasional sensation of numbness in the right foot. The mind was not, apparently, at all impaired. He continued, up to the period of my being consulted, fully competent to discharge all his commercial duties, attended to his accounts, and wrote letters of business with his usual ability and clearness. His brother informed me that, at times, he was greatly *abs*tracted and *dis*tracted; that, whilst engaged in conversation, he would suddenly pause, put his hand to his head, and appear vexed with himself at having lost all consciousness of what he was saying. This symptom was observed *two* years before any question arose, or suspicion existed, as to the state of the brain! The family, judging from the subsequent progress of the case, were of opinion that the cerebral disorder was first exhibited by the sudden lapses of thought, to which he was subject for many years previously to the manifestation of other and more unequivocal symptoms of brain disease. Such, also, was my opinion. In a few weeks I lost sight altogether of this case, as the patient was removed to the continent, under the idea of trying the effect of one of the Spa waters. In about a year and a half from my being consulted, I was informed that this patient died quite paralytic. Considerable organic disease of the brain is said to have been discovered after death.

A member of the Irish bar, who became insane whilst at Paris, during the autumn of 1856, and died three months after his return

---

[1] The *post-mortem* examination of King Oscar revealed extensive disorganization of the brain.

to England, complained to his friends, and subsequently to the surgeon who attended the family, *three years* previously to his attack, of an inability to collect his thoughts whilst addressing the courts of law. He was, occasionally, observed to stop whilst speaking, as if his ideas were momentarily paralyzed. So marked was this symptom that a professional friend, often associated with him in the conduct of legal matters, considered it his duty to direct the attention of the gentleman's wife to the fact, considering that such attacks of distraction, on occasions when it was of essential importance for the mind to be in a state of continuous activity, looked suspicious, and, according to his judgment, were not consistent with a healthy state of the brain.

This patient, about two years after this morbid abstraction, or transient loss of consciousness was observed, had a slight *epileptiform* seizure whilst at his chambers, during a very hot day in the month of July. As this attack was considered to have been one of syncope, and to be caused by the then high state of temperature, little or no notice was taken of it. Previously to proceeding on the continent, he had been working unusually hard, eating and drinking very sparingly, sitting up late at night, and rising early in the morning. In fact, he acted with great indiscretion and imprudence, and the result was, an acute attack of brain disease affecting the mind, a fortnight after his arrival in Paris. There was found, after death, chronic disease of the membranes of the brain, supposed to have been of long existence.

CHAPTER XIII.

MORBID PHENOMENA OF MEMORY.

THIS section will embody an analysis of,

1. *Acute Disorders of Memory.*
2. *Chronic (Modified) Affections of Memory.*
3. *Perversion of Memory.*
4. *Exaltation of Memory.*
5. *Memory of the Insane.*
6. *Psychology and Pathology of Memory.*

The memory may, as the effect of natural decay, accident, or disease, be,

α. *Disordered.*
β. *Weakened.*
γ. *Lost.*
δ. *Perverted.*
ε. *Exalted.*

I propose to consider in this section, somewhat in detail, not only the impairment and aberration of memory which may properly be considered symptomatic of acute disease of the brain and disorder of the mind, but those singularly obscure, and inexplicable cases of total and modified paralysis of the faculty, consequent upon injuries inflicted on the delicate nerve vesicle, either by inflammation resulting in adventitious depositions in the substance, or on the surface of the brain and its membranes, mechanical violence to the head, or by atheromatous changes in the structure of the cerebral vessels (fatty degeneration), disordered states of the cranial circulation, and conditions of mal-nerve nutrition.

This division of the subject will involve a consideration of,

1. *Acute Disorders of the Memory.*
2. *Chronic (Modified) Affections of the Memory.*

What is memory?   How are we enabled by an effort of volition to reproduce previous mental conceptions, revive past states of consciousness, and recall to the mind a long and complex train of apparently obliterated and forgotten thought?

Are the ideas carefully housed, registered, and classified in hidden and mysterious cells, vesicles, or chambers of the brain? If so, what is, to adopt the language of Cicero, the nature of this " *thesaurus omnium rerum ;*" where the situation of the vesicular mental repository and cerebral treasure-house, destined to garner, preserve, and protect from injury the myriads of ideas that obtain an entrance into the mind through the media of the senses?

Is memory a distinct sovereign power, exercising independent autocratic authority, or, is it one of the results of a *combined* or *complex* operation of several of the mental faculties?

The facts to be detailed, and principles enunciated in the subsequent pages will, I hope (to a limited extent), satisfactorily answer the important preceding interrogatories in relation to the metaphysics, or psychology of memory.[1]

Before analyzing in detail the morbid phenomena of memory, as illustrating the incipient symptoms of obscure diseases of the brain and mind, it will be necessary to consider the natural order in which various classes of ideas stand in relation to each other, not only as to the *priority* of their admission into the mind, but *durability* of their impression on the sensorium.

Metaphysicians agree in the opinion, that *qualities* of objects and *events*, are more easily retained in the mind than *dates* and

---

[1] When speaking of this faculty we should fully recognize the philosophical distinction between what is termed, the *automatic* operations of the mind involved in the spontaneous and involuntary reproduction to the consciousness of former mental impressions, and that condition of the intellect connected with the revival of ideas by an *act of volition*, the former state being properly termed *memory*, and the latter *recollection*.

" Memory," says an able logician, " is not au original power of faculty. It is made up of two ingredients, the thing remembered and the idea of having seen it. The last ingredient, however, consists of three component parts, our present remembering self, our past remembering self, and these being united by certain trains of consciousness, unite the two selfs, which form a compound, called by metaphysicians personal identity."—(*James Mill.*)

names; in other words, that the intellect takes a more tenacious grasp of *adjectives*, than of *substantives.*

Gratiolet considers that the ideas of things are more or less allied to the notions we have of ourselves, and that they are effaced the more easily the less they are thus associated and identified. General ideas disappear from the mind only after those that are *particular* and *contingent.* An object, he affirms, has two names; one *generic* and the other *specific.* The former is more easily retained than the latter. When a man is seen for the first time, a certain distinct idea is formed of him, from his *aspect* and *qualities,* before his name is known. He is a particular man, *great* or *little, blond* or *dark,* before he becomes to the observer, *John, Peter,* or *Thomas.* The relation of names to things is often accidental and arbitrary. There is not in this respect a general order, it is a fortuitous association of a *sign* and of a *thing.* That alone remains readily in the memory which is conceived according to a natural order. If the memory becomes enfeebled, it is with regard to proper names that this enfeeblement is first apparent. There are in this respect many differences among men, according to the degree of importance with which words are appreciated. One man investigates particularly facts, from whence results a spontaneous definition of things, and the name of objects or persons will be but of accessory 'importance. Another will touch slightly on the *fact,* and pre-occupy himself with the *name.* This is witnessed constantly among naturalists.[1] Some are best acquainted with objects, others with names.

---

[1] "I cannot help," says an eminent metaphysical philosopher, "taking this opportunity of expressing a wish that medical writers would be at more pains than they have been at hitherto, to ascertain the various effects which are produced on the memory by disease and old age. These effects are widely diversified in different cases. In some it would seem that the memory is impaired in consequence of a diminution of the power of attention; in others, that the power of recollection is disturbed in consequence of a derangement of that part of the constitution on which the association of ideas depends. The decay of memory, which is the common effect of age, seems to arise from the former of these causes. It is probable that as we advance in years the capacity of attention is weakened by some physical change in the constitution; but it is also reasonable to think that it loses its vigor partly from the effect which the decay of our sensibility and the extinction of our passions have in diminishing the interest which we feel in the common occurrences of life. That no derangement takes place in ordinary cases in that part of the constitution on which the association of ideas depends is clear from the distinct and circumstantial recollection which old men retain of the transactions of their youth. In some diseases

If (according to the same authority) the memory becomes enfeebled in two men of this character, he who has the most vivid image of facts, will lose the memory of words before that of things, whilst the other, contented with the sign, will forget everything in losing the memory of names. But in both the one and the other the first result of an enfeeblement of the memory will be a species of dissociation between the ideas of things in themselves and of the arbitrary names which designate them.

"A distinguished *savant*," says Gratiolet, "connected with one of the continental academies, is unable to designate his *confrères* by their names, and he characterizes them by their *works*. If he speaks of one of them, he expresses himself thus: 'My *confrère* who has written *such a book;* who has made *such* a discovery.' He designates him, in short, not by his *name*, but by a *quality*. Things are first known to us by a certain number of *qualities* which affect us, the ideas of qualities being generators of the ideas which we have of things considered as *substances*. In the order of acquisition of ideas, the substance predominates over the accident, and the accident predominates over the foundation. Thus the general idea of being, united to the particular idea of a certain number of properties, suffices for a definition, and in practice these spontaneous definitions precede the names. 'What is this called?' we say every day. 'What is the name of this round object? of this green object?' The arbitrary name comes but afterwards; the name is then secondary and added; it is then less essential, and ought to be lost first in this process of interior dislocation, in which the ideas separate themselves with greater or less difficulty, the one from the other, on account of the degree of their reciprocal affinities."

This theory, Gratiolet affirms, enables us to understand why proper names disappear first, then substantives, which are the proper names of things. Adjectives or qualificatives disappear last, and everything disappears with them, because we cannot have an idea of a thing independently of its qualities. We recall

this part of the constitution is evidently affected. A stroke of palsy has been known while it did not destroy the power of speech, to render the patient incapable of recollecting the names of the most familiar objects. What is still more remarkable, the name of an object has been known to suggest the idea of it as formerly, although the sight of the object ceased to suggest the name."—*Dugald Stewart's " Elements of the Philosophy of the Human Mind."*

things, and the names of things, in the ratio of their necessity. In the order of thought, the *coincident* is more easily forgotten than the *correlative*, the consequence *remote* more readily than the consequence *immediate*.[1]

Dr. Itard observes, that the loss of memory that generally accompanies attacks of apoplexy occurring in advanced life, follows in the subjoined order: there is first a forgetfulness of *names*, then of *substantives*, then of *verbs*, and next of *adjectives*. Adjectives appear to retain their hold with the firmest tenacity upon the mind. It is a well-known fact, says Dr. Itard, that many idiots have had a memory only for adjectives.

Some light may be, perhaps, thrown upon this subtle question, by considering the mode in which the understanding is built up, the intellectual superstructure reared; in other words, the relation in which ideas are admitted into the mind. "The order of learning," says Vives, as translated by Sir W. Hamilton, "is from the senses to the imagination, and from this to the intellect. Such is the order of life and of nature. We thus proceed from the *simple* to the *complex*, from the *singular* to the *universal*. This is to be observed in children, who first of all express the several parts of different things, and then conjoin them. Things general they call by a singular name; for instance, they call all Smiths by the name of that individual *Smith* whom they have known; and all meats *beef* and *pork*, as they happen to have heard the one or the other first when they began to speak. Thereafter the mind collects universals from particulars, and then again reverts to particulars from universals." The same doctrine, without any knowledge of Vives, is maintained by Locke. He says: "There is nothing more evident than that the ideas of the persons children converse with (to instance them alone), are like the persons themselves, only particular. The ideas of the nurse and the mother are well framed in their minds, and, like pictures of them, represent only those individuals. The names they first gave to them are confined to those individuals, and the names of *nurse* and *mamma* the child uses, determine themselves to those persons. Afterwards, when time and a larger acquaintance have made them observe that there

---

[1] "Anatomie comparée du Système Nerveux considéré dans ses Rapports avec l'Intelligence." Par Fr. Leuret et P. Gratiolet; tome 2, par M. P. Gratiolet, Paris, 1839–1857.

are a great many other things in the world that in some common agreement or shape, and several other qualities, resemble their father and mother, and those persons they have been used to, they frame an idea which they find those many particulars do partake in, and to that they give with others, for example, the name *man*. Thus they come to have a general name and a general idea."[1]

[1] Locke, on the "Human Understanding."

CHAPTER XIV.

ACUTE DISORDERS OF THE MEMORY.

In estimating the condition of the memory in relation to a suspected state of cerebral or mental disease, it is important to remember that, as age advances, the power of recalling to the mind, by an effort of the will, recent events, becomes much impaired, and is sometimes altogether destroyed. Horace says, when alluding to the sad infirmities that sometimes accompany old age :—

> "Multa senem circumveniunt incommoda, vel quod
> Quærit et inventis miser abstinet, ac timet uti;
> Vel quod res omnes timidè gelidèque ministrat,
> Dilator, spe longus, iners, avidusque futuri,
> Difficilis, querulus, laudator temporis acti."

In a few instances, however, in very advanced life, the faculty of memory exhibits an extraordinary degree of elasticity, and a surprising amount of vigor.[1] There is undoubtedly much differ-

[1] A charming illustration of the tenacity with which the mind retains early impressions occurs in the life of Niebuhr the celebrated Danish traveller. When old, blind, and so infirm that he was able only to be carried from his bed to his chair, he used to describe to his friends the scenes which he had visited in his early days with wonderful minuteness and vivacity. When they expressed their astonishment at the vividness of his memory, he explained, "that as he lay in bed, all visible objects shut out, the pictures of what he had seen in the East continually floated before his mind's eye, so that it was no wonder he could speak of them as if he had seen them yesterday. With like vividness, the deep intense sky of Asia, with its brilliant and twinkling hosts of stars, which he had so often gazed at by night, or its lofty vault of blue by day, was reflected, in the hours of stillness and darkness, on his inmost soul."

"The angels of youth leave the deepest footmarks on the rocks of Memory, and the long ago and distant past is more often and more deeply imprinted on the soul than the distant future. In the same manner the first ornamental letters of our existence, like those in illuminated writings, carry on their beautiful emblazonments all round the four sides of the manuscripts."—*Jean Paul F. Richter.*

"The *young*," says Aristotle, "live forward, *in hope*, the *old* live backwards, *in memory*."

> "Hoc est
> Vivere bis, vita posse priore frui."—*Martial.*

ence among the aged as to their ability to revivify *recent* mental impressions. We sometimes, however, witness in old persons, great power of reproducing these as well as former and long antecedent ideas. This state of healthy psychical activity depends partly upon natural strength of the faculty or original vigor of mind, early educational discipline, freedom from a great strain upon the functions of the brain, and absence of any lengthened worry and mental anxiety. Temperate habits, an immunity from those youthful excesses which so frequently sap and undermine the physical and mental constitution, and sow the seeds of premature psychical impairment and bodily decrepitude, are essential to the preservation of the memory.

"Strange infirmities of the memory there are associated with cerebral disease, and justly to be regarded among its symptoms: large blanks in the backward gaze, fitful suspensions of the re-membering power; partial glimpses of the past; resurrections of thoughts long buried in oblivion! I speak not of that natural decay of the memory which is noticeable in most persons as age creeps on, and which is one of the most affecting of the many warn-ings then vouchsafed to us that the bodily frame is suffering dilapi-dation.[1] Even of this natural decay there are some curious things

---

[1] "The imbecility of age is not so painful to the old as it is to those who stand by and observe its condition. With the return of our second childhood, we lose the con-sciousness of our prime. The loss of any of our senses is accompanied with the obli-vion of its enjoyment. Thus, the blind are cheerful, the deaf happy, and the old con-tent. So that we are tempted to conclude, that those exquisite lines of Goethe, so ably rendered into English by their noble translator, express a poetic fiction rather than a reality:—

> 'Give me the active spring of gladness,
>   Of pleasure stretched almost to pain;
>   My hate, my love, in all their madness,—
>   Give me my youth again!'

Although the sight of the angelic Margaret, as

> 'She sat by the casement's chequered glass,
>   The clouds fly by, and she watches them pass
>   Over the city wall,'——

meditating on her love, were sufficient to enkindle a spark of passion even in the icy veins of an old dotard. But no: in the really old, the flame is extinct, the ashes have been burnt out, and no spark can ever fire them again. An aged gentleman, during the stunning and damaging effect of an apoplectic seizure, lost all his money by the failure of a bank. On recovering his senses, he could never, fortunately, be awak-

to be noted. Recent events are retained with difficulty and soon forgotten; while those of older date are easily and accurately recalled. This has been referred, and rightly, I believe, to the differing degree of interest, and therefore of attention, which the same objects excite in the young and in the old. It would seem as if the effort of attention stamped characters upon the material fabric which are deep and lasting in the youthful brain, faint and soon effaced in the aged. But disease may revive things long forgotten; a language long unspoken and unthought in; or blot out entirely all traces of definite portions of time gone by."[1]

An accomplished writer, when discussing the subject of "Human Longevity," makes the subjoined remarks respecting the impairment of memory consequent upon that gradual physical decadence so often witnessed in advanced life. He says: "The memory is undoubtedly the mental faculty which is first and most obviously affected by old age. This wonderful intermedium between body and mind, varying so greatly in different individuals, and so strangely capricious in the same individual; from the accidents of the day or hour, would seem to partake more of mere mechanism than any other of the intellectual powers. It undergoes changes more explicitly from physical causes, and both its excellences and defects are marked by peculiarities which appear to belong to conditions of an organic kind. The anomalies of memory in advanced life are familiar to every one, especially so, the facts of the early forgetfulness of names, and the frequent retention of things long past, while recent events flit away like shadows, leaving scarcely any trace behind.[2] Or, more strangely still (though never, perhaps,

---

ened to the feeling of poverty, nor the embarrassing consciousness of being a poor dependent on the bounty of his friends. Another gentleman, during a fit of apoplexy and its tedious consequences, lost two of his dearest relatives by death, and came into possession of some considerable property besides. On his recovery, he neither regretted the loss he had sustained, nor rejoiced at his own good fortune."—*Psychological Journal.*

[1] "Practice of Physic," by Thos. Watson, M.D.

[2] How sad is the picture which Lord John Russell has drawn of his friend Rogers's state of memory in advanced life! When speaking of this illustrious poet's decay of intellect, he says:—

"In his ninetieth year his memory began to fail him in a manner that was painful to his friends. He was no longer able to relate his shortest stories, or welcome his constant companion with his usual complimentary expressions. He began to forget familiar faces, and at last forgot that he had ever been a poet. It was impossible, however, even when memory had at length deserted the poet who had sung her

without some morbid changes of brain), the obliteration of certain classes of events or certain subjects of memory, as if by a sort of mechanical separation from everything else abiding in this mysterious receptacle.

" The importance of preserving memory in its integrity, as long and so far as it can be done, will probably be admitted. Some may urge that an oblivion of things past is the best security for a tranquil old age. But this virtually reduces man to a mere moiety of existence; and the same reasoning might be used to prove that utter imbecility of mind is a blessing in this latter stage of life; such imbecility from natural causes often occurs; but we have no title to consider it a good, or to neglect any means which may obviate or retard it. We will not venture to say that these means are many or certain. As regards memory in particular, all that can be done at this period of life is to aid in giving it the direction which circumstances make desirable, and to spare it those painful efforts at recollection which seem to weaken the very faculty they exercise. *The latter remark we believe to be of valu-

charms, to look upon him without a feeling of veneration. Faces of other times seemed to crowd over him as he sat, and what that now vacant mind had once known, what those now lifeless eyes had once seen, and what that now faltering tongue could once relate so well, were the thoughts uppermost in the minds of all who saw and knew him."

Another authority (*Edinburgh Review*, 1856) observes :—

" Till near ninety, Rogers was a striking exception to the rule ' of the decay of the mind before that of the body.' He then gradually dropped into that state, mental and bodily, which raises a reasonable doubt whether prolonged life be a blessing or a curse—

> 'Omni
> Membrorum damno major dementia, quæ nec
> Nomina servorum, neo vultum agnoscit amici,
> Cum quo preteritâ cœnavit nocte, nec illos,
> Quos genuit, quos eduxit.'—JUVEN. Sat. x.

" Although his impressions of long past events were as fresh as ever, he forgot the names of his relations and oldest friends, whilst they were sitting with him, and told the same stories to the same people, two or three times over in the same interview. But there were frequent glimpses of intellect in all its original brightness, of tenderness, of refinement, and of grace. ' Once driving out with him,' says a female correspondent, ' I asked him after a lady whom he could not recollect. He pulled the check-string, and appealed to his servant. ' Do I know Lady M——?' The reply was, ' Yes, sir.' This was a painful moment to us both. Taking my hand, he said, ' Never mind, my dear, I am not yet reduced to stop the carriage and ask if I know you ?' "

able application to other periods, long antecedent to old age ; but especially, perhaps, to that time when the faculty is first felt to decline in clearness and power.[1] Recollection—that is the effort of the will to combine or extricate what is laid up in the memory—cannot be carried beyond a particular point without inducing a certain confusion of mind hurtful to the faculty itself, and probably to others also.   The consciousness of every one will give proof as to these occurrences ; and at the time, if duly consulted, afford warning to avoid them.''[2]

The memory is often the power of the mind that first exhibits, in the acute and chronic affections of the brain and intellect, as well as disturbances of the cerebral circulation, symptoms of disorder, impairment, and decay.

In many of the organic diseases of the encephalon, some modification or weakness of the memory is usually observed, and in cases of red and white softening, cerebral tumors, as well as in those morbid changes in the nerve matter, its membranes or vessels, associated with general paralysis, this mental power shows, frequently, marked symptoms of early senescence.   Instances, however, of extensive organic disease of the brain occur, without, in a marked degree, deranging this faculty.   In some cases of tumor, abscess, and even extensive pulpy softening of the brain, I have known the memory to continue, intact, up to the moment of death! Inexplicable phenomenon ! Impairment of the memory is, however, often one of the earliest symptoms, attracting notice, and exciting apprehension at the commencement of cerebral disease. The patient, conscious of his failing, defective, or impaired power of retention, feels anxious as to the state of his brain and mind, and it often occurs, when he first consults his physician, that this is the only recognized and appreciable *psychical* sign detected by

---

[1] According to the theory of Dr. Lordat (Professor of Physiology in the University of Montpelier), a weakened memory does not always indicate a decadence of the intellectual principle. Memory (or the preservation of ideas in their full integrity), according to this authority, and the recollection of these ideas, are complex functions executed in concert by two principles. The remembrance of a fact is usually composed of two elements, the one *concrete*, the other *abstract*. The first of these is rather the offspring of the *vital* force than of the *intellectual* principle. It is not therefore surprising, that the aged condition of the former should manifest itself, while the latter power preserves its full integrity.

[2] *Edinburgh Review*, vol. cv, p. 75.

himself and noticed by others, of any disorder of the great nervous centre.

Previously to attacks of apoplexy and paralysis the patient is heard to complain of a stunned, inactive, confused, and sluggish state of the faculty, indicated by a difficulty in recalling with facility, ideas to the recollection. The attempt to revivify former states of consciousness, is accompanied by a severe effort, and sensations of physical distress clearly referrible to the head. This impairment of the memory is often connected with a condition of *hyperæmia* of the brain, and is occasionally premonitory of apoplexy, congestion, inflammation, softening, delirium, and other forms of acute cerebral disease.

The loss of memory that frequently precedes and accompanies disease of the brain is generally so insidious in its advances, that it occasionally for a period altogether escapes observation. This mental symptom is often associated with headache, vertigo, slight loss of sensation, and unrecognized hidden *epileptiform*, or even *epileptic* seizures. Occasionally, however, it exists for some time before any serious disturbance of the psychical, motorial, or sensorial functions is detected.

In the incipient stage of cerebral softening, as well as in those organic disintegrations of the delicate nerve vesicle observed in what is termed progressive, general, and cerebral paralysis, the patient often exhibits a debility of memory (long before disease of the brain is suspected) in regard to the most ordinary and trifling matters connected with the every-day occurrences of life. He forgets his appointments, is oblivious of the names of his particular friends, mislays his books, loses his papers, and is unable to retain in his mental grip for many consecutive minutes, the name of the month, or day of the week. He sits down to write a letter on some matter of business, and the attention being for a second diverted from what he is engaged in, he immediately loses all recollection of his correspondence, and leaves the letter unfinished. In this condition of mind he will be heard constantly inquiring for articles that he had carefully put aside but a few minutes previously. He neglects his dress and person, walking about the house in an unwashed condition, with his clothes most carelessly arranged, not from any indisposition to attend to his personal appearance, but from an unhealthy forgetfulness of, as well as morbid indifference to, the common courtesies, amenities, and decencies of life.

Sudden, transient, and paroxysmal attacks of loss of memory ought to be regarded as most important symptoms when considered in relation to a questionable state of the brain.   These temporary and apparently trifling conditions of impaired retention are often the preludes to serious manifestations of cerebral disease, the dark and threatening clouds that occasionally envelope, obscure, and often eclipse the mind previously to fatal attacks of paralysis, softening, apoplexy, and insanity !

A clergyman, a few weeks prior to an attack of cerebral hemorrhage, experienced on several occasions, whilst preaching extemporaneously, a sudden and momentary paralysis of all his ideas. This occurred on four or five occasions, causing great embarrassment in the exercise of his ministerial duties.   Instead of immediately recognizing this to be a symptom of disorder of the brain, imperatively demanding that he should obtain medical advice, and temporarily retire from anxious and active clerical work, he indiscreetly and obstinately persisted in preaching twice on the Sabbath-day, and also occupying himself during the week in parochial duties, until he discovered that he was utterly incapable of an act of continuous thought, and unable to preserve the current of his ideas, or even to connect together two consecutive sentences !   This patient died six months subsequently of softening of the brain ! Fatal result, may I not add, of an inexcusable neglect of urgent head symptoms ?

A man, about fifty years of age, forgot his own name.   He was from time to time convinced that he was dead.   He no longer recognized his immediate relatives.   He continued fifteen days in this state, when he died of an attack of apoplexy.   The *post-mortem* examination revealed an extravasation of blood within one of the hemispheres of the brain.   There was no other important cerebral lesion.[1]

A gentleman who had for many years been engaged in an arduous and painfully anxious contest for professional position and political advancement, struggling at the same time with great pecuniary embarrassments, whilst addressing one of the judges, suddenly lost all recollection of the facts embodied in his brief.

[1] Andral's " Clinique."

He was immediately obliged to retire from the court and return to his chambers. Severe headache ensued, accompanied by distressing nausea, terminating in a violent paroxysm of vomiting. Other symptoms denoting considerable head disorder then appeared. Under prompt treatment he recovered, and was able to resume, in a few weeks, his professional duties. On *three* subsequent occasions he experienced the same sudden loss of memory. This gentleman eventually died of softening of the brain, causing imbecility of mind.[1]

Cases, however, occur of loss of memory connected with slight sympathetic disturbances of the cerebral functions, dependent upon disorder of the general health, which are amenable to judicious remedial treatment. John Hunter was subject to an affection of the kind. Sir Everard Home says, of this illustrious physiologist and surgeon, " that he was, on one occasion, on a visit at the residence of a friend. He did not know in what part of the house he was, nor even the name of the street when he was told, nor where his own home was. He had not a conception of anything existing beyond the room in which he was, and yet he was perfectly conscious of his loss of memory. He was sensible to various kinds of impressions, and therefore looked out of the window, although rather dark, to see if he could be made conscious of the situation of the house. The loss of memory gradually subsided, and in a few hours it was perfectly restored."

In some cases, temporary attacks of loss of memory are caused by excessive animal indulgences, self-abuse, intemperance, debaucheries, injudicious use of mercurials, exhausting discharges, and in one instance that came under my observation, the impairment of memory was clearly the result of arsenical medicine incautiously administered for the cure of an obstinate cutaneous disease.

Intemperance in eating has been known to impair the memory. It is said by Suetonius that the Roman Emperor Claudius lost his

---

[1] "*Amnesia* always indicates preceding disorders of the brain, especially of the anterior lobes, or very depressed powers. In acute disorders, it generally betokens a fatal termination, if not an instantaneous crisis; in chronic diseases, for the most part, it indicates incurability; or, when it occurs suddenly in epileptic and hysterical patients, an immediately approaching violent paroxysm. Partial amnesia (forgetfulness of some things) indicates a probably violent, but not always permanent, effect on the brain."—Feuchtersleben's " *Medical Psychology*," p. 194.

memory so entirely from this cause, that he not only forgot the names and persons of those to whom he wished to speak, but even of what he intended to say when attempting to engage in conversation.[1]

A lady, after a protracted labor, suffered a severe attack of uterine hemorrhage, and her life, for nearly a week, was despaired of. The loss of blood that occurred reduced her to a condition of extreme vital prostration and mental depression. It was necessary for the nurse to feed and attend to her like a child. When she was able to articulate, her husband was astonished to find that her memory was paralyzed! She had forgotten where she was residing, who her husband was, how long she had been ill, the names of her children, and in fact, her own name was obliterated from her recollection! She was unable to call anything by its right appellation. In attempting to do so she made the most singular mistakes. She had been in the habit, previously to her illness, of talking in French more than English (her husband being a native of France), but whilst in the state of mind described, she appeared to have lost all knowledge of French, for when addressed by her husband in that language she did not appear to have the slightest comprehension of what he was saying, although she could speak English without much difficulty. A period of nearly seven or eight weeks elapsed before the memory began to improve, and it was not until the expiration of some months that her mind appeared to regain its original strength.

Sir H. Holland refers to his own case, as an example of transient failure of memory resulting from bodily fatigue. He says: "I descended on the same day, two very deep mines in the Harz Mountains, remaining some hours underground in each. While in the second mine, and exhausted both from fatigue and inanition, I felt the utter impossibility of talking longer with the German inspector who accompanied me. Every German word and phrase deserted my recollection, and it was not until I had taken food and wine, and been some time at rest, that I regained them."[2]

A gentleman whose mental and physical powers had been

---

[1] By an old Spanish law no person was admitted into the witness-box to give evidence in a disputed legal case, who was proved to indulge in habits of intemperance, as an excessive use of stimulants was considered to weaken and destroy the memory.

[2] "Mental Pathology," by Sir H. Holland, Bart., M.D., D.C.L., p. 167.

20

severely exercised, suddenly lost all recollection of recent events. His memory appeared to be paralyzed. Whilst engaged in active conversation he was able, by a strong effort of the will, to retain possession of the ideas suggested by others to his mind, but if there were the slightest interruption, even to the extent of a minute, in the conversation, he lost all recollection of what he had previously been saying! This gentleman had been living for some weeks below par, with the view of enabling him to perform an amount of urgent mental work, requiring for its execution the lengthened concentration of a clear and vigorous intellect. He had been in the habit of drinking a fair portion of wine, but had unwisely abandoned the use of stimulants, fancying that by so doing he would be better fitted for clear-headed mental occupation. Under my advice he lived generously, took iron tonics, quinine, and zinc, and resumed his daily quantity of wine. This treatment eventually restored his memory to a state of health.

I have known other instances of temporary loss of memory cured within a short period by a free exhibition of tonics and stimulants. In these cases the brain is generally in a starved and impoverished condition (owing to poverty of blood), and suffers from a state of innervation and inanition. A gentleman, well known for his intense passion for field-sports (living, it may be said, upon the saddle during the greater part of the year), frequently complained of transient attacks of loss of memory after a hard day's run with the hounds. His remedy for this affection was half-a-pint to a pint of port wine, *which he was in the habit of occasionally drinking at a draught!* The effect of this heroic stimulating dose upon the depressed energy of the brain was magical. The memory immediately recovered its vigorous activity.

In more chronic cases of loss of memory, a persevering use of iron, combined with small doses of strychnine, the sulphate of copper, cod-liver oil, quinine, minute doses of phosphorus, the shower-bath, electricity applied locally to the head, as recommended by Dr. Darwin in his "*Zoonomia*," all, according to circumstances, are found beneficial, provided no serious extent of acute organic lesion has taken place in the brain, or the attack of loss of memory has not followed paralysis or apoplexy. But, even in these apparently hopeless cases, much good may be accomplished, when all *active* head symptoms have subsided, by a course of tonic and stimulating treatment.

A clergyman, between forty and fifty years of age, was actively employed in reading with two young gentlemen who were preparing for their university examinations and degrees. He had been so engaged for eight continuous weeks, working laboriously at the rate of from eight to ten hours *de die in diem*. One afternoon, whilst busily engaged in explaining a subtle mathematical problem to his pupils, he was suddenly seized with an attack of severe *vertigo* (unaccompanied by any convulsive symptoms). This was succeeded by a complete loss of memory. He could retain nothing in his mind. On the following day he was brought to London, and I saw him. He complained of dull, heavy headache, and great depression of spirits. His general health was sadly vitiated. The cerebral symptoms being somewhat active, and congestion diagnosed, a few leeches were applied to the head, followed by a blister to the nape of the neck. A state of complete *brain* and mind quietude, repose, and inaction were enjoined. He had also administered to him mercurial alteratives, with occasional warm and aromatic purgatives. In the course of a few weeks he decidedly improved. He then took mineral acids with the extract of taraxacum. I then sent him abroad for the purpose of diverting his attention from the anxieties of home, but more with the view of removing him from all temptation to mental work. He returned to England, after the lapse of a few months, quite restored in mind and body. He has had no return of the loss of memory. He, however, found it necessary to abstain from severe mental application, and consequently, in deference to my advice, declined receiving pupils.

An eminent provincial surgeon, of large and anxious practice, was seized with a sudden failure of memory. He forgot all his appointments, and to such a degree was the faculty of retention impaired, that he was obliged to make memoranda of every trifling and minute circumstance which it was important for him to remember, and to these he was constantly referring in order to refresh his memory. This attack was preceded by headache, of which he had complained for nearly a fortnight. Up to the period of the case being brought under my notice, no suspicion was entertained as to the existence of any prior state of cerebral ill-health sufficient to account satisfactorily for his apparently *sudden* loss of mental power. I, however, ascertained that about eight weeks, or nearly three months previously, he was seized, whilst in the act of applying the stethoscope to the chest of a patient, with severe epileptic vertigo. He lost consciousness for a minute. This was succeeded by an attack of distressing sick headache. Three days subsequently he had a second paroxysm of vertigo, and nearly fell out of the carriage in which he was sitting at the time. His spirits subsequently became much depressed, but in a few days he again rallied, and flattered himself that he had quite recovered. He made no mention of these attacks to any member of his family, and carefully avoided all conversation on the subject of his health with his medical brethren. When I saw this gentleman the only appreciable mental symptom was an inability to retain in his mind, for many consecutive minutes, any recent impressions. His pulse was feeble, face pallid, and general health shattered. His spirits were, however, at times buoyant, and the prognosis which he formed of his own case was favorable! Alas! as the result established, he proved to be a false prophet. I had a consultation with this medical gentleman's partner, and gave it as my opinion that the attacks of vertigo were clearly of an *epileptiform* character, and consequent upon subtle structural changes taking place in the brain. Two weeks after his return home he had an epileptic fit. He then became rapidly worse, and ten months subsequently died in a deplorable state of mental imbecility !

A patient, connected with a large commercial house as confidential traveller, consulted me the year before last, complaining of impairment of memory. He had occupied a position of great trust and unceasing anxiety for a continuous period of *fifteen* years, always exhibiting a remarkable degree of intelligence, acute sagacity and capacity for business. For about six months previously to my being consulted, he had foolishly undertaken *extra* evening work, as one of the principal clerks in the house with which he was connected was obliged to leave England to visit a near relative residing abroad, who was in a state of alarming illness. This additional brain work was the "straw that broke the camel's back." This gentleman continued under my care for nearly twelve months, by which time he entirely recovered the use of his memory. I found small doses of the acetate of strychnia, combined with iron and quinine, of great benefit. He had, however, previously taken, with much advantage, cod-liver oil and the phosphate of iron, and had used the shower, and, eventually, the *douche* bath to the spine, with evident service.

A member of the bar complained some years ago of occasional attacks of enfeebled memory. He attributed this mental impairment to the fact of his having been engaged as counsel the previous year in several anxious and severely contested election cases. I advised an entire cessation from all professional work. I had great difficulty in persuading this gentleman to recognize the necessity for a complete abstinence from mental occupation. He promised a guarded acquiescence in my strict injunctions, but finding himself relieved, after an interval of a few weeks he returned, in opposition to my solicitations, to his chambers, and recommenced active practice. As I predicted, he soon broke down, and I was once more conferred with. He then recognized it to be a matter of vital necessity that he should give his mind prolonged rest, and agreed, unreservedly, to do so. I kept him for a period of *two years* from all anxious and severe mental occupation, and by that time his powers of mind had rallied to a surprising extent; in fact they became, according to his own impression, more vigorous than they were prior to his attack of illness. For many years this patient has continued steadily at work, never having had a return of loss of memory. I should premise that I exacted from him a promise that he would read no briefs after dinner. He has rigidly adhered to this understanding; but being an early riser, and a man of remarkable quickness of apprehension, he is able to master a large amount of work before breakfast. I also made it a *sine qua non* that he should go abroad every year for a period of two months, thus insuring for him a complete diversion and relaxation of the mind from all injurious pressure. He has scrupulously complied with my instructions, and the result is, an entire freedom from all symptoms of mental impairment and cerebral disorder.

A commercial traveller, anxious to accomplish with expedition a particular portion of his journey, travelled in an open gig during a severely cold night in the month of February, 1857. On his arrival at daylight at a wayside inn, he felt extremely benumbed. He drank a glass of hot brandy and water, and then partook of some solid refreshment. In the afternoon of that day he complained of severe headache. The pain was of so intense a character, that the patient screamed during the paroxysms of cephalalgia. This headache was succeeded by a violent attack of vomiting, and great impairment and confusion of sight. In the evening he became extremely lethargic. A local surgeon was summoned to the case, and the treatment adopted was, as the result established, extremely judicious. The acute brain mischief was arrested, and the man, at the expiration of a fortnight, was able to return apparently well to London. A few months after this attack of cerebral disease he was brought under my notice in consequence of *the memory being nearly paralyzed.* He had previously been an active man of business, and had always exhibited great shrewdness in matters of account; but he complained, when I saw him, of a total inability to retain in his mind the most trifling matters, particularly in relation to *figures.* He was unable to add up, with his usual facility, a long account, and could not recollect for one second the result of the calculation. His general health was impaired; the action of the heart feeble, the pulse weak and irregular, secretions depraved, and the renal functions unhealthy. I advised a total absence from business for a lengthened period. He continued, near London, under my care for some weeks, during which period he took the mineral acids, taraxacum, mild mercurial alteratives, and subsequently small doses of sulphate of zinc and copper combined with the extract of nux vomica. He had blisters applied to the nape of the neck and behind the ears, and used the tepid as well as the cold shower-bath.

He then, by my advice, removed into the country, and remained in a passive cerebral and mental state for nearly nine months, attending to no matters of business, but taking regular horse exercise. At the expiration of twelve months he came back to London nearly well. He soon resumed his ordinary occupation, and since then has had no return of cerebral symptoms. His memory is sufficiently strong for all business purposes, but not so tenacious as it was previously to his illness.

A tradesman fell down a trap-door at the back of his shop into a cellar, and received a severe blow upon his head. He was partially stunned. He was able, however, in the course of the afternoon of that day, to go to the country and join his family. For some days after the accident he complained of considerable uneasiness in the neighborhood of the right parietal bone. The sensation was not one of pain, but that of *weight* and *heaviness.* I saw him in consequence of unusual manifestations of irritability, sleeplessness, and damaged memory. His pulse was quick and sharp, the action of the heart laborious, and there was a want of uniformity in the movement of the pupils. The symptoms indicated somewhat active head disturbance. I ordered him to be cupped to the extent of ten ounces, and to be well purged by means of drastic cathartics. The loss of blood proved decidedly beneficial. The feeling of weight and heaviness in the head materially diminished after the cupping. In the course of five days, the brain again exhibited signs of morbid activity, and the patient was a second time cupped. This was followed by more decided results than the first local depletion. I enjoined the strictest quietude, and abstinence from both physical and mental excitement. After all evidence of acute cerebral mischief had subsided, he went through a course of mineral tonics, and subsequently took quinine with decided advantage. He, eventually, was able to return to business with his memory but slightly impaired. This patient has for some years occupied a trying commercial position, free from any recurrence of active and anxious cerebral symptoms.

A solicitor was thrown out of a hansom cab, and fell upon his head. He was removed into a chemist's shop, and a neighboring surgeon sent for. I am informed that there were at the time slight symptoms of cerebral concussion. He was confined to his bed for a few days, and to the house for some weeks. He was able after that time to return to his professional duties, apparently quite restored to his original health. Seven months after the accident he called upon me respecting the state of his memory. I found it extremely defective, particularly as to *dates* and *names*. There were no other mental symptoms denoting mischief in the brain, or mind, independently of occasional attacks of severe mental depression. I had this case under my observation, at varying intervals, for nearly eighteen months, but no treatment I adopted appeared to give more than temporary relief. This gentleman eventually exhibited great general mental impairment, and in the course of the fourth year from the accident, became hemiplegic, and ultimately died in a severe attack of convulsions. The brain after death exhibited evidence of long-existing chronic white softening in both hemispheres. There was also considerable fatty degeneration of the vessels of the brain.

An officer in the Hon. East India Company's service, returned to England with a singular loss of memory, caused by what was alleged to be a *moon stroke*, he having incautiously slept one night for several hours exposed to the rays of a full moon. When he awoke his mind was much confused.   He then had headache and great gastric irritation.   He recovered from the acute cerebral symptoms, with his memory, however, much affected.   In consequence of this state of mind, he was obliged to leave India and return home on sick leave.   His father brought him to me, and placed him under my care.   I treated him by means of counterirritants and tonics, after attending particularly to the condition of the liver, which was in a state of great engorgement.   Cod-liver oil, combined with phosphorus and iron, was eventually exhibited with decided advantage.   This gentleman, after the lapse of eighteen months, returned to India, apparently quite restored.   I regret to hear that, some months after his arrival there, the memory again manifested symptoms of impairment.   He has, unfortunately, been placed in an anxious and trying position since his return to military duty, and this may account for the recurrence of his enfeebled powers of retention.

A gentleman left London for the seaside, accompanied by his wife, who was a serious invalid.   He had for some months been in an anxious state of mind respecting her health.   Independently of the mental distress he experienced in consequence of the alarming character of his wife's indisposition, his own mind had been for many years most zealously, actively, and continuously occupied in literary, political, and professional pursuits.   A few days after his arrival his wife became dangerously ill.   This gave rise to additional worry and anxiety.   Subsequently to her acute attack he felt indisposed, and complained slightly of his head. He said to a member of his family, that he was going to take a hot sea-water bath.   He did so, and on his return home he went to his bedroom, where he was found, some hours afterwards, in a profound state of lethargic sleep.   Upon being roused he awoke, but was evidently in a confused state of mind.   He asked where he was, and many other absurd questions respecting himself and family.   He appeared to be suffering from a complete paralysis of the memory.   I was requested to see him, and accordingly left London for that purpose.   I found his memory as to recent events seriously damaged.   He was under no kind of delusion, or in fact any form of aberration, neither were his perceptive faculties or reasoning powers at all affected.   He conversed with great sagacity, fluency, and acuteness on every subject, but if I permitted a second to elapse in the conversation, he entirely forgot what he had been previously talking of. ' Beyond this period he could not retain in his mind a suggested idea or train of thought. He never rallied from this state of intellect. For a few months he exhibited mental powers of a high order. He could discuss at short intervals, the most subtle and abstruse political, professional, and literary matters, with apparently unimpaired mental vigor. His memory, however, never recovered its healthy tenacity. This gentleman's intellect subsequently became much weakened, as the effect of several paralytic seizures which he has suffered from of late years. I am informed that up to the day of using the hot sea bath, his memory was not appreciably affected. Had he a fit immediately after coming out of the water, or on his return home? It appears that the bath was taken after an early dinner, and at the time of his complaining of uneasy cerebral sensations ! [1]

A tradesman, who died at the age of fifty-four of softening of the brain, exhibited four years previously symptoms of undoubted cerebral disorder, which were considered at the time to depend upon disease of the liver. He had for a period of nearly thirty years a great strain upon his mind, having to conduct, without any material assistance, a large and complicated commercial business. He eventually engaged with a partner, but not until his friends recognized symptoms that made them anxious as to the state of his brain. He was at times unusually agitated and flurried. He would sit up late at night looking through accounts and reading letters relating to matters long since settled. He could not be persuaded of the absurdity of this proceeding, and when expostulated with would say, "I know my own affairs best ; it is necessary I should acquaint myself with the state of my business." On one occasion he carried a letter about with him for the whole of the day. It was of long antecedent date, and related to a matter that had been arranged many years previously. He appeared puzzled respecting the letter, and frequently asked whether it was all right ? It was with difficulty he was persuaded that it was not of the slightest importance. On another occasion he insisted upon going most minutely and unnecessarily into his banker's account, without saying anything that would justify a

---

[1] According to the authority of the ancients, the warm bath is most destructive to voluptuaries, by producing fatal attacks of paralysis and apoplexy, particularly when used *turgide epulis.* "*Hinc subita mortes atque intestata senectus,*" says Juvenal.

suspicion that he thought any error had been committed. He was
restless and fidgety, anxious to be actively engaged, without having
any clear conception as to what he was doing, or wished to do.
At this time there was no perceptible aberration of mind, failure
of memory, or positive symptoms of cerebral paralysis. He continued in this condition for two years, during which time he was
occasionally better in mind. His memory eventually showed
signs of great impairment. This was considered as the first
decided symptom of brain disease. His agitation of manner, restlessness, disposition to read old letters, and annoy himself respecting unimportant matters of business, were considered at the time
as a state of simple "nervousness," dependent upon hepatic and
gastric derangement. The result, however, established the error
of diagnosis that had been committed, for at this period it was
evident disease of the *brain* had commenced.

In many forms of brain disease and psychical disorder, the
memory, in the incipient stage, is not so much impaired as it is
confused and erratic in its manifestations. The patient recollects
with sufficient clearness what he desires or wishes to recall to mind,
but the images so reproduced are disjointed and in a state of *mêlée*.
He complains of his brain and intellect being in a muddled and
addled state. I attended a patient who suffered, principally from
this symptom, four weeks prior to his death from apoplexy.

In inflammatory as well as in white softening of the brain, this
confused condition of the memory is a prominent and common
symptom in the early periods of the disease. A literary gentleman of some position died at the age of fifty-nine, of non-inflammatory ramollissement of the brain, complicated with epilepsy.
For many years previously to his death, his mind had become
manifestly impaired. He complained of a loss of mental vigor
and tone, but with these symptoms his memory, for a time, exhibited no obvious sign of actual weakness. It was, however, occasionally very much confused. He was in the habit, for some
period previously to the development of serious head symptoms,
of comparing his mind to a *kaleidoscope!* There was no want of
vivid ideas, or capacity to revive, by an effort of the will, past
states of consciousness, but the images so reproduced were, to use
his own expression, in a " confused and entangled condition."

In certain states of perturbed and agitated thought, the ideas
appear to lose their coherence and connection, the mental faculties

(particularly the memory) becoming quite confused. This ofteñ occurs to persons in health who are subject to paroxysms of violent passion and ill-governed emotion. Similar phenomena are observable in cases of insanity. They have been compared to the distorted reflections observed in a troubled piece of water. "*Les idées se rétablissent par le repos et la tranquillité, comme une eau qui cesse d'être agitée, représente des images fidèles.*" [1]

[1] "Dict. des Scien. Méd." tome xii, p. 99.

CHAPTER XV.

CHRONIC (MODIFIED) AFFECTIONS OF THE MEMORY.

REMARKABLE modifications in the operations of the memory are occasionally seen connected with the early symptoms of brain disease, such as recollecting only the Christian name of relations and intimate friends, confounding one name with another, being able only to pronounce words of a certain sound; an inability to remember or articulate (arising from the effects of paralysis and other diseases of the brain) particular letters of the alphabet.

A patient, who had several paralytic seizures, always knew when his attack was approaching by forgetting his own Christian name. When asked to sign a letter, he could only write his surname, and occasionally only half of that. A gentleman, subject to severe attacks of epilepsy, some days before his attack, invariably signs half of his name, not being able to do so in full!

A lady, in consequence of an attack of acute disease of the brain, lost, for some time, all recollection of her own name, and never could pronounce it unless she saw it in writing.

A gentleman of rank, when in the incipient stage of white softening of the brain, occasionally forgot his name when walking in the public streets, and sometimes lost all notion of his address. He was in the habit of stopping strangers, and saying, "I live so-and-so, what is my name?" or, "I am Sir So-and-so, where do I reside?"

A gentleman injured his head by a fall from his horse. He was confined to his bed for several weeks in a state of imperfect consciousness. On his recovery, it was found that all recollection, not only of the accident, but of the circumstances which for some time preceded it, had been obliterated entirely from his mind! A considerable period elapsed before the lost ideas began gradually to recur to the memory. The circumstances of his journey returned by degrees to his recollection. As he repeatedly rode over that part of the country where the accident occurred, the sight of surrounding objects gradually recalled the evanescent trains of ideas with which they had been connected, to his recollection. He afterwards remembered nearly the whole transaction.

Mr. Abernethy has recorded the case of an injury of the head, which happened to a foreigner, twenty-seven years of age, who spoke English perfectly well; during his illness this man could only answer in French, and said he was but sixteen years old.

A man was brought into St. Thomas's Hospital who had received considerable injury of the head, but from which he ultimately recovered. When he became convalescent, he spoke a language which no one about him could comprehend. However, a Welsh milk-woman came one day into the ward, and immediately understood what he said. It appeared that the patient was a Welshman, and had been absent from his native country about thirty years. In the course of that period he had entirely forgotten his native tongue, and acquired the English language. But when he recovered from his accident he forgot the language he had been so recently in the habit of speaking, and regained the knowledge of that which he had originally acquired and lost.

A French countess, during the Revolution, left her country and resided in England. She had a severe attack of fever, in the course of which she became completely delirious. At this time she was frequently heard to talk and cry out in a jargon, which at first was quite unintelligible to everybody, and seemed to consist of mere sounds without meaning. However, there happened to be in the house a Welsh domestic, who declared that she understood the countess, and affirmed that she spoke correctly the Welsh language. When the lady recovered from her illness, and again spoke to her friends in an idiom intelligible to them, they related the fact to her, which had excited no small surprise and curiosity. They were then informed, that during her infancy she had been taught the dialect of Lower Britanny, by a nurse who was a native of that country, but had totally forgotten it many years before the attack of fever, which in so curious a manner revived the impressions that had been so long obliterated.[1]

A lady, fifty-one years of age, of sanguine complexion and ple-

---

[1] The language of Lower Britanny is well known to be a dialect of Welsh.

thoric habit, after a fit of apoplexy, which induced a state of unconsciousness, which continued for three or four days, was found to have her faculties in some respects impaired. The remarkable circumstance was, that she had lost the power or aptitude to speak in her native language, which was English. This continued a month, and her nurses and servants were obliged to employ a person to interpret for them. The lady herself spoke to them in French.

An old gentleman was seized with hemiplegia of his right side, associated with profound sleep. The same side was convulsed on the second day. On the ninth day he recovered from the state of stupor, but his faculties were gone. After several weeks he began to know his intimate friends; then to remember words, to repeat the prayers of his church, and read a few words of *German* (instead of *French*, his native language), every day. While making slow advances in knowledge, he died suddenly of an acute cerebral attack.[1]

The following facts form good illustrations of that modified condition of memory, of which I am now speaking. After an attack of brain disease, a man had at his command only the first syllable of names, that is to say, he could not finish the pronunciation of one word, although he knew the first syllable of it. An old man forgot the names of persons, but appeared to recollect very correctly, every evening, a remarkable epoch of his life, although it had occurred a long time previously. When sitting with his wife he imagined he was at the house of a lady with whom, many years previously, he was in the habit of spending his evenings. He would then, addressing his wife, say, "Madam, I cannot stop any longer with you, for when one has a wife and children, we owe them a good example—I must return home." After this compliment he endeavored to depart.

There is upon record the particulars of a remarkable case of a patient who had, in consequence of an injury to the brain, forgotten how to *read*, but who was still able to *write* fluently and correctly. After two attacks of apoplexy, a man forgot his own name as well as that of his wife, children, and all his friends. He became restless, suspicious, and very irritable. Eventually, his

---

[1] A few of these illustrations are transcribed from Dr. Prichard's treatise "*On the Diseases of the Nervous System.*"

memory was partially restored. He was enabled, however, to repeat only the following expressions: "Yes," "no," "much," "very well," "not at all," "it is true," "it is just," "it is wonderful." These words, which he generally applied with tolerable accuracy, were almost the only ones he knew how to use.

After an attack of hemiplegia, a lady suffered from a singular defect of memory. In speaking she only used the infinitive of verbs, and did not employ any pronouns. For example, instead of saying, "I wish you good day; stop, my husband has just come," she would remark, "To wish good day, to stop husband to come." For a long time this patient could not count beyond the number three, but eventually was able to go as high as forty. She also succeeded in obtaining a knowledge of pronouns without being able to make a proper application of them.

A very intelligent and highly respectable young lady, after much painful and prolonged family altercation, married a man whom she passionately loved. After her first confinement, she suffered from an acute bodily affection, which was followed by protracted and distressing debility. After her apparent recovery, it was found that she had lost altogether the recollection of the time that had elapsed since the day of her marriage. She remembered, with remarkable vividness, every previous event of her life; but, from the day of her marriage, every idea appeared to have been obliterated from the mind. When her husband made advances, she repudiated all knowledge of, or relation to him. She acted in the same way with regard to the child. Her parents and her friends by their authority succeeded in persuading her that she was in reality married, and had given birth to a son. She attached some degree of faith to their assurances, because she would rather believe that she had lost the recollection of her wedding-day, than entertain the notion that her friends and relations were lying impostors. She, however, beheld her husband and her child without being able to imagine by what magic she had acquired possession of the one, and given birth to the other![1]

"In August, 1785," says Dr. Hertz, "I was called to an officer of the artillery, a man about forty years old, who, as I was informed, was seized with a palsy in consequence of cold and violent anger. His tongue, hands, and feet were paralyzed by the attack.

[1] Vide Art. "Mémoire," *Dict. des Sciences Méd.*, tom. xxxii, p. 5.

He was under the care of one of our first physicians, at whose desire I was consulted concerning the propriety of applying electricity. From the time that this remedy was first employed until the following year, I never saw him; but he then sent for me again, as his own physician, he said, had deserted him. I found him so much recovered as to have the complete use of his feet; his hands, also, were stronger, but in regard to his speech the following very remarkable circumstance was to be observed: he was able to articulate distinctly any words which either occurred to him spontaneously, or when they were slowly and loudly repeated to him. He strenuously exerted himself to speak, but an unintelligible kind of murmur was all that could be heard. The effort he made was violent, and terminated in a deep sigh. On the other hand, he could *read aloud with facility*. If a book, or any written paper, was held before his eyes, he read so quick and distinctly, that it was impossible to observe that there was the slightest fault in his organs of speech. But if the book or paper were withdrawn, *he was then totally incapable of pronouncing one of the words which he had read the instant before*. I tried this experiment with him repeatedly, not only in the presence of his wife, but of many other people. The effect was uniformly the same."[1]

Dr. Osborne, who has published an interesting paper on the loss of the faculty of speech and memory, in connection with disease of the brain, considers that there are two kinds of loss of memory of language; the first he believes to be usually connected with softening of some portion of the brain, and is most frequently witnessed in advanced age. This is characterized by an imperfect recollection of dates, names of places, as well as of persons; but as far as the muscular powers of articulation have not been impeded by paralysis, the faculty of language remains unimpaired, and the individual speaks with his usual facility, until all the faculties become involved in the disease, and total fatuity results.

The other imperfection, he believes, involves language in all its parts nearly in an equal degree, except in the slighter forms, when proper names, or other words of less frequent occurrence, are alone affected. It does not consist in want of memory of the word to be pronounced, but in a loss of recollection of the mode

[1] "Psychological Magazine," vol. viii.

of using the vocal apparatus so as to pronounce it. This peculiar affection comes on during all ages. Although appearing to arise from disease of the brain, yet it is not necessarily the precursor of any serious cerebral affection.

Defective or perverted memory is one of the common results of concussion of the brain, and even follows some of the slighter forms of mechanical injury to the head. Numerous cases illustrative of this fact are upon record.

A soldier, who was trepanned, lost in the operation some portion of the brain. It was afterwards discovered that he had forgotten the numbers *five* and *seven*, and was not able until some time to recollect them. A man of scholastic attainments lost, after an attack of acute fever, all knowledge of the letter F. A gentleman who was thrown from his horse, and who suffered from a severe concussion of his brain, for some months after the accident entirely lost all memory of his own children's names.

Sir B. Brodie mentions the case of a groom who was cleaning a horse, and was kicked so as to produce concussion of the brain. He quickly recovered from the shock, and having quite forgotten what he had been about, he informed those near him, that he must " go and get the horse out of the stable to clean him."

Wepfer relates the case of a gentleman who, after having received a partial injury to the head by a fall from his horse, found that he had entirely lost the knowledge of a particular language with which he had been well acquainted, although his memory in other respects remained uninjured.

A young man, about twenty years of age, a miner by profession, fell from a height of a dozen feet, alighting upon his heels, but receiving such a shock that he was insensible for half an hour, and unable to articulate distinctly. At the expiration of a couple of years he was taken to the Hôtel Dieu, being supposed to labor under hemiplegia.

The patient was carried into the operating theatre, and examined by Baron Dupuytren, under whose care he was placed. He was emaciated, pale, and rather embarrassed in his manner, but not presenting the least appearance of idiotcy or feebleness of intellect.

" What is your profession ?" asked the Baron.

"*Mine*—" answered he, with considerable difficulty, and it was only after repeated efforts that he was able to articulate "*mineur*."

" What age are you ?"

21

"*Ving—t—t—d—eux—ans.*"

" Your name ?"

"*Jacques Col—in—Col—as—Col—ard.*"

" Have you any brothers and sisters ?—*Oui.* How many brothers ?—*Un.* How many sisters ?—*Trois.* What is your father ?—*Peintre.* What profession is the husband of your eldest sister ?—*V—V—Ver—.* Vitrier (a glazier) ? asked M. Dupuytren.—He shook his head. Does he make bottles ?—Sign in the negative; and *V—V—Ver—*was all he could pronounce.

" Do you understand what I am asking you? said the surgeon.—*Oui.* Strike the table—he struck it; lift up your foot; put it back upon the ground; turn your head to the right side, to the left; walk forwards; return; put on your cap, &c. He was obeyed with the most military precision. The muscular motions of the tongue were free enough, and it was evident that nothing like paralysis or hemiplegia existed.

" On being ordered to repeat *sa, se, si, so, su,* he was unable to articulate the two latter, and merely pronounced the *o* and *u.* Instead of *mon père*, he could only answer *pè—*; for *ma mère*, he answered *mè—.* The examination was completed, and the patient walking off without a salutation, when M. Dupuytren called him back, and told him to doff his cap. He did as he was required. Bid the gentlemen *adieu.* *Ad—d—eu*, said he, and walked away.

" On a subsequent day, experiments were made to ascertain whether the tongue, as the organ of *taste*, continued perfect in its functions. Salt, sugar, and pepper were the substances employed; the first of which he recognized, the second he confounded with the first, and the pepper he called rum. On giving him some water, he knew and drank it without the slightest difficulty.

" The patient evinced no signs whatever of feebleness of intellect, and the muscular motions of the tongue were free and unembarrassed. M. Dupuytren considered the affection as resembling what occasionally occurs after apoplexy, or chronic affections of the brain, where the patient suffers loss of the memory of things, or particular words, as proper names, substantives, or adjectives. In some individuals the power of judging and comparing objects is destroyed. An old lady, after an attack of hemiplegia, preserved the general use of her intellectual faculties, but could only answer to whatever question she was asked: ' *Saint Antoine, Saint Antoine !*' M. Dupuytren considered, in the case previously recorded, the affection of the tongue (both as an organ of articulation and of taste), as rather depending on a general affection of the brain, than on a local lesion of the two sets of nerves which endow the organ with the sense of taste and the power of motion."[1]

A French soldier was struck at the battle of Waterloo by a bullet, at the exterior of the forehead, six or eight millimetres from the left eyebrow, and in the point corresponding to the curved line on the temporal fossa. He fell senseless, and remained two days and nights on the field of battle. He was subsequently conveyed to Brussels, and although many attempts were made to extract the ball, they proved fruitless. Bleeding and other remedies were adopted to remove the paralysis of the side and other existing symptoms of brain compression. After some months he was received into the military hospital at Paris. The wound, on examination, presented an inflamed circumference, and in the centre the ball was imbedded in the substance of the *os frontis* to that depth that the half of it must have projected into the cranial cavity. After a period he was fit for active service, but it was discovered that he had lost the memory of proper names and of some substantives, although all his powers of reasoning were unimpaired.

He eventually died of phthisis, the singular mental defect referred to continuing up to the time of his death. M. Larrey, who related the case at the Academy of Medicine, exhibited the skull, with the ball firmly fixed in the previously mentioned place, the internal table of bone having been fractured and forced inwards at the moment of the accident.

A gentleman after an attack of paralysis, when attempting to pronounce words, always transposed the letters. For example, in endeavoring to say the word *flute* he said *tufle*, *puc* for *cup*, *gum* instead of *mug*.

A case is upon record of a young woman who, at each periodical change in her health, forgot entirely all that occurred to her during the interval. On one occasion, at the time of the intermission, she inflicted a serious injury upon a person with whom she had a dispute. The case came into court a few days afterwards, when she denied the fact upon oath. The plaintiff being condemned to

[1] " Clinique."

costs, brought witnesses to corroborate her charge, and establish that the defendant had denied upon oath what was the fact, but without any bad object in view.

Thucydides records, that after the plague of typhus fever which followed (in the Dorian war) the famine at Athens, many who recovered from the effects of this epidemic, entirely lost their memories. So completely was such the case, that they not only forgot the names of their friends and relations, but their own.[1]

A somewhat similar impairment of memory has been observed to follow all great epidemics and severe national disasters. Dr. Gase, in his "*History of the Epidemic of Wilna*," refers to this phenomenon. Sydenham remarks, that after the epidemic fever that prevailed in 1673, the memory of those who had been ill was singularly affected.

Prolonged exposure to a low, as well as to a high degree of temperature, has been known temporarily and permanently to paralyze the memory.

A gentleman who had made a successful ascent of one of the high Alps, records, that for some weeks subsequently he found his memory considerably impaired, particularly as to *dates* and *figures*. He made the most singular mistakes in this respect, rarely being able to name accurately the day of the week or month. He also found himself unable, with his usual facility, to calculate his daily and weekly expenditure, and made the most odd mistakes in addition, as well as in figures, writing 7 for 5 and 3 for 1. This aberration of memory was, happily, not of long duration.

In an account published many years back, of the wreck of a ship in the Pacific Ocean, it is recorded, that the crew and passengers suffered from extreme privations, fatigue, and lengthened exposure to anxiety of mind and intense cold. The unhappy crew and passengers were fortunately rescued from death by a whaler. Several of the seamen subsequently died, three became deranged, and a few who escaped death and madness found that their intellects were much impaired, particularly as regards the faculty of memory. One man lost all recollection of the antecedents of his life. The memory as to recent painful events was singularly accurate and vivid, but he could give no information as to where he was born, whether he had any family, or where they resided.

---

[1] "Thucydides," lib. ii, cap. 49.

The past history of his life appeared like a blank,—a *tabula rasa*.

In the retreat of the French from Moscow, during Bonaparte's Russian campaign, many of the soldiers and officers found that their minds were greatly enfeebled, consequent, as it was supposed, upon their exposure to great mental anxiety, physical privations, and intense cold.   Bonaparte's own memory became temporarily affected, particularly as to names and dates.   For a time he was constantly confusing one person with another, and making odd mistakes in dates.[1]   This impairment was, however,

---

[1] Count Philip de Segur has published, in his "*History of the Expedition to Russia by the French Army under the Command of the Emperor Napoleon, in* 1812," some interesting details of the effects of the terrible calamities and severe sufferings that overwhelmed that heroic band of soldiers, upon the sensitive mind of their illustrious chief.   When these facts are philosophically considered, we need not feel surprised at the influence they exercised, not only upon the intellect of the Emperor, but upon the minds of the marshals who fought so gallantly by his side.   During the battle of Semenowska, when Ney sent an aide-de-camp to the Emperor for instructions, Count Segur says, "He merely made some gestures of melancholy resignation, on every occasion, when they came to inform him of the loss of his best generals.   He rose several times to take a few turns, but immediately sat down again.   Every one around him looked at the Emperor with astonishment.   Hitherto, during these great shocks, he had displayed an active coolness; but here it was a dead calm, a mild and sluggish inactivity.   Some fancied they traced in it that dejection which is generally the follower of violent sensations; others that he had already become indifferent to everything, even to the emotion of battles.   Several remarked, that the calm constancy and *sangfroid* which great men display on these great occasions, turn, in the course of time, to phlegm and heaviness, when age has worn out their springs.   Those who were most devoted to him, accounted for his immobility by the necessity of not changing his place too much, when he was commanding over such an extent, in order that the bearers of intelligence might know where to find him.   Finally, there were others, who, on much better grounds, explained the whole by the shock which his health had sustained, and his violent indisposition."

At another period of the day, during the same battle, Murat sent Belliard to the Emperor for advice.   Belliard informed the King of Naples that "he had found Napoleon still seated in the same place, with a suffering and dejected air, his features sunk, and a dull look; giving his orders languishingly, in the midst of these dreadful warlike noises, to which he seemed completely a stranger!"   Ney expressed in strong and unguarded language, his sentiments as to the apathy of the Emperor, but, as Count Segur observes, "Murat was more calm; he recollected having seen the Emperor, the day before, as he was riding along observing that part of the enemy's line, halt several times, dismount, and with his head resting upon the cannon, remain there some time in the attitude of suffering.   He knew what a restless night he had passed, and that a violent and incessant cough cut short his breathing.   The King guessed that fatigue, and the first attacks of the equinox had shaken his weakened frame, and that, in short, at that critical moment, the action of his genius was, in a

only of short duration. One of his *aides-de-camp* suffered from a severe attack of loss of memory for several years. His intellect was, in other respects, unclouded.

Sir Jos. Banks relates a case of sudden paralysis of memory occurring to a fireman, who, in an heroic attempt to rescue some children from the interior of a house enveloped in flames, exposed himself for some time to an intense degree of heat.

Boerhaave mentions the particulars of the case of a Spanish tragic author, who in consequence of an attack of acute fever so completely lost all memory, that he forgot not only the languages he had formerly learnt, but even their alphabets. His own poems and compositions were shown to him, but it was impossible to convince him that they were his production. He afterwards, however, began again to compose verses, which had so striking a resemblance to his former writings, that he at last became convinced of his having been the author of them.

Numerous cases are recorded of sudden temporary failure of the memory, from an undue exercise and illegitimate straining of this faculty.[1]

manner, chained down by his body; which had sunk under the triple load of fatigue, of fever, and of a malady which, probably more than any other, prostrates the moral and physical strength of its victims."

When referring to the temporary mental prostration of Napoleon during the calamitous retreat of the French army, Count Segur remarks, the "Russian autumn had triumphed over him; had it not been for that, perhaps the whole of Russia would have yielded to our arms on the plains of the Moskwa; its premature inclemency was a most seasonable assistance to their empire. It was on the 6th of September, the very day before the great battle! that a hurricane announced its fatal commencement. Ever since the night of that day a burning fever had dried up the Emperor's blood, and oppressed his spirits; he was quite overcome by it during the battle, and the state of suffering he endured for the five following days arrested his march, and bound up his genius. This it was which preserved Kutusof from total ruin at Borodino, and allowed him time to rally the remainder of his army, and withdraw it from our pursuit."—(Vol. i, pp. 838–9, 342–3, 363.)

[1] "It is a fact well attested by experience, that the memory may be seriously injured by pressing upon it too hardly and continuously in early life. Whatever theory we hold as to this function of our nature, it is certain that its powers are only gradually developed, and that if forced into premature exercise, they are impaired by the effort. This is a maxim indeed of great import, applying to the condition and culture of every faculty of body and mind, but singularly to the one we are now considering, which forms, in one sense, the foundation of intellectual life. A regulated exercise short of fatigue is improving to it, but we are bound to refrain from goading it by constant and laborious efforts in early life and before the instrument is strengthened to its work, or it decays under our hands."—*Sir Henry Holland's Mental Pathology.*

A man of rather weak intellects, who held an office, the sole duty of which consisted in signing his own name to a number of papers, had so weakened his memory, that he at last was incapable of recollecting the word he ought to sign. Mr. Von B——, formerly envoy to Madrid, and afterwards to St. Petersburg, a man of a serious turn of mind, yet by no means hypochondriacal, went out one morning to pay a number of visits. Among other houses at which he called there was one where he suspected the servants did not know him, and where he consequently was under the necessity of giving in his name, but this he had at that moment entirely forgotten. Turning round immediately to a gentleman who accompanied him, he said with much earnestness, "For God's sake tell me who I am?" The question excited laughter, but as Mr. Von B—— insisted on being answered, adding that he had entirely forgotten his own name, he was told it, upon which he finished his visit.

Occasionally in certain morbid conditions of the brain, connected with organic alterations or disordered conditions of the cerebral circulation, the patient loses for a period all knowledge of his native tongue. Patients in a state of delirium have been known to address their physician in the Latin language. It is said that Dr. Johnson, when dying, forgot the words of our Lord's Prayer, in English, but attempted to repeat them in Latin. Dr. Scandella, an Italian gentleman of considerable scholastic abilities, resided in America. He was master of the Italian, French, and English languages. In the beginning of the yellow fever, which terminated his life in the city of New York, in the autumn of 1798, he spoke *English* only ; in the middle of his disease he spoke *French ;* but on the day of his death he spoke *Italian*, the language of his native country.

Dr. Rush says, that the Reverend Dr. Muhlenberg, of Lancaster (U. S. A.), when alluding to the German emigrants over whom he exercised pastoral care, observes, "People generally pray, shortly before death, in their native language. This is a fact which I have found true in innumerable cases among my German hearers, although hardly one word of their native language was spoken by them in common life and when in health !"

Dr. Hutchinson refers to the case of a physician who had in early life renounced the principles of the Roman Catholic Church. During an attack of delirium which preceded his death, he prayed only in the forms of the Church of Rome, whilst all recollection of the prescribed formulæ of the Protestant religion were effaced and obliterated from the mind by the cerebral affection.[1]

A gentleman was thrown from his horse while hunting. He was taken from the field to a neighboring cottage in a state of unconsciousness, and was subsequently removed to his own residence. For the period of a week his life was considered in imminent danger. When he was restored sufficiently to enable him to articulate, he began to talk *German*, a language he had acquired in early life, but had not spoken for nearly *twenty-five* years !

Dr. Rush cites a case of paralysis in which the premonitory symptom was forgetfulness how to spell the most common and familiar words. A gentleman, after an attack of paralysis, forgot the names of all his friends, but designated them correctly by mentioning their ages, with which he appeared to be well acquainted.

A man, aged sixty-five, in consequence of an attack of apoplexy, forgot how to read, or even to distinguish one word or letter from another, but if a name or phrase were mentioned to him, he was able to write it immediately, and that, too, with the greatest accuracy. He was, however, incapable of reading or distinguishing what he had written, for if asked what a letter was, or how the letters were combined, it became evident that the writing had been performed *mechanically*, without any exercise of the reflection or judgment. In this case none of the means which were employed were successful in restoring the knowledge of letters to his mind.[2]

A gentleman had a serious attack of illness. When restored, it was found that he had lost all recollection of *recent* circumstances, but had a lucid memory as to events that had occurred in *early life:* in fact, impressions that had long been forgotten were again revived. As this patient recovered his bodily health, a singular alteration was observed in the character of his memory. He again recollected *recent* ideas, but entirely forgot all the events of an *antecedent* period !

"A gentleman between fifty and sixty years of age, of temperate habits, nervo-bilious temperament, and with the moral sentiments and intellect predominating over the propensities,

---

[1] " *Biographia Medica.*"   [2] "*Ephemerides Curiosæ.*"

besides his professional duties as a clergyman, had been for several years engaged in writing a voluminous county history. One day, in the month of September, 1839, he had been working without intermission in the compilation of an index for a volume of his history, then about being published. Feeling drowsy, he laid himself down on a sofa, and slept for some time. On awaking he felt extremely cold, and, seeing a female in the room, he asked her who she was, not knowing his own wife. He afterwards became giddy and drowsy, but recovered from his disposition to sleep by medical treatment. Since that time he can seldom remember rightly the *name* of any article, place, or person, neither can he recollect numbers. Though he recognizes persons he was previously acquainted with, he can seldom mention their names. In talking on any subject he constantly calls one thing by the name of another, so as to render his conversation nearly useless. On attempting to read, a dull pain attacks the region of his perceptive organs, and particularly the organ of language: he becomes giddy, and before he can get to the end of a line, the whole appears a blank. His sight he considers not so good as previously to the attack; complains much of a cold head; remembers better when his eyes are closed, or when stooping. He often showed absence of mind in conversation and in reading for many years previous to the attack. His reflective, moral, and animal organs appear unaltered; his appetite is good, his general health improved, and he enjoys bodily exercise. In conversation he reasons on his malady, and gives a clear account of the attack. When he was a boy at school he suffered occasionally from a dull pain in the region of the perceptive organs, and it has frequently recurred during his subsequent life."[1]

Wepfer relates the particulars of the case of a man, who, after recovering from the effects of an attack of apoplexy, was found to know nobody and remember nothing. After several weeks, he began to observe his friends, remember words, repeat our Lord's Prayer, and to read a few words of Latin rather than German, which was his native language. When urged to read more than a few words at a time, he said, with a heavy sigh, "I formerly understood these things, but now I do not." After some time he began to pay more attention to what was passing around him, but, while

---

[1] *The Phrenological Journal*, vol. xiv, pp. 55–56.

thus making slight and gradual progress, he, after a few months, suddenly died of an attack of apoplexy.

Willis refers to the case of a man, who, in recovering from an attack of putrid fever, was found to have so entirely lost his mental faculties that he recognized no one, remembered and understood nothing. "*Vix supra brutum saperet.*"

A gentleman whom Dr. Abercrombie attended, after recovering from an apoplectic attack, knew his friends perfectly, but could not name them. Walking one day in the street, he met a gentleman to whom he was very anxious to communicate something respecting a mutual friend; after various ineffectual attempts to make him understand whom he meant, he at last seized him by the arm and dragged him through several streets to the house of the gentleman of whom he was speaking, and pointed to the nameplate upon the door. A lady, after an apoplectic attack, recovered correctly her ideas of things, but could not name them. In giving directions respecting family matters she was quite distinct as to what she wished to have done, but could make herself understood only by going through the house and pointing to the various articles.

A man, after an accident, could not recall to mind the names of his relations; another could recollect no proper names without the assistance of his friends.

"A young woman," says Dr. Shapter, "of weak intellect, subject to headaches and '*mal réglée*,' at the age of twenty-one experienced an attack of apoplexy. In her convalescence it was observed that she had lost all recollection of persons and occurrences. She early recollected her mother, without the power of calling her by name; at the end of a month she pronounced some words, though but very imperfectly, and her efforts to express herself involved her in almost unintelligible periphrases."

A man whilst grooming a restive horse received a kick on the head. He was in an unconscious state for six hours. He recovered with a singular perversion of speech. For some weeks the only words he could utter were "stable," "horse," "kick." He used these epithets whenever he wished to communicate with those about him. An effort was made to induce him to use other words, and to connect his ideas, but without effect. He eventually recovered the use of language, but for nearly a year his memory was in a very impaired state.

A well-known pugilist entirely lost his memory after a severe contest with a man who had severely punished him about the head.

A lady of rank experienced a severe shock consequent upon the receipt of the melancholy intelligence of the sudden death of an only and much-beloved child. She continued for several days in a stunned and apparently dying state. She, however, recovered. For many months afterwards, her memory exhibited a singular defect. She appeared to have no recollection of the cause of her illness, and of the severe loss she had sustained. When she was informed of the death of her son, for the period of a minute she appeared to realize the melancholy fact; but the impression almost instantly passed away. About nine months from this time she was found dead in her bed. Disease of the heart and brain was said to have been discovered after death.

A French soldier received a compound fracture of the cranium, opening the superior longitudinal sinus. There were, in the first instance, symptoms of compression. When in the hospital of Antwerp, he understood all that was said to him, and seemed quite intelligent. But he could only reply *ba-ba* to interrogatories. It was rather singular to observe his evident vexation at his inability to give expression to his ideas.

Dr. Shapter, of Exeter, has published the following very interesting case, illustrative of the morbid phenomena of memory.

" *Case.*—Pietro Gillio, LL.D., aged forty, a native of Italy, is, or rather was, a man possessing great comprehensiveness of mind, much vigor of intellect, of extensive acquirements, deeply read in metaphysics and general literature, and the perfect master of several languages.

" In consequence of having been a prominent agent in the insurrection of Piedmont, he was condemned to death. Fortunately he effected his escape, and, since that period, has been a solitary wanderer, for some years in Spain and the Channel Islands, but latterly in England, where he supported himself by teaching the Italian and Latin languages.

" Having been exposed to anxiety of mind, study, night-watchings, fastings, and cold and damp, he became affected on the night of the 14th of April, 1835, with headache, vertigo, and vomiting, succeeded by an indescribable confusion, after which these symptoms subsided.

" On the 15th, Dr. Shapter was called to him, in company with Mr. Froom.

"We found him in a state of great excitement and irritability, pacing hastily up and down his chamber with unequal steps. He was incapable of articulation, and there was an almost total loss of the memory of language ; for though his attention was readily attracted by speaking to him, yet the purport of what was said appeared to be in no way understood ; if there were any indistinctness of hearing, it must have been but very slight. Deglutition difficult. The pupil of the right eye dilated, and but slightly answering to the impulses of light ; the sight distant and indistinct ; that of the left eye natural ; the general expression of the eyes restless, and watching with anxious quickness those in the room. Pain in the back part of the head, but apparently not acute. Pulse rapid, unequal, 120 ; on the right side strong, full, and vibrating, especially pronounced in the right subclavian and carotid arteries ; on the left side, the arterial action small and weak. General weakness of the left side, but not amounting to paralysis, excepting for the first hour or two after the attack. His landlady says, that at breakfast this morning he was silent, irritable in manner, and looking anxious ; that suddenly he made some effort as if to speak, and then rushed hastily from the house.

" The usual antiphlogistic treatment indicated was pursued, such as bleeding, blisters, and purgatives. We early found, however, that he had not stamina to permit such means to be carried to any great extent.

" On the 6th of June, the arterial action of the right side was still tumultuous in the extreme. He could recollect *portions* of a few words, and, after repeated trials, could write some of the shortest ones correctly, without the assistance of a dictionary ; but words of three or four syllables were far beyond his powers of concentration ; his efforts at composing a sentence were unavailing, as well as the understanding one addressed to him : he had no command of tongue. He commenced studying, with the most feverish anxiety, the English lexicon, and, in great measure, managed to explain himself by pointing to particular words ; but his capacity for re-learning language appeared limited and confined.

"After this he had an excessive secretion from the membrane of the nose and fauces. In October he complained of some tenderness on pressure over the lumbar vertebræ, which was relieved by the application of leeches and a blister. He then took to reading various books on diseases of the brain, as well as on worms, to which he said he had been prone. He occasionally drew up reports of his symptoms, and one, which he received about Christmas, is transcribed by Dr. Shapter. In the beginning of December, he sent a memorandum, in which he took a comparative view of his symptoms, stating the whole number as one hundred, and then giving each symptom its relative proportion according to his estimate of its intensity and importance. The following is the report alluded to.

"'Sir dear—have a symptom of illness—viz. 1, spit in night and day—2, dry cough—3, an unequal pulse—4, no sleep—5, uninclination to go to stool and non-evacuate thing *quite*—6, swoon —7, loathing of food and other times a voracious appetite—8, a privation of speech—9, foot, hand bad, a hinde right—paleness of the face and times red of the face—11, whitish color urine (teeth, nose—throat).

" 'In first attack 15 April, I had swoon in stool, not evacuate quite the bowels; and was sleep and was awaken and privation.

" '(Mr. Duval.)

" 'In child in is pains of worm—medicine—rue and wormwood.

" 'In 15 year, the same pains, medicine, oil, &c.

" 'in jersey—no medicine except rhubarb; in Guernsey—medicine—calomel; in Plymouth—no medicine; in Exeter is privation of speech.

" 'Mrs. —— non speak true to Dr. Shapter, viz. 1, 2, 4, 5.

" '(non speak—write.)   *P. Gillio.*'"

In September, 1836, having received a free pardon from the King of Sardinia, and being about to return to Vico, his native place, Dr. Shapter took the subjoined final note of his condition.

"Has now a nearly perfect recollection of facts, of ideas, and of his past life generally; and has also recovered the recollection of many words when written before him, and to a lesser extent when spoken to him: this difference does not depend on any deafness. His powers of reading are soon exhausted; and he has, for the most part, lost the faculty of properly arranging and constructing his sentences, and is now almost totally incapable of articulating with correctness the few words he has with difficulty reacquired. His general irritability is much decreased, and the pain on pressure of the spinal column has subsided entirely; but he complains much of painful pulsations in the posterior part of the head and neck, occurring especially during the night and towards morning. Pervigilia; pulse 104, in right side strong, left weak; the general strength of the right side restored; pupil of right eye still dilated, the sight rather more distant than that of the left; the indistinctness of vision almost recovered from; habit of body costive; appetite good only towards evening. General health from the period of the first attack, though slowly, yet progressively improves.''

Dr. Shapter referred the proximate cause of the symptoms in this case to the rupture of a bloodvessel at the base of the brain, or the superior portion of the spinal column. He considered that some coagulum had been formed near that part where the glossopharyngeal and lingual nerves arise. The eyesight was not particularly affected, but there was some loss in the powers of adaptation of the right eye. He therefore concluded that the optic nerve was intact, but that the motor nerves of these parts were disordered.

The late eminent Dr. Baillie[1] describes a curious case of impaired memory produced by paralysis. A gentleman, aged fifty-six, was seized with symptoms of compression of the brain, and became completely paralytic on the right side. It was found that he had lost the recollection of the words of his own language, except a very few, which he pronounced with the greatest distinctness, and with a variety of tones to express pleasure and displeasure, joy and sorrow, to explain the circumstances of his disorder, and to give directions about what he wanted, without being aware they were not the proper words to express his meaning.

A gentleman, forty-six years of age, who had always enjoyed a good state of health, after experiencing great uneasiness of mind, and being exposed to severe bodily fatigue, was seized with apoplexy, followed by hemiplegia. The apoplexy was slight, but the hemiplegia was complete. The power of speech was entirely lost, so that he could only utter the sounds ee-o, which, however, he so varied, that with the assistance of expressive gestures, he was able to convey to those about him his meaning very distinctly upon ordinary subjects. He perfectly comprehended everything that was said to him, and clearly understood what he meant to answer, but was able only to utter the previously-mentioned sounds. Believing, however, that he actually employed the words adapted to

---

[1] "Medical Transactions of the College of Physicians," vol. iv.

the communication of his ideas, he often appeared surprised and displeased when he was not understood. He sometimes endeavored to explain his meaning by writing on a slate; but he generally substituted one word for another, and almost always erred in spelling what he wrote.[1]

Dr. T. K. Chambers has published the following interesting case of loss of language following acute disease of the brain:—

"Harriet C., aged twelve, had typhus fever in December, 1845; she had much delirium and low symptoms, but, as is usual with children, soon got about again, and was able to return to school. However, after a few days' attendance, she was one evening, on returning thence, taken with a fit, of an undecided epileptic character, had rigors, and was again delirious. The delirium was monotonous, and remarkable for her constant repetition of the word 'sinner' with every variety of intonation. Wine and bark were, as during her former attack, resorted to, but symptoms of slight effusion in the brain caused its suspension. She recovered after a few weeks, so as to be up and dressed, but with the loss of power to pronounce any word except the one she had so often repeated during her fever. This she made serve to express all her ideas; for denial she shook her head, and said 'sinner:' assent was expressed by the same word, and bread and butter was called 'sĭn-ŭn-sĭnnĕr.' She perfectly understood all that was said to her, and appeared capable of reading her usual lessons. Blisters were applied behind her ears, and small doses of mercury administered, and at the same time her mother and family were instructed to teach her as they would an infant to talk. I also took opportunities of showing her, by exaggerated motions of my mouth and throat, the way of forming the letters, in the manner in which the born deaf and dumb are instructed, and found her intelligent and ready. She soon acquired the word 'yes,' and other elementary expressions, and by the end of the spring was able, as her mother told me, 'to talk like an old woman.' Symptoms of consumption had, however, appeared, and she died this last summer under the care of another medical man, whose kind efforts to obtain a post-mortem examination for me were unavailing."

"A farmer in the county of Wicklow, in comfortable circumstances, when fifty years of age, had a paralytic fit. Since that

---

[1] "On Nervous Diseases," by Dr. Cooke.

time he has never recovered the use of the affected side. The attack was succeeded by a painful hesitation of speech. His memory was good for all parts of speech except noun-substantives and proper names; the latter he could not at all retain. This defect was accompanied by the following singular peculiarity: He perfectly recollected the initial letter of every substantive or proper name for which he had occasion in conversation, though he could not recall to his memory the word itself. Experience had taught him the utility of having written in manuscript a list of the things he was in the habit of calling for or speaking about, including the proper names of his children, servants, and acquaintances: all these he arranged alphabetically in a little pocket dictionary, which he used as follows: If he wished to ask anything about a cow, before he commenced the sentence he turned to the letter C, and looked out for the word 'cow,' and kept his finger and eye fixed on the word until he had finished the sentence. He could pronounce the word cow in its proper place, so long as he had his eyes fixed upon the written letters; but the moment he shut the book it passed out of his memory, and could not be recalled, although he recollected its initial, and could refer to it when necessary. In the same way when he came to Dublin, and wished to consult Dr. Graves, his physician, he came with his dictionary open to the hall-door, and asked to see Dr. Graves; but if by accident he had forgotten his dictionary, as happened on one occasion, he was totally unable to tell the servant what or whom he wanted. He could not recollect his own name unless he looked out for it, nor the name of any person of his acquaintance; but he was never for a moment at a loss for the initial which was to guide him in his search for the word he sought.

"His was a remarkably exaggerated degree of the common defect of memory observed in the diseases of old age, and in which the names of persons and things are frequently forgotten, although their initials are recollected. It is strange that substantives or proper names, words which are the first acquired by the memory in childhood, are sooner forgotten than verbs, adjectives, and other parts of speech, which are a much later acquisition."[1]

[1] *Dublin Quarterly Journal of Medical Science;* a case recorded by Dr. Graves.

CHAPTER XVI.

PERVERSION AND EXALTATION OF MEMORY. MEMORY OF THE INSANE.

PERVERSION OF MEMORY.—Andral refers to a curious modification of the memory, connected with a sudden or gradual loss of the remembrance of everything save one object, which " becomes to the person so afflicted the universe." " There is," says Andral, " a very singular perversion of the memory, which consists in the patient remembering everything except himself. He has, as it were, forgot his own existence, and when he speaks of himself, it is in the third person, the words I or ME are not in his vocabulary."[1]

M. Leuret has related the case of a woman who, in speaking of herself, always said, " *La personne de moi même.*" An old soldier who was in the Asylum of Saint Yon, named Lambert, believed that he was killed at the battle of Austerlitz. When he spoke of himself, he was in the habit of saying, " This machine, which they thought to make like me, is very badly manufactured." When he spoke of himself, he did not use the personal pronoun I, but the demonstrative pronoun THAT, as if speaking of some inanimate object.

A man seventy years of age was suddenly seized with lockjaw and formication over the surface of the body. This was succeeded by vertigo, and a strange alteration in his language. He spoke with ease and fluency, but often made use of odd words which nobody understood. He appeared to have coined new phrases in the place of others which he had forgotten. Occasionally he mixed numbers instead of words in his conversation, and in this respect the memory appeared to have been altered in its mode of action.

John Hunter was in the habit of relating in his lectures a sin-

[1] Andral's " Clinique Médicale."

gular case of perversion of the memory, succeeding an attack of acute disease of the brain. In this instance the gentleman, who, besides referring the circumstances of his early life to the present period, had to such an extent lost all idea of the connection between the *past* and the *present*, that although his mind could direct him as to what was to be done in consequence of certain impressions, and would direct him rightly as to the part of the body affected by them, he was in the habit (having apparently lost all notion of his own identity) of constantly referring his own sensations to those immediately about him. Thus he would tell his nurse and the bystanders that he was certain that *they* were hungry or thirsty; but on offering him food or drink, it was evident by his eagerness that the idea had arisen from a sense of hunger and thirst, and that the word *they* referred to himself and not to others.

He was subject to a violent cough, and after each paroxysm he would, in very appropriate and sympathetic terms resume the subject on which he had been conversing, previously, however, expressing his feelings of distress from having witnessed the sufferings of his friend, adding, "I am sorry to see that *you* have so troublesome and harassing a cough."

A gentleman, who was in the habit of indulging in "potations pottle deep," whenever he became intoxicated invariably referred his own perverted sensations in a similar way to those immediately about him. Hence, upon going home, he imagining all the family to be in the lamentable state to which he had reduced himself, would insist on undressing them and putting them to bed, declaring that they were all too drunk to do so for themselves!

Mr. Combe records the case of an Irish porter, who forgot when sober what he had done when drunk, but being drunk again, distinctly recollected the transactions that had occurred during his former state of intoxication. On one occasion he had mislaid a parcel of some value, and in his sober moments could give no account of its *locus in quo*. He again became intoxicated, and then clearly recollected that he had left the parcel at a certain house, and, having no address on it, it had remained there safely, and was immediately given to the party who claimed it.[1]

The following remarkable cases of erratic memory, evidencing

[1] " System of Phrenology."

itself in certain morbid conditions of brain disorder, are deserving of notice.   They are supposed to form striking illustrations of the phenomena of "double or divided consciousness," or, as suggested by Mr. Combe, "*double personality* manifesting itself in the exhibition of two separate and independent mental capabilities in the same individual; each train of thought and each capability being wholly dissevered from the other, and the two states in which they respectively predominate, subject to frequent interchanges and alterations."

The patient was a girl of sixteen: the affection appeared immediately before puberty, and disappeared when that state was fully established.   It lasted from the 2d of March to the 11th of June, 1815, under the eye of Dr. Dyce.   The first symptom was propensity to fall asleep in the evenings.   This was followed by the habit of *talking* in her sleep on these occasions.   One evening she fell asleep in this manner, imagined herself an Episcopal clergyman, went through the ceremony of baptizing three children, and gave an appropriate *extempore* prayer.   Her mistress took her by the shoulders, on which she awoke, and appeared unconscious of everything except that she had fallen asleep, of which she showed herself ashamed.   She sometimes dressed herself and the children while in this state, or, as Mrs. L—— called it, "dead asleep;" answered questions put to her in such a manner as to show that she understood what was said; but the answers were often, though not always, incongruous.   One day in this state she set the breakfast with perfect correctness, with her eyes shut.   She afterwards awoke with the child on her knee, and wondered how she got on her clothes.   Sometimes the cold air awakened her, at other times she was seized with the affection while walking out with the children.   She sang a hymn delightfully in this state, and from a comparison which Dr. Dyce had an opportunity of making, it appeared incomparably better done than she could accomplish when well.

In the meantime a still more singular and interesting symptom made its appearance.   The circumstances which occurred during the paroxysm were completely forgotten by her when the paroxysm was over, but were perfectly remembered during subsequent paroxysms.   Her mistress said, that when in this stupor on subsequent occasions, she told her what was said to her on the evening on which she baptized the children.   Other instances of this kind are

given. A depraved fellow-servant understanding that she wholly
forgot every transaction that occurred during the fit, clandestinely
introduced a young man into the house, who treated her with the
utmost rudeness, while her fellow-servant stopped her mouth with
the bed-clothes, and otherwise overpowered a vigorous resistance
which was made by her, even during the influence of her complaint.
Next day she had not the slightest recollection even of that transaction, nor did any person interested in her welfare know of it for
several days, till she was in one of her paroxysms, when she related
the whole facts to her mother. Next Sunday she was taken to
the church by her mistress while the paroxysm was on her. She
shed tears during the sermon, particularly during the account
given of the execution of three young men at Edinburgh, who had
described in their dying declarations the dangerous steps with
which their career of vice and infamy took its commencement.
When she returned home, she recovered in a quarter of an hour,
was quite amazed at the questions put to her about the church
and sermon, and denied that she had been in any such place; but
next night on being taken ill, she mentioned that she had been at
church, repeated the words of the text, and, in Dr. Dyce's hearing,
gave an accurate account of the tragical narrative of the three
young men, by which her feelings had been so powerfully affected.
On this occasion, though in Mrs. L——'s house, she asserted that
she was in her mother's.[1]

The particulars of the following case are detailed by Dr.
Mitchell :—[2]

Miss R——, possessing naturally a very good constitution,
arrived at adult age without having it impaired by disease. She
possessed an excellent capacity, and enjoyed fair opportunities of
acquiring knowledge. Besides the domestic arts and social attainments, she had improved her mind by reading and conversation,
and was well versed in penmanship. Her memory was capacious,
and stored with a copious stock of ideas. Unexpectedly, and
without any forewarning, she fell into a profound sleep, which
continued several hours beyond the ordinary term. On waking,
she was discovered to have lost every trait of acquired knowledge.
Her memory was a *tabula rasa*—all vestiges, both of words and
things, were obliterated and gone. It was found necessary for her

---

[1] Combe's "Phrenology," p. 225.   [2] Medical Repository.

to learn everything again. She even acquired, by new efforts, the art of spelling, reading, writing, and calculating, and gradually became acquainted with the persons and objects around, like a being for the first time brought into the world. In these exercises she made considerable proficiency. But, after a few months, another fit of somnolency invaded her. On rousing from it, she found herself restored to the state she was in before the first paroxysm; but was wholly ignorant of every event and occurrence that had befallen her afterwards. The former condition of her existence she called the old state, and the latter the new state; and she was as unconscious of her double character as two distinct persons are of their respective natures. For example, in her old state she possessed all her original knowledge; in her new state, only what she acquired since. If a gentleman or lady were introduced to her in the old state, and *vice versâ* (and so of all other matters), to know them satisfactorily she had to learn them in both states. In the old state, she possessed fine powers of penmanship, while in the new she wrote a poor, awkward hand, having not time or means to become expert. During four years and upwards she underwent periodical transitions from one of these states to the other. The alternations were always consequent upon a long and sound sleep. Both the lady and her family were capable of conducting the affair without embarrassment. By simply knowing whether she was in the old or new state, they regulated the intercourse and governed themselves accordingly.[1]

EXALTATION OF MEMORY.—In some cases during the early period of brain disease, the memory is in a state of morbid exaltation, the patient having a vivid recollection of occurrences that happened many years previously, and which had, apparently, been long forgotten. In the cerebral diseases of early life, this symptom is frequently observed, and should never pass unnoticed. In some cases of insanity we also observe an acute condition of this faculty.

In fever accompanied by an active state of the cerebral circulation, the patient has been known to exhibit to an intense degree this symptom. Any sudden and unnatural exaltation of the faculty of memory, or of any other mental power, should (particularly if associated with other symptoms indicative of brain disorder) immediately excite attention.

[1] Combe's " System of Phrenology," p. 173.

A gentleman returned home from his counting-house late in the evening. He had been occupied for nine continuous hours in going carefully through his books, with a view of finally arranging a partnership with a gentleman with whom he was in treaty. Soon after his arrival home, he was observed to be unusually talkative. He spoke of what he had been occupied in during the day, making no complaint of fatigue. He then referred to the state of his accounts, and boasted of his ability to recollect with great accuracy the most minute details connected with the monetary and commercial transactions of the house, extending over a period of many years. He then referred to several matters of business and calculation, evidencing an extraordinary power of memory. This was about nine o'clock. At eleven, whilst sitting near the fire engaged in conversation with his wife, he complained of sickness, and immediately afterwards vomited the dinner he had eaten about two hours previously. His wife administered some restoratives, which appeared to be productive of relief, and therefore no medical man was sent for. About twelve o'clock he complained of severe headache over the occipital region, and had a second attack of vomiting. About half an hour after he became drowsy, and eventually sank into a state of profound coma. He died in the course of the night, never having recovered from this state of unconsciousness. The *post-mortem* examination revealed an aneurismal tumor of the middle cerebral artery (which was never suspected), with a state of general sanguineous congestion of the brain.

Romberg refers to the case of a girl who, when very young, had a severe attack of small-pox. She lost her sight, but acquired an extraordinary memory. She repeated perfectly on her return home a long sermon she had recently heard. "It is well known," adds Romberg, "that the scrofulous, and frequently the rachitic diathesis in childhood, is accompanied by this phenomenon."

In the incipient state of brain disease of early life connected with acute fevers, disturbed conditions of the cerebral circulation and vessels, and in affections of advanced years, there is often witnessed a remarkable exaltation of the memory. Events that have occurred many years previously, and which were, apparently, obliterated from the mind, have been distinctly reproduced, and that too, with extraordinary accuracy and vividness.

A sudden "lighting up" and improvement of the memory, occurring to persons in advanced life, are occasionally precursory of

death and fatal apoplexy.   Hippocrates notices this phenomena.
A gentleman, aged seventy-six, exhibited, with other signs of
brain disorder, a remarkably vivid recollection of a complicated
transaction previously entirely forgotten, that had taken place
thirty-five years before.   On the following day he had an attack
of apoplexy, of which he died.[1]

Portal has observed among the incipient symptoms of cerebral
hemorrhage and paralysis, a disposition to talk garrulously respecting events that have long since been apparently forgotten.   An
old gentleman surprised his family by recounting the minute particulars of an eventful epoch that had occurred in early life, known
only to himself, as if the circumstances were familiar to those
about him, and were of recent date.   Two days subsequently he
was found in bed in a state of apoplectic coma, from which he
never rallied.

An intelligent American was travelling in the State of *Illinois*,
and suffered the common lot of visitants from other climates, in
being seized with a bilious fever.   "As very few live," he remarks, "to record the issue of a sickness like mine, and as you
have requested me, and as I have promised to be particular, I will
relate some of the circumstances of this disease.   And it is in my
view desirable, in the bitter agony of such diseases, that more of
the symptoms, sensations, and sufferings should be recorded than
have been, and that others in similar predicaments may know that
some before them have had sufferings like theirs, and have survived them.   I had had a fever before, and had risen and been
dressed every day ; but in this with the first day I was prostrated
to infantile weakness, and felt with its first attack that it was a
thing very different from what I had yet experienced.   Paroxysms
of derangement occurred the third day, and this was to me a new
state of mind.   That state of disease in which partial derangement
is mixed with a consciousness generally sound, and a sensibility
preternaturally excited, I should suppose the most distressing of
all its forms.   At the same time that I was unable to recognize my
friends, I was informed that my memory was more than ordinarily
exact and retentive, and that I repeated whole passages in the
different languages which I knew with entire accuracy.   I recited,
without losing or misplacing a word, a passage of poetry I could
not so repeat after I had recovered my health, &c."[2]

[1] Hagendorn, "Observations Médicale." Paris.
[2] Flint's "Recollections of the Valley of the Mississippi," Letter xiv.

MEMORY OF THE INSANE.—In ordinary cases of insanity the memory is not, as a general rule, impaired or lost. Dr Haslam appears to think that this faculty is the first mental power that decays in insanity. I doubt this. It is true that in many cases the patient has but a feeble and confused recollection of the transactions of recent date, but is able, vividly, to recall to the mind the scenes of early life. It is, undoubtedly, a fact, that the conversations of old, incurable lunatic patients relate principally to the events of past years, but, at the same time, they do not manifest that utter obliviousness and forgetfulness of recent circumstances that Dr. Haslam and others appear to believe.

I have witnessed some singular instances among the insane, of extraordinary retentiveness of memory, relating to recent transactions, but I am bound to admit, as a general *postulate*, that this faculty is found, in the majority of cases, in an impaired and muddled state.

According to Shakspeare, one of the essential elements, in all cases of insanity, is an inability to revive past impressions, to "re-word" that which he says

<blockquote>"Madness would gamble from."</blockquote>

But this Shakspearian test has been long exploded.

I have, in a previous part of this work, spoken of the exaltation of memory often observed in cases of cerebral disorder. The same phenomena is remarkably characteristic of many forms of insanity, particularly of the hysterical types. In these cases, the organic and psychical sensibility is in a condition of extreme exaltation, and the memory generally exhibits marked evidence of activity.

CHAPTER XVII.

PSYCHOLOGY AND PATHOLOGY OF MEMORY.

IT is difficult to suggest a physiological or metaphysical hypothesis which satisfactorily explains those remarkable conditions of
mental paralysis, singular manifestations and aberrations of memory (to which I have previously referred), as preceding, accompanying, and following acute and chronic affections of the brain,
unless we espouse the doctrine of the *indestructibility of ideas*, and
subscribe to the notion that no impression made upon the mind is
ever destroyed.

If we accept this as an established philosophical theory, we can
easily understand how subtle microscopic changes in the delicate
nerve-vesicle (*gray* matter of the brain) may cause great eccentricity and singular irregularity in the exercise of the memory, and
occasionally, in certain morbid as well as healthy conditions of
cerebral exaltation, awaken into active consciousness ideas imagined either to have no existence, or long since supposed to be
buried in oblivion.[1]

Annihilation exists but in the fancy. It is an illusion of the
imagination, a dream of the poet, the wild and frigid phantasy of
the sceptic. Nothing obvious to sense admits of destruction. This
is a well-established axiom in physics. It is not in the power of
man to destroy the slightest particle of matter. What is termed
"destruction," as applied to material substances, is nothing but a
change in their elementary composition, or alteration of their con-
stituent atoms. The good and wise Benefactor, the Beneficent

---

[1] Is the permanent character of the pictures traced upon the memory dependent
(as Locke surmises) on the "*temper*" of the brain, as if some impressions were made
upon *marble*, others on *freestone*, and some on little better than on *sand?*

"*Cur seniores amplius mente valeamus, juniores citius discimus?*" asks Aristotle; why
is it that in youth we learn more quickly, and wherefore is it, as age advances, the
intellect becomes more powerful?

Creator of the universe, has not delegated to poor puny man the power of destroying any portion of the physical universe by which he is surrounded, and which ministers so bountifully and mercifully to his every necessity. He may, by chemical or other scientific processes, alter and rearrange the existing combinations of organic matter, but, when disintegrated by such means, the particles so dissipated and apparently destroyed, enter into new and different forms, and assume other types and organisms, but are, in their *original* nature and elements, never annihilated.

What is true with regard to *material*, holds good, *à fortiori*, respecting *psychical* phenomena. Hence the tonic, permanent, and indestructible character of the impressions made upon the *cerebrum*, and *received* and *registered* in the *mind* during infancy and childhood, as well as in adult age, as established by their resuscitation in advanced and at other periods of life during certain normal and abnormal conditions of the vesicular brain structure and cerebral circulation.[1]

[1] I use the phrase "*received*" advisedly, for it must be admitted that there are many impressions which impinge themselves transiently on the mind—ideas that are evanescent in their character, and therefore obtain no settled hold upon the consciousness —which cannot philosophically be deemed as *received* and *registered* in the memorial archives. Such are the fugitive notions which do not become objects of *perception*, that so frequently float upon, and pass like shadows over the surface of the mind, in early as well as in matured life, when the brain is not anatomically and physiologically organized or fitted for the facile perception, reception, and registration of ideas. There can be no doubt that the defective memory which so often accompanies old age, is mainly dependent upon certain (as yet unexplained) modifications in the physical nutrition or chemical constitution of the brain interfering with that *vital, organic*, and I may add *psychical sensibility*, so essentially necessary for its ready adaptation to mental impressions. It may be that the ideas are in reality received, but that the faculty of *reminiscence* being either originally defective, or enfeebled by age or disease, it ceases to obey the commands of the will. The atrophy, as well as diminution in the depth and complexity of the convoluted surface of the brain, so often witnessed after death, in aged persons, undoubtedly impairs that organic cerebral susceptibility and sensibility so necessary for the rapid and permanent reception of mental impressions.

I had an opportunity, last year, of observing two remarkable illustrations of this fact. I was present at the *post-mortem* examination of the body of a gentleman who died of visceral disease, at the advanced age of 84. Up to this period he had been remarkable for great vigor of intellect, and for extraordinary elasticity and retentiveness of memory. He appeared to have forgotten no impression that ever had been made upon his mind, in early as well as in advanced life. During the examination of the brain I was remarkably struck with its anatomical appearance. The gray matter was by no means diminished in quantity or consistence. The sulci were well marked. and both as to volume, character, and depth of its convolutions, the brain

"The images," says an illustrious English moralist, "which memory presents are of a stubborn and untractable nature. The objects of remembrance have already existed, and left their signature behind them impressed upon the mind, so as to defy all attempts at erasure or of change. Whatever we have once deposited, as Dryden expresses it, in the 'sacred treasures of the past,' is out of the reach of accident or violence, nor can it be lost, either by our own weakness, or another's malice.[1]

> " Non tamen irritum
> Quodcunque retro est efficiet; neque
> Diffinget, infectumque reddet
> Quod fugiens semel hora vexit."
>   HORACE, lib. iii, ode 29.

"The seeds of immortal truth," remarks an eminent writer, "are not sown to perish, even in the loose soil where they have long laid disregarded."[2]

Goethe embodies the same idea in the following transcendently beautiful passage :—

> " Kein Wesen kann zu nichts zerfallen,
> Das Ew'ge regt sich fort in allen,
> Am Seyn erhalte dich beglückt!
> Das Seyn ist ewig, denn Gesetze
> Bewahren die lebend'gen Schätze
> Aus welchen sich das All geschmückt."[3]

How, it may be asked, can the physiologist and pathologist reconcile with this latency and indestructibility of psychical conceptions, the fact of the constant wear and tear, destruction and construction, waste and reparation, absorption and deposition of nerve-brain matter ? Can the doctrine of the *individuality* and

---

presented an aspect similar to what a pathologist would expect to detect in a person dying in full intellectual power at the age of 30 or 40. In another case, I examined the brain of a gentleman whose mind had become prematurely enfeebled for six years previously to his death. He died at the early age of 56. The convolutions of the brain had greatly diminished in depth as well as in complexity, and the encephalic mass also presented a general shrunken or atrophied appearance. The brain was unusually pale, and there was also (without softening) a want of coherence in its texture.

[1] " The Rambler." Dr. Johnson.
[2] " Amenities of Literature," by Isaac Disraeli, vol. ii, p. 365.
[3] Goethe's " Wilhelm Meister's Wanderjahre."

indivisibility of mind, and the metaphysical theory of the *unity of the consciousness*, be established on a philosophical basis, if these physical laws are acknowledged thus materially to alter the structural organization of the brain, and to produce modifications in its recognized intellectual and emotional manifestations?

Is not the gradual development of the mind from childhood to adult age, and its steady and melancholy decadence from a condition of youthful vigor and advanced maturity, to that of second childhood and senile imbecility, connected with those subtle changes in the composition of the cerebral matter and modifications in the organization of the gray nerve-vesicle, which we know to be in constant progression?

How can we explain the expansion and discipline which the mind undergoes as the effect of a system of educational training? By what physiological and psychical processes are the memory, attention, and reasoning faculties developed and invigorated by exercise? What is the rationale of the judgment being improved by judicious and careful cultivation, the moral sense elevated, the taste disciplined and chastened, the volitional power increased? Are not these various psychical changes the results of some new, and as yet inexplicable, law regulating the action of nerve-matter? Is it possible to suppose that changes similar to those previously referred to, in the manifestations of the thinking principle, can be consequent upon any alteration in the mind *per se?* May not these developments and modifications in the physical attributes of the cerebrum, and gradual unfoldings of the mind which we perceive through the various epochs of life, be mysteriously connected with and dependent upon that waste and repair of nerve-matter which all physiologists recognize to be in constant operation?

Are these *psychical* phenomena more inexplicable and inscrutable to the philosopher than the physical facts that the physiologist is daily making matter of observation and reflection? How can we account for the transmission of particular types of disease, certain modifications and eccentricities of physical organization from generation to generation? Are these phenomena less occult than the descent of mental idiosyncrasies, modulations of the voice, and expressions of the countenance, from father to son, mother to daughter? Slight distortions in the feet, peculiar malformations in the fingers, singular defects in the development of the muscles regulating the movements of the eyes, moles, mother's marks, have all been known to be physical defects, or, more properly speaking, arrests of structural development that have existed in families for generations! How can we reconcile these physical facts with our notions of the organic revolutions occurring in the animal economy!

Again, if we turn to the consideration of pathological phenomena, the physiologist is still more bewildered in his attempt to penetrate behind the veil that conceals from finite understandings the incomprehensible laws regulating the operations of life, as dependent upon and connected with the organization of the body. I refer to those subtle changes in the character of the blood effected in infancy by the introduction into it of minute portions of morbific matter with a view of protecting the body from the influence of noxious and often deadly poisons. I allude to the effect of the vaccine virus upon the blood in producing a *permanent and organic change in its constitution and character, which continues to exercise a protective influence against small-pox, in the great mass of cases, through a long life, during which time the blood must have undergone many thousands, if not millions, of changes and modifications!* If we could imagine a person so armed, by means of the introduction into the system of healthy vaccine matter, under favorable bodily conditions for its reception, to be drained of nearly his last drop of blood, and subsequently restored to his original vascular condition, we should find no diminution in the force of its sanitary effect upon the vital fluid in early life; in other words, he would continue protected, certainly for many years, from the influence of the small-pox poison.

How can this assimilative power of the blood be explained? Is the phenomenon less mysterious and inscrutable than the permanent and indestructible character of all psychical impressions?

Mr. Paget refers to these phenomena without attempting their elucidation. When alluding to the blood's own assimilative power, he remarks: "After the vaccine and other infectious or inoculable diseases, it is most probably not the tissues alone, but the blood as much or much more than they, in which the altered state is maintained, and in many cases it would seem that, whatever materials are added to the blood, the stamp once impressed by one of these specific diseases is retained; the blood, by its own formative power, exactly assimilating to itself, its altered self, the materials derived from the food.

"And this, surely, must be the explanation of many of the most inveterate diseases; that they persist because of the assimilative formation of the blood. Syphilis, lepra, eczema, gout, and many more, seem thus to be perpetuated; in some form or other, and in ever varying quantity, whether it manifests itself externally or not, the material they depend on is still in the blood; because the blood constantly makes it afresh out of the materials that are added to it, let those materials be almost what they may. The tissues once affected may (and often do) in these cases recover; they may have gained their right or perfect composition ; but the blood, by assimilation, still retains its taint, though it may have in it not one of the particles on which the taint first passed : and hence, after many years of seeming health, the disease may break out again from the blood, and affect a part which was never before diseased. And this appears to be the natural course of these diseases, unless the morbid material be (as we may suppose) decomposed by some specific; or be excreted in the gradual tendency of the blood (like the tissues) to regain a normal state ; or, finally, be, if I may so speak, starved by the abstraction from the food of all such things as it can possibly be made from.

"In all these things, as in the phenomena of symmetrical disease, we have proofs of the surpassing precision of the formative process, a precision so exact that, as we may say, a mark once made upon a particle of blood, or tissue, is not for years effaced from its successors. And this seems to be a truth of widest application; and I can hardly doubt that herein is the solution of what has been made a hindrance to the reception of the whole truth concerning the connection of an immaterial mind with the brain. When the brain is said to be essential, as the organ or instrument of the mind in its relations with the external world, not only to the perception of sensations, but to the subsequent intellectual acts, and especially to the memory of things which have been the objects of sense—it is asked, how can the brain be the organ of memory when you suppose its substance to be ever changing? or, how is it that your assumed nutritive change of all the particles of the brain is not as destructive of all memory and knowledge of sensuous things as the sudden destruction by some great injury is ? The answer is,—because of the exactness of assimilation accomplished in the formative process: the effect once produced by an impression upon the brain, whether in perception or in intellectual act, is fixed and there retained; because the part, be it what it may, which has been thereby changed, is exactly represented in the part which, in the course of nutrition, succeeds to it. Thus, in the recollection of sensuous things, the mind refers to a brain in which are retained the effects, or rather the likenesses, of changes that past impressions and intellectual acts had made. As, in some way passing far our knowledge, the mind perceived, and took cognizance of, the change made by the first impression of an object acting through the sense-organs on the brain, so afterwards it perceives and recognizes the likeness of that change in the parts inserted in the process of nutrition."[1]

How fraught with interest of the most sublime and exalted character to the metaphysical philosopher, physician, and theologian, is the theory (previously referred to) of the indestructible character of all mental impressions?

The subjoined singularly interesting facts *illustrate*, if they do not *demonstrate*, the truth of this theory. In the present imperfect state of our knowledge of the intimate character and composition of nerve structure, admitted ignorance of the nature of the *vis nervosa*, as well as of the laws governing the operations of thought, as connected with and dependent upon recondite alterations in the vesicular neurine of the brain, it would be useless to speculate as to the cause of the psychical phenomena to which I am about to refer. Much light may yet be thrown upon this important and intricate subject, as the result of a closer study of mental dynamics as well as of *chemico-cerebral* pathology. Morbid phenomena of mind, incomprehensible to the physiologist, and inscrutable to the pathologist, may be intimately dependent upon minute changes (out of the range of the microscope, and only to be detected in the laboratory) in the organic chemical constitution of brain matter affecting not only the *quantity*, *quality*, but distribution of the *nerve* and *psychical* force, not, in the existing state of our knowledge of physiological and dynamical science, susceptible of demonstration.[2]

---

[1] "Lectures on Surgical Pathology." By J. Paget, Esq., F.R.S. Vol. i, p. 52.

[2] Much has been said by phrenological authorities, as well as by physiological writers, disposed to favor, to some extent, the theory of Gall and Spurzheim, as to the relation between the *volume* of the brain and the *degree* of psychical power manifested. A

A vast and unexplored region of scientific inquiry is open to the zealous, courageous, and enterprising philosopher, who investigates the subject of *chemico-cerebral pathology*.   Much untrodden ground exists in association with this deeply interesting and hitherto neglected subject.   Any attempt to unravel, by the aid of chemical science, psychical and nervous phenomena so abstruse, may prove, for a time, unproductive of any practical results, nevertheless, some advantage must accrue from these investigations. Lord Bacon, when referring to the persevering efforts of the ancient alchemists to discover the philosopher's stone, remarks, that although they did not succeed in obtaining the immediate

few of the opponents of phrenology have rather overstepped the bounds of prudence by attempting, in their mistaken zeal to establish as a first principle, that there is no clearly established *organic* connection between the brain and mind, that as far as the intellect is concerned we could have done as well without as with a brain!

> Quis furor iste novus; quo nunc, quo tenditis? inquam
> Heu miseri cives!

I am astonished to find an acute and profound thinker like the late Sir W. Hamilton countenancing this extreme view of an important dynamical and physiological question. He observes: " There is no good ground to suppose that the mind is situate solely in the brain, or exclusively in any one part of the body. On the contrary, the supposition that it is really present wherever we are conscious that it acts—in a word, the Peripatetic aphorism, the soul is all in the whole and all in every part— is more philosophical, and, consequently, more probable than any other opinion. It has not been always noticed, even by those who deem themselves the chosen champions of the immateriality of mind, that we materialize mind when we attribute to it the relations of matter. Thus, we cannot attribute a local seat to the soul, without clothing it with the properties of extension and place, and those who suppose this seat to be but a point, only aggravate the difficulty. Admitting the spirituality of mind, all that we know of the relation of soul and body is, that the former is connected with the latter in a way of which we are wholly ignorant; and that it holds relations, different both in degree and kind, with different parts of the organism. We have no right, however, to say that it is limited to any one part of the organism ; for even if we admit that the nervous system is the part to which it is proximately united, still the nervous system is itself universally ramified throughout the body ; and we have no more right to deny that the mind feels at the finger-points, as consciousness assures us, than to assert that it thinks exclusively in the brain. The sum of our knowledge of the connection of mind and body is, therefore, this,—that the mental modifications are dependent on certain corporeal conditions ; but of the nature of these conditions we know nothing. For example, we know, by experience, that the mind perceives only through certain organs of sense, and that, through these different organs, it perceives in a different manner. But whether the senses be instruments, whether they be media, or whether they be only partial outlets to the mind incarcerated in the body,—on all this we can only theorize and conjecture."—*Lectures on Metaphysics*, vol. ii, p. 127.

object of their search, much good resulted from the investigations they pursued. They did not, it was admitted, succeed in discovering the philosopher's stone, but they accomplished by their efforts what might be considered almost tantamount to it in value. By the processes that were adopted, and persevering attempts made, to find the hidden treasure, they turned up and pulverized the soil, thus rendering it better fitted for the purposes of vegetation.

Sir W. Hamilton distinguishes *three* kinds of *latent* mental impressions.[1] 1. Where the greater part of our spiritual treasures lies beyond the sphere of consciousness, and hidden in the obscure recesses of the mind. 2. When the mind contains certain systems of knowledge or certain habits of action which it is wholly unconscious of possessing in its ordinary state, but which are revealed to consciousness in certain extraordinary exaltations of its powers. 3. Consists in ordinary mental modifications, *i. e.*, mental activities of which we are unconscious, but which manifest existence by effects of which we are conscious. This last appears a somewhat ambiguous proposition, for, as Sir W. Hamilton asks, "How can we know that to exist which lies beyond the one condition of all knowledge, —consciousness ? how can knowledge arise out of ignorance, consciousness out of unconsciousness,—the cognizable out of the incognizable ? *i. e.*, how can one opposite proceed out of another ?" "There are many things," says Sir W. Hamilton, "which we neither know nor can know in themselves,—that is, in their direct and immediate relation to our faculties of knowledge, but which manifest themselves through the medium of their effects. Consciousness cannot exist independently of some peculiar modification of the mind ; we are only conscious as we are conscious of a determinate state. To be conscious, we must be conscious of some particular perception, remembrance, imagination, or feeling. We have no general consciousness. As consciousness supposes a special mental modification as its object, it may be remembered that this modification or state supposes a change—a transition from some other state or modification. But as the modification must be present before we have a consciousness of the modification, it is evident that we can have no consciousness of its rise or awakening, for its rise and awakening is also the rise or awaken-

_____
[1] *Lectures on Metaphysics*, vol. i, p. 348.

ing of consciousness." Sir W. Hamilton cites the following illustration of such subtle mental phenomena. "When we look," he observes, "at a distant forest, we perceive a certain expanse of green. Of this, as an affection of our orgasm, we are clearly and distinctly conscious. The expanse of which we are conscious is evidently made up of parts of which we are not conscious. No leaf, perhaps no tree, may be separately visible. But the greenness of the forest is made up of the greenness of the leaves, that is, the total impression of which we are conscious is made up of an infinitude of which we are not conscious? When we hear the distant murmur of the sea, what are," says Sir W. Hamilton, "the constituents of the total perception of which we are conscious? This murmur is a sum made up of parts, and the sum would be zero if the parts did not count as something."[1]

[1] Latent *psychical* are certainly not more singular and inexplicable than latent *physical* phenomena. The subjoined interesting facts relative to *light* illustrate the matter in question.

" M. Niepce de Saint-Victor has been pursuing with much diligence his investigations into the influence of solar light on organic and inorganic bodies. An extensive series of experiments has been communicated by M. Chevreul to the Académie des Sciences. Many of these experiments were merely confirmatory of his former results, or tended to show that the property of absorbing the solar rays and giving them out again in darkness was common to a very large number of dissimilar bodies. It will be remembered by many of our readers, that M. Niepce, in a former communication, stated that a tube of paper or metal, white on the inside, being exposed directly opposite the sun for an hour, absorbed a large quantity of light, which could, by closing the end of the tube, be preserved and employed at some future time in producing a photographic copy of a picture on tissue paper upon a piece of chemically prepared paper placed to receive it. That, indeed, the solar radiations could be bottled up for a future day. M. Niepce has since proved *that if a cylinder of white card-board, which has been exposed to sunshine, be carefully closed up in a tin case,* '*it is active* six *months after its insulation,*' and if there is placed at the end of the tube a transparent print, and then a piece of photographic paper, the radiations from the inside of the tube will act precisely as if the arrangement had been exposed to the solar rays. After these absorbed radiations have once effected the decomposition of any of the salts of gold or silver they are powerless; that is, they are expended in producing this change. M. Niepce has been carrying his investigations still farther, and he has approached the confines of that territory between physics and physiology, which has hitherto been but a bewildering problem. Earth—agricultural soil—has been taken from a considerable depth and spread upon a plate in darkness, a piece of paper covered with chloride of silver has been placed above it, and no effect has been produced. The same soil has *been exposed to sunshine*—one half of it being covered by an opaque screen. It has then been taken into a dark room, and a piece of similar photographic paper placed as in the former experiment. All that *part of the paper over the soil which had been exposed was darkened,* but that portion which had been

The theory of the persistent and indestructible character of psychical impressions is *countenanced* (I will not say *established*), by phenomena observed during various abnormal *mental* and disordered *cerebral* conditions. I refer,

1. *To the state of the intellect as manifested in certain forms of asphyxia, caused by drowning and hanging.*
2. *To the condition of the mind as exhibited previously to death.*
3. *To the morbid mental phenomena observed to result from injuries inflicted upon the brain, or to follow particular types of encephalic disease.*

It has occurred, that persons in the act of drowning (I presume during the *asphyxia* caused by the circulation of *venous* instead of *arterial* blood in the brain, consequent upon the suspension of the respiratory process), have had presented to their minds, whilst in the agonies of death, a series of striking *tableaux* of the most minute and remarkable occurrences of their past lives! Events associated with the period of childhood have been, under these circumstances, recalled to the mind, and presented to it like so many exquisitely executed artistic photographic representations. These phenomena have occurred not exclusively during the act of drowning, and at the moment of death, but in analogous conditions of morbidly asphyxiated and affected brain.[1]

A gentleman, during an attack of acute mental depression, hung himself. A short period only elapsed before he was cut down. He was subsequently brought to me for advice, and placed for a time under my medical supervision. He ultimately recovered. He often related to me the strange mental visions that floated before

covered produced no effect. Here we have evidence of the absorption of the solar rays by the surface soil, and of the continuation in obscurity of that action which has commenced under the influence of sunshine. The researches of M. Niepce de Saint-Victor confirm in a remarkable manner the views entertained by his uncle, M. Niéphoré Niepce, who, in December, 1829, wrote thus : ' Light, in its state of composition and decomposition, acts chemically upon bodies. It is absorbed, *it combines with them, and communicates to them new properties.*' We shall anxiously wait the extension of these researches upon vital organisms, in the direction indicated by M. Chevreul."—*Athenæum*, January 8, 1859.

[1] Müller says, " We know that every idea is a permanent, immutable impression in the brain, which may at any moment present itself anew, if the mind be directed to it—if the ' attention' be turned to it—and that it is merely the impossibility of the attention being occupied by many objects simultaneously that causes each to be forgotten. All these latent ideas must be regarded as impressions on the brain which cannot be effaced. Lesions of the brain may annul a part or all of these ideas."

his mind during the few minutes, or (in all probability) seconds, he continued suspended, and temporarily deprived of consciousness. They were of the most pleasing character. The scenes of his early life were, in their minutest particular, revived. He was taken to the cottage in which he was born, interchanged tokens of affection with his beloved parents, gambolled once more with the companions of his childhood on the village green, and again

> " Whispered the lover's tale,
> Beneath the milk-white thorn, that scents the evening gale."

Incidents connected with the school in which he received his early instruction were reproduced to his mind.   He once again renewed acquaintance, and shook hands with the loved and dearly cherished companions of his boyhood !   The remembrance of faces (*known when a child*) that had been (as he supposed) entirely obliterated from his memory, was restored to his recollection in a most remarkably truthful and vivid manner.   During that critical second of time (when he might almost have been considered struggling with death), every trifling and minute circumstance connected with his past life was presented to his mind like so many charming pictorial sketches and paintings.[1]

"I was once told," says De Quincey, author of the '*Confessions of an English Opium Eater*,' "by a near relative, that having in her childhood fallen into a river, and being on the very verge of death, but for the critical assistance which reached her, she saw in a *moment* her whole life, in its minutest incidents, reflected before her, as in a mirror."

[1] A person who was hung, but cut down on the arrival of a reprieve, upon being asked, " what his sensations were whilst hanging ?" replied, that " the preparations for his execution were dreadful and horrible beyond all expression ; but that, upon being dropped, he instantly found himself *amid fields and rivers of blood*, which gradually acquired a greenish tinge.   Imagining that if he could reach a certain spot he should be easy, he seemed to himself to struggle forcibly to attain it, and then consciousness and all feeling were completely suspended."

" I remember to have heard of a certain gentleman that would needs make trial. in curiosity, what men did feel that were hanged ; so he fastened the cord about his neck, raising himself upon a stool, and then letting himself fall, thinking it should be in his power to recover the stool at his pleasure, which he failed in, but was helped by a friend then present.   He was asked afterwards what he felt ; he said he felt no pain, but first he thought he saw before his eyes a great fire, and burning ; then he thought he saw all black and dark ; lastly, it turned to a pale blue, or sea-water green ; which color is also often seen by them which fall into swoonings."—*History of Life and Death*," *by Lord Bacon.*

How often the mind, during the last struggle with life, is busily occupied in the contemplation of pastoral imagery and pleasant early remembrances, associated with the innocent recreations and unmatched beauties of country life!   All the unsophisticated aspirations and fond reminiscences of the youthful fancy appear, occasionally, at this awful crisis, to gush back to the heart in all their original beauty, freshness, and purity!

"A young man," says Dr. Symonds, "who had been but little conversant with any but rural scenery, discoursed most eloquently, a short time before his death, of sylvan glen, and bosky dell, purling streams, and happy valleys, 'babbling of green fields,' as if his spirit had been always luxuriating itself in the gardens of Elysium."   Shakspeare alludes to this phenomenon in his account of the death of Falstaff, in the play of Henry V.

A gentleman fell accidentally into the water, and was nearly drowned.   After being rescued, he continued in a state of apparent death for nearly twenty minutes.   After his restoration to consciousness, he thus described his sensations whilst in the act of drowning: "They were the most delightful and ecstatic I have ever experienced.   I was transported to a perfect paradise, and witnessed scenes that my imagination never had, in its most active condition, depicted to my mind.   I wandered in company with angelic spirits through the most lovely citron and orange groves,

> 'Roseate bowers,
> Celestial palms, and ever-blooming flowers,'

basking in an atmosphere redolent of the most delicious perfumes. I heard the most exquisite music proceeding from melodious voices and well-tuned instruments.   Whilst in this world of fancy my mind had recalled to consciousness the scenes and associations of my early life, and the memory of the companions of my boyhood. All the knowledge I had acquired during a long life recurred to my mind.   Favorite passages from Horace, Virgil, and Cicero, were revived, and pieces of poetry I had been fond of repeating when a boy, came fresh to my recollection."[1]

[1] The late Professor Clarke, of Cambridge, thus described his state of mind when in the act of being drowned: "After being immersed in the water," he says, "I saw my danger, but thought the mare would swim, and I knew I could ride when we were overwhelmed.   It appeared to me that I had gone to the bottom with my eyes open.   At first I thought I saw the bottom clearly, and then felt neither apprehen-

Analogous phenomena occur sometimes immediately before death. The delirium that occasionally accompanies the act of dying, is often marked by a singular and significant reference to the minute circumstances of the past life; and aged persons have been heard, like Falstaff, not only to "babble about green fields," but (in imagination) to converse with, and of the companions of their youth, and to talk of particular events that had occurred at the period of their early childhood! An elderly lady, whilst in a state of delirium immediately preceding death, addressed those about her on the subject of marriage, and requested them to arrange her bridal dress, and gave other instructions respecting an event that had occurred, under unusually peculiar romantic circumstances, nearly *fifty* years previously!

A lady, who died of obscure visceral disease, became delirious three hours before death. She then began to talk, in what appeared to those about her, to be the "unknown tongue." No one understood a word she uttered. It was eventually surmised that she was conversing in German, a language she had acquired in early life, but which she had apparently forgotten. A native of that country, who was at the time on a visit at a friend's house, was sent for, and conversed with the patient in German. The relations of the lady assured the medical gentlemen in attendance, who were much struck by the singular phenomenon, that she had not spoken the foreign language since she was *ten* years of age! Five years previously to her fatal illness she accompanied some friends to Frankfort, but whilst there never attempted, although frequently

sion nor pain; on the contrary, I felt as if I had been in the most delightful situation; my mind was tranquil and uncommonly happy. I felt as if in paradise, and yet I do not recollect that I saw any person; the impression of happiness seemed not to be derived from anything around me, but from the state of my mind. And yet I had a general apprehension of pleasing objects; and I cannot recollect that anything appeared defined, nor did my eye take in any object, only I had a general impression of a green color, as of fields or gardens. But my happiness did not appear to arise from these, but appeared to consist merely in the tranquil—indescribably tranquil state of mind. By-and-by I seemed to awake, as out of slumber, and felt unutterable pain and difficulty of breathing; and now I found I had been carried by a strong wave, and left in very shallow water on the shore, and the pain I felt was occasioned by the air once more inflating my lungs and producing respiration. How long I had been under water I cannot tell; it may, however, be guessed at by the circumstance that, when restored to the power of reflection, I looked at the mare, and saw her walking leisurely down shore towards home, then about half a mile distant from the place where we were submerged."

urged, to converse in the language of the country. It was then supposed that all the knowledge she had acquired of German when a child had been effaced from her mind.

Dr. Rush alludes to a patient subject to attacks of recurrent insanity, whose paroxysms were always indicated by her conversing in a kind of Italian *patois*. As the disease advanced, and had reached its culminating point, the lady could only talk in *French*, at the decline of her illness she spoke only *German*, and during the stage of convalescence she addressed those about her in her *native tongue*. This lady when quite well rarely spoke any but her own language, and if she attempted to do otherwise, always did so with extreme diffidence and difficulty. During her attack of insanity she spoke with great fluency, never apparently being at a loss for words to convey her ideas. It is said that, with the exception of the Italian, the other languages, German and French, were singularly accurate.

Lord Monboddo relates the following singular case : "A gentleman well known both to the learned and political world, who did me the honor to correspond with me upon the subject of my first volume of metaphysics, says, ' that about six-and-twenty years ago, when I was in France, I had an intimacy in the family of the late Maréchal de Montmorenci de Laval. His son, the Compte de Laval, was married to Mademoiselle de Maupeaux, the daughter of a lieutenant-general of that name, and the niece of the late Chancellor. This gentleman was killed at the battle of Hastenbeck ; his widow survived him some years, but is since dead.

" ' The following fact comes from her own mouth. She has told it to me repeatedly. She was a woman of perfect veracity, and very good sense. She appealed to her servants and family for the truth ; nor did she, indeed, seem to be sensible that the matter was so extraordinary as it appeared to me. I wrote it down at the time, and I have the memorandum amongst my papers.

" ' The Comtesse de Laval had been observed by servants, who sate up with her on account of some indisposition, to talk in her sleep a language that none of them understood ; nor were they sure, or, indeed, herself able to guess, upon the sounds being repeated to her, whether it was or was not gibberish.

" ' Upon her lying-in of one of her children, she was attended by a nurse who was of the province of Britanny, and who immediately knew the meaning of what she said, it being in the idiom of the natives of that country : but she herself, when awake, did not understand a single syllable of what she had uttered in her sleep upon its being retold to her.

" ' She was born in that province, and had been nursed in a family where nothing but that language was spoken ; so that in her first infancy she had known it and no other ; but, when she returned to her parents, she had no opportunity of keeping up the use of it ; and, as I have before said, she did not understand a word of Breton when awake, though she spoke it in her sleep.

" ' I need not say that the Comtesse de Laval never said or imagined that she used any words of the Breton idiom more than were necessary to express those ideas that are within the compass of a child's knowledge of objects, &c.' "[1]

A patient of Sir H. Holland's was attacked by hemiplegia at an advanced age. He passed, a few days before death, into a state of low, rambling delirium. He then spoke only in French, a language he had not been known to speak for *thirty* years before. " This continued," says Sir H. Holland, " until utterance ceased altogether to be intelligible."[2]

The following circumstance occurred in a Roman Catholic town in Germany, a year or two before Mr. Coleridge arrived at Gottingen. It was at the time a frequent subject of conversation. " A young woman, of four or five and twenty, who could neither read or write, was seized with a nervous fever, during which, according to the asseverations of all the priests and monks of the neighborhood, she became possessed, as it appeared, by a very learned devil. She continued incessantly talking Latin, Greek, and Hebrew, in very pompous terms, and with the most distinct enunciation. This possession was rendered more probable by the known fact that she was or had been a heretic. Voltaire humorously advises the Devil to decline all acquaintance with medical

---

[1] " Ancient Metaphysics."

[2] " *Mental Pathology*."

" It is in vain," says Dr. Carpenter, " to speculate as to the nature of the change by which sensory impressions are thus registered." He, however, considers that they are in some way dependent upon the *nutrition* of the brain. In cases like those previously cited, there can be no doubt, he says, " that some alterations either in the circulation of the blood or in the quality of the fluid, was the cause of changes which, operating in the substance of the sensorium, reproduced the former sensations, just as a disturbance of the circulation in the retina occasions the sensations of flashes of light or other visual phenomena."—*Principles of Human Physiology*, p. 358.

men, and it would have been more to his reputation if he had taken this advice in the present instance.   The case had attracted the particular attention of a young physician, and by his statement many eminent physiologists and psychologists visited the town, and cross-examined the case on the spot.   Sheets full of her ravings were taken down from her own mouth, and were found to consist of sentences coherent and intelligible each for itself, but with little or no connection with each other.   Of the Hebrew, a small portion of the whole could be traced to the Bible, the remainder seemed to be the rabbinical dialect.   All trick or conspiracy was out of the question.   Not only had the young woman ever been a harmless, simple creature, but she evidently was laboring under a nervous fever.   In the town in which she had been resident for many years as a servant in different families, no solution presented itself.   The young physician, however, determined to trace her past life from step to step, for the patient herself was incapable of returning a rational answer.   He at length succeeded in discovering the place where her parents had lived, travelled thither, found them dead, but an uncle surviving, he learned from him that the patient had been charitably taken by an old Protestant pastor at nine years of age, and had remained with him some years, even till the old man's death.   Of this pastor the uncle knew nothing, but that he was a very good man.   With great difficulty, and after much search, our young medical philosopher discovered a niece of the pastor's who had lived with him as his housekeeper, and had inherited his effects.   She remembered the girl, related that her venerable uncle had been too indulgent, and could not bear to hear the girl scolded; that she was willing to have kept her, but that after her patron's death the girl herself refused to stay.   Anxious inquiries were made concerning the pastor's habits, and the solution of the phenomenon was soon obtained.   It appeared that it was the old man's custom for years to walk up and down a passage of his house, into which the kitchen door opened, and to read to himself with a loud voice out of his favorite books.   A considerable number of these were still in the niece's possession.   The pastor was a learned man, and a great hebraic scholar.   Among the books were found a collection of rabbinical writings, together with several of the Greek and Latin authors, and the physician succeeded in identifying so many passages with those taken down at the young woman's bedside, that no doubt could remain in any rational mind concerning the true origin of the impressions made on her nervous system."

Analogous phenomena are observable in some forms of somnambulism as well as of catalepsy. Sir W. Hamilton quotes a singular illustration from a German book by Abel, entitled, "*A Collection of Remarkable Phenomena from Human Life.*" "A young man had a cataleptic attack, in consequence of which a singular change was effected in his mental constitution. Some six minutes after falling asleep, he began to speak distinctly, and almost always of the same objects and concatenated events, so that he carried on from night to night the same history, or rather, continued to play the same part. On awakening he had no reminiscence whatever of his dreaming thoughts, a circumstance, by the way, which distinguishes this as rather a case of somnambulism than of common dreaming. Be this, however, as it may, he played a double part in his existence. By day he was the poor apprentice of a merchant; by night he was a married man, the father of a family, a senator, and in affluent circumstances. If, during his vision, anything were said in regard to his waking state, he declared it unreal and a dream."

But, reverting more particularly to the phenomena of memory, I would ask, how are we to explain physiologically the *modus operandi* of attention in fixing certain impressions on the mind? Is the fact referable to a *mechanical* or *psychical* law?

It is deemed of importance that a certain idea or aggregation of ideas should, to use colloquial phrases, be permanently *impressed, fixed,* or *stamped* upon the mind, in other words, be susceptible, by an effort of the will, of being *remembered.* In ordinary understandings, unless the attention be continuously directed and concentrated to the subject immediately under consideration, the impression made upon the brain, the material recipient of the mental image, is faint, transient, and evanescent. If it be necessary to commit any piece of prose or poetry to memory, we repeat it without intermission, until we are *conscious* that a durable effect is made upon the mind. Such continuity and concentration of the attention satisfactorily accounts for the tenacity of certain conceptions, healthy as well as morbid, in which the mind has taken a deep and abiding interest, and explains the fixed character of a particular type of ideas (*delusions ?*) which implicate in their operations, the emotions, passions, imagination, as well as reasoning and reflective faculties ?

A circumstance occurs which greatly interests and involves the feelings. A loved object dies in a particular room, or is accidentally deprived of life in a certain locality. The attention of the unhappy survivor is painfully alive and vividly concentrated to all the *physical* as well as *moral* and *emotional* associations connected with the severe loss sustained, and an impression is thus made upon the memory, which is rarely, if ever, effaced. Again, the activity and accuracy of the memory are greatly dependent upon the laws regulating the association of ideas.[1] This faculty is noticed in various conditions of manifestation or states of development, according to educational training, and original and connate vigor of mind. In a few understandings it is observed to be altogether absent, in others it operates sluggishly, and in some it is in a most painfully *morbid* and *sensitive* state of activity. The most trifling and insignificant allusion, the faintest reference to a particular subject, in a certain type of healthy as well as of disordered mind, recalls immediately and vividly to the recollection a complicated chain of past conceptions.[2]

[1] The faculty of memory, reproduction, or to use Sir W. Hamilton's phrase, "re-suscitation," is considered by metaphysicians to be regulated by the laws which govern the general association of our ideas. Aristotle, who flourished more than 2000 years ago, has left behind him a masterly philosophical analysis of these laws. Thoughts, he maintains, which have once coexisted in the mind are afterwards associated, and never can, except by disease, be disassociated. This is what is termed the law of the "disintegration." In what way, asks Aristotle, does the presence of one thought determine and produce another? All our thoughts are said to have a well-defined relation to each other. The laws governing the association of ideas Aristotle reduces to four, viz, Contiguity in time and space, Resemblance, and Contrariety. "It has been established," says Sir W. Hamilton, "that thoughts are associated; that is, are able to excite each other, 1, if co-existing, or immediately successive in time ; 2, if their objects are conterminous or adjoining in space ; 3, if they hold the dependence to each other as cause and effect, or of mean and end, or of whole or part; 4, if they stand in a relation either of contrast or of similarity ; 5, if they are the operations of the same powers, or of different powers conversant about the same object ; 6, if their objects are the sign and the signified, or, 7, even if their objects are accidentally denoted by the same sound."—*Vide Aristotle's Essay, entitled,* " Περὶ Μνήμης καὶ Ἀναμνήσεως."

[2] Lord Kames refers to this fact, and ascribes this mental condition to a " bluntness of the discerning faculty." He says, " A person who cannot accurately distinguish between a slight connection and one that is more intimate is equally affected by each ; such a person must necessarily have a great flow of ideas, because they are introduced by any relation indifferently ; and the slighter relations being without number furnish ideas without end."

A look—a word carelessly and thoughtlessly spoken; the sight of some trivial object, perhaps, token of affection; the melancholy wail of the wind among the trees; murmur of the ocean's dash upon the beach; sound of distant village bells floating upon the evening breeze; the strains of a plaintive melody associated with the sad reminiscences of the past, "strike the electric chain," which so mysteriously encircles, and binds the mind, and suggests a long forgotten succession, it may be, of agonizing, burning, and, alas! maddening thoughts!

A lady at some distance from town was in the last stage of an incurable disorder. A short time before her death she requested that her youngest child, a girl about four years of age, might be brought to visit her. This was accordingly complied with. The child remained with her about three days. Thirty years afterwards this young lady had occasion to go to the same house. Of her visit when a child she retained no trace of recollection, nor was the name of the village even known to her. When she arrived at the house, she had no memory of its exterior, but on entering the room where her mother had been confined, her eye anxiously traversed the apartment, and she said, "I have been here before; the prospect from the window is quite familiar to me, and I remember that in this part of the room there was a bed and a sick lady, who kissed me and wept." On minute inquiry none of these circumstances had ever occurred to her recollection during this long interval, and in all probability they would never have recurred, but for the locality, which revived them.

Are the ideas conveyed to the mind productive, at the time of their conception, of a molecular change in the *physical* tissue of the brain, and are the impressions so made on the *material* instrument of thought, subsequently, by an effort of the will, revived, and only made objects of consciousness, by the application of a *specific* kind and degree of stimuli, physical, mental, objective, or subjective, applied to the special cerebral registering-ganglia upon which the mental pictures are supposed to be traced?

Do the following ingenious experiments (as detailed by Dr. Draper),[1] with reference to impressions made upon *material* sub-

[1] "*Human Physiology, Statical and Dynamical*," by John W. Draper, M.D. Pp. 288. New York, 1856.

stances cognizable to sense, throw any light upon the *physical* or *psychical* phenomena of memory ?

- " If, on a cold polished piece of metal, any object, as a wafer, is laid, and the metal then be breathed upon, and, when the moisture has had time to disappear, the wafer be thrown off, though now upon the polished surface the most critical inspection can discover no trace of any form, if we breathe upon it, a spectral figure of the wafer comes into view, and this may be repeated again and again. Nay, even more; if the polished metal be carefully put aside where nothing can deteriorate its surface, and be so kept for many months, even for a year, on breathing again upon it, the shadowy form emerges; or, if a sheet of paper on which a key or other object is laid, be carried for a few moments into the sunshine and then instantaneously viewed in the dark, the key being simultaneously removed, a fading spectre of the key on the paper will be seen, and if the paper be put away where nothing can disturb it, and so kept for many months, at the end thereof, if it be carried into a dark place and laid on a piece of hot metal, the spectre of the key will come forth. In the cases of bodies more highly phosphorescent than paper, the spectres of many different objects which may have been in succession laid originally thereupon, will, on warming, emerge in their proper order. These illustrations show how trivial are the physical impressions which may be thus registered and preserved. A shadow is said never to fall upon a wall without leaving thereupon its permanent trace, a trace which might be made visible by resorting to proper processes. All kinds of photographic drawing are, in their degree, examples of this kind. Of the moral consequences of these phenomena, it is not my object here to speak. The world would be none the worse if every secret action might thus be made plain. But if on such inorganic surfaces impressions may in this way be preserved, how much more likely is it that the same thing occurs in the purposely-constituted ganglion ! Not that there is any necessary coincidence between an external form and its ganglionic impression, any more than there is between the letters of a message delivered in a telegraphic office and the signals which the telegraph gives to the distant station, yet these signals are easily re-translated into the original words—no more than there is between the letters of a printed page and the acts or scenes they may chance to describe; but those letters call up with clearness in the mind of the reader

the events and scenes. Indeed, the quickness with which the
mind interprets such traces or impressions in its registering ganglia is illustrated by the rapidity with which we gather the sense
it contains, or as a skilful accountant runs his eye over a long
column of figures, and seems to come by intuition at once to the
correct sum. The capability which we thus possess of determining a final perception or judgment of results, without dwelling on
the intermediate traces or steps, is also illustrated by our appreciation of music without concentrating our thoughts on the time
and intensities of vibration or interferences of the notes, though
these mathematical relations are at the very bottom of the harmony; and conspicuously does the Supreme Intelligence, God,
reach with unerring truth to every final result without any necessary concern in the intermediate steps."

"From the preceding considerations, we may infer that there
is a necessary limitation of the amount of impressions capable of
being registered in the organism, and, therefore, in this regard,
all human knowledge is finite. Yet its term is much farther off
than might at first sight appear. A library of a given size may
only be able to contain a given number of books upon its shelves,
but the amount of information it is capable of containing may
be made to vary with the condensation and perspicuity of the
books."

In many cases of want of sequence in the ideas, or defective
continuity of thought, the cerebral nerve channels, considered to
be the media for the transmission of impressions to and from the
brain, are either impervious to their free passage, or there exists
a loss of *efferent* conducting power in the central nerve fibres,
arising (most probably) from some subtle and as yet unexplained,
mal-nutrition, morbid change in the molecular portion of their
tissue, abnormal condition of what is termed the *polarity* of the
nerve force, or change in the *chemical* constitution of brain matter
not yet discovered in the laboratory, and at present inexplicable
to the physiologist and pathologist.

Comparing the aggregations of gray matter on the hemispherical
surface of the brain to a galvanic battery placed at the extremity
of, or in connection with a number of *electric* wires (the white or
medullary cerebral matter), we can easily understand, if any of
these should become deranged, and not be in healthy condition, or

the *battery* (the brain) itself be out of order, that the ideas cannot be freely transmitted (in consequence of a breach of continuity in the channels of communication, conducting, or *efferent* nerve-tubes) in obedience to the mandates of vòlition, originating in the primary *dynamical* centre of the *cineritious* portion of the cerebral mass, or that the impressions made by the feeble (*disordered?*) efforts of the mind upon the motor and sensor powers may be faint, confused, or altogether unintelligible.[1]

Can we explain by any other hypothesis the singular anomalies in the operations of the mind to which I am about to refer ?

A man loses all knowledge of a language acquired in early youth, in consequence of a severe blow upon the head, or as the effect of a serious derangement of the cerebral circulation or alteration of the molecular structure of the brain associated with an attack of fever, paralysis, or apoplexy. He recovers from the illness, but with an entire forgetfulness of a language with which he was previously familiar. He is advised, when restored to health, to relearn it. He commences with the grammar, and makes an attempt to acquire the rudiments of the lost tongue. Whilst so doing, he painfully realizes the mortifying fact that all recollection of what he had formerly so well known and highly valued is entirely obliterated from his memory. He endeavors to translate some elementary classical work, and during a determined effort to resuscitate his dormant, and, to all appearance, lost ideas, and revive former impressions by attempting to construe a difficult Latin sen-

---

[1] An attempt has been made by carefully-executed experiments to estimate the rapidity with which the electric current passes along the nerve-tubes. M. Helmholtz has, by means of an ingenious and delicately-constructed galvanic apparatus, ascertained that in a nerve of 50 to 60 millimetres length, the time required for the transmission of nerve force was from 0·0014 to 0·0020 of a second ! (*Vide Comptes Rendus*, vol. xxx, 1850. *Article* " *Sur la Vitesse de Propagation de l'Agent dans les Nerfs Rachidiens.*")

" If mental action be electric, the proverbial quickness of thought—that is, the quickness of the transmission of sensation and will—may be presumed to have been brought to an exact measurement. The speed of light has long been known to be about 192,000 miles per second, and the experiments of Wheatstone have shown that the electric agent travels (if I may so speak) at the same rate, thus showing a likelihood that one law rules the movements of all the 'imponderable bodies.' Mental action may accordingly be presumed to have a rapidity equal to 192,000 miles in a second, a rate far beyond what is necessary to make the design and execution of any of our ordinary muscular movements, apparently identical in point of time, which they are." · (" *The Vestiges of the Natural History of Creation,*" p. 342.)

tence, he is conscious of a physical change taking place in the brain—

"Quick as Ithuriel's spear,"

all his critical knowledge of the apparently forgotten language rushes like a torrent back to the mind. The preceding illustration is *not* a hypothetical one. The following is an analogous case :—

Rev. J. E——, a clergyman of rare talent and energy, of sound education, while riding through his mountainous parish, was thrown violently from his carriage, and received a violent concussion of the brain. For several days he remained utterly unconscious, and at length when restored, his intellect was observed to be in a state like that of a naturally intelligent child, or like that of Caspar Hauser, after his long sequestration. The good man again, but now in middle life, commenced his English and classical studies under tutors, and was progressing very satisfactorily, when, after several months' successful study, the rich storehouses of memory were gradually unlocked, so that in a few weeks his mind resumed all its wonted vigor, and its former wealth and polish of culture. For several years he has continued his labors as a pastor, and has suffered no symptom of cerebral disturbance. The first evidence of the restoration of this gentleman's memory was experienced whilst attempting the mastery of an abstruse Greek author, an intellectual effort well adapted to test the penetrability of that veil that so long had excluded from the mind the light and riches of its former hard-earned possessions.

A clergyman, about thirty years of age, a man of learning and acquirements, at the termination of a severe illness, was found to have lost the recollection of everything, even the names of the most common objects. His health being restored, he began to re-acquire knowledge like a child. After learning the names of objects, he was taught to read, and after this, began to learn Latin. He had made considerable progress, when, one day in reading his lesson to his brother, who was his teacher, he suddenly stopped, and put his hand to his head. Being asked why he did so, he replied, "I feel a peculiar sensation in my head ; and now it appears to me that I knew all this before." From that time he rapidly recovered his faculties. A state of the mind somewhat analogous occasionally occurs in diseases arising from simple exhaustion.

Many years ago, Dr. Abercrombie attended a lady who, from a severe and neglected diarrhœa, was reduced to a state of great weakness, followed by a remarkable failure of memory.   She had lost the recollection of a particular epoch of her life extending over the period of about ten or twelve years.   She had formerly lived in another city, and the time of which she had lost the recollection was that during which she had lived in Edinburgh.   Her ideas were consistent with each other, but they referred to things as they stood before her removal.   She recovered her health after a considerable time, but remained in a state of imbecility resembling the dotage of old age.

It is a well-established fact that idiocy, apparently irremediable, connate imbecility, has been *cured by a blow upon the head !*   Who can fathom the depths, unravel the intricate labyrinths, and penetrate into the secret arcana of the nervous system !   " *Omnia exeunt in mysterium,*" exclaims an old schoolman.

A child up to the age of thirteen was idiotic, giving evidence either of a total deficiency of intelligence, or of a stunted intellect of the lowest grade and order.   He fell from a height upon his head, and was stunned.   He rallied from this state of unconsciousness, and was, *Credat Judæus?* found to be in full possession of his intellectual faculties.

A somewhat similar case is recorded by Louyer-Villermay.   A man suffered from a paralysis of memory, following a severe blow upon the head.   He was fortunate enough (as the result established) to have a repetition of the physical injury, and, as the effect of this accident, his memory was immediately restored to its original strength.[1]

Petrarch records that Pope Clement VI found his memory wonderfully strengthened after receiving a slight concussion of the brain.

" I have been informed," says Dr. Prichard, " on good authority, that there was, some time since, a family, consisting of three boys, who were all considered as idiots.   One of them received a severe injury of the head : from that time his faculties began to brighten, and he is now a man of good talents, and practises as a barrister.   His brothers are still idiotic or imbecile." [2]

[1] " Dictionnaire des Sciences Médicale," vol. xxxii, p. 321.

[2] " Treatise on Diseases of the Nervous System," by J. C. Prichard, M.D., 1822.   I was relating these and other analogous and inexplicable facts, illustrative of the sin-

Father Mabillon is said to have been in his younger days an idiot, continuing in this condition until the age of twenty-six.   He then fell with his head against a stone staircase and fractured his skull.   He was trepanned.   After recovering from the effects of the operation and injury, his intellect fully developed itself.   He is said to have exhibited subsequently to the accident and operation " a mind endowed with a lively imagination, an amazing memory, and a zeal for study rarely equalled."

Mrs. M——, aged twenty-six, ten days after confinement, resumed her usual household labors, and being a feeble woman, and of an irritable nervous temperament, she had the misfortune to have an attack of acute puerperal mania.   She was not often violent, but being constantly tormented with the most terrific panophobia, she frequently made vigorous attempts to escape from her countless imaginary adversaries.   This state of things continued for one week, when she leaped from a window of her apartment, in the second story, upon the pavement below.   This act she repeated on several successive days, and on each occasion she was immediately secured and quieted in her room.   Again she repeated her efforts to escape; she leaped into the street, ran several blocks, entered a large warehouse, ascended to the third story, and fancying herself still hotly pursued by her foes, she leaped from a small ventilating aperture, through which she could scarcely press her way, and the narrowness of which served to break her leap, and cause her partly to fall upon a low shed beneath.   She was severely stunned by the force of the fall—says that she " saw stars and

gular vagaries and wonderful eccentricities of the nervous system, to a medical sceptic, when he emphatically exclaimed, " I don't believe that such things can occur!" " Why?" I asked.   He immediately replied, "Because I cannot understand the nature of the phenomena."   "Are we," I asked, "to discredit, disbelieve, and put aside everything that is not susceptible of mathematical demonstration, and a satisfactory psychological and physiological explanation?   If so, how much valuable knowledge must we entirely ignore?"   That eminent Christian, John Newton, was once told by a zealous Unitarian (proceeding on the principle adopted by my medical friend, that we are not required to believe what we cannot prove, understand, and explain) that he had carefully read the New Testament, but could find no proof there of the doctrine of the Trinity.   Newton knew with whom he was talking, and answered by saying, " Do you know what happened to me last night?"   " Well," replied his opponent, "what?"   "Why," said Newton, "when I was going to my bedroom, I wondered what ailed my candle, that I could not light it, and on examination I found that *I had been attempting to do so with the extinguisher on!*   Is it not better to believe too much than too little, on the principle that "a man may breathe (according to Dr. Johnson) in foul air, who would die in an exhausted receiver."

felt very dizzy;" she was for a few moments insensible, but in a short time became perfectly conscious, and returned to her home restored to her right mind.

It was immediately after this daring hegira that the writer first saw this patient, when he found her very much exhausted, timorous, but not particularly excitable; the countenance was placid, and the expression of the eye full of life. She expressed great joy and devout gratitude for her safe escape from the great perils of her frenzied flight and leaps, as well as for her delivery from the dreadful panophobia which had driven her to such heroic daring. Her restoration to health was speedy and complete, and there has been no recurrence of any symptom of mental aberration.[1]

The previous illustrations establish: 1, *To what degree the mental operations are under the dominion and control of the nervous matter of the brain ;* 2, *how trifling, in some cases, is the* PHYSICAL *obstruction that interferes with the healthy* ACTION OF THOUGHT ; *and* 3, *how fine and fragile is the line that separates the* SANE *from the* INSANE *man, the babbling, drivelling* IDIOT *from the man of transcendent* GENIUS. Well may it be said,

> " Great wit to madness nearly is allied,
> And THIN PARTITIONS do their bounds divide."

What is the solution of the preceding phenomena? Have the blows upon the head suddenly removed a *mechanical* entanglement or derangement of the molecular portion of the brain structure, thus dislodging any obstructions that may have existed in the *afferent* and *efferent* nerve-tubes, interfering with the free and unfettered *current* of psychical, sensorial, and motor force, as well as with the reception of *peripheral* and transmission of *mental* impressions?

Analogous singular inexplicable psychical phenomena are observed in affections of the brain associated with insanity. A man is seized with mental derangement whilst engaged in some manual employment, or when occupied in the contemplation of a particular idea or class of ideas. He recovers, and contemporaneously with his restoration to mental health, the mind recurs immediately to the train of thought or business in which it was engaged when seized with insanity, all notion of *duration* being annihilated, the

---

[1] Dr. Elisha Harris, in " *New York Journal of Medicine*," for September, 1854.

interval between the first moment of seizure and the restoration of reason appearing like a blank, or analogous to a troubled and distressing dream.

Bergmann relates the case of a man, aged ninety, who became insane when he was eighteen, and was always under an impression that he continued of a juvenile age. I have seen several interesting cases similar to the one just referred to.

I attended a lady who was reduced by pernicious physical habits to a sad state of apparently hopeless and incurable imbecility. She exhibited little or no evidence of intelligence, was incapable of any degree of rational conversation, and manifested other symptoms of imbecility. This patient having been placed under strict supervision for some time, gradually recovered her intelligence. The first symptom which she manifested of a return of reason, was her going to her work-box and taking out a piece of work in which she was engaged twelve months previously, at which time it was supposed her mind had first exhibited symptoms of derangement.

Phenomena of a somewhat analogous kind are observed in connection with conditions of sleep, and temporary states of morbid unconsciousness resulting from injuries of the head.

A person of the name of Samuel Chilton, a laborer, of Timsbury, near Bath, in the year 1696, is said to have slept for *seventeen* continuous weeks, from the 9th of April to the 7th of August. Life was sustained by the daily exhibition of small quantities of wine. When he awoke he dressed himself and walked about the room, being, as the narrator observes, "perfectly unconscious that he had slept more than *one* night. Nothing could make him believe that he had been asleep for so lengthened a period, until, upon going into the fields, he saw crops of barley and oats ready for the sickle, which he remembered were only sown when he last visited them."[1]

It is recorded of a British captain at the battle of the Nile, that he was giving an order from the quarter-deck of his vessel, when a shot struck him on the head, depriving him immediately of speech. As he survived the injury, he was taken home, and remained, deprived of sense and speech, in Greenwich Hospital for *fifteen* months ! At the end of that period, during which he

[1] " Fraser's Magazine."

is said to have manifested no sign of intelligence, an operation was performed on the head, which almost instantaneously restored him to consciousness.   He then immediately rose from his bed, and not recognizing where he was, or what had occurred, expressed a desire to complete the order which had been so abruptly interrupted when he received his injury during the battle *fifteen* months previously!

A farmer, of fair character, who resided in an interior town in New England, sold his farm with an intention of purchasing another in a different town.   His mind was naturally of a melancholy cast.   Shortly after the sale of his farm, he was induced to believe that he had sold it for less than its value.   This persuasion brought on dissatisfaction, and eventually a considerable degree of melancholy.   In this situation one of his neighbors engaged him to enclose a piece of land with a post and rail fence, which he was to commence making the next day.   At the time appointed he went into the field, and began with a beetle and wedges to split the timber out of which the posts and rails were to be prepared.   On finishing this day's work he put his beetle and wedges into a hollow tree, and went home.   Two of his sons had been at work through the day in a distant part of the same field.   On his return he directed them to get up early the next morning, to assist him in making the fence.   In the course of the evening he became delirious, and continued in this situation several years, when his mental powers were suddenly restored.   The first question he asked after the return of his reason, was whether his sons had brought in the beetle and wedges?   He appeared to be wholly unconscious of the time that had elapsed from the commencement of his delirium.   His sons, apprehensive that any explanation might induce a return of his disease, simply replied that they had been unable to find them.   He then immediately arose from his bed, went into the field where he had been at work a number of years before, and found the wedges and the rings of the beetles where he had left them, the beetle itself having mouldered away.   During this delirium his mind had not been occupied with those subjects with which it was conversant in health.[1]

Mrs. S——, an intelligent lady, belonging to a respectable family in the State of New York, some years back, undertook a

---

[1] Dr. Prichard on " The Diseases of the Nervous System."

piece of fine needlework. She devoted her time to it, almost un-
ceasingly, for a number of days. Before she had completed it she
became suddenly insane. In this state, without experiencing any
material abatement of her disease, she continued for about *seven*
years, when her reason was suddenly restored. One of the first
questions which she asked, after her sanity was restored, related
to her needlework! It is a remarkable fact that, during the long
continuance of her mental aberration, she said nothing, so far as
was recollected, about her needlework, nor concerning any of the
subjects that usually occupied her mind when in health.

In the Transactions of the French Academy of Sciences for
1719, there is published a statement illustrative of the subject
under consideration It is as follows:—

A nobleman, residing at Lausanne, whilst giving orders to a
servant, suddenly lost his speech and senses. Various modes of
treatment were adopted to restore his intellect to a sound state,
but for a very considerable time without effect. For *six* months
he appeared to be in a deep sleep, apparently unconscious of everything. At the end of that period a surgical operation was decided
upon and performed. The effect was to restore him to the use of
his speech and consciousness. When he recovered, the servant to
whom he had been giving orders upon entering the room, was
asked by him if he had done what he was requested to do at the
commencement of his illness, not being aware that any interval,
except perhaps a very short one, had elapsed during his attack.[1]

A girl, aged six years, while indulging in a game with her play-
mates, tossing and catching playthings on the pavement, failed to
notice something that was thrown to her, and while hurriedly seeking for, and inquiring about it, made a false step and fell upon the
pavement. The cerebral concussion appeared to have been violent, and she was watched with much anxiety for about ten hours
after the accident. She then, for the first time, opened her eyes
and manifested signs of consciousness. She then immediately
jumped to the margin of her bed, exclaiming, "Where is it?
where did you throw it?" and immediately commenced throwing
little articles from her dress, exclaiming, "Catch these!" By
these acts, she was manifestly continuing those physical operations

[1] The Academy received this statement from Crousaz, Mathematical Professor at
Lausanne, and author of a Treatise on Logic, &c.

and train of thought which had been so suddenly arrested by her fall.   No marked vascular reaction occurred in this case ; the pupil was very much contracted during the first six hours of the period of concussion, the pulse soft and hurried ; she vomited much, but did not open her eyes at any time, until the moment of her sudden restoration to consciousness.   Her recovery was perfect from that moment.

A clergyman was, one wintry day, employed in snipe-shooting with a friend.   In the course of their perambulations, a high hedge intervened between the companions ; the friend fired at a bird which sprang unexpectedly up, and lodged a part of the shot in the forehead of the clergyman.   He instantly fell, and did not recover the shock for some days, so as to be deemed out of danger. When he was so, it was perceived that he was mentally deranged. He was to have been married two days subsequently to that on which the accident happened.   From this peculiar combination of circumstances, the phenomena of the case appeared to arise, *for all sanity of mind seemed to make a full stop, as it were, at this spot of the current*, and he soon sank into a state of inoffensive lunacy. All his conversation was literally confined to the business of the wedding.   Out of this circle his mind never deviated.   He dwelt upon everything relating to it with minuteness, never retreating or advancing one step further for *fifty years*, being, ideally, still a young, active, expecting, and happy bridegroom, chiding the tardiness of time, although it brought him, at the age of eighty, gently to his grave !   He was never known to complain of heat or cold, although his windows were open all the year round.[1]

A gentleman, on the point of marriage, left his intended bride for a short time.   He usually travelled in the stage-coach to the place of her abode.   The last journey he took from her was the last of his life.   Anxiously expecting his return, she went to meet the vehicle.   An old friend announced to her the death of her lover.   She uttered an involuntary scream and piteous exclamation, "He is dead !"   From that fatal moment, for *fifty years*, has this unfortunate female daily, in all seasons, traversed the distance

---

[1] Gall saw, in an asylum at Vienna, a lunatic, whose insanity had reduced him to a state of almost complete idiocy.   His only occupation was that of counting, but he never could count to one hundred.   At the figure ninety-nine he invariably stopped. Gall tried frequently to induce him to say *one hundred*, but it was useless ; he always began again to count from the figure one.

of many miles to the spot where she expected her future husband to alight from the coach, uttering, in a plaintive tone, "He is not come yet—I will return to-morrow."[2]

Garrick's King Lear is said to have been this great tragedian's masterpiece. His delineation of the acute mental sufferings of the unhappy monarch, consequent upon a recognition of his daughter's ingratitude, is recorded as one of the most terrible and natural pieces of acting ever witnessed upon the stage. Garrick admitted that he owed his success in Lear to the following fact :—

A worthy man, whilst playing with his only child at an open window, accidentally let it fall upon the pavement beneath. The poor father remained at the window, screaming with agony, until the neighbors delivered the child into his arms a corpse! He instantly became insane, and from that moment never recovered his understanding. He passed the remainder of his long and wretched life in going to the window, and there playing in fancy with his child, then appearing to drop it, immediately bursting into a flood of tears, and for a while filling the house with his wild and unearthly shrieks. He then became calm, sat down in a state of profound gloom, his eyes fixed for a long time on one object, and his mind intensely absorbed in the contemplation of a fearful image. Garrick was often present at this heartrending scene of misery; and "thus it was," he said, "I learned to imitate madness."

A young gentleman having £10,000 undisposed of and unemployed, placed it, for business purposes, in the hands of his confidential broker. This sum he invested in a stock that had an unexpected, sudden, and enormous rise in value. In a fortunate moment he sold out, and the £10,000 realized £60,000. An account of the successful monetary speculation was transmitted to the fortunate owner of this large sum. The startling intelligence produced a severe shock to the nervous system, and the mind lost its equilibrium. The poor fellow continued in a state of mental alienation for the remainder of his life. His constant occupation until the day of his death, was playing with his fingers, and continually repeating without intermission, and with great animation and rapidity, the words, "Sixty thousand! sixty thousand! sixty thousand!" His mind was wholly absorbed in this one idea, and at this point the intelligence was arrested and came to a full stop.

[1] This case is related in the "Monthly Mirror," for August, 1799.

CHAPTER XVIII.

MORBID PHENOMENA OF MOTION.

THIS function of the Cerebro-Spinal system may be,

α. *Impaired.*
β. *Lost.*
γ. *Exalted.*
δ. *Perverted.*

Under the head of impairment, I propose to consider all those exceedingly subtle and insidious cases of paralysis which are preceded for a length of time by a deficiency of motor force and an enfeebled state of the muscular power. This condition of motility is often confounded with general physical debility, and attracts no special notice until more obvious cerebral symptoms appear, or the paralytic affection is quite localized.

In the second division of the subject are classified those cases of lesion of motion in which the volition ceases to exercise any influence over the paralyzed limbs, as in well-developed cases of hemiplegia and paraplegia. In states of motor exaltation we have a condition of spasm, tonic and clonic, and in perverted conditions of the motility, we observe as types of the affection, epilepsy, tetanus, convulsions, and chorea.

It is important, in considering paralytic affections either in their incipient or advanced stage, to recognize the threefold division of which the subject is susceptible. These affections of motility may in their origin be,

α. *Cerebral.*
β. *Spinal.*
γ. *Peripheral.*

In other words, paralysis may commence in the *brain, spinal cord,* or in the *peripheral* ramifications of the nerves. It may be a *centric* or an *eccentric* affection. How important it is, when investigating practically this subject, to recognize this *physiological* and *pathological* classification of the lesions of the motor power, with a view to accuracy of diagnosis, and success of treatment.

Dr. Marshall Hall points out with his usual discrimination, the distinction between paralysis of spontaneous and voluntary motion arising from the removal of the influence of the *cerebrum* from parts in communication with it, and the lesions of motility which result from an arrest of the supply of nervous influence from the spinal marrow. In *cerebral* paralysis, there will be always found augmented irritability, and in *spinal* paralysis the irritability is either diminished or altogether lost.

"We may conclude," says this distinguished physiologist, "that in cerebral paralysis, the irritability of the muscular fibre becomes augmented from want of the application of the stimulus of volition; in paralysis arising from disease of the spinal marrow and its nerves this irritability is diminished, and at length becomes extinct from its source being cut off. We may further deduce from the facts which have been detailed, that the spinal marrow, and not the cerebrum, is the special source of the power in the nerves of exciting muscular contraction, and of the irritability of the muscular fibre; that the cerebrum is, on the contrary, the exhauster, through its acts of volition, of the muscular irritability."

GENERAL MUSCULAR DEBILITY.—For some period before any positive *lesion* of motility is perceptible, the patient complains of a *general* failure and loss of muscular power. He is easily tired; is obliged, if engaged in a walk, to frequently sit down, complaining of fatigue. This condition of muscular debility is observed to precede, for some length of time, any *local* or *specific* form of paralysis.

As the affection of the brain, involving a disordered state of the motor *force* advances, the patient's feet slip on one side. He is observed frequently to stumble whilst walking, as if the ligaments of the ankle-joint were weakened or elongated. He cannot put his foot or leg forward without an *obviously conscious effort.* Succeeding this general deficiency of muscular power, there is occasionally noticed a want of *local specific* motor strength in one of the limbs.

"The patient experiences a greater difficulty in executing forced and limited movements, than those in which he merely follows the impulse of his inclinations; he finds it much more laborious to walk slowly, with a measured step in a given direction, than to let his feet take their own course; rising from the chair, or going up stairs, is more difficult than sitting down or descending; the next difficult matter is to turn round in walking."[1]

In the early stage of cerebral disease, complaints are made of a weakness in the arms, hands, legs, or in one side of the body.[2] Objects cannot be grasped, or firmly held steadily or comfortably. There is often in these cases an awkwardness in using one or both hands.

In a case related by Andral, for some months before an attack of paralysis which ended fatally, there was a loss of power in the right *hand*, and to such an extent, that the patient could not hold his pen when in the act of writing.   There was no impairment of sensibility, affection of the motility in the right *arm*, or in any other part of the body.   Andral says, "In cases of incipient paralysis, the patients perceive that one of the extremities has less strength than the other, one of the hands can hold objects less strongly than the other; one of the arms appears insensible to them, or the patients' legs drag a little in walking."   He continues, and the observation is of great practical significance, "this commencement of paralysis *may remain stationary for a long time,* then it is seen progressively to increase, or else it becomes all at once more considerable."[3]

A gentleman who had previously manifested no symptom of decided illness, was observed frequently to drop his stick, as well as his umbrella, in the street.   This was the first loss of motility

---

[1] Romberg. Dr. Sieveking's translation.

[2] Dr. Fuch states a sudden loss of power in the extremities of one side while walking, so that the patient is compelled to sit down or fall, without suffering any loss of consciousness, to be an important and diagnostic symptom of softening of the brain. Among the early symptoms of this disease, is a slight degree of facial paralysis. Occasionally it affects the eyebrow and the mouth. The patient appears to have lost power over one of the eyelids, as if it were too heavy to be completely raised. One eyebrow is more elevated than the other. The mouth is occasionally seen to be drawn on one side. When these symptoms are present, Durand-Fardel says, *we may almost predict with certainty that softening of the brain is threatening or has already commenced.* These apparently slight attacks of paralysis, the same authority observes, are accompanied with an astonished look, or one of stupor, indifference, or idiocy.

[3] Andral's "Clinique."

observed for some weeks prior to an apparently sudden and acute attack of apoplexy, followed by paralysis.

A patient, aged sixty, previously to an attack of cerebral hemorrhage of which he died, exhibited in the incipient stage, indistinctness of speech and loss of recollection. He appeared, at times, to have a weakness of the right arm, being occasionally observed to drop things from the right hand, but did not admit that he felt any muscular weakness. He made no complaint in this stage of headache or giddiness, but admitted that he was weak and in an exhausted condition, and did not feel himself able to bear much fatigue. Eighteen days afterwards he exhibited confusion of thought, and when endeavoring to write a letter, was obliged to relinquish the attempt. He complained that he could not make sense of what he was engaged in writing. "The words as he wrote them appeared," he said, "to run one into the other." The letter when finished was scarcely legible, and the lines were very crooked. He died nine days afterwards of apoplexy.

The loss of motor power in incipient diseases of the brain is occasionally confined to *one* of the fingers, this being the only appreciable symptom calculated to excite alarm. These are curious and inexplicable cases. A partial affection of this kind has been recognized as one of the first threatening symptoms of paralysis and apoplexy. A gentleman, *for some months* before he had an attack of cerebral hemorrhage, complained of loss of motion in the little finger, and called the attention of his physician to the fact. There was no marked headache at the time, but about a week or ten days after this premonitory symptom of paralysis was observed, the patient said his head felt as if it were "a lump of lead." There was also a slight defect in the hearing; but these symptoms were not considered at the time of any consequence.

For two months before an attack of paralysis a patient was unable to swallow with facility or put any liquid into his mouth without slabbering himself, or spilling a portion on the table or on his clothes. This caused much irritation at the time, but it was not considered a symptom of any importance. It was, however, the first appreciable sign, and, in fact, the commencement of a morbid affection of the motor power. Three weeks afterwards the right hand became so weak that the patient could not hold anything steadily in it. Subsequently he was seized, whilst dressing for

dinner, with an attack of paralysis, and continued for a short time
in a state of unconsciousness, out of which he eventually rallied,
but with his mind much enfeebled. A paralysis of the powers of
deglutition is often observed as an incipient symptom of disease of
the brain.

" I have known a person first lose the strength of his legs, then
talk childishly, fiddle with his knife and fork during dinner, to
the confusion of his family, attempt in vain to direct the morsel
to his mouth, and at length carried to bed several hours before he
became apoplectic."[1]

Inability to hold the pen when writing, to draw on the boots
(in consequence of morbid loss of motor power in the muscles of
the arm), to handle the razor steadily when shaving (in consequence of defective muscular strength in the fingers), to play the
piano with the usual vigor and facility, have been observed (in
several cases) to be the first warnings of approaching paralysis.

Dr. Ulric, of Berlin, has detailed an exceedingly interesting
case illustrative of this incipient stage of paralysis. It is also
valuable as pointing out the gradual, insidious, stealthy, and progressive march of cerebral disease, when once established within
the cranium.

In this particular instance, the first symptom of disease of the
brain was observed at *eighteen*, the patient dying at the age of
twenty-six!

The progress of the malady was as follows : " For *six* years a
condition of *muscular sluggishness existed*. This gradually increased. The limbs became heavy, and the motor power began
to fail. At the end of six years, the *sight* became obscured, and
the patient had *diplopia* and *strabismus*. Then followed great
difficulty of walking. The gait subsequently became *vacillating*,
and the feet appeared *glued* at every step to the ground." Important and significant incipient symptom of paralysis ! "The
patient was then attacked with a general numbness and paraplegia. He next was subject to cramps affecting the extensor
muscles of the great toes. A year afterwards he had tetanic
spasms of the muscles of the back, and the paraplegia was converted into paralysis of the upper and lower extremities. The

[1] *On Nervous Diseases*, in 2 vols. ; vol. 1, *On Apoplexy*, &c. ; by John Cooke, M.D.,
1820.

paralysis ultimately became general, deglutition and respiration were impossible, and the patient is said to have died with his intellectual faculties unimpaired!'' The *post-mortem* examination revealed a state of softening of the *pyramidal* and *olivary bodies*, as well as of the left half of the *pons varolii.* The restiform bodies were slightly colored red.

MUSCULAR TREMOR.—In the precursory stage of disease of the brain, a tremulous state of the muscular fibre is occasionally observed. In one remarkable case, for nearly a fortnight previously to the manifestation of any *acute* head symptoms, the patient was observed to have a tremulous state of the hand. He appeared at the time otherwise in good health. This condition of the muscles was succeeded by violent paroxysmal attacks of headache, causing the patient to scream from the intensity of the pain. He subsequently died paralytic. When examined, after death, a malignant tumor was found in the substance of the brain.

A tremulous state of the tongue has been noticed as the forerunner of acute cerebral attacks. A military gentleman, who had for many years honorably served his Queen and country in a tropical climate, returned to England invalided. He had, when in India, suffered from two strokes of the sun. The effect of these attacks, however, rapidly subsided, and he was soon able to do duty in the field. Several months after his arrival home he complained of feeble memory and general want of muscular vigor. The symptoms, however, which caused most alarm, and induced him to obtain my opinion, were, an extreme state of tremor of the tongue whenever he protruded it from his mouth, and an almost unceasing state of agitation when retained within the lips. It required, on the part of the patient, a resolute effort of the will to keep the tongue at all quiescent for many consecutive minutes. These symptoms continued with slight intermissions for nearly three months. One morning, whilst dressing for dinner, he was seized with extreme vertigo, and fell down in a violent epileptic convulsion. He had a succession of epileptic fits, at varying intervals, for a period of twelve months, when his mind became deranged, and in this state of mental alienation he died, about two years subsequently to the first epileptic seizure. In this case, the extreme tremor of the tongue was certainly the first significant symptom of existing, or approaching lesion of the brain. I have observed in the incipient stage of cerebral disease this tremulous state of the tongue in several cases of acute and chronic softening of the brain, as well as in general paralysis.

In some cases the patient complains for some time before decided symptoms of paralysis exhibit themselves, of suffering from a *spasmodic* affection of the muscles of the leg and arm, but particularly of the former. In other instances the legs are stiff, and show a want of suppleness, independently of any loss of sensibility, or actual want of muscular power. These symptoms often precede paralytic attacks, but they are generally associated with other characteristic evidences of cerebral mischief. I have known a patient, for some months before an attack of hemiplegia, complain of acute spasm of muscles of the calf. Occasionally the spasm seizes hold of the whole of the leg, which becomes quite *tetanic*. This symptom is observed in the early stages of acute cerebral *irritation*, connected in some cases, but not always, with organic disease of the nature of inflammatory softening of the brain. A sensation of slight stiffness of the limbs, combined with pain, analogous to that of rheumatism, spasm, and convulsive twitching of the muscles, if accompanied by headache, mental confusion, vertigo, &c., should never escape careful medical observation.

IRREGULAR MUSCULAR ACTION.—In the second stage of disordered motility, the patient exhibits an inequality and unsteadiness in the action of the muscular system. There is an absence of co-ordination in the motility, a want of consentaneousness in the motor movements, "a disturbance," to quote the language of Romberg, "either in the antagonism, or in the symmetrical muscular balance." This condition of the motor power is analogous to that affection, termed by the French pathologists, *Paralysie croisée.*

The patient, in walking, always crosses one leg over the other. For example, he places the right foot invariably before the left, and the latter again before the right; in doing this, the front of the foot is turned inwards, the individual generally stepping upon his toes, and but rarely upon the external margin of the entire sole; the large toe of one foot strikes against the Achilles tendon of the other.

Romberg has described with great accuracy these affections of motility. When alluding to the incipient signs of brain disease, he says: "The gait becomes tottering and insecure, especially when the patient is walking slowly. When he wishes to walk from one place to another, he is obliged to give himself an impulse repeatedly, which renders his mode of progression the more peculiar. When complicated movements, such as climbing or jumping, are attempted, the exertions made to achieve them bear no relation to the result attained. When the patient has fairly commenced to advance, he can accelerate his movements, and even run; when lying in bed, so that the trunk is supported, he has no difficulty in moving his feet. As the disease advances, articulation becomes still more limited, and very indistinct; it is almost necessary to guess the words; the legs are almost deprived of their power to support the body. When the insane person rises from his chair and walks, he rests his hands upon the back of his chair; raises himself up slowly, and, like a child that is measuring its first steps, bends to the right, and bends to the left, then makes an attempt and drags himself slowly along in a zigzag direction. He stumbles over the most trifling impediment, and is constantly tumbling down."[1] These affections of the motility may exist for a long period before symptoms of a more decided and alarming character awaken attention and excite apprehension.

Romberg candidly admits that he is unable to satisfactorily explain these phenomena. The irregular action of the motor power, he observes, occurs in hemiplegic subjects, and especially in cases of cerebral hemorrhage. The patient, when in active locomotion, advances with the healthy foot, which forms the fulcrum of the body, while the paralyzed extremity, with the toes pointed downwards, performs circular or semicircular movements slowly, and with a sort of slide. The other is met with in hydrocephalic patients, before the supervention of complete immobility, and has been accurately described by Gölis.

When engaged in walking, the patient drags one of his legs, as if it were heavier than the one on the opposite side. This symptom occasionally exists to so slight a degree that it may be present for some time and be unnoticed, unless the attention were particularly directed to the state of the muscular system and powers of locomotion.

The patient is often seen to roll himself about like a drunken man, as if he had entirely lost his balancing power. In cases of approaching general paralysis, this symptom is often observed in

---

[1] "A Manual of the Nervous Diseases of Man," by M. H. Romberg, M.D. Translated from the German by E. H. Sieveking, M.D. London, 1853.

a remarkable degree.   The gestures, gait, and walk closely resemble that of a man slightly inebriated.   These irregular actions
of the muscular system are allied to the phenomena observable in
the earlier as well as in the more advanced stage of *Chorea.*

CONVULSIVE ACTION.—I have now to consider those irregular
and morbid states of the motor power or muscular fibre generally
grouped under the head, convulsion.   Among this class of affections, epilepsy, in all its varied types and degrees of manifestation,
occupies a prominent position.

This disease admits of a threefold division, viz. :—

a. Epilepsy.
(With violent muscular movements.)
β. Epilepsy.
(Nocturnal in its character, and accompanied with slight muscular
convulsion.)
γ. Epileptic Vertigo.
(Without muscular convulsions.)

This affection is generally divided by writers into two classes,
viz. : *epileptic vertigo,* without convulsive action, or the *Petit-mal,*
and epilepsy with convulsions, or, the *Grand-mal ;* but there exists
a modified type of epilepsy occurring generally at night with slight,
and often unobserved, convulsive muscular action (termed by the
late Dr. Marshall Hall " Hidden Seizures,") which is distinct (not
in its *nature,* but in its form of *manifestation*) from the true epileptic convulsive paroxysm.

The important phase of epilepsy, designated " epileptic vertigo,"
or "epileptiform seizures," will be fully considered in the succeeding chapter on the " Morbid Phenomena of Sensation."

The attacks of epilepsy that occur at night, are generally accompanied by little or no marked disturbance or irregular action of the
muscular system.   Occasionally the convulsive movement, when it
takes place, is analogous to an attack of simple *spasm,* and in
many cases the epileptic fit closely resembles an apparently unimportant " twitching" of the muscular fibres generally observed to
occur during sleep.   How many cases of insidious epilepsy I have
detected, particularly among children, by these symptoms !

This obscure type of what Dr. Trousseau terms, "nocturnal
epilepsy," may exist for months, and in some cases for years,

25

without attracting observation, until the bodily health has been seriously undermined, and the mental powers fatally and irremediably impaired.

Patients suffering from these hidden, and for a time unobserved, attacks, complain of great muscular, vital, and nervous debility, disturbed and unrefreshing sleep, depression of spirits, and headache, particularly on first waking in the morning.

If the epileptic seizures that occur at night are undetected, and allowed to proceed without any remedial treatment being adopted to arrest their fatal progress, the physical health generally becomes seriously impaired, and the mind soon sinks into a condition of senile imbecility. The incipient psychical manifestations are, mental lassitude, weakened powers of attention, impaired memory, enfeebled volition, and marked indifference to all the important concerns and business of life.[1]

[1] I have referred, in the previous pages, to the acute affections of the memory accompanying various types of epilepsy. Dr. Russell Reynolds, when speaking of the impairment of this faculty generally associated with what he terms " Interparoxysmal (Epileptic) Phenomena," observes : " By far the commonest and earliest change is *loss of memory*. At first it is noticed only with regard to the trivial matters of the day, whilst those long since passed are readily recalled. Subsequently, the patient forgets the earlier elements of his knowledge, and his mind then becomes an utter blank. The progress of deterioration resembles, in many respects, that which is natural to the decay of human life ; often, as it were, anticipating the work of time, and hurrying a just opening life into a premature old age, with all its feebleness, and more than all its gloom. Failure of memory (except when occurring only as the immediate sequel of severe attacks) is commonly attended with diminished power of apprehension ; and this is at first most marked with regard to new ideas, but subsequently appears to affect the mind in relation to previous knowledge, diminishing the power of applying past experience to the new circumstances of daily life. The patient cannot, or frequently does not, concentrate his thoughts upon any subject. Ideas follow one another, it may be in very rapid succession, as they are accidentally suggested by one another, or by surrounding events. When this power is only slightly deteriorated, the mind may be recalled by a strong effort, or a powerful impression ; but when the intellectual disease has advanced further, this becomes impossible, and incoherence of expression indicates but too plainly the incoherence of thought, which may pass still further into utter fatuity.

" These earlier mental changes resolve themselves mainly into defective volition. The first failure of memory is due to want of attention rather than to anything else. The individual does not sufficiently attend to what is going on for deep impressions to be made, and consequently there is no power which can recollect them. Attention appears to be simply the direction of consciousness by an effort of volition ; and in this first failure there is the first indication of diminished will. Probably the loss of apprehension has its origin in the same cause ; it is the consequence of neglected or not properly exercised attention. By simple disuse, the power becomes diminished.

This mischievous form of epilepsy, Trousseau thinks, may continue for eight or ten years without any one, not even the patient himself, being aware of its existence. "There are," he says, "two principal diagnostic signs in such a case, viz., the *biting of the tongue*, and the *involuntary emission of urine*, especially in women. If the person who comes to consult you complains of waking with headache, if the lateral parts of the tongue are lacerated, and if you can ascertain that urine has been passed unconsciously, do not hesitate to declare that there has been a nocturnal attack of epilepsy. Moreover, in a very great number of cases, you may observe on the forehead, and especially below the eyes, myriads of petechiæ, the size of a pin's head, which are never produced under other circumstances. In possession of these details, the diagnosis of this form of the disease becomes certain, while without their aid it is almost always impossible."[1]

The premonitory symptoms of ordinary attacks of epilepsy vary according to the proximate cause of the disease as well as constitutional temperament. Many patients have clear intimations of the approaching convulsive attack. These warnings I have known to occur for several days prior to the accession of a paroxysm. Some patients have disturbed dreams for many nights previously to the attack; others are subject to spectral illusions; occasionally patients complain of singular and perplexing trains of thought a

---

The same thing is to be observed with regard to thought. The associations, which in mental health form the basis of correct judgment and logical appreciation, from having their ground in the truest relations which we can discover between separate ideas, are lost altogether, or are replaced by associations of a merely accidental or inessential character; and thought becomes incoherent, or 'wandering,' from the deficiency of voluntary power exercised in its direction and control. Thus, with deficient volition, and with increased readiness of emotional disturbance, the epileptic is reduced to a mere machine, played upon by every external impression, or suggested feeling, and without any power to appreciate, account for, or control his state."—*Lancet*, Aug. 4 and 11, 1855.

[1] A young man aged twenty-two years, condemned to five years' imprisonment by a court of assizes for having struck, without provocation, one of his best friends a blow which nearly killed him, was subject to attacks of epilepsy during sleep. I have been able to verify this fact in the prison where this unhappy man was confined, who was descended from a family among whom might be counted epileptics, insane persons, and individuals who had died of cerebral hemorrhage. He had no clear recollection of the criminal offence for which he was incriminated, neither did he show the least regret for it. This apparent insensibility, the consequence of his disease, did not contribute a little to his condemnation.—"*A Treatise on Mental Diseases*," by Dr. B. A. Morel. Paris, 1860, p. 695.

few hours before the fit. I have known epilepsy to be preceded by remarkable affections of the motor power, lesions of sensibility, peculiar sounds within the head, resembling the tinkling of bells, roar of the sea, bleating of sheep, and in one case the patient said that for two days previously to his usual epileptic paroxysm, he heard distinctly sounds like those proceeding from a number of persons quarrelling.

In one case, the mental faculties, particularly the memory, exhibited great and unnatural exaltation a few hours anteriorly to the fit. The patient's sense of hearing and seeing also became painfully acute. A child who is subject to epilepsy becomes extremely agitated in body and excited in mind for several hours before the paroxysm. He rushes about the house in a state of great terror and alarm, and if an attempt be made to control his movements, he strikes and struggles with those who interfere with him. In some cases, the incipient stage is characterized by great depression of spirits. This often occurs in the hysterical types of epilepsy. A patient whom I saw, always barked like a dog a few hours before the attack. In another case the fit was preceded by intense irritability, occasionally amounting to violent passion. A young lady subject to epilepsy, is always able to indicate the approach of the convulsion by the appearance of a bright halo surrounding every object she gazes at. A youth, who has for five years been afflicted with the disease, informs me that for an hour prior to the epileptic seizure he hears a sound in his head resembling the ticking of a watch. A patient, for a few hours before his epileptic attack, affirmed that he distinctly heard the voice of a deceased relative speaking to him in terms of affection. This symptom invariably precedes the convulsive fit. A young boy subject to acute and violent epilepsy is always conscious of the approach of his attacks by a curious perversion of the sense of smell. Everything that he comes in contact with has a putrid odor, similar, as he describes it, to "a dead body in an advanced state of putrefaction." In another case, the sense of touch is painfully acute, arising from an exalted condition of the functions of sensibility preceding the epileptic seizure.

" On the eve of a fit," says Dr. Radcliffe, " confirmed epileptics are noticed to sit or move about in a moping and listless manner; to complain of chills and shiverings, or of faintness and sickness. The respiration is interrupted by frequent sighs; the pulse is weak, irregular, and slow. Occasionally, there are headache, dazzling of the eyes, singing in the ears, and other excitements of sensation; slight flushing of the face, dilatation of the pupils, and extreme irritability of temper. In some rare instances, there is, immediately before, or at the commencement of the attack, a phenomenon of a more specific nature."

Foville, when speaking of the premonitory signs of epilepsy, remarks, that "a peculiar sensation, it may be of cold, pain, heat, or itching, is developed suddenly in a toe, a finger, a limb, in the belly or the back, and from the point whence it originates, mounts gradually to the head. When it arrives there, the patient immediately falls (as if struck), and the convulsions break forth at once. This sensation has received, from the earliest times, the name of *aura epileptica*. It is rare, so much so, that by many its existence is doubted or ignored, and by others explained in a different manner." Dr. Herpin considers this aura as nothing more than the commencement of a tonic spasm of the muscles of the limb.

Dr. Radcliffe asserts that premonitory symptoms are constantly to be observed in this disease. Professor Romberg notices them in about one-half of his patients. M. Herpin states the proportion to be about one-fourth. M. Georget affirms that not more than four or five per cent. of those attacked with an epileptic seizure have any premonition; M. Beau gives the proportion of seventeen per cent. M. Foville, Esquirol, and Dr. Cheyne give no numerical ratio, but state that in much the greater number of cases of epilepsy there are no precursory symptoms.

"A young epileptic at the moment of invasion of his fit perceived, exclusively with the left eye, a toothed wheel, the centre of which was occupied by a hideous figure. In some cases of epilepsy there may be a special premonition. In one of my patients, the fit is invariably preceded by an intense feeling of hunger. In another patient, since insane, a little blue imp perched upon the table, and moped and mocked at him as he lost his consciousness. In a third, a guitar seemed to have been roughly grated near the ear."[1]

"Remarkable intellectual activity has sometimes signalized," says Morel, "the commencement of epilepsy among the young.

[1] Dr. Radcliffe on "Epilepsy, and other Convulsive Affections," 1858, p. 144.

A wonderful aptitude to conceive things quickly, to examine them under their most brilliant and poetical aspects, has been exhibited by many of them. History has transmitted to us the names of several men of great genius who have been epileptics; but, as the late Dr. G. M. Burrows remarks, these individuals have been the victims of the most tyrannical passions. The full and entire preservation of the faculties of epileptics, the possibility of applying them in a continuous manner to the execution of designs remarkable for their grandeur and continuity, are facts excessively rare." "There are, however," says M. Sandras, "some exceptions to this rule, such as Cæsar, Mahomet, Petrarch, &c."

"The first changes," continues the same authority, "that are remarked in the character of epileptics threatened with insanity is, a very great irritability, which takes place without, and even at the least, contradiction, under the most varied, and sometimes most compromising forms. In the first period of their affection, it is natural to see that the diseased preoccupations of epileptics have a *point d'appui* in the elements which constitute the great diversity of temperament and character. Hypochondriasis and hysteria have an undeniable action in the delirium which begins to systematize itself in the mind of the patients. Preoccupations on the subject of their health, unjust complaints, recriminations without foundation, decided venereal tendencies, are facts which awaken the just solicitude of families."[1]

Dr. Sieveking, in his able treatise on epilepsy, has described at considerable length, and with great accuracy, the premonitory symptoms of the disease. He says: "Of fifty-eight cases of epilepsy which have been under my own care, and of which I have preserved careful notes, thirty showed some indication of the approaching paroxysm. It must not, however, be concluded that because a patient at one time is made aware of the event about to take place that therefore it will always be so. This Protean disease varies in this as in many other features; still it is most commonly the case that a patient habitually experiences a premonitory symptom, or that he is uniformly seized without any indication whatever.

"The sensations which the patients describe as preceding the fit are extremely various. But even after hearing the details of a

---

[1] "*A Treatise on Mental Diseases*," by Dr. B. A. Morel. Paris, 1860, p. 695.

small number, it cannot fail to suggest itself that they may, without an effort, be ranged in two classes: those that are referred to the trunk and extremities, and those that appear at once to affect the head; in the former case the sensation is always described as mounting towards the head, and in the majority of cases the paroxysm appears to strike down the patient on its reaching that part: in the latter the sensation commonly takes the form of some strange illusion, which, however, the patient is able to recognize as such.

"Tissot, whose works may yet be consulted as models of close observation and clear reasoning, quotes from Peiroux the case of a young man who, when his fits came on, thought he saw a carriage drive up at a gallop and with great noise, containing a little man in a red bonnet; fearing to be *écrasé* by the carriage, he fell down stiff and without consciousness. In Tissot's work we find that even in sleep, during which epilepsy frequently supervenes, peculiar dreams may indicate the approaching paroxysm. He gives the case of a man who dreamt that he was pursued by a bull, and soon after waking was seized with a fit.

" These are, however, rather the curiosities of epilepsy, the sensations of the patient not generally acting upon the sensorium in such a way as to produce illusions of the fantastic kind just described. With this exception, we may say that there is scarcely an impression referrible to the nerves of common or muscular sense, or of the special senses, which does not occasionally indicate the approach of an epileptic fit. The premonitory symptom is generally accompanied by a sense of fear and terror. One of my patients described the sensation, which in him passed from the stomach to the head, as of a pleasing character. Children particularly show the alarm they experience by running to and clinging to their nurses or mothers. The aura may be an undefined sense of indisposition or discomfort; it may be a definite pain, giddiness, or suffocating feeling; or it assumes the more classical form described as an aura, which is characterized by the passage of a peculiar sensation from some part of the body to the throat or head. In the case of the last we would specially observe that authors commonly state that when the aura or sensation reaches the head, the insensibility ensues; it has rather appeared to us that the patients refer the termination to the throat. With some patients the premonitory symptoms assume a more tangible form, and one that makes itself perceptible to bystanders.

"Dr. Cooke relates a case in which the approach of a paroxysm was indicated by a peculiar blue color of the lips. 'Frank,' as related by Dr. Copland, 'saw the paroxysm preceded by an eruption over the whole body except the face, of the vitiligo alba.' The same author states 'that in twenty-one epileptics treated in the clinical wards of the hospital at Wilna, vomiting announced the paroxysm in seven.' Symptoms that may be termed objective have presented themselves to me in the form of tremors, cough, sickness, rigors, and a shaking of one hand.

"Schenck relates a case of epilepsy which came under his own observation, in which the patient, before the seizure, was repeatedly turned round in a circle, and then fell to the ground in an ordinary paroxysm, 'magna astantium commiseratione.' Peiroux (quoted by Tissot) mentions a man who, before becoming unconscious, was compelled to run backwards ten steps; the unconsciousness was very brief, and he at once rose up again as if nothing had occurred. In Schenck we also find the account of a man, aged thirty, of whom it is said in rather quaint Latin, "Solebat, quum duos vel tres passus progressus esset, sese inflectere quasi in circulum, idque continenter facere compulsus erat." This patient subsequently became epileptic, and the peculiar movements then ceased. Such cases as those related by Schenck and Peiroux have received the name of "epilepsia cursiva," under which term Dr. Andree[1] details two well-marked instances, which were both cured by venesection, antiphlogistic remedies, and antispasmodics. They are instructive and well told, so as to justify our inserting one of them briefly here: "Rebecca Cole, ætatis 16, before her seizures first perceives a weight in her head, which makes her hang it down; then a tremor all over ensues, and a sense of faintness; she then runs till she meets with some resistance, then falls down, struggles at first, after which she lies still, and gradually recovers. The fit being over, she trembles, is faint, sick at stomach, and dizzy; and now, by frequent returns of them, is almost become stupid."[2]

AFFECTIONS OF THE TONGUE, AND MUSCLES OF THE MOUTH.—In the premonitory stage of paralysis, the tongue often gives evi-

---

[1] "Cases of Epilepsy, Hysteric Fits, and St. Vitus's Dance," by John Andree, M.D. London, 1746.

[2] "On Epilepsy and Epileptiform Seizures," by E. H. Sieveking, M.D. 1858.

dence of a deficiency of muscular strength. The patient is observed to have lost, to a degree, the power of protruding it rapidly and freely from the mouth, and, occasionally, he cannot do so at all. I have frequently noticed this symptom in connection with other signs of flagging motility, as precursory of severe attacks of cerebral disease, particularly of softening. Occasionally the tongue is observed to be tremulous, and turned *slightly* on one side. How often this symptom has been observed as the *avant courier* of fatal attacks of apoplexy, softening, and paralysis!

In the early stage of general paralysis, the tongue occasionally presents an hypertrophied appearance. It looks large and flabby. I have often noticed this symptom associated with softening, and other organic lesions of the brain, but it is more particularly characteristic of cerebral paralysis.

How apparently slight and insignificant are occasionally the most important of the early signs of organic disease of the brain! An inability to forcibly eject saliva from the mouth, in consequence of a slight paralysis of the *orbicularis oris* and *buccinator* muscles preceding more marked and decided symptoms of cerebral disorder, has been known to indicate serious alterations in the structure of the brain!

Dr. Watson details at length a deeply interesting case of paralysis connected with cancer of the brain, in which the following were the incipient symptoms: "The patient found, when he came down stairs on the morning after he was taken ill, *that he could not spit as usual*, and his friends observed an unusual state of his features. He had no fit, nor loss of consciousness, but he thought his memory was failing. At the time when the paralysis was first noticed, he had some numbness and tingling in the right arm, extending to the last two fingers. He was deaf in the right ear.[1]

A celebrated player on the flute, who died of softening of the brain, exhibited, fifteen months prior to the manifestation of more alarming signs of cerebral disease, an inability to use the instrument with his accustomed facility, owing (as was supposed) to incipent paralysis of the muscles of the mouth and cheek.[2]

---

[1] "Practice of Physic," by Thomas Watson, M.D. 1857.

[2] Softening of the cerebral hemispheres, according to Andral, induces alteration in *motion* much more constantly than in *intelligence*. However, even this rule is not, he says, without its exceptions. He cites some cases in which there was not observed, in reference to *motility*, any appreciable modification. In four instances of this kind

HANDWRITING.—A remarkable peculiarity in, and singular variation from, the ordinary character of the handwriting, have been observed as the first signs of approaching general paralysis, softening of the brain, and apoplexy. The patient has not been able to write in a straight line or to form his letters correctly. Occasionally he singularly misplaces his words, and appears to have lost all power of correct spelling. When writing, the patient substitutes one word for another; his letters are flighty, full of eccentricities, blunders, and erasures! How often have these symptoms been observed for months before a suspicion has existed as to the healthy state of the brain.

A gentleman connected with the mercantile world (who died of softening of the brain, at the age of fifty-four) for *two* years before his state of cerebral ill-health attracted attention, exhibited in his correspondence and accounts remarkable peculiarities and eccentricities. In looking back at his books and letters, after he was

---

which Andral has recorded, the softening occupied the most different seats. In one case it was limited to a portion of the convexity; another time it occupied at the base of the anterior lobe of one of the hemispheres a space large enough to contain a pullet's egg. In two other cases it occupied several points of the two hemispheres. Several cases, however, are on record in which softening of the brain existed without any disturbance of motion having been observed.[a] "When this does happen," says Andral, "it is probable that the softening takes place very slowly. Such cases remind us of those in which the brain, subjected to a gradual compression by tumors developed around it or in its substance, does not announce its suffering by any paralysis or other disturbance in locomotion.

"When motion is affected (and this case may be regarded as nearly constant), it is very far from being always affected in the same way. It has been laid down much too generally, that softening of the brain produced, in the greater number of cases, a flexion (contracture) of the limbs. Observation has satisfied us that this flexion may be as often absent as it is present; but it is very true that when it does occur, it becomes an excellent sign to distinguish a softening of the brain from any other affection of this organ. Let us not, however, regard such a sign as pathognomonic; for it has been found in other cases where there was no softening. It has been often noticed, for instance, in the cases of congenital atrophy of the brain published by MM. Bouchet and Casauvielh.[b] The modifications which motion undergoes in cases of softening of the brain, are far from being always of the same nature. These modifications most usually consist either in simple paralysis, flexion of the limbs, or in convulsions. There are other cases then, in which motion is modified in quite a different way."[c]

---

[a] "Répertoire d'Anatomie et de Physiologie Pathologique," par Breschet. Tom. i, p. 116. Also, "Journal Hebdomadaire," tom. iv, p. 270.
[b] "Archives Générales de Médecine," tom. ix.
[c] "Clinique Médicale," by M. Andral.

obliged to retire from all active business, this patient's written communications with various persons presented the most conclusive proof of the *long existence of undetected premonitory symptoms of cerebral softening.* The letters in question were full of erasures, and the words were misspelt and wrongly used. The lines were written crookedly, and his calculations were remarkable for their inaccuracy. Occasionally his letters were singularly well and correctly written, without evidencing a blunder, but, after the interval of a week, he again lapsed into a careless, inaccurate, and, I may say, *morbid* style of penmanship.

PARALYSIS AGITANS.—Any analysis of the incipient morbid phenomena of the *motor* power would be incomplete which did not embody a description of the premonitory symptoms of that singular disorder of the nervo-muscular system, termed paralysis agitans.

Mr. Parkinson has entered more fully than any other writer into a history of the precursory stage of this disease, and to his treatise I am indebted for the subjoined accurate and graphic *resumé.*

"So slight and nearly imperceptible are the first inroads of this malady, and so extremely slow is its progress, that it rarely happens that the patient can form any recollection of the precise period of its commencement. The first symptoms perceived are a slight sense of weakness, with proneness to trembling in some particular part; sometimes in the head, but most commonly in one of the hands and arms. These symptoms gradually increase in the part first affected; and at the end of an uncertain period, but seldom in less than twelve months or more, the morbid influence is felt in some other part. Thus, assuming one of the hands and arms to be the first attacked, the other at this period becomes similarly affected. After a few more months, the patient is found to be less strict than usual in preserving an upright posture: this being most observable whilst walking, but sometimes whilst sitting or standing. Sometimes, after the appearance of this symptom, and during its slow increase, one of the legs is discovered slightly to tremble, and is also found to suffer fatigue sooner than the leg of the other side: and, in a few months, this limb becomes agitated by similar tremblings, and suffers a similar loss of power.

"Hitherto, the patient will have experienced but little inconvenience; and, befriended by the strong influence of habitual endurance, would, perhaps, seldom think of his being the subject of disease, except when reminded of it by the unsteadiness of his hand, whilst writing or employing himself in any nicer kind of manipulation.   But as the disease proceeds, similar employments are accomplished with considerable difficulty, the hand failing to answer with exactness to the dictates of the will.   Walking becomes a task which cannot be performed without considerable attention. The legs are not raised to that height, or with that promptitude which the will directs, so that the utmost care is necessary to prevent frequent falls.

"At this period, the patient experiences much inconvenience, which unhappily is found daily to increase.   The submission of the limbs to the directions of the will can hardly ever be obtained in the performance of the most ordinary offices of life.   The fingers cannot be disposed of in the proposed directions, and applied with certainty to any proposed point.   As time and the disease proceed, difficulties increase : writing can now be hardly at all accomplished ; and reading, from the tremulous motion, is accomplished with some difficulty.   Whilst at meals, the fork, not being duly directed, frequently fails to raise the morsel from the plate ; which, when seized, is with much difficulty conveyed to the mouth.   At this stage, the patient seldom experiences a suspension of the agitation of his limbs.   Commencing, for instance, in one arm, the wearisome agitation is borne until beyond sufferance, when, by suddenly changing the posture, it is for a time stopped in that limb, to commence, generally in less than a minute, in one of the legs, or in the arm of the other side.   Harassed by this tormenting round, the patient has recourse to walking, a mode of exercise to which the sufferers from this malady are in general partial, owing to their attention being thereby somewhat diverted from their unpleasant feeling, by the care and exertion required to insure its safe performance.

"But, as the malady proceeds, even this temporary mitigation of suffering from the agitation of the limbs is denied.   The propensity to lean forward becomes invincible, and the patient is thereby forced to step on the toes and fore part of the feet, whilst the upper part of the body is thrown so far forward as to render it difficult to avoid falling on the face.   In some cases, when this state of the malady is attained, the patient can no longer exercise himself by walking in his usual manner, but is thrown on the toes and fore part of the feet; being, at the same time, irresistibly impelled to take much quicker and shorter steps, and thereby to adopt unwillingly a running pace. In some cases it is found necessary entirely to substitute running for walking; since otherwise the patient, on proceeding only a very few paces, would inevitably fall.

"The sleep now becomes much disturbed. The tremulous motions of the limbs occur during sleep, and augment until they awaken the patient, and frequently with much agitation and alarm. The power of conveying food to the mouth is at length so much impeded that he is obliged to consent to be fed by others. The bowels, which had been all along torpid, now in most cases demand stimulating medicines of very considerable power : the expulsion of matter from the rectum sometimes requiring mechanical aid. As the disease proceeds towards its last stage, the trunk is almost permanently bowed, the muscular power is more decidedly diminished, and tremulous agitation becomes violent.

"The patient walks now with great difficulty, and unable any longer to support himself with his stick, he dares not venture on this exercise unless assisted by an attendant, who, walking backwards before him, prevents him falling forwards by the pressure of his hands against the fore part of his shoulders. His words are now scarcely intelligible, and he is not only no longer able to feed himself, but when the food is conveyed to the mouth, so much are the actions of the muscles of the tongue, pharynx, &c., impeded by impaired action and perpetual agitation, that the food is with difficulty retained in the mouth until masticated, and then as difficultly swallowed. Now also, from the same cause, another very unpleasant circumstance occurs : the saliva fails of being directed to the back part of the fauces, and hence is continually draining from the mouth, mixed with the particles of food which he is no longer able to clear from the inside of the mouth.

"As the debility increases, and the influence of the will over the muscles fades away, the tremulous agitation becomes more vehement. It now suddenly leaves him for a moment; but even when exhausted nature seizes a small portion of sleep, the motion becomes so violent as not only to shake the bed-hangings, but even the floor and sashes of the room.

"The chin is now almost immovably bent down upon the sternum.

The fluids with which he is attempted to be fed, with the saliva, are continually trickling from the mouth.

" The power of. articulation is lost.   The evacuations are passed involuntarily ; and at the last constant sleepiness, with slight delirium, and other marks of extreme exhaustion, announce the fatal result."

AFFECTIONS OF THE SPINAL CORD.—As a general rule, the motor power is affected in all cases of softening of the spinal marrow, but there are exceptional cases on record.

Dr. Janson, of Lyons, has published the particulars of a case in which the spinal marrow was for the most part in a state of *bouillie*, yet the patient had no impediment in the power of motion.   M. Velpeau cites a case in which the cervical portion of the spinal cord was morbidly softened without impairing the motor power.   In animals the spinal cord has been damaged without interfering with the movements.   Andral, when addressing himself to this subject, observes : " Do all not know that the fœtus, during uterine life, has free power of motion, although its spinal cord at that period is far from having that consistence which it acquires subsequently."   M. Rullier relates a case where there was considerable softening of the spinal cord, but communication was maintained between the upper and lower portions of the cord, merely by a slight though firm slip ; there was no relation between the part of the cord affected and the parts of the body capable of being moved ; the patient could walk, but his arms were paralysed and contracted.

There is a form of acute softening of the spinal marrow which developes itself very suddenly, progresses with great rapidity, and speedily terminates in death.   These cases of acute ramollissement of the spinal cord resemble, in many of their features, those of cerebral hemorrhage.   The patient in the first instance appears to have an attack of lumbago ; this is succeeded by great muscular debility in the spinal column, as well as in the lower extremities. Coma then speedily supervenes, the limbs become forcibly contracted, and the patient dies in a state of tetanic spasm.   In many cases, however, even in acute softening of the spinal cord, the mind often continues unclouded until the moment of death.

PERIPHERAL PARALYSIS.—I have not yet spoken of those lesions of the motor and sensorial power which commence in the peripheral extremities of the nerves, and which are occasionally seen to progress upwards from the lower limbs, and ultimately involve the great nervous ganglia, and eventually the brain itself.

I have seen several remarkable cases of this kind. The early symptoms of this affection are occasionally altogether overlooked, in consequence of their great obscurity. A patient complains of a general failure in the muscular tone of his feet and legs. He (if accustomed to active walking) is conscious of his inability to take his usual amount of exercise. He notices for some time no other alteration in the motor power. The loss of muscular strength is confined to the foot and leg. This state of local partial paralysis may exist for years before the patient has any apprehension of danger, or feels under the necessity of obtaining medical advice. In one remarkable case that came under my notice, I was informed that this failure of muscular power had been progressing gradually for *six* years. It was first observed in the foot, it then extended to the legs and arms, and it was not until the expiration of *seven* years that the brain became involved ! Occasionally the paralysis is confined to the legs, and appears to be *arrested* there, in the course of its progress upwards towards the brain.

CHAPTER XIX.

MORBID PHENOMENA OF SPEECH.

THIS division of the subject will be considered in the following order :—

1. *Cerebral Localization of Speech.*
2. *Irregular Action of Articulation.*
8. *Impairment and Loss of Speech.*
4. *Morbid Imitative Movements of Articulation.* *Involuntary Articulation.*

Various attempts have been made to localize the organs of speech, and to ascertain by carefully executed *post-mortem* examinations, as well as by accurately observed physiological experiments made upon animals during life, the precise portion of the brain influencing and regulating this faculty.

The following distinguished physiologists, Gall, Serres, Pinel, Grandchamp, Belhomme, and Bouillard, maintain that the *anterior* lobes of the brain preside over the organ of speech, and a number of cases of total and partial loss of this function have been cited, in which this portion of the encephalon has been discovered, after death, in a state of organic disease.

In 1845, at l'Académie Royale de Médecine, M. Belhomme read a memoir " On the Localization of Speech in the anterior lobes of the Brain," in which, by a reference to ten cases which he narrates, he endeavored to prove that the cerebral organ which regulates speech was seated in the anterior lobes of the brain. M. Belhomme arrived at the following conclusions :—

1. " Affection of the faculty of speech depends either on a cerebral affection, or on a lesion of the organs of communication between the brain and the organs of speech.

2. "The sudden loss of speech depends on a hemorrhagic or other lesion of one, or more frequently of both, anterior lobes of the brain.

3. "It is necessary to guard against confounding convulsive and paralytic disorders which affect the power of speech, with that sudden loss of memory of words, and consequently difficulty of speech, depending on affection of the anterior lobes of the brain.

4. "In disorder or partial destruction of the anterior lobes of the brain, the speech is suddenly arrested, and it is only after a cicatrix has formed in the brain, that the organ recovers more or less of its former function."

Out of thirty-seven cases carefully observed and analyzed by Andral, as well as by other pathologists, relative to hemorrhage and other cerebral lesions, in which the morbid affection resided in one of the anterior lobes, or in both, speech was abolished *twenty-one*, and retained *sixteen* times.

On the other hand, the particulars of fourteen cases were collected by Andral, where the speech was abolished without any alteration in the anterior lobes. Of these fourteen cases *seven* were connected with diseases of the middle, and *seven* with diseases of the posterior lobes.

The loss of speech is not then, as Andral concludes, the *necessary* result of the lesion of the anterior lobes. It may take place in cases where examination does not reveal any alteration at all in the structure of these lobes.[1] M. Lallemand has cited a case in which no other change was detected than softening of the white substance of the left lobe of the cerebellum. In this case the faculty of speech was completely lost.[2]

In M. Olivier's work on the spinal cord,[3] he records the particulars of a patient, in whom occurred the phenomenon of loss of speech, at first partial, and then complete. In this case there was organic disease of the *pons varolii*, but no affection of the anterior lobes. The former part of the brain was found softened at its lower surface to an extent equal, at least, to the size of a filbert.

Cruveilhier cites some remarkable cases of extensive disorganization of the anterior lobes of the brain, the functions of speech

---

[1] Andral's " *Clinique Médicale*," p. 119.   [3] Letter ii, p. 134.
[2] Tom. ii, p. 614.

remaining intact.   Other modern pathologists have placed upon
record similar illustrations.   I have, in fifty-four cases, detected,
after death, a considerable amount of organic disease of the anterior cerebral lobes, without being accompanied during life with any
perceptible loss of speech.   In one case of softening of the cerebellum, the principal symptom was great perversion of the faculty
of speech without complete loss of power over this function.   The
anterior lobes were free from all organic alteration.   In another
case, a large encysted abscess was discovered at the base of the
brain, which produced, during life, the most singularly remarkable
modification in the faculty of speech.   The patient's misplacement
of words was at times most eccentric and grotesque.   He occasionally, however, appeared to have lost all power of articulation.
In a third case a tumor of a malignant character was found in the
cerebellum, which produced a complete loss of speech.

Undoubtedly cases occur of loss of, or serious alterations in, the
faculty of speech, clearly associated with structural changes in
the anterior lobes of the brain; but to prove anything like a physiological and pathological relationship between the phenomena, it
will be necessary to establish a greater uniformity of cause and
effect than the researches of morbid anatomists at present appear
to justify.

I recollect one remarkable instance of general paralysis associated with considerable imbecility of mind, which (like many other
cases of this disease) was accompanied, in the incipient stage, by
considerable loss of power of speech and defective articulation, in
which, after death, the only morbid lesion of the brain detected
was a piece of circumscribed softened brain of the *size of a shilling*
on one of the anterior lobes.   The most careful examination of the
brain was made without discovering any other organic change!
In another case of softening of the cerebellum, the speech was remarkably impaired for some time previously to death without any
perceptible lesion of the anterior lobes of the brain.

A gentleman had an attack of apoplexy, consequent upon extravasation, the effect of a rupture of one of the cerebral vessels.   He
rallied.   He had a second attack, and again recovered.   At the
expiration of eighteen months he experienced a third attack, and
this eventually proved fatal.   He became hemiplegic, and entirely
lost his speech.   He continued in this state for two months, never
uttering a vocal sound!   After death, a small patch of softened

brain was found in the *pons varolii*, surrounding a clot which had been deposited on that ganglion. The other portions of the cerebral mass were apparently in a healthy condition, with the exception of some of the vessels being closed by depositions of bony matter.

In a work recently published, an attempt is made to establish a close physiological and pathological connection between the functions of articulation and speech and the *corpora olivaria*. Professor Schrœder Van der Kolk was led to this conclusion in consequence of the anatomical connection existing between the two previously-mentioned cerebral ganglia and the nuclei of the hypoglossus.[1] "Speech," he observes, "and the articulation of words require such a multitude of peculiar motions of the tongue, and such an infinite number of varying combinations of its muscular movements, that two auxiliary ganglia should be required for the performance of these functions." Professor Van der Kolk cites numerous cases in illustration of his hypothesis. His friend, Dr. Röell, allowed him to examine the *medulla oblongata* of a woman, aged fifty, who had been for twenty-five years insane and completely demented, and could only indistinctly utter the single word "snuif" (snuff). There was paralysis of the right side of the face. In the medulla there was very decided fatty degeneration; the right *corpus olivare* was more slender and somewhat smaller than the left, although both were slender and atrophied. In the *corpora pyramidalia* were numerous wide vessels of 0·276 mm. in the raphe = 0·305. There was no vascular dilatation in the other parts.

Dr. Martini, physician to, and director of, the Leubus Institution for the Insane in Silesia, met with a case of total loss of speech connected with induration of the *corpora olivaria*. Olivier relates a remarkable case of paralysis and dementia of long standing, where eventually the voice was all but wholly lost. The patient could scarcely utter a few articulate sounds. After death, the *corpora olivaria* and *pyramidalia* were found softened and changed into a gray semi-fluid pulpy state. Cruveilhier relates the following case :—

[1] "On the Minute Structure and Functions of the Spinal Cord and Medulla Oblongata, and on the Proximate Cause and Rational Treatment of Epilepsy," by Professor Schrœder Van der Kolk. Translated by W. D. Moore, A.B., M.B., 1859. (New Sydenham Society.)

A child, of four years, had fallen into a state of such general weakness that he could not stand, and had to be carried or laid on a bed; he could, however, move all his limbs, but could not guide his movements with precision, nor could he exercise any force. Deglutition was very difficult, especially of fluids, only a small quantity of which reached his stomach, while the rest was rejected by the mouth, and sometimes through the nose. The articulation of sounds was exceedingly slow; the voice was low and stammering; the little patient still articulated distinctly, but only syllable by syllable; the respiration was slow, often oppressed and sighing, and in a recumbent position was impossible, even when the head was supported by several pillows. The intellectual powers of the child were developed very much beyond his time of life; nutrition was perfectly well performed, the patient being even stout and fat. The illness was the result of convulsions, with which the child had been attacked three years previously, and which had since returned repeatedly at irregular intervals, causing him to be considered epileptic. Five or six months later, he died asphyxiated, although in the full possession of his intellect, but no longer able to utter a sound.

On examining the body, Cruveilhier found the *corpora olivaria* as hard as cartilage; in other respects they exhibited no change, nor was there any abnormity of color or extent; one of the *crura cerebelli* (the author had forgotten which) and the *tubercula mammillaria* participated in the induration; the entire of the remaining cerebral mass was sound. He was able to examine only so much of the *medulla oblongata* as could be taken out by the *foramen magnum;* the *medulla* was perfectly healthy below, and at the sides of the *corpora olivaria*.[1]

' Dr. Maudt, officer of health in the Dutch Indies, relates the case of a native gunner under treatment in the hospital, who was bitten by a serpent called by the natives Oeloer. Severe vertigo immediately ensued, followed by syncope, and in about ten minutes he lost the power of swallowing. These symptoms were associated with total loss of speech, but unimpaired consciousness. Whenever he was spoken to, he applied his hand to his throat, as if to signify that the part was constricted. He died from the effects of the bite. The principal symptoms observed at the post-mortem exa-

---

[1] Cruveilhier, l. c., livr. xxxv. "Maladies de la Protubérance Annulaire," p. 2.

mination were, great congestion of the *medulla oblongata* under the
arachnoid, especially between the *corpus olivare* and *corpus resti-
forme.* There was also a hyperæmia and tension of the cervical
muscles which are supplied by the accessory and hypoglossal
nerves.   Professor Kolk, commenting on this case, says "that he
can scarcely avoid inferring that the *corpora olivaria* were affected,
whereby the *nuclei* of the two nerves (accessory and hypoglossal)
were injured, particularly in their bilateral relations, consequently
the powers of speech and deglutition were completely lost."

A woman under the care of Professor Schrœder Van der Kolk,
aged twenty-eight, became epileptic and quite silly.   She was able
to speak, but there was in the tone and accent of her voice something strange which she could not control.   The vocal sound varied, without any reason, nearly an octave up and down, and often
ended in a sharp, high, discordant tone.   Latterly both speech and
deglutition were difficult, apparently from paralysis of the right
side of the tongue.   After death, there was found atrophy of the
right *corpus olivare,* and dark ganglionic cells were scattered in
and around the *nuclei* of the *hypoglossi,* especially that of the right
hypoglossus.   The entire *medulla oblongata* had fallen into a state
of decided fatty degeneration.   In the fits, the patient often bit
her tongue.   It is not probable, says Professor Schrœder Van der
Kolk, that the dark degeneration of the ganglionic cells was of
very recent occurrence, though this would certainly closely correspond with the symptoms above detailed.

Pinel says, that as alterations in speech are characteristic of
general paralysis, and changes in the *corpora olivaria* are equally
constant, the latter organs must be connected with the articulation
of the sounds formed in speech, and consequently with the development of voice.[1]

IRREGULAR ACTION OF THE ARTICULATION.—In the early stage
of cerebral disease we occasionally observe a *perversion* of the
faculty of articulation.   There is a want of co-ordination in the
action of those portions of the nervous centres necessary for the
production of articulate sounds, or, more correctly speaking, as
suggested by Romberg, "there exists an interruption (caused by
various morbid states of the brain) in the pre-established harmony
which should obtain between the subjective intelligence and the

---

[1] *Vide* Professor Schrœder Van der Kolk's Work, p. 164.

organs of speech, giving rise to those singular anomalies in the co-ordinating faculty of articulation, occasionally witnessed in connection with organic cerebral conditions."

The power of expressing our thoughts in suitable language depends, as Dr. Todd observes, upon "the due relation between the centre of volition and that of intellectual action. The latter centre may have full power to frame the thoughts, but, unless it can prompt the will to a certain mode of sustained action, the organs of speech cannot be brought into play."

"A loss of the power of speech is frequently a precursor of more extensive derangement of sensation and motion. In some cases, the intellect seems clear, but the patient is utterly unable to express his thoughts; and in others there is more or less of mental confusion. The want of consent between the centre of intellectual action and of volition is equally apparent in cases of this description, from the inability of the patients to commit their thoughts to writing."[1]

In the incipient stage of disease of the brain, the patient, if he has not lost all power of articulation, will be observed, occasionally to stammer, and his words are sometimes half-formed, and *clipped*. He also shows signs of great embarrassment when speaking. He commences a sentence without finishing it, either forgetting what he intended to say, or having a difficulty in using the right word to express the conceptions originating in his mind. How frequently does this paralysis of *ideas* precede for a length of time all the other evidences of vocal muscular loss of power? This cerebral affection is considered by some to arise from a failure of memory; but such, I think, is not the fact. It is a paralysis of *ideas*, which I have seen to exist for a long period antecedently to any actual and noticeable loss of muscular or sensorial power. The patient has, however, in many cases, a clear notion of what he *wishes* and *means* to say, but is either unable to, or has extreme difficulty in pronouncing the words characteristic of his thoughts.

This singular want of co-ordination between the mental conceptions and the act of articulation is distinct in its character from those partial losses of memory, of which I have spoken in the chapter on chronic affections of this faculty, consequent upon organic cerebral lesions or mechanical injuries to the head.

<hr>

[1] "Physiology," by Todd and Bowman, vol. i, 1845.

Dr. Watson relates the particulars of an interesting case, in which this forgetfulness of certain words was a prominent symptom, associated with an apoplectic condition:—

"I received, on the 3d of September, a note, written in a remarkably clear and neat hand, desiring that I would call upon the writer, as he had had a severe attack of apoplexy a day or two before. I concluded that the note had been penned by some member of the patient's family, and I expected to see him in his bed, paralytic probably, or manifestly ill. But I found a stout active gentleman walking about in his drawing-room, apparently in perfect health, and declaring that he felt so. He showed me, however, a paper written by a surgeon, who on the previous day had brought him to town from a distance, and who had been obliged to return immediately. The paper stated that Mr. —— had suffered a sudden and decided fit of apoplexy on the 30th of August; that he was then freely bled; that perfect consciousness was not restored, nor the force of the pulse subdued, till twenty ounces of blood had issued from his arm; and that on the evening of the same day sixteen ounces more were drawn. My patient spoke of going down to his country house, where he had, he said, 'a good deal of shooting to do.' I dissuaded him from this, and enjoined perfect quiet for at least a fortnight to come. The next day, after a long and imprudent conversation with a friend, he suddenly lost the thread of his discourse, and could not recover it. Then he became confused, and misapplied words. I asked him how he felt. He answered, 'Not quite right,' and this he repeated very many times, abbreviating it at first into 'not right,' and at length into 'n'ight.' Wishing to mention 'camphor,' he called it 'pamphlet.' I mention these as specimens. On the 5th, it was evident that his right arm and leg were weak, in comparison with the others; but their sensibility was unimpaired. By slow degrees the weakness degenerated into complete palsy, and the right side of the face became motionless. Gradually, also, he grew heavy, stupid, comatose, unable to swallow, with a fixed pupil; and so, on the morning of the 15th of September, he died. We examined his head the next day. On the left side, the dura mater adhered to the skull-cap with morbid firmness. During the endeavors made to detach it, a teaspoonful or more of a dirty-looking, greenish, very offensive pus spurted forth. This was found to have proceeded from an abscess, which must have contained two ounces of pus, and which was situated in the upper part of the left hemisphere of the cerebrum. The walls of the abscess looked as if they were coated with a layer of yellowish plaster. In the centre of this cavity was a small, fibrous, tough mass, of a dull red color; the coagulum, doubtless, of blood effused on the 30th of August. In front of the abscess, the brain seemed natural, but its consistence was that of liquid custard."[1]

An attorney, says Dr. Crichton, much respected for his integrity and talents, had many sad failings to which our physical nature too often subject us. In his seventieth year he married an amiable lady much younger than himself, and indulged in great venereal excesses. The reproductive organs are not to be unduly exercised with impunity at the age of seventy. He was consequently suddenly seized with great prostration of strength, giddiness, forgetfulness, insensibility to all concerns of life, and every symptom of approaching fatuity. When he wished to ask for anything, he constantly made use of some inappropriate term. Instead of asking for a piece of *bread*, he asked for his *boots*. If he wanted a tumbler, he would call for a decanter, and *vice versâ*. He was evidently conscious that he pronounced wrong words, for when the proper expressions were used by another person, and he was asked if it were not such a thing he wanted, he always appeared aware of his mistake, and corrected himself by adopting the appropriate expression. This gentleman was cured of his complaint by large doses of valerian and other nervine medicines.

Professor Gruner, of Jena, relates the history of a learned friend of his, whose articulation was affected in a singular manner. After recovering from an acute fever, one of the first things he desired to have was coffee (*kaffee*), but instead of pronouncing the letters *ff*, he substituted in their place a *t* and *z*, and therefore asked for a cat (*katze*). In every word which had an *f* he committed a similar mistake substituting a *z* for it.

Van Goens says that the wife of Mr. Hennert, professor of mathematics at Utrecht, who, like her husband, was also a mathematician and astronomer, was affected with a remarkable defect of articulation. When she wished to ask for a chair she asked for a table, and when she wanted a book she demanded a glass. But what was singular in her case was, that when the proper expression of her thought was mentioned to her she could not pro-.

---

[1] "On the Principles and Practice of Physic," vol. i, p. 512, by T. Watson, M.D.

nounce it. She was angry if people brought her the thing she had named instead of the thing she desired. Sometimes she herself discovered that she had given a wrong name to her thoughts. This complaint continued several months, after which she gradually recovered the right use of her faculty of speech. It was only in this particular point that her memory seemed defective, for Van Goens says, that she conducted her household matters with as much regularity as she ever had done.

A man, aged seventy, was seized with a kind of cramp in the muscles of the mouth, accompanied with a sense of tickling all over the surface of the body, as if ants were creeping over it. After having experienced an attack of giddiness and mental confusion, a remarkable alteration in his speech was observed. He articulated easily and fluently, but made use of strange words which nobody could understand. When he spoke quickly, he pronounced numbers, and now and then he employed common words in an improper signification. He was conscious that he spoke nonsense. What he wrote was equally wrong with what he spoke. He could not write his name. The words he wrote were those he spoke, and they were always written conformably to his manner of pronouncing them. He could not read, and yet many external objects appeared to awaken in him the idea of their presence.

The articulating movements in these cases of incipient disease of the brain are produced, Romberg remarks, like movements of locomotion, in single sounds, or in a certain series, as syllables or words, without any mental act, or even against the will of the patient. He has observed the phenomenon accompanying cerebral hemorrhage, in which the patient intends to utter a certain sound, but emits a different one. A gentleman, distinguished by rank and education, once assured Romberg that of the various inconveniences and troubles following an apoplectic seizure, none were so painful to himself as the fact of his applying wrong terms (such as water for wood and the like) to express his meaning, and the suspicion of insanity which he thus excited among his friends.

Dr. Bright describes the case of a girl of eighteen years of age, who, in consequence of depressing mental emotions, was obliged to sigh involuntarily and very frequently. This passed into a spasm, during the continuance of which she every three seconds uttered a sound like *heigh-ho*, which she sometimes changed into *heigh*. She was only able to control the sound for a short time, if, for instance, she wanted to say a short sentence, but she was unable to combine two or three sentences without being interrupted by that exclamation.[1]

A patient has been observed to entirely lose the memory of certain words while preserving the integrity of his reasoning powers. If any were pronounced before him, he seized them in an instant, but in conversation he was obliged to employ a paraphrase to designate the objects, the names of which had escaped him. An epileptic could not pronounce spontaneously a single word, but he repeated them and wrote them without difficulty when they were pronounced to him.

A patient attacked with cancer of the uterus, which completely prostrated her, was suddenly seized in the middle of the night, and without any known cause, with an almost complete dumbness, which only enabled her to say, "Yes! yes!" to all questions, whether they were contradictory or not. She, however, retained possession of her intelligence, for she was neither paralyzed or insane. If she were requested to write what she had to communicate, she traced an assemblage of letters on the paper, to which no meaning could be attached.

Patients at the commencement of an attack of apoplexy, congestion, and softening, lose the use of almost all the vocabulary, and only retain a knowledge of few words, which, in their estimation, have all possible kinds of signification. When they are not understood the patients are moody, impatient, and repeat with more or less vehemence the words they have coined. Such persons have apparent possession of their reason. This is easily manifest by the expression of their eyes, and especially by their gestures, and by the air of satisfaction which they show when one has guessed their meaning. This state often exists for a long time, even to the period of death itself.[2]

Dr. Beddoes knew a gentleman who, previously to an attack of epilepsy, misplaced his words in a singular manner. He was constantly committing blunders of the kind in his letters, and when talking he was in the habit of substituting one word for another, bearing, however, some resemblance in sense as well as in sound. For example, he would say: "*Everybody feels very languid this* WET *weather—I mean this* HOT *weather;*" or, "*Come, who will sit*

[1] "Reports of Medical Cases," vol. ii, p. 458.
[2] "Traité des Maladies Mentales," par le Docteur B. A. Morel. Paris, 1860.

down to supper? here is only cold meat and pudding—I mean pie."

A gentleman connected with commerce, and whose mind had been for several weeks severely on the strain, in consequence of some urgent and anxious matters, was observed one day, when in his counting-house, singularly to misplace his words. He was able, however, to continue in his business for several days, and attended a meeting of the firm, when matters of a complicated character were under discussion and consideration. Three days afterwards he complained of great giddiness, and one morning whilst shaving was seized with a fit of vomiting. Two hours subsequently he was on his back in a state of profound *coma*. He, however, recovered from a very unpromising state of cerebral disorder.

A clergyman experienced the same difficulty whilst preaching, but he was able, by a strong effort of the will, to conquer the difficulty. He, however, eventually became paralyzed. A patient, a few hours before an attack of apoplexy, called his children by their wrong names, reversing the sexes, addressing "Sarah" by the name of "John," and "Emma" as "Thomas," and *vice versâ*. This misplacement of names has been observed in many cases among the incipient symptoms of acute brain disease.

In some types of insanity the same morbid phenomenon is observed. A lady deeply imbued with religious feelings, became the subject of a severe nervous and mind affection, not, however, amounting to alienation. Occasionally, while in the act of repeating the Lord's Prayer, instead of saying, "Our Father which art in *Heaven*," she was obliged by an irresistible impulse to say, "Our Father which art in *Hell*." This was the cause of great mental agony. She did not conquer the difficulty until restored by appropriate remedies to a state of cerebral health.

Alterations of speech sometimes present very curious phenomena most difficult of explanation. A woman suffering from chronic softening of the brain, could not speak without, at the end of three or four words, saying: "*par le commandement.*" . . . . . This woman exhibited the same phenomenon for several years. The only symptoms which revealed the existence of an organic lesion of the brain were the doltishness of the physiognomy, and the torpid state of her intelligence. A woman aged sixty-eight years, could only make incoherent sounds, always the same, and which formed the word *sinona* or *chinona*. She heard and understood perfectly well, and she answered everybody by this single word, only varying the inflexion of her voice, according to the idea she wished to express. The right arm was rigid and flexed, deprived of motion and painful in its articulations. The sensibility had quite vanished in that part.

There was at the infirmary of·the Salpêtrière a woman of forty years of age, quite hemiplegic, and who could only say : " *Madame été !*" . . . . "*Mon Dieu !*" . . . . "*Est-il possible ?*" . . . . "*Bonjour, Madame !*" . . . . Her intelligence was perfectly preserved ; she laughed at jokes which she heard, and cried when she wished to testify her thankfulness for the care that was taken of her. She pronounced perfectly the few words which she could say, and these she repeated incessantly ; but, however, it was impossible for her to utter anything else.[1]

IRREGULARITY AND IMPAIRMENT OF SPEECH. LOSS OF SPEECH. —Associated with the slight loss of power over the muscles of the tongue and mouth previously referred to, there is in the early stage of brain disease an inability on the part of the patient to give, with his usual clearness, perspicuity, and facility, expression to the ideas. He speaks in a *slow* and *measured* intonation, as if he were cautiously and critically selecting his phrases, and carefully considering what he is saying. He drawls out his words. The voice is often *thick* and *husky*, giving rise to the impression that the patient is suffering from the effects of a cold, or has some extraneous body in the mouth, interfering with his freedom of speech. He talks with what may be termed a muffled (*voilée*), veiled, or clouded voice, like a man slightly under the influence of stimulants, strong emotional excitement, or as if he were even partially intoxicated.

Slowness of speech, feebleness of voice, mistakes in accentuation, hesitation in pronunciation, and disorder in the succession of words, are phenomena of great diagnostic value. They point out, says Dr. Guislain, correctly very grave cases of cerebral disturbance. The tremor of the tongue, hesitation of speech, are the most characteristic signs of general paralysis. It is almost impossible, says Morel, to mistake the embarrassed speech, sympto-

[1] " Traité du Ramollissement du Cerveau," par Max. Durand-Fardel, M.D., Paris, 1843.

matic of the commencement of general paralysis, with the tremor of the tongue, which under the impression of quick emotion sometimes attacks persons with very decided nervous dispositions.

Occasionally, when in this incipient state of brain disease, the patient is observed to make repeated but ineffectual efforts to utter articulate sounds. He is seen to open and close his lips, as if trying to speak, but cannot do so. The attempt thus made produces a singular movement of the lips, similar to that seen in the action of smoking a pipe, conveying to those who notice the phenomenon the idea of the patient having, in a slight degree, a symptom hitherto described and considered as pathognomonic of a serious and fatal state of cerebral coma, designated by French pathologists, " *Le malade fume la pipe.*"

These symptoms of failing vocal power may exist for several months before the attention is directed to them. Such morbid affections of articulation are to be found among the most insidious signs of incipient centric brain disease.

The speech, says M. Durand-Fardel, is almost constantly altered in acute softening. When the symptoms develope themselves gradually, derangement of the pronunciation is a usual accompaniment of the disease. There is a kind of heaviness of the tongue, which is observed to increase daily as the malady progresses. In general, when doltishness and hemiplegia have become complete, the articulation of sounds is quite impossible. This happens at the commencement of softening, when the malady is announced by a sudden loss of knowledge, accompanied with paralysis. At a later period patients usually recover the power of articulating a few words, making themselves a little understood. This obtuseness of the faculty of speech occasionally remains a permanent condition.

Delirium, or agitation, joined or not to paralysis, is accompanied sometimes with difficulty or impossibility of articulation : this gives place to the use of very curious language, in the midst of which one often distinguishes syllables or words, but as though produced at random. Sometimes patients have lost, not the faculty of articulation, but the consciousness of the *sense of words*. They pronounce them with volubility, without order, connection, and meaning. Usually the same words or the same phrases recur almost incessantly to the mind. Sometimes such patients speak at random. At other times they struggle as though they really wished to express an idea, but without being able to find it, or even appearing able to discover the right mode of expression.

Sometimes they appear to have lost not only the faculty of articulation, but that of uttering even a sound: not a whine is heard to escape from them, and they live in the most absolute silence. This phenomenon does not exhibit itself exclusively among patients plunged into a state of coma.[1]

LOSS OF SPEECH.[2]—The first evidences of approaching apoplexy and paralysis are often recognized by sudden loss of speech. A gentleman, previously in a state of excellent health, had conveyed to him abruptly a painful piece of intelligence. He at first exhibited in his physiognomy an expression of great terror and alarm: he subsequently appeared to be stunned. When spoken to, he tried to reply to the questions addressed to him; but his efforts to speak were fruitless. His power of articulation was perfectly paralyzed. He died that evening of apoplexy!

I have seen several cases of a similar kind, as well as numerous instances of aphonia, from mental shocks, and great and prolonged anxiety. A lady, pending the prosecution of a protracted and expensive suit in chancery, which caused great mental distress, entirely lost her voice for eighteen months. In another case, a lady was informed of the accidental death of a son, which gave rise to an intense degree of mental agony, reducing her to a state of insensibility, which continued for several hours. When consciousness was restored, it was found that she could only speak

[1] *Vide* Drs. Morel, Guislain, and Durand-Fardel.

[2] Loss of voice is occasionally dependent upon pressure or change of structure at the origin of, or in the course of the lingual and glosso-pharyngeal nerves. Dr. Copland relates a case of the kind in which the aphonia preceded some months a fatal attack of apoplexy. The patient was fifty years of age. He had for many months lost all power of uttering the most simple articulate sound. He swallowed substances with great difficulty, and sometimes he was unable to do so at all, unless they were conveyed over the base of the tongue. The tongue could not be protruded, and was incapable of action. This gentleman had neither headache, or any other ailment. No other part of the body was paralyzed. He attended regularly to the duties of his profession during the usual hours of business, but was obliged to write down all he wished to say.

Aphonia is, in many cases, as observed by Dr. Copland, a *laryngeal affection*. In its nature and consequences it is distinct from those morbid affections of the *articulation* which so commonly are precursory of paralysis and apoplexy. The loss of voice, dependent upon disease of the larynx, its tendons, muscles, and cartilages, is easily distinguished from the affection of the vocal organs, symptomatic of disease of the brain.—(*Vide* Dr. Copland's admirable treatise "*On Palsy and Apoplexy.*")

in the faintest whisper: this state of aphonia continued for six months.

A gentleman, subject to periodical attacks of epilepsy, invariably loses all power of speaking in his usual intonation for some hours before the convulsive attack supervenes.

A clergyman, whilst reading the litany, became suddenly speechless, without losing his consciousness. He was obliged to leave the church. He continued in this state for an hour, being perfectly sensible of everything that was going on about him, and being able to write on a piece of paper a request for a certain physician to be immediately telegraphed for. Two hours after the loss of speech he was in a state of apoplectic coma, in which he died! Alas! for the interests of science, no *post-mortem* examination was permitted!

It is a most unusual circumstance for this sudden loss of speech to exist without being immediately followed by acute cerebral symptoms.

A patient, having exhibited these premonitory signs of paralysis for a short period antecedently to the development of more decided signs of cerebral disease, informed me that he was distinctly conscious of something "snapping" in his brain before he was sensible of his inability to speak. He had been overworking his mind during the previous week, and had been riding some distance on horseback. He felt, on the day previously to the attack, a sensation of "throbbing" and "metallic tinkling" (as he described it) in his head, *and these were the only warnings he had of an approaching attack of hemiplegia.*

A literary gentleman, whose vocation in life was that of a public lecturer, noticed, for nearly *eight weeks* before he was seized with paralysis, that occasionally, whilst speaking, he lost for a second or two all power of articulation. This occurred on five or six occasions previously to an attack of decided hemiplegia. This patient had taxed his powers of mind to their utmost, by lecturing twice, and often thrice, a day; but independently of this amount of literary labors, he had been exposed to much anxiety respecting family matters, and this had produced restless, and, in some instances, sleepless nights.

A gentleman, aged thirty-five, while standing in the street conversing with a friend, suddenly lost his speech; he recovered it after a few minutes, walked home, and made no particular com-

plaint of indisposition.   In the evening of the same day he suddenly fell from his chair, speechless, and paralytic on the right
side, but without coma; being sensible of what was said to him,
and answering by signs.   He was then confined to bed for several
weeks without any change in the symptoms.   At the end of three
months he had recovered so far the motion of his leg as to be able
to walk a little, dragging forward the leg by a motion of the whole
right side of his body.   He afterwards improved considerably in
bodily strength, so that he could walk for several miles; but his
thigh and leg continued to be dragged forward by the same kind
of effort, without any farther improvement.   He never recovered
any degree of motion of the arm or hand; he could not even move
the fingers; his speech was very inarticulate, and his countenance
expressive of great imbecility.   In this state he continued without
relapse, or any farther improvement, for fifteen years, when he
died at the age of fifty.   Dr. Abercrombie saw him about four
days before he died, and found him in a state resembling typhus;
his pulse frequent and weak, his tongue very foul and dry in the
middle; he had no other complaint.   He was not then in bed, but
was confined to it next day, and died in three days more, of rapid
sinking without *coma*.[1]

A young man, aged sixteen, bathed twice, in the month of June,
in the river Tweed.   After coming out the second time he lay down
on the bank, and fell asleep without his hat, with his head exposed
to the direct beams of a hot sun!   On awaking he was *speechless;
but walked home, and seemed to be otherwise in good health!*   He
was bled and purged, and the next day recovered his speech, but
lost it again at intervals several times during the three or four following days.   He was forgetful, and his look was dull and heavy:
he made little complaint, but, when closely questioned, said he had
a dull uneasiness at the back of his head.   In a few days more he
had squinting and double vision, and a very obstinate state of
bowels, and his pulse was 60.   After further bleeding, the pulse
rose to 86; but he gradually sank into coma, and died on the 30th.

The substance of the brain in general was found highly vascular, and a very considerable extent of it was in a state of softening
mixed with suppuration.   The ventricles were distended with fluid,
and the membranes in many places were much thickened.   One

[1] "On Diseases of the Brain," p. 261.

very curious circumstance (affording, perhaps, some explanation of the readiness with which the inflammation was produced) was, that the cranium was of very unequal thickness at its upper part. In one spot, as big as a sixpence, it was as thin as writing paper, and transparent.[1]

Loss of speech has been known to occur without any previously existing premonitory symptom of brain or nervous disorder; in other words, there has been no headache, vertigo, noise in the ears, loss of sensibility, depression of spirits, affection of vision, or any other symptom to excite suspicion as to the presence of any abnormal state of the structure of the brain or condition of cerebral circulation.

Dr. Graves cites the following interesting illustrative case: "A barrister was walking up and down the hall of the Four Courts, waiting for a case to come on, and chatting with one friend and another; as the hall was rather crowded and hot, he went out into the area of the Courts for the sake of the air, and had not remained there more than ten minutes when an old friend from the country came up and spoke to him. He was pleased to see his friend, and wished to inquire about his family, when he found, to his great surprise, that he could not utter a single audible sound; he had completely lost his voice. He recovered the use of his tongue in about three weeks, but not completely, for some slowness of speech remained. When the loss of speech was first perceived, his friend brought him home in a carriage; and during the day he had several attacks of vertigo, and afterwards hemiplegia. For several hours, however, before distortion of the face, or any of the usual symptoms of paralysis had commenced, the only existing symptom was loss of speech. This gentleman died of apoplexy in about two months."[2]

A lady after an attack of paralysis, lost all power of speaking, but was able to communicate in writing her wishes. When, however, doing so, she invariably wrote *no* when she meant *yes*, and *vice versa*. When she wrote, "I wish you to do so," it was construed conversely. This patient, I am informed, is still living, the singular defect alluded to remaining unaltered.

A gentleman, after many premonitory warnings, which were dis-

---

[1] Dr. Abercrombie, " *On Diseases of the Brain.*"
[2] "A System of Clinical Medicine," by R. J. Graves, M.D., Dublin, 1843, p. 688.

regarded, fell down in a fit. It was a combination of epilepsy and apoplexy. For two days his life was in imminent danger. He, however, partially recovered, but with an inability to give anything like a clear expression of his wishes. He could speak, but what he said, without a key to its interpretation, was quite unintelligible. He was able to pronounce words with great clearness, but they were sadly misplaced and transposed. What he said was written down, and the words placed in their proper order. By adopting this course, his family were able clearly to comprehend his wishes. This state of brain and impairment of speech continued with slight intermissions for nearly a fortnight, accompanied by acute pain in the occipital region. In consequence of this and other symptoms of local congestion, the gentleman, at my request, was cupped. The abstraction of blood was followed by a decided mitigation of the symptoms. Mercurial purgatives were exhibited, the head was shaved, and counter-irritation applied behind the ears. In the course of five days from the time the cupping-glasses were applied, he was able to converse coherently for a few minutes, but if he continued in conversation beyond that time, he again began to jumble and misplace his words. Minute doses of bichloride of mercury were subsequently administered in combination with tincture of cinchona, with the greatest benefit. This gentleman, in the course of a few months, entirely recovered, and has been for four years free from all symptoms of brain disease.

A military gentleman, who had resided for many years in Canada, suffered from somewhat similar cerebral symptoms, supervening upon two attacks of apoplexy. His conversation was a singular intermixture of words to which no meaning could be attached; but the remarkable feature in this case was, that he was able to write coherently, and with perfect lucidity, whatever he wished to communicate to others, but when he tried to talk, his conversation was quite unintelligible. I saw this patient on two occasions, and suggested a course of remedial treatment, but in consequence of his removal to America, where the family were obliged to go on urgent family business, I have lost all knowledge of the progress of the case. I was not, however, sanguine of his recovery, as there were symptoms of general paralysis associated with the case, dependent, as I conceived, upon some subtle organic changes in the vesicular neurine of the brain.

The wife of an eminent dissenting minister lost, in consequence of a cerebral affection, all knowledge of the distinction of sex. This lady invariably addressed men as women, and *vice versa*.

Napoleon Joubert, aged twenty-three years, sailor of the third class, was admitted into the principal marine hospital at Toulon, on the 31st October, 1855, under the care of M. Reynaud.

Joubert, on the 28th April, 1855, had been wounded in the trenches before Sebastopol. A ball pierced the upper portion of the forehead, a little to the left of the median line, and after passing beneath the skin for a distance of three centimetres, issued to the left of the first aperture. The projectile carried along with it a small fragment of the external table of the frontal bone, which remained adherent to the bullet.

In consequence of this wound, Joubert was for four months a patient in one of the hospitals on the Bosphorus. In the month of September, he was sent to Toulon, and on his arrival there, he received sick leave, which he did not avail himself of.

On the 31st October, 1855, he was suddenly seized with vertigo, followed by syncope, in consequence of which he was compelled to enter the hospital again. At this time the wounds on the forehead were not cicatrized, and they were covered with fungosities, beneath which the probe encountered denuded osseous surfaces. However, a very considerable tumefaction was remarked towards the external angle of the left eye, due apparently to a lesion of the malar bone. Fistulous tracts opening beneath this point indicated that the locality had been the seat of previous abscess.

In the night of the 31st October, or 1st November, the wounded man was seized with vertigo and subsequent syncope. On the evening of the 1st of November, he was again attacked in a similar manner. This ended in a true epileptiform seizure. On the 2d, in the morning, he had heaviness of the head, was torpid, had difficulty in articulating words, no appetite, a regular pulse, and the bowels had not acted for twenty-four hours.

In the night, the epileptic attacks recurred five times; the bowels acted abundantly from the effects of a purgative.

In the night of the 3d there were many epileptiform seizures; articulation became more and more difficult, and finally the power of speech was entirely lost.

On the morning of the 4th the patient still remained torpid; he awoke up at intervals for a few moments, but he was not able to

articulate a word.   In the evening there was an epileptic seizure;
in the night he was calm.

In the morning of the 5th there was a brief seizure; contractions
of the face and of the limbs, particularly of the right superior
member; foam on the lips.   As in the preceding seizure, the contractions persisted but a few moments; they terminated promptly,
and the patient fell into his habitual torpor.   The *mutism* continued.
There was no other seizure during the day.   The pulse was full
and regular, the tongue a little white.

On the 6th November, 1855, the comatose state of the patient
was a little less profound than on preceding days; hearing persisted, because the eyes were fixed upon any one who spoke to
him; but he did not appear to comprehend what was said, and he
did nothing that he was commanded.   He was still incapable of
answering questions put to him.   His attention could not be fixed,
or it was very quickly fatigued: a bottle of ammonia placed
beneath the nostrils excited the pituitary membrane; the sensibility of the skin was very obtuse, a needle plunged into the in-
tegument of the limbs occasioned scarcely any movements.   Voluntary motion was abolished; when the limbs were raised, they
fell as if inert; the patient had only automatic movements; defecation and micturition were involuntary.

At eight o'clock, A.M., it was decided to trepan.   A T incision
having been made in the integuments of the cranium, and the bone
exposed, a medium-sized trepan was applied to the superior portion
of the frontal bone, to the left of the median line, in the interval
which separated the wound of entrance and the wound of exit of
the ball.   The osseous ferule having been raised by the elevator,
there was seen a splinter of the internal table of the frontal bone.
This splinter was rather more than a centimetre in diameter, it
was entirely detached, exhibited the commencement of necrosis,
with thinning, and compressed the dura mater on a level with the
anterior lobe of the brain.   This splinter being removed, a jutting
point of the frontal bone, which might have induced further mischief, was re-sected; after which no other detached splinters were
discovered, neither any suppuration under the dura mater.

Soon after the operation the aspect of the patient became better;
the physiognomy appeared more open, the eye showed more attention, and some movements of the lips were distinguished.   About
two hours after noon the patient responded *Yes* to the surgeon in

charge, who questioned him; and about five, P.M., he uttered some connected words.

On the 7th, the wounds gave neither pain nor trouble; there had been no epileptic seizure since five, A.M. No sleep in the night, a little agitation, disturbing dreams, some incoherent words, involuntary stools. At eight, A.M., the tongue was natural, pulse full and regular, heat of the skin normal; the patient responded by some words to questions addressed to him; he executed in part certain movements at command.

On the 8th tactile sensibility returned, the movements were more regular, but the intelligence was still sluggish, the responses were slow and confused, but there was a gradual and marked improvement. On the 13th, the eighth day after the operation, as well as on the 15th the tenth day, he exhibited manifest signs of marked intelligence.

On the 21st, the sixteenth day, he raised himself a few moments. On the 27th, the twenty-second day, of all the functions the vision alone is still changed, the left eye cannot distinguish objects but at a little distance and in a confused manner; the speech is precise. On the 29th, a splinter was removed from the zygomatic arch. On the 16th December, several small-pox pustules appeared on the arm and visage (the patient had been vaccinated). The wound was cicatrizing well.

On the 28th December, 1855, fifty-three days after the operation, Joubert left the hospital cured, enjoying the whole of his faculties, speaking sanely, and having no more disturbance of the vision.

This man, after some weeks' rest in the barracks, obtained sick-leave for six months. On his return, about ten months after the operation, he presented himself anew before the *conseil de santé*; his intelligence was perfectly clear, and the speech entirely free. He declared that all his functions were executed as regularly as before the operation; he read and wrote as well as before; and a depressed cicatrix was alone visible at the point where the trepan had been applied.[1]

Fagan, a pipe-maker, was wounded in the head with a dragoon's sword. The skull was fractured, the membranes wounded, and the brain protruded. On the eighth day he was attacked with convulsions, followed by stupor. A portion of the bone was removed

[1] Reported by M. Lalluyeaux. (*Gazette Médicale de Paris*, 1857, p. 567.)

by Hey's saw. The convulsions gradually passed away, but fungus cerebri appeared on the tenth day. In twenty-four days this had disappeared, and in eleven days after this the wound was healed. In a fortnight more, Fagan was discharged, and resumed his employment. He was unable to remember the names of things. At this point the last report ended.

After this man was discharged he led a very irregular life, suffering after each debauch from severe pain in the head. On the 22d of August (he was discharged on the 15th May) he nearly lost all power in the right arm and hand, and the right side of the face was paralyzed. On the 24th he was readmitted.

The following statement is abridged from the hospital journal: "John Fagan, readmitted August 24th, complaining of severe pain in the seat of the original wound ; and although his head pain is not constant, the paroxysms recur several times in an hour, and last for two or three minutes ; vomits occasionally ; vision indistinct ; pupils dilated, and very sluggish ; strength and sensibility of the right arm and leg much diminished ; pulse 100, soft and easily compressible ; tongue clean ; bowels free ; memory very defective, particularly with respect to names and recent events ; but the defect is not confined to the faculty of memory, as, with few exceptions, he cannot repeat proper names, but miscalls almost everything ; although he can perfectly describe the use of it, he calls, for instance, a watch, a gate ; a book, a pipe, &c. ; a pipe is the word that he pronounces most frequently ; it is remarkable, however, that the moment he employs a wrong word he is conscious of his mistake, and is most anxious to correct it. The cicatrix of the wound, which is six inches long, and half an inch broad, is *raised*, particularly at its centre, above the level of the scalp ; it is of a purplish red color, tense, and shining, and very painful to the touch ; and at the centre, which is the softest and most prominent part, there is a strong pulsation, obviously synchronous with the radial pulse.

"26th. Had several severe paroxysms of pain, accompanied with grinding of the teeth and contortions of the features, and succeeded by complete insensibility, which lasted for five or six minutes, during which time the pulse fell to fifty in a minute. Twenty leeches were applied round the cicatrix, a blister to the nape of the neck, and a cold lotion to the head ; purgative pills.

"27th. No return of paroxysms ; pain relieved.

"28th. Several paroxysms of convulsion, followed by stupor; cicatrix more tense and red, but the fluid which it covers disappears on pressure, and returns when the pressure is removed; pulse seventy-two, and regular; tongue foul; bowels open. Continued to improve; paroxysms becoming less frequent until the 4th of September, when he had violent vomiting followed by convulsion, after which he remained insensible for several hours; pupils dilated; pulse fifty-four; respiration natural; a small opening was made into the prominent part of the cicatrix, and two drachms of healthy pus were discharged; the pulse immediately rose to sixty-eight: he sat up in the bed, answered questions rationally, and said he was quite free from pain."

7th. Continued free from pain or convulsion; the little opening is healed, and the tumor is as large as before; a larger opening was made into it, and a small quantity (about half a drachm) of bloody serum was discharged.

Oct. 9th. Has had no pain or convulsion since the 4th of September, when the abscess was opened; he appears in perfect bodily health, with the exception of some remaining weakness in the right arm and hand, and some slight confusion of vision; the cicatrix is perfectly on a level with the head, and there is no sensible pulsation in the seat of the former abscess; the mental phenomena are as before described, and are most remarkable; he speaks correctly, and even fluently; describes his sensations with great clearness, but avoids all proper names; he says (for example), "I have a great weakness and numbness here" (pointing to his shoulder), "and along here" (drawing his finger along the arm to the palm of the hand), "but no pain. When I sit up suddenly I don't see rightly; but I soon see as well as ever." He counted five on his fingers, but could not say the word "finger," though he made many attempts to do so. He called his thumb, "friend." When desired to say "stirabout," he said, and invariably says, "buttermilk;" but was immediately conscious of his error, and said, "I know that's not the name of it." Sometimes the association of ideas could be traced through which he was led to the misnomer; stirabout and buttermilk being connected in the mind of every man of his class in this country; but in the greater number of instances no such association could be traced; but this should excite no surprise, as the disturbing cause, which was of sufficient force to dissociate the idea of the *name* from the *thing*, would, naturally enough, be sufficient to disorder the faculty of "association."[1]

Dr. Osborn has detailed the following remarkable illustration of the morbid phenomena of speech, which deserves to be quoted *in extenso*.[2]

A gentleman of about twenty-six years of age, of very considerable literary attainments, a scholar of Trinity College, and a proficient in the French, Italian, and German languages, about a year ago was residing in the country, and indulged the habit of bathing in a neighboring lake.

One morning, after bathing, he was sitting at breakfast, when he suddenly fell in an apoplectic fit. A physician was immediately sent for; the patient was bled, and after being subjected to appropriate treatment, he became sensible in about a fortnight. Although restored to the use of his intellects, he had the mortification of finding himself deprived of speech. He spoke, but what he uttered was quite unintelligible, although he labored under no paralytic affection, and uttered a variety of syllables with the greatest apparent ease. When he came to Dublin his extraordinary jargon led to his being treated as a foreigner in the hotel where he stopped; and when he went to the college to see a friend, he was unable to express his wish to the gate-porter, and succeeded only by pointing to the apartments which his friend had occupied.

Dr. Osborn had ample opportunities of observing the peculiar nature of the deprivation under which the patient labored; and the circumstance of his having received a liberal education, enabled him to ascertain some peculiarities in this affection, which would not otherwise have come to light. They were as follows :—

1. He perfectly comprehended every word said to him; this was proved in a variety of ways unnecessary to describe.

2. He perfectly comprehended written language. He continued to read a newspaper every day, and, when examined, proved that he had a very clear recollection of all that he read. Having procured a copy of Andral's Pathology in French, he read it with

---

[1] "Dublin Quarterly Journal of Medical Science," for 1833. A case under the care of the late Sir P. Crampton, M.D

[2] *Ibid.* vol. iv, p. 157.

great diligence, having lately intended to embrace the medical profession.

3. He expressed his ideas in writing with considerable fluency; and when he failed, it appeared to arise merely from confusion, and not from inability, the words being orthographically correct, but sometimes not in their proper places. Latin sentences he translated accurately. He also wrote correct answers to historical questions.

4. His knowledge of arithmetic was unimpaired. He added and subtracted numbers of different denominations with uncommon readiness. He also played well at the game of draughts, which involves calculations relating to numbers and position.

5. His recollection of musical sounds could not be ascertained, not knowing the extent of his knowledge of music before the apoplectic seizure; but he remembered the tune of " God save the King ;" and when " Rule Britannia" was played, he pointed to the shipping in the river.

6. His power of repeating words after another person was almost confined to certain monosyllables; and in repeating the letters of the alphabet, he could never pronounce *k, q, u, v, w, x*, and *z*, although he often uttered those sounds in attempting to pronounce the other letters. The letter *i* also he was very seldom able to pronounce.

7. In order to ascertain and place on record the peculiar imperfection of language which he exhibited, Dr. Osborn selected and laid before the patient the following sentence from the by-laws of the College of Physicians, viz. : " *It shall be in the power of the College to examine or not examine any Licentiate previous to his admission to a Fellowship, as they shall think fit.*"

Having set him to read, he read as follows: " *An the be what in the temother of the trothotodoo to majorum or that emidrate ein einkrastrai mestreit to ketra totombreidei to ra fromtreido as that kekritest.*" The same passage was presented to him in a few days afterwards, and he then read it as follows : " *Be mather be in the kondreit of the compestret to samtreis amtreit emtreido and temtreido mestreiterso to his eftreido tum bried rederiso of deid daf drit des trest.*"

Dr. Osborn observes that there are several syllables in the above of frequent occurrence in the German language, which probably had made a strong impression on the patient's memory. But the most remarkable fact connected with the case was, that although he appeared generally to know when he spoke wrongly, yet he was unable to speak correctly notwithstanding, as is proved by the preceding specimen. He was completely free from any paralytic affection of the vocal organs.

MORBID IMITATIVE MOVEMENTS OF ARTICULATION.—I have not yet spoken of a singular affection of the imitative movements of articulation which is sometimes witnessed in the early, as well as advanced, stage of cerebral disease. Romberg refers to the phenomenon, and terms it the "echo" sign. The patient exhibits this symptom by repeating, in a monotonous tone of voice, the words and sentences spoken, not only by persons near him, but by those with whom he is immediately engaged in conversation.

I have often observed this symptom at the commencement of acute attacks of disease of the brain, particularly of inflammatory softening. The physician says "Good morning;" the patient echoes the question, without giving any kind of response to the interrogatory. "The pulse is weak," observes the physician to an anxious bystander; "The pulse is weak," echoes the invalid. "Let me see the tongue," asks the physician; "Let me see the tongue," repeats the patient, at the same moment protruding it from his mouth.

I recollect a remarkable illustration of this morbid condition of the imitative movements of articulation, in the case of a gentleman to whom I was called, suffering from many of the alarming symptoms premonitory of paralysis. He repeated every question I put to him, as well as the remarks made by others. This symptom is often observed in chronic conditions of imbecility and insanity.

"A lady," says Romberg, "who died of softening of the brain, invariably repeated my questions, as 'Show me your tongue,' or 'Will you lift up your arm?' without doing as she was bid. I am acquainted with an idiot of eleven years, who in this way mimics music in a remarkable manner. The same phenomenon has occurred to me in two young girls laboring under typhus fever, when the disease was at its height."

A gentleman, who had suffered acute mental distress, and whose mind was never remarkable for its vigor, exhibited symptoms of softening of the brain. I examined him. He had, to a singular degree, the "echo" symptom, repeating almost every question I addressed to him. His friends, who accompanied the patient to my house, were themselves struck with this symptom, although they had never before observed it. This patient subsequently had an attack of decided paralysis, and, after death, there was found extensive softening in the whole of the right hemisphere of the brain.

I presume the "echo" phenomenon may, to some extent, arise from that sluggish and abstracted state of thought amounting to reverie, which is so often seen in cases of long-existing and un-detected, because obscure, affection of the brain. The mind ap-pears incapable, under these circumstances, of apprehending the most simple questions, and parrot-like repeats them. I have no-ticed this symptom in other conditions of depressed vital and nerv-ous power, but it more particularly accompanies softening of some portion of the brain.

INVOLUNTARY ARTICULATION, OR THINKING ALOUD.—Whilst referring to the morbid phenomena of speech, it will not be out of place to direct attention to a precursory symptom, not only of ap-proaching paralysis, but of insanity. I allude to the practice of many patients, suffering from incipient brain and mind disease, of talking aloud, when alone. A distinguished physician observed this symptom to precede an attack of paralysis, in the case of a nobleman who for many years ruled the destinies of this country.

In many conditions of brain irritation and disease, the patient is observed to talk to himself, and the commencement of insanity is often detected by this symptom. I am fully aware that this eccentric habit is quite consistent with a perfect state of health of body and mind ; but, nevertheless, it is a symptom that should be carefully regarded in all cases of *suspected* disease of the brain, coming on at a critical period of life, particularly if conjoined with other signs of cerebral disorder.

MORBID VOCAL PHENOMENA ACCOMPANYING INSANITY. — In some cases of insanity all power of speech appears, for a consider-able period, to be lost. Insane patients have been known to con-tinue for years without uttering a vocal sound. This does not generally arise from any paralysis of the organs of speech, al-though this affection sometimes exists, but it is owing to the mind being intensely absorbed or preoccupied in the contemplation of predominant insane ideas.

Dr. Brierre de Boismont relates the case of a man who was for fifty-two years insane, but who had not spoken for *thirty* years !

When perseveringly interrogated, he gave a kind of grunt, and
ran away. About fifteen days before his death, this patient recovered the use of his speech, and answered perfectly well all
questions put to him.

There are certain peculiarities characteristic of the voice and
speech of the insane, and these are occasionally recognized in the
incipient stage of the malady. I am acquainted with a gentleman
subject to attacks of recurrent insanity, whose paroxysms are always preceded by singular alteration and eccentricity of voice.
For a week or ten days, and occasionally for a fortnight, before the
mind exhibits symptoms of aberration, the voice becomes remarkably *sharp* and *shrill*. This warning of the approaching relapse
is immediately appreciated by the family, and steps are at once
taken to prevent any mischief that might ensue from the violence of
a sudden maniacal outbreak. In another case, a lady, who has had
repeated attacks of insanity, begins to clip her words and leave her
sentences half-finished in the early period of the attack. Some
patients, in the incipient stage, speak snappishly, sharply, and
quickly. In other forms of insanity, the voice assumes a solemn
and grave character. These latter alterations are observed to precede attacks of acute melancholia. I have known the voice to
undergo very remarkable modifications, and sometimes a complete
metamorphosis, in the incipient stage of insanity.

A lady, some years ago, consulted me respecting her husband,
who had, according to the observation of her friends, exhibited
symptoms of mental unsoundness. She had not, however, herself
noticed any remarkable change in his mental condition, such as to
justify her entertaining a suspicion of approaching aberration of
mind. She, however, admitted she had remarked a singular alteration in the character of his voice, which was attributed to a cold
which she presumed he was suffering from. She could not accurately describe his voice to me. "It sounded (she observed) hollow, as if it came through a large empty tub." Two months subsequently to this consultation, the gentleman was in confinement
as a dangerous lunatic.

M. Morel refers to a case of insanity, in which the patient was
subject to dangerous periodical attacks of violent homicidal delirium. His relations always knew when the maniacal crisis was
about to occur, from a singular alteration that took place in his
voice. It had at these periods a bell-like sound. He spoke in

what is designated by French pathologists, "*Voix de Polichinelle*," or, Punch's voice.

Guislain, when alluding to the subject of morbid vocal phenomena as associated with insanity, observes:—

"The speech is altered from the natural tone and style; the articulation becomes embarrassed. It is not so distinct as usual, or it is clipped, or hurried, or weak, or too emphatic, or prosy, or drawling. Some words are cut short like a drunken man's, or single words are repeated hastily, or a syllable of a word is repeated, or there is a difficulty in uttering certain letters, such as T's and R's, or words requiring an emphasis, or when several consonants come together. At times the patient stammers, and seems to be at fault in finding the proper word, expletive, epithet, or phrase, which in health he was both apt and fluent in using; or, it may be, that instead of being cautious and studied in his speech, he is all of a sudden voluble, redundant, and profusely garrulous. But at other times the speech is perfectly natural in utterance and rational in what is said, and yet the patient is deeply attainted with insanity all the time. There shall not be a single unreasonable or ill-spoken word uttered. But at the same time there is a retired, reserved manner, a slinking out of sight, a refusal to speak to an old friend, or answer the queries of the medical man; an ill-temper or sulkiness, that is worse than imperfect articulation. At length he speaks with irritation : 'I know *their* designs —he is not *my* friend; he has been informed of everything. I am surrounded with freemasons, or papists, or tories, or dissenters. I know there is a God,' &c. &c. Such a person is still insane in spite of his good articulation."

CHAPTER XX.

MORBID PHENOMENA OF SENSATION.

THE sensibility is very frequently affected in organic disease of the brain, and exalted, depressed, or perverted states of this important function are to be found among the early and premonitory symptoms of all cerebral affections. The sensation may be,

　　α. *Exalted.*
　　β. *Impaired or lost.*
　　γ. *Vitiated.*

EXALTATION OF SENSATION (HYPERÆSTHESIA).—In many affections of the nervous system unconnected with organic disease of the brain, the sensibility exhibits great acuteness; and to such a degree do we occasionally witness this state of morbid exaltation, that the slightest touch of the skin, or puff of cold air, has been known to throw the patient into a paroxysm of convulsive agony. In hydrophobia this condition of acute sensibility is observed, perhaps, in its highest degree of development, and it is frequently seen to exhibit itself for some time after death has apparently taken place.

　　In these cases, such is the morbid peripheral acuteness of sensibility, that the minimum portion of cold wind, or even a faint puff of air from the mouth, coming in contact with the cutaneous surface of the hydrophobic patient, has often induced a fearful paroxysm of spasmodic suffering. In cases of acute visceral inflammation involving some of the ganglia of the great sympathetic nerve, the general sensibility has become keenly acute. In certain hysterical affections of women the sensation is often intensely manifested. To such a degree has this hyperæsthesia been observed, that the patients have been known to scream violently when the skin has been only touched. The faintest whisper, sudden opening of a door, or ruffle of a newspaper, has been known, in such cases, to induce severe conditions of violent convulsive spasm. It is difficult satisfactorily to explain this phenomenon, but as described here, it is frequently observed in practice.

Occasionally, in the incipient stage of inflammation of the encephalon, an exalted condition of sensation is noticed. The same phenomenon is apparent in cases of tumors interfering with the *corpora restiforma, pons varolii, processus cerebelli, corpora quadragemina.* An exaltation of sensibility, both special and general, has been frequently observed in diffused neuralgic conditions, and when connected with cephalalgia of long continuance, and associated with morbid psychical phenomena, it should always command attention in cases of supposed disease of the brain and spinal cord.[1] Hyperæsthesia of the special sensorial ganglia will be more particularly referred to when I proceed to a consideration of the exaltations of special sensibility, viz. :—

      a. Vision.
      β. Hearing.
      γ. Taste.
      δ. Touch.

Epileptic Vertigo.—Physiologists have described various types of vertigo. 1. When the body appears to move backwards and forwards. 2. In which the movement seems to be on one side. 3. When the illusory sensation is rotatory. It is not my intention to consider in detail these various phases of vertiginous sensation.

In all affections of the brain, the sensation of illusory move-

---

[1] Spinal softening is often connected with a profound pain occupying the depth of the limb or following the course of the great nervous trunks. Exalted sensibility is, as Andral observes, liable to be mistaken for neuralgia. In other cases these pains do not exist. The limb is merely benumbed, the extreme parts are cold and less sensible than they should be. The patient, says Andral, treats these incipient symptoms with neglect, but the disease marches on, the *engourdissement* and insensibility gradually increase, and then paralysis ensues. Andral refers to the particulars of a case in which the chief symptom for two consecutive months was nothing more than a sensation of cold—of intense cold—occupying the extremities of the fingers and toes. This symptom continued without any change for eight weeks. It was suddenly changed to a pricking kind of feeling in the same part. After a short time the extremities were seized with a brusque convulsive movement, "des mouvements saccadés." These latter symptoms continued to progress until followed by characteristic signs of spinal softening.

ments termed vertigo, or giddiness, stand prominently forward among the significant and important incipient symptoms. In some respects it is more characteristically diagnostic of serious cerebral disease, organic and functional, than that of headache, even in its more acute form of manifestation. If the vertigo be clearly an idiopathic encephalic affection, and not, as is often the case, symptomatic of some form of stomach, heart, hepatic, visceral, renal, or blood disease, we may infer that the state of the brain is entitled to careful pathological analysis, and earnest therapeutic consideration.

This phase of disordered sensibility, when not obviously arising from the above causes, or connected with states of poisoned blood, resulting from retained excretions, or presence of a toxic agent in the vital fluid, generally indicates serious disturbance of the cranial circulation, and is frequently dependent upon a want of normal balance in the amount of blood distributed to the various sinuses as well as to the venous and arterial cerebral vessels.

The cerebral type of vertigo is easily diagnosed by the absence of those affections of other organs which sympathetically disorder the brain, such as gastric and hepatic derangement, loss of blood, and long-continued, exhausting discharges from various parts of the body.[1]

[1] " Vertigo or giddiness," says Dr. Clutterbuck, " though unattended with pain, is, in general, of a more dangerous nature than the severest headache. Vertigo consists in a disturbance of the *voluntary power*, and in some degree of *sensation*, especially of *vision ;* and thus it shows itself to be an affection of the brain itself; while mere pain in the head does not necessarily imply this, it being for the most part an affection of the membranes only. In *vertigo*, objects that are fixed appear to be in motion, or to turn round, as the name implies. The patient loses his balance, and is inclined to fall down. It often is followed immediately by severe headache. *Vertigo* is apt to recur, and thus often becomes frequent and habitual. After a time the mental powers become impaired, and complete idiocy often follows, as was the case in the celebrated Dean Swift. It frequently terminates in apoplexy or palsy, from the extension of disease in the brain.

" Vertigo is induced by whatever is capable of disturbing suddenly the circulation of the brain, whether in the way of increase or diminution : thus the approach of *syncope*, whether produced by loss of blood, or a feeling of nausea ; blows on the head, occasioning a concussion of the brain ; stooping ; swinging; whirling ; or other unusual motions of the body, as in sailing, are the ordinary exciting causes of the disease. *Vertigo* is exceedingly frequent at an advanced period of life, and generally indicates the approach and formation of disease in the brain. Accordingly, it is a frequent forerunner of *apoplexy* and *palsy*.

" The immediate or *proximate* cause of giddiness or vertigo, that is, the actual con-

The most important form of vertigo is undoubtedly that associated with obscure and often hidden types of epilepsy, and it is to this form of neurosis of sensibility I am particularly desirous of directing special attention.

This type of epilepsy has been termed by the French pathologists, the *Petit-mal*, and, by English writers, epileptic vertigo. It is observed, at all periods of life, in various degrees of severity. It is a common affection of childhood, and often, before its existence is suspected, fatally damages the bodily health and undermines the intelligence. Much of the defective and enfeebled intellect observed among children, associated with great disorder of the general health and impaired vital and nerve-force arises from this subtle and mischievous phase of epilepsy.

In the majority of cases, particularly in adults, these attacks of *pseudo* epilepsy are unassociated with any form of convulsive action. The patient never falls down in a characteristic fit, neither is he deprived for any length of time of consciousness. The malady exhibits itself at all periods of the day, and in all possible positions of the body. The fit occurs in the middle of the night, during the transition state between sleeping and waking, early in the morning on first rising, during meals, whilst engaged in conversation, and when walking in the streets. The patient, for a second or two, and occasionally for a longer period, is seized with severe vertigo, and momentarily loses his consciousness. This disorder of sensation often developes itself whilst the patient is actively engaged in his accustomed vocation. I have known clergymen attacked whilst preaching in the pulpit, merchants when engaged at the desk, or on the Stock Exchange, barristers whilst

dition of the brain at the moment, is probably some partial disturbance in the circulation there; which all the *occasional causes* mentioned are obviously calculated to produce. It is more or less dangerous, according to the cause inducing it, and the state of the brain itself, which may be sound or otherwise. And as this cannot be certainly known, nor the extent of it when actually present, the event is of course uncertain. At all times, your *prognosis* should be guarded; because *vertigo* seldom occurs under favorable circumstances of age and general health; unless when produced by so slight a cause as *bloodletting*, or a trifling blow upon the head. Whenever *vertigo* recurs frequently, and at an advanced period of life, and more particularly when it is accompanied with drowsiness, weakness of the voluntary muscles, impaired memory or judgment, or, in short, any other disturbance or imperfection in the state of the *sensorial* functions, an unfavorable result is to be expected; because all these afford decisive evidence of a considerable degree and extent of disease in the brain."

28

addressing courts of law. I have in many cases traced the
malady back for a period of some years, manifesting itself under
all conceivable physical and mental conditions. This affection is
rarely considered of an important character, until the bodily
health and mental condition of the patient begin to be affected.
It is then discovered that the invalid has been subject for a lengthened time to undetected and unobserved attacks of epileptic
vertigo, which have been considered either as symptomatic of a
disordered state of the stomach or liver, or as simple fits of ordinary syncope.

"It is scarcely possible," says Trousseau, "to describe these
epileptic attacks except by examples. In childhood, when it is
especially common, it may manifest itself thus: The child stops
short in the middle of its play, remains motionless, with fixed eye
and suspended respiration, returning to itself after seven or eight
seconds, and sometimes hardly two. We may observe analogous
examples in the adult. A person while playing at cards finds the
movement of his hand suddenly arrested when about to play, the
card remaining in his hand as if affixed to it. A deep inspiration
occurs, the suspended movement is completed, and the vertigo has
passed away. At other times the patient rises, walks he knows
not where, striking against objects, and stops short at the instant
he returns to himself. At others he mumbles some unintelligible
words, or repeats the same word, as his own name, obstinately,
during seven or eight seconds. In all these cases the individual
is completely without the external world. Sensation is abolished,
and we may shake or pinch him without his feeling anything. In
certain cases, as in a patient now in the wards, the vertigo is announced by a peculiar sensation, to which authors have given the
name of *aura*, and which, in the great majority of cases, consists
in the feeling of a current, that mounts up from one of the limbs,
or some other point of the surface, towards the head. At other
times there is a sensation of pain, of formication, or of little imperceptible convulsive shocks. In a great number of cases these
phenomena constitute the entire affection, and deserve the name
of epileptic vertigo. At others, they go on increasing until the
fit itself occurs, and then it is usually by the thumb that the
aura commences. But the fit is only preceded by the aura quite
exceptionally."

A child, five years of age, was brought for M. Trousseau's ad-

vice. Several times a week, and more than once a day, the child
became the subject of hiccough, which, accompanied by remarkable paleness, lasted for several seconds, and never more than a
minute, headache and hebetude succeeding. M. Trousseau, alone
in his opinion, pronounced this epilepsy, and a year after the
child had regular epileptic fits. "At other times," says the same
authority, "epilepsy manifests itself by a marked sensation of
cardiac suffocation. The patient, seized with most violent palpitations, becomes extremely pale, and loses all consciousness. In
ordinary palpitation, consciousness is always preserved; and it is
well to be aware of these palpitations in the epileptic, since the
patient complaining only of his heart, an erroneous idea of the
nature of the disease may be easily formed.

"Disturbances of the intellect are very frequent after the epileptic fit, and they are also met with subsequent to the vertigo.
The head is heavy and aching, the patient being morose and taciturn, and as if stupefied for a while,—for a half or whole hour.
For the purpose of diagnosis, it is of extreme importance to observe these changes; for we find them as a consequence of no
other nervous spasm, however violent it may have been. There
may be exhaustion after a violent fit of hysteria, but the intellect
always remains very clear. This relative confusion of the mental
powers may escape the physician's attention, but it is very rare
for it to escape that of the patient or his relatives, so that they
should be always interrogated upon this point.

"There is nothing special in the vertiginous form, as it depends
upon the same causes as the fit; and very often we observe alternations of the vertigo and the fits in the same subject. It is by no
means rare, however, to find, after from one to ten years' time,
the fits entirely displace the vertigo."

There is no type of epilepsy so fearfully and fatally destructive
to the intelligence as that previously described. It is generally
associated with obscure and not easily detected or defined changes
in the cerebral tissue. These pathological alterations are more
particularly diagnosed in the advanced stage of the affection.
Hence the grave importance of an early recognition of this subtle
and insidious form of vertigo, and the necessity for a speedy administration of remedies for its cure.

HEADACHE.—This type of hyperæsthesia of the brain will be
considered more in detail when, in the concluding section of the

work, I address myself particularly to an analysis of the general principles of diagnosis. It may be affirmed, as a *postulate*, that all organic diseases of the brain are accompanied by vertigo, headache, acute and chronic, or by some abnormal physical sensation within the cranium. Cephalalgia, however, may be considered as an almost invariable accompaniment of all cerebral affections. This symptom is rarely absent, particularly in the early or acute stage of the encephalic disease. In some forms of tumor, and in those obscure alterations of tissue connected with general paralysis, the patient often positively denies that he has headache, or ever was subject to any cerebral pain or uneasiness. I have, however, after minute inquiry, generally ascertained that cephalalgia has existed, but been forgotten by the patient, arising in many instances from an impairment of intelligence and loss of memory. In cases of advanced general paralysis and chronic softening of the brain, the patient stoutly maintains that he is quite free from all headache, and will not admit that he suffers from vertigo, or any description of uneasiness within the cranium, but his actions clearly demonstrate that there exists a hyperæsthesia of the brain.

" With the exception of atrophy," says Romberg, "none of the diseases of the brain occur unaccompanied by headache." Nasse affirms that pain of the head is one of the most constant symptoms associated with cerebral tumors. It always exists, particularly in central softening of the brain involving the corpus callosum, septum lucidum, fornix, and the ventricular parietes. Dr. Todd says, that disease of the corpus striatum and optic thalamus is attended with little or no localized pain pointing out the exact seat of the lesion.

In abscess of the brain, headache, paroxysmal in its character, is rarely absent. In all the affections of the encephalon consequent upon chronic otorrhœa, the same symptom is generally present. Apoplexy is almost invariably preceded by either severe vertigo, noises in the head, confusion of intellect, or severe paroxysms of cephalalgia. In cerebral hemorrhage, the patient is often heard to complain, immediately prior to the attack, of a sensation in the head giving rise to the impression that an actual laceration of the cerebral substance has taken place.

Pain of the head does not always denote the character of the cerebral lesion. It may accompany, as Andral remarks, the most varied morbid condition of the contents of the cranium, bones, membranes, injection of their tissue, formation of concretions on the free surface of the arachnoid, purulent infiltration of the pia mater, or effusion of pus or serum into the ventricles.

According to the opinions of some authorities, this symptom of organic disease of the brain has been somewhat exaggerated.[1] It

[1] "Cephalalgia is a symptom of less frequent occurrence than we might have anticipated—a fact which negatively demonstrates the necessity of additional care in attending to other signs indicating disturbance of the nervous centres. The analysis of authentic cases of this description also shows that there is no definite relation except in the instance of the cerebellum, between the site of the lesion and the site of the previous pain. With a view to determining these points, I have gone through the cases recorded in Dr. Abercrombie's work on diseases of the brain, and Andral's fifth volume of that monument of talent, industry, and logical induction, the 'Clinique Médicale.' The results of the experience of the British and the French physician are numerically wider apart than we should have expected, though they coincide in proving that undoubted cerebral mischief frequently is unassociated with cephalalgia.

"We take first—by the laws of courtesy—the foreign author. He gives one hundred and eight cases in which death was manifestly due to intra-cranial disease, as confirmed by *post-mortem* examination; or in which, though the fatal issue was immediately due to other causes, the cadaveric section demonstrated coincident cerebral disorganization.

"In conformity with the observations of Andral, the ratio in which headache accompanies intra-cranial mischief is as forty-five to sixty-one, or nearly as two to three: if we subtract the apoplectic cases, in which this symptom is comparatively of less import, we obtain a ratio of thirty-nine to forty; in other words, the frequency and absence of headache are almost equal, or, to use a sporting phrase, it is an even chance whether the intra-cranial disease is or is not accompanied by cephalalgia.

"According to the analysis of Dr. Abercrombie's one hundred and thirty-nine histories of intra-cranial diseases, the ratio in which headache is a concomitant of organic disease of the brain is as ninety-two to thirty-eight, or nearly three to one; while by eliminating the apoplectic cases, we obtain the still higher ratio of seventy-four to fifteen, or nearly five to one.

"We cannot stop to inquire into the causes that determine so great a want of accordance between the two authors; it certainly is not due to any bias on one side or the other, because both are eminently impartial observers, and neither upholds any peculiar theory in regard to cerebral affections; nor can we suppose that the national constitution of the French and English habit of body is so different as to afford an adequate explanation of the discrepancy. Still the numbers given demonstrate that headache is an important symptom in the local affections of the cerebral system, while they also show that its absence must not be regarded as trustworthy evidence of the immunity of the cranial contents. When we examine into the occurrence of headache in the individual varieties of cephalic disease, we see that the ratio varies considerably; it is comparatively rare, as we have already seen, in apoplectic disorders; here the cerebral tissue itself is commonly primarily involved. The cases of cerebral softening in which headache is absent also predominate largely over those in which it occurs; while the reverse is the case in meningeal disease, where the frequency of cephalalgia to its absence is, according to Andral's observations, as four

has been asserted that headache is not invariably present in encephalic affections.   Cases undoubtedly occur where the patient
makes no complaint of headache, but it would be unsafe to infer,
from this repudiation of the symptom, that it has not, at any stage
of the disease, existed.   I have never carefully examined a case
of clearly developed disease of the brain, without having assured
myself that vertigo, headache, or some form of abnormal cerebral
sensation, pain, or uneasiness, has not been referred to by the
patient.

ANÆSTHESIA (loss of sensation) is more closely connected with
certain morbid cerebral states than the condition previously referred to.   •

These lesions of sensibility occur occasionally a few days and
hours before acute attacks of brain disease; sometimes, however,
the loss of sensation has been noticed to exist for years prior to
anything like active cerebral symptoms manifesting themselves.
This impairment of sensation is often most obscure in its origin,
as well as insidious in its progress.   For some time before the
patient complains of any diminution of sensibility, he is conscious

---

to three. This is in harmony with what we observe in all the organs of the body;
for, it is a rule almost without exception, that disease affecting the envelopes is accompanied by pain in a severer form and more frequent ratio than when it seizes upon
the actual parenchyma of the viscera. This point is also one that may be made
available in estimating the probable locality affected in the chronic or periodical forms
of cephalalgia. The relation of the envelopes of the brain, in a physiological point
of view, to their contents, is even of more importance, if such a remark is justifiable,
than in the cases of most other viscera, since they serve not only for protection and
for the facilitation of change of form and place, but are, at least in part, eminently
the medium of nutrition. The liver, the kidneys, the spleen, the heart, the lungs, and
the muscles, receive their supplies of the nutrient fluid by conduits that enter directly into their structure, by immediate vascular connection with the nearest arterial
trunk. The great bulk of the blood conveyed to the brain is, as it were, filtered
through the ramifications contained in the pia mater, while it quits the organ in a less
indirect course, though still in a much more circuitous manner than commonly prevails
elsewhere. Both the pia mater, therefore, as the arterial membrane, and the dura
mater, sit venia verbo, as the venous membrane, claim our attention in a point of view
distinct from that presented by the epithelial, serous, or fibro-serous membranes occurring elsewhere. I am far from asserting that we are able to localize every case
of headache in any one of the intra-cranial tissues; but it is the more necessary to
establish all the elements which may enter into the determination of the question, as
it is one upon which we are comparatively ignorant; and the whole history of medicine teaches us that we can only arrive at positive results by minute attention to all
the items constituting a complex of morbid phenomena."—Dr. Sieveking, Medical
Times and Gazette, August, 1854.

of the cutaneous surface of some part of his body being in an abnormal state.   He is observed to be rubbing his hands, arms, legs, or scalp, for the purpose of giving activity to the circulation of the blood in these parts.   The sensation at this period is simply that of numbness, in its first or earliest stage of manifestation. The patient recognizes this symptom, and eventually directs attention to it.   I attended a gentleman with hemiplegia who was annoyed by this feeling of slight numbness for *several years* before an attack of cerebral hemorrhage.   He was often seen to be apply-ing friction to his hands, arms, as well as the scalp, by means of a flesh-brush, with a view of reviving the sensibility of these portions of the body.[1]

I attended, a few years ago, a gentleman slightly insane.   He was melancholic, and imagined, without any valid reason, that his pecuniary circumstances were in an embarrassed state.   Six months before his death, he complained of numbness in his left hand and arm.   I examined him carefully, but could detect no other symp-tom of threatening acute cerebral disease.   He left London for the country, and, whilst residing there with his family, had an apo-plectic fit.   The lesion of sensibility referred to, existed for some months as the only premonitory symptom of the approaching attack.

The mucous membrane of the conjunctiva exhibits, occasionally, in the early stage of disease of the brain, a remarkable state of insensibility.   Andral remarks, that under these circumstances, the end of the finger may be passed over the entire surface of the globe of the eye without causing any irritation in the part sufficient to produce even an approximation of the eyelids.   The patients manifest no sign of pain or insensibility of the eyes even when there is no diminution of sensation in other parts of the body.

In some apoplectic cases, the same physiologist has observed a

[1] " When we read the history of trials for witchcraft," says Dr. Michéa, " we observe that the inquisitors attached a high value to the existence of *cutaneous anæsthesia* as a sign of demoniacal possession.   When an individual was charged with the alleged crime, the experts, after having bandaged the eyes, passed a magnifying glass over all parts of his body, previously shaved, with a view of discovering the mark of Satan, '*stigmata diaboli*.'   The slightest spot on the skin was probed with a needle. If the puncture did not cause a painful sensation, if it provoked no cry or movement, the poor creature was a sorcerer and condemned to be burnt alive.   If, on the con-trary, he felt the wound he was acquitted : Satan had not impressed his claw upon him."—(P. Gray, " Chirurgia," 1609, lib. vii, c. 10.)

decided impairment of sensation in one of the halves of the mucous
membrane of the nasal fossæ. In some cases, prior to an attack
of acute disease of the brain, there has been noticed a loss of sensibility on one side of the mouth. This symptom is apparent when
the patients are taking their food.

Andral relates a case of apoplexy in which a complete loss of
sensation was observed some time previously to the attack in isolated parts of the thorax. There existed in this case five or six
portions of skin, about the size of a five-franc piece each, where it
showed no signs of sensibility even when pinched or pricked with
a sharp instrument. In other parts of the thorax, the sensibility
of the skin continued intact. These circumscribed states of cutaneous insensibility were not continuous in their manifestation,
sensibility and insensibility appearing to be alternate conditions.

Decided loss of sensation is frequently preceded, in some cases
for many years, by states of numbness, which are considered unimportant, and, in fact, in many cases, are altogether neglected.
I have known several cases of apoplexy and paralysis where slight
degrees of cutaneous anæsthesia have existed for many years previously to the fatal attacks. In some instances this diminution of
sensibility has been associated with a feeling of intense cold in one
of the extremities.

Andral, Romberg, and other pathologists, have noticed this incipient symptom of apoplexy, paralysis, and softening. Among
the premonitory symptoms of cerebral hemorrhage, the former
authority has observed odd sensations confined to the tips of the
fingers, resembling a feeling of intense cold in those parts. "The
tips of the fingers," he says, "appear as if they had been plunged
into iced water." Dr. Cooke refers to a case of apoplexy where
the patient complained, some weeks before the attack, of a painful
sensation of cold in one of his feet. There was no apparent diminution of sensibility in the leg or any other part of the body. In
other cases, the anæsthesia has been confined to a side of the face,
one of the fingers, to the scalp, and in some remarkable cases on
record, the feeling of numbness has been restricted altogether to a
lateral half of one of the fingers. This was a remarkable symptom
in the case of a nobleman who died several years ago of paralysis.

These circumscribed states of impaired sensation are often valuable diagnostic signs of the commencement of softening of the brain,
particularly when the feeling of defective sensibility is limited to

one side of the body, and there exists vertigo, headache, impairment of the intelligence, or confusion of mind.

I attended a case of a gentleman who died of this disease, who, for five years before he was suspected to be suffering from ramollissement, felt a partial paralysis of sensibility in his left arm and leg. This symptom was observed, but was never considered to be cerebral in its origin. The affection was viewed as of a local character, and treated accordingly.

In other cases I have remarked, among the incipient symptoms of acute diseases of the brain, an impaired state of the function of taste consequent upon a loss of sensibility in the tongue as well as fauces. In one remarkable instance the defect of sensation was confined to one lateral half of the tongue. This symptom was only occasionally manifested, and at one period appeared altogether to subside. After the lapse of two years it recurred. The patient at this time suffered also from great general muscular debility, occasional headaches, severe attacks of vertigo, and depression of spirits. He eventually died at Berlin of well-marked symptoms of softening of the brain.

This morbid state of the nervous system is occasionally diagnosed by a sensation, not of numbness or actual anæsthesia, but a feeling of *weight* and *heaviness* in the affected part. The patient will be heard to complain of one leg, arm, or the side of the body being heavier than the other. I have observed this premonitory symptom in several cases of acute as well as chronic disease of the brain. This symptom is occasionally associated with a sensation of stiffness in the limbs and joints, as well as with spasmodic muscular contraction, deep-seated pain, and coldness in the part. Durand-Fardel refers to these symptoms when speaking of the incipient stage of cerebral softening. He remarks that they are, particularly the deep-seated pains in the limbs, significantly diagnostic of the commencement of chronic softening of the brain.

There has been much written on the subject of the insensibility of the insane, and an attempt made by several authorities to establish that a state of anæsthesia exists in the majority of cases of mental disease. Such an opinion could only have been expressed by writers practically unacquainted with the ordinary phenomena of insanity. Insane patients, as a general rule, are not reduced to a condition of anæsthesia. In many cases the sensibility, *psychical* as well as *physical*, is most acutely and painfully manifested.

Impairment of sensibility is, however, one of the characteristics of certain types and stages of insanity. This state of anæsthesia admits of a *psychical* and a *physical* explanation. In many cases the disease of the brain causing the insanity induces a paralysis throughout the whole of the body of the nerves of sensation, consequently their special function is weakened, benumbed, or entirely paralyzed. This condition of anæsthesia is observed in various degrees of manifestation, in proportion to the nature and degree of the mental alienation, or cerebral organic change.

In the early stage of general paralysis, this impairment of sensibility is well marked. The phenomenon is observed in many cases of this disease, long before it is suspected to have commenced. Deficient sensibility is occasionally manifested in many types of disease of the brain, previously to any decided and perceptible loss of motor power. Such patients are not ordinarily susceptible to the influence of marked alternations of temperature. They have been known to wander about during the most severely cold nights in a state of nudity, without exhibiting the slightest physical pain, discomfort, or uneasiness.

They often resist, when in bed, the application of any extent of bed-clothes. Occasionally it is necessary for their protection to mechanically fix the blankets to the bed-posts ; but this is often resisted, even in very severely cold weather. This state of insensibility prevails throughout the whole of the body, internally as well as externally. The mucous membrane of the stomach and intestinal canal participate in the anæsthesia. The peristaltic action of the intestines either altogether ceases, or is considerably impaired. All the organic functions of animal life are altered in tone and vigor. Hence large and active doses of cathartic medicine produce no salutary stimulating effect upon the lining membrane of the bowels, and opium in heroic proportions is administered without in the slightest degree influencing the brain or nervous system. In these cases there appears to be a general sluggish state of mind and body, mental and physical stimuli making no impression upon the one or the other. This condition of insensibility may arise from the preoccupation of the mind in an intensely morbid contemplation of fixed, engrossing insane delusions or hallucinations. Pinel, speaking of the insensibility of the insane, says :—

" Their insensibility is so great, that instances occur of patients with comminuted fractures of the lower extremities tearing off their bandages and splints, and trying to walk with their broken limbs, without betraying the slightest feeling of pain ; and of others who, with broken ribs, sing and dance without showing the slightest sign of suffering. Patients, in short, who have been operated on for hernia, have introduced their fingers into the wounds, and in the coolest manner amused themselves by pulling out their intestines, as if they were manœuvring on a dead body."

A patient in Bethlem Hospital some years ago attempted suicide in the most determined manner. He watched his opportunity whilst the attendants were out of the ward, and then went and deliberately laid the back of his head upon the fire, and held it there, without flinching or apparent suffering, until a large portion of the scalp was burnt away. Very extensive sloughing and exfoliation of the bone ensued. The patient recovered from the effects of the injury without appearing to suffer any particular pain, and lived twelve or thirteen years afterwards. His skull, in the museum, St. Bartholomew's Hospital, shows the whole of the parietal bones exfoliated. The brain was protected by a tough dense membrane stretched across the opening.[1]

An insane gentleman, aged thirty-two, suffering from suicidal melancholia, succeeded, during the temporary absence of the servant who was employed to watch him, in thrusting his foot into a bright, blazing fire. He voluntarily held it in this position until the flesh was nearly burnt to the bone. He was never heard to complain of a sensation of pain until he recovered from his mental disorder. He then alleged he felt great uneasiness in the injured limb.

A French dragoon became insane from the effects of a *coup de soleil* during the Peninsular war. In a paroxysm of delirium he obtained access to the kitchen of the hospital, seized hold of a vessel that was on the fire, and drank at a draught about a pint of boiling water. He then quietly returned to bed, without complaining of the slightest pain or discomfort.

Insane patients have been known to expose themselves to the

---

[1] " Lectures on Insanity," by Sir A. Morison, M.D.

severest degrees of cold in the depth of winter without apparent suffering. Lunatics, influenced by religious delusions, have scooped out the eyes, cut away the tongue, and even emasculated themselves without exhibiting any consciousness or evidence of pain. An insane woman deliberately put her hand in the fire, and held it there until it nearly dropped from the wrist, without feeling (as she said) any sensation. She laughed at the idea of the suggestion made to her that she must have undergone great torture whilst voluntarily holding her hand in the burning flame.

A mistress of Robespierre became insane, and was sent to the Salpêtrière. She would not lie down in bed till she had drenched it with a bucketful of water. Pinel mentions the case of a man confined in the Bicêtre, who, in the depth of winter, when the thermometer stood at twenty, twenty-five, and even thirty degrees below the freezing-point, had such a sensation of heat in his system that he could not bear a single blanket, but remained seated all night on the frozen pavement of his cell, and scarcely was the door open in the morning, when he ran out in his shirt, and applied quantities of snow to his chest, and allowed it to melt with a delight like that experienced by persons when breathing cool air in the dog-days.

M. Verga has published in one of the Italian journals a case to illustrate the extreme insensibility of the insane to suffering. A deranged person ate and drank heartily to the last day of his life; he died during a violent paroxysm of asthma. Upon examination after death, it was found there was a most extensive ulceration of the stomach. The disorganization had advanced to a striking extent without its having apparently had the slightest effect upon the sensibility of the patient.

In speaking of the anæsthesia of the insane, Dr. Browne says: "This torpidity of the nervous system is chiefly manifested in melancholic females. Suicide and self-mutilation, of the most cruel and appalling kinds, have been practised; the religious fanatics, called the Convulsionaires of St. Medard, bore with pleasure and relief to the hysteric ecstasy into which they were thrown, the infliction of every species of torture. Cases occur in every asylum of complete anæsthesia, in which operations have been performed, and pain induced therapeutically by blisters, cupping, &c., and no cry or confession of uneasiness been elicited; where diseases attended by suffering, even by excruciating agony, have advanced to a fatal issue unnoticed, perhaps unknown to the victim, showing that even the ganglionic feeling, which is exalted in many other examples of melancholia, is here suspended or impaired.   There is among the melancholic patients a case of experimental suicide, who has tried upon his own person various means to extinguish life, partly to determine the comparative merits of the different physical modes of escaping from moral disquietude, and who was only prevented from accomplishing his purpose by strangulation with his own hands, in consequence of the loss of consciousness."

This destruction of sensibility is most frequently observed among the class of the insane termed monomaniacs.   Dr. Haslam refers to the case of a woman who seriously mutilated herself by grinding into powder with her teeth a quantity of glass.   She appeared to suffer no pain.   Esquirol observes that he has applied blisters, setons, moxas, and actual cautery, to patients strongly disposed to suicide, with a view of testing their sensibility, but has not been able to produce a sensation of pain.   A woman, suffering from religious delirium, injured herself very severely.   She only expressed one single regret, viz., that of not having succeeded in destroying herself.   A young lunatic, a prey to religious exaltation, steeped his arm in boiling water.   He never ceased, during this paroxysm of delirium, in singing loudly the praises of God.   He appeared quite insensible to pain.   The injury was followed by enormous suppuration.   His skin fell into shreds, leaving the bones almost bare.   The physical wound appeared for the time to master and overpower the delirium, and the patient then suffered acutely from the self-inflicted injury.   His mind at this time was exclusively absorbed with the idea of undergoing the amputation of the arm, which the surgeon considered necessary to perform for the safety of his life.[1]

In many cases of insanity, incurable and fatal structural disease has been known to originate and progress unobserved, owing to this condition of vital and organic insensibility.   The lungs, stomach, liver, kidneys, heart, bladder, and intestines have occasionally exhibited after death serious lesions, the existence of which was never suspected during the life of the patient.   Organic structures appear in insanity to undergo important and often unobserved material modifications; hence the grave necessity of watching closely the

---

[1] "Traité des Maladies Mentales," par le Docteur B. A. Morel.   Paris, 1860.

pathological state of the insane, with the view of detecting, at the earliest possible period, the presence of certain physical complications often seriously interfering with the mental recovery of the patient, and proving perilous to his life.

I have known patients suffering from active inflammation of the pleura as well as lungs, repudiate all idea of indisposition. A gentleman, who had a large calculus in his bladder, declared that it gave him no kind of uneasiness. Had he been sane, exhibiting an abnormal degree of sensibility, I am satisfied his agony would have been intense. I have witnessed operations of a very painful character performed upon the insane without giving rise to any apparent disturbance of their sensibility.

I have not yet referred to the anæsthesia of the insane resulting from the preoccupation or intense absorption of the imagination, in some fearful hallucination of the mind, or all-engrossing monomaniacal illusion of the senses. I have no doubt that much of the apparent physical insensibility of the insane arises from this cause. Insanity often effectually masks and obscures all evidence of organic sensibility, the greater malady effectually paralyzing the functions of the sensor nerves.

When Lear, Kent, and the Fool are standing alone on the wild heath, exposed to the raging of the pitiless storm, Kent affectionately and feelingly implores the king to seek shelter in an adjoining hovel from the "tyranny of the open night." In answer to this appeal, Lear exclaims:

> " Thou think'st 'tis much, that this contentious storm
> Invades us to the skin : so 'tis to thee ;
> But *where the greater malady is fixed,*
> *The lesser is scarce felt ;*
> . . . . *The tempest in my mind*
> *Doth from my senses take all feeling else,*
> *Save what beats there.*"

Analogous psychical and physical phenomena are exhibited in certain conditions of morbid exaltation of the conscience in connection with the religious and superstitious observances of barbarous and uncivilized nations. Persons have been known, after having excited themselves to the highest pitch of enthusiastic ecstasy, to burn, cut, and maim their bodies in the severest possible manner, without exhibiting the slightest symptom of sensibility.[1]

VITIATED SENSATION.—In the incipient stage of various forms of cerebral disease, the sensibility is not only heightened, impaired, and paralyzed, but it shows marked evidence of being vitiated. The patient complains of the existence of pricking sensations in various parts of the body, as well as of the existence of formication, particularly at the extremities of the fingers and toes. For some time previously to the development of well-marked symptoms of cerebral disease, a patient remarked that everything he touched was extremely cold. In some cases a gritty body, like that of sand, and a piece of cloth, appeared to be interposed be-

[1] Mr. Catlin, in his "*Notes on the North American Indians*," vol. ii, p. 170, refers (and the facts he records afford a good illustration of the effects of intense mental preoccupation in blunting the sensibility) to the self-imposed tortures of the Mandan Indians, for the purpose of qualifying themselves for the honored rank of warriors. "One at a time the young fellows, already emaciated with fasting, and thirsting, and waking, for nearly four days and nights, advanced from the side of the lodge, and placed himself on his hands and feet, or otherwise, as best adapted for the performance of the operation, where he submitted to the cruelties in the following manner. One inch or more of the flesh of each shoulder was taken up between the finger and thumb by the man who held the knife in his right hand, and the knife, which had been ground sharp at both edges and then hacked and notched with the blade of another, to make it produce as much pain as possible, was forced through the flesh below the fingers, and being withdrawn, was followed by a splint or skewer from the other, who held a bundle of such in his left hand, and was ready to force them through the wound. There were then two cords lowered down from the top of the lodge, which were fastened to these splints or skewers, and they instantly began to haul him up: he was thus raised until his body was just suspended from the ground where he rested, until the knife and a splint were passed through the flesh or integuments in a similar manner on each arm below the shoulder, below the elbow, on the thighs, and below the knees. In some instances they remained in a reclining posture on the ground, until this painful operation was finished, which was performed in all instances exactly on the same parts of the bodies and limbs, and which, in its progress, occupied some five or six minutes.

"Each one was then instantly raised with the cords, until the weight of his body was suspended by them, and then, while the blood was streaming down their limbs, the bystanders hung upon the splints each man's appropriate shield, bow, quiver, &c., and in many instances the skull of a buffalo, with the horns on it, was attached to each lower arm and each lower leg, for the purpose, probably, of preventing, by their great weight, the struggling which might otherwise take place to their disadvantage whilst they were hung up. When these things were all adjusted, each one was raised higher by the cords, until these weights all swung clear from the ground. . . . . The unflinching fortitude with which every one of them bore this part of the torture surpassed credibility."

tween the patient's fingers and whatever they came in contact with. Other invalids have affirmed, that whatever they touched felt like a piece of *velvet*. Andral notices this phenomenon.[1] Six weeks before a paralytic attack, a patient complained of one-half of the scalp feeling like a piece of leather. In the case of a gentleman who died of apoplexy, there was for some time previously to his illness a feeling in both hands as if the skin were covered with minute and irritating particles of dust or sand. He repeatedly complained of this symptom, and was frequently observed to wash his hands with the view of removing the imaginary annoyance. Impairment of sensibility in the arm, preceded first by a feeling of intense cold in the part, and subsequently of numbness, followed this perverted state of the sensation. The patient had also slight paroxysmal attacks of headache, and, occasionally, considerable confusion of thought. In another case, some time prior to a paralytic seizure, the patient imagined that he had extraneous particles of dirt and stones in his boots, or inside his stockings, irritating his feet, and interfering with his personal comfort, as well as freedom of locomotion. This perverted state of the sensation was observed for *two months* previously to his attack of acute cerebral disorder.

---

[1] He terms it the "*velvet-like sensation*" accompanying the alterations of sensation preceding attacks of paralysis and softening.

CHAPTER XXI.

THIS section of the subject will be considered in the following order :—

    a. Sight.
    β. Hearing.
    γ. Taste.
    δ. Touch.
    ε. Smell.

In estimating the value of all morbid evidences of the special senses, supposed to be symptomatic of brain disease, we must carefully consider their normal state, making proper allowances for any previously existing idiosyncrasies in their mode of action. The sense of vision, of hearing, &c., is occasionally seen extraordinarily acute. I have known individuals in whom the sense of smell and taste was so exquisitely developed, that certain substances and odors produced a severe degree of mental torture, when brought in contact with the gustatory and nasal organs. The slightest particle of ipecacuanha has caused violent vomiting in certain nervous temperaments. In other instances, the smell of rhubarb has produced a severe action upon the bowels, and the faintest odor of aloes has affected, in a marked manner, the lower portion of the bowels. It is literally true that a person may

        "Die of a rose in aromatic pain,"

for there exists among the North American Indians a tribe whose mode of punishment consists in subjecting their prisoners to the influence of the odors of certain plants. This produces the most exquisite mental distress and bodily pain; and occasionally, if the

29

prisoner be exposed long to its influence, death has been known to ensue.

It is said that in some portions of China, and in the South Sea Islands, the natives are in the habit of exposing their victims as a punishment to what Falstaff terms, the "rankest compound of villanous smells."

We occasionally observe unnatural manifestations and exquisite conditions of the sense of seeing, hearing, touch, and taste, quite apart from disease of the brain. In some persons the sense of hearing is in an exalted state of manifestation, the slightest sound coming from remote distances being at once perceptible. Celebrated musicians, owing in the first place to the natural vigor and acuteness of the sense of hearing, and, secondly, to the careful education and long-continued exercise of this faculty, have had this special sense in a high state of activity. It is said of Mozart that, during the performance of a most complicated piece of concerted music, he was able, among several hundred musicians, to detect with wonderful precision and quickness the slightest deviation from the correct score. He was able also to name the instrument that was at fault. Any aberration of harmony produced the most painful sensations in the nervous system of this wonderful musical genius.

Among blind persons we often notice an extraordinary capacity of recognizing objects by the sense of touch. A person who became blind at an early period of life, was able to distinguish individually, by means of the touch, a number of botanical plants, and to single them out with wonderful accuracy. We occasionally witness, as the effects of certain diseases, particularly of the nervous system, a great acuteness in the capacity of the special senses, as well as positive perversion in their modes of action.

I have known instances in which the sense of hearing and smell have become painfully sensitive after recovery from attacks of fever, conditions of nervous debility and exhaustion. In other cases the various special senses have been perverted, or their functions either diminished in power, or entirely lost.

Dr. Heberden records the particulars of the following case: "A man about forty years old had in the spring a tertian fever, for which he took too small a quantity of bark, so that the returns of it were weakened without being removed. Three days after his last fit, being then employed on board a ship in the river, he

observed at sun-setting that all objects began to look blue, which
blueness gradually thickened into a cloud; and not long after, he
became so blind as hardly to perceive the light of a candle. The
next morning, about sun-rising, his sight was restored as perfectly
as ever. When the next night came on, he lost his sight again in
the same manner, and this continued for twelve days and nights.
He then came ashore, where the disorder of his eyes gradually
abated, and in three days was entirely gone. A month after he
went on board another ship, and after three days' stay in it the
night blindness returned as before, and lasted all the time of his
remaining in the ship, which was nine nights. He then left the
ship, and his blindness did not return while he was upon land.
Some little time afterwards he went into another ship, in which he
continued for ten days, during which time the blindness returned
only two nights, and never afterwards." It appears, however,
that this individual had previously labored under an affection
produced by the use of lead, which had left him in a state of much
nervous debility. Notwithstanding this circumstance, this' case
clearly proves that the affection is liable to be increased and
brought on by local influences.

A lady of advanced age, lodged on the eastern coast of Kent,
in a house that looked immediately upon the sea, and exposed to
the glare of the morning sun. The curtains of her room were
white, a circumstance which added to the intensity of the light.
When she had been there about ten days, she observed one evening, at the time of sunset, that first the fringes of the clouds
appeared red, and soon after the same color was diffused over all
the objects around her, especially if they were white. This lasted
the whole night, but in the morning her sight was again perfect.
This alternation of morbid with sound sight prevailed the whole of
the time the lady resided on the coast, which was three weeks;
and for nearly as long after she left it, at which time it ceased
suddenly of its own accord.

Some remarkable instances are recorded of want of power in
distinguishing colors. These facts are important to bear in mind
when testing the healthy condition of the organs of vision. In
some cases a morbid condition of this sense (symptomatic of
centric disease of the brain) consists in the patient not being able
to distinguish one color from another, as well as in their observing
certain objects surrounded by a halo, variously colored and tinted.

Dr. Priestley has published a curious case of error of color in five brothers and two sisters, all adults. One of the brothers could form no idea whatever of colors, though he judged very accurately of the form and other qualities of objects; hence he thought stockings were sufficiently distinguished by the name of stockings, and could not conceive the necessity of calling them white or black. He could perceive cherries on a tree; but only distinguished them, even when red-ripe, from the surrounding leaves by their size and shape. One of the brothers appeared to have a faint sense of a few colors, but still a very imperfect notion; and upon the whole, they did not seem to possess any other distinguishing power than that of light and shade, into which they resolved all the colors presented to them—so that dove, or straw color, was regarded as white; and green, crimson, and purple, as black or dark. On looking at a rainbow, one of them could distinguish that it consisted of stripes, but nothing more. Dr. Nicholl relates the case of a boy who confounded green with red; and called light red and pink, blue. His maternal grandfather and one uncle had the same imperfection.

CHAPTER XXII.

MORBID PHENOMENA OF VISION.

In diseases of the brain the visual power may be,

α. *Impaired,*
β. *Lost,*
γ. *Exalted,*
δ. *Perverted.*

IMPAIRMENT AND LOSS OF VISION.—These are common and important symptoms of organic disease of the brain. The impairment of vision may come on gradually or occur suddenly. The sight is occasionally lost in one eye before the defect is observed, but, as a general rule, the disordered function of the eye, is of slow and progressive growth, proceeding, *pari passu*, with the development of subtle structural changes in the delicate tissue of the brain, its membranes and vessels, more immediately connected with the origin, course, and distribution of the optic nerves.

Impairment of vision is often symptomatic of gastric, hepatic, and intestinal derangement. It is of importance not to overlook this fact, when diagnosing a suspected condition of brain disease, associated with what may be considered, symptoms of cerebral amaurosis.

This affection of sight arises, occasionally, from general debility, hemorrhage, morbid states of the blood, and exhausting and debilitating discharges. Sudden loss of vision has been known to succeed a severe mental shock. It is observed as one of the consequences of typhus fever, and frequently succeeds blows upon the head, after the acute cerebral symptoms so induced have subsided. This condition of vision may also be the effect of lead poison, syphilis, the effect of tabes dorsalis, arthritis, or be consequent upon great and long-continued anxiety, and distress of mind, inter-

fering with the nutrition, and causing atrophy of those portions of
the brain more immediately connected with the optic nerve.

Dr. F. Hawkins, when speaking of the inflammatory affections
of the brain, says: "It is well known that sympathy with the
nerves of the digestive organs will give rise to various affections
of vision, from the slightest dimness up to temporary amaurosis,
from the occasional appearance of a luminous spot, up to that of
forms and spectra which are shaped by the imagination into distinct
apparitions. It is difficult, therefore, to arrive at any certain
conclusion with respect to the existence of cerebral disease from
the indications afforded by the organs of vision; and numerous
cases of affection of the optic nerves have been considered as only
sympathetic, which, in fact, were symptoms of disease acting at
once on the origin of those nerves of the brain. A gentleman
came to town about two years ago on discovering suddenly, with
surprise and alarm, that the sight of one eye had utterly failed
him. He consulted all the oculists and surgeons chiefly celebrated
for the treatment of such cases, and most of them were of opinion
that this partial defect of vision was purely sympathetic, and
would be removed by the use of senna and blue pill, and in fact it
was, to a certain extent, so removed: but as he died soon afterwards
in Ireland, with the symptoms, as I have been informed, of disease
of the brain, and as he inherited, and himself evinced, a tendency
to cerebral disorder, which appeared to be hereditary (his mother
being at this moment afflicted with hemiplegia), I think there can
be little doubt that his temporary loss of sight was a symptom, not
merely, as it was supposed, of dyspepsia, but of a morbid state then
existing in the brain. In a recent case of paralysis, the occurrence and fatal termination of which the friends of science everywhere deplore, it appeared from the result that a singular affection
of the optic nerves, which had previously been attributed to
derangement of the stomach, indicated with too much truth the
existence of irritation or pressure, affecting the origin of one of
those nerves."[1]

In the early stages of cerebral amaurosis, termed amblyopia, or
incomplete amaurosis, the patient complains of his vision becoming
gradually indistinct, objects appearing either lighted up by a bright
flame, or surrounded by a fog or mist. These symptoms are

[1] "Croonian Lectures on the Inflammatory Affections of the Brain," by F. Hawkins, M.D.

somewhat analogous to those described by Romberg as symptomatic of *gutta serena.*

"The outlines of objects," says Romberg, "appear not only indistinct, but also broken, and thus disfigured. The light of the candle appears rent; while reading, the patient misses single syllables, words, and lines, and he is forced to follow them by moving his eye, head, or entire body. At times, the upper or lower, the right or left half, the circumference or centre of the object only is seen; at others the loss of vision is still more partial, and is confined to different spots of small extent, and with differently shaped outlines. Instances also occur in which the object is only seen when it bears a definite relation to the eye, and it vanishes on the slightest movement of the eye or head."

Let me consider briefly some of the more characteristic symptoms of centric cerebral amaurosis connected with organic diseases of the brain, and disturbances of the cerebral circulation. The ordinary premonitory or associated symptoms, by means of which we may be facilitated in our diagnosis of *cerebral* from *sympathetic* conditions of morbid vision are as follows:—[1]

In all cases of centric cerebral amaurosis, the patient complains of vertigo and headache. The cephalalgia is sometimes acute in character, but occasionally of so mild a type as altogether to escape observation. The headache is associated occasionally with sympathetic affections of the other organs of sense, such as the hearing, smelling, &c. The mind in many cases also exhibits symptoms of disorder. The patient complains at times of great depression of spirits, is occasionally suicidal, and frequently troubled with hallucinations.

The cephalalgia of centric cerebral amaurosis, is, according to the experience of all authorities, not generally of a permanent and stationary kind; it occasionally entirely disappears, but is extremely liable to recur in violent paroxysms. "The remissions," says Dr. Copland, "from this severe suffering are often so remarkable as to lead a superficial observer to the belief, that it is merely

[1] Mr. Jabez Hogg has called professional attention to an extremely ingenious instrument, termed the "*Ophthalmoscope*," by means of which the more obscure diseases of the eye are easily detected, and diagnosed. This discovery will effectually aid the physician in distinguishing *cerebral* from those amaurotic affections, the effect of organic changes in the delicate structure of the eye itself.—(*Vide* Mr. Hogg "*On the Use of the Ophthalmoscope in the Exploration of Internal Diseases of the Eye.*" London, 1859.)

periodical headache connected with dyspepsia."[1]   The character
of the headache differs remarkably in various cases.   Sometimes
it is acute and lancinating; in other instances it is oppressive and
obtuse.   The pain is frequently referred to a particular spot.
During the severe paroxysms, the headache is aggravated to perfect torture by the slightest motion, is greatly increased by mental
application, aggravated when the patient stoops, and becomes
acute under the influence of stimulants.

Dyspeptic symptoms, often accompanying a pain and sickness of
the stomach, occur occasionally during the severer paroxysms of
cephalalgia.   When alluding to these symptoms, Dr. Abercrombie
observes, " After some continuance of fixed headache, the organs
of sense become affected, as the sight, the hearing, the taste, and
smell, and occasionally the intellect."   The loss of sight generally takes place gradually, being first obscured, and, after some
time, entirely lost.

Double vision soon supervenes.   This condition may either be
permanent or occur at intervals.   A remarkable case is on record
in which blindness took place rather suddenly, and, after it had
continued some time, sight was restored by an emetic.   The vision
was distinct for an hour, and then, alas! was permanently lost.
The intellect is frequently impaired in these cases, and sometimes
the speech is lost.   The morbid appearances after death present
no uniformity.

" In two cases there were tumors so situated as directly to com-
press the optic nerve; in another, a large tumor pressed upon the
corpora quadrigemina; in a third, the disease was situated at the
lower part of the anterior lobe; and in another, in which the right
eye was affected, it was in the substance of the left hemisphere,
near the posterior part.   In a case by Drelincurtius, the disease
was an enlargement of the pineal gland; and in another case, in
which there were both blindness and deafness, a large tumor was
found, situated between the brain and the cerebellum."[2]

Amaurosis is occasionally the effect of local pressure on the
optic nerve, or on some portion of the brain in its immediate
neighborhood.   This affection arises from organic disease of the
cerebellum, as well as the cerebrum, and from lesions in parts of

[1] Med. Dict.   [2] " Abercrombie on Diseases of the Brain," p. 318.

the brain remote from the origin of the nerves of sight. The impairment of vision is often the consequence of white softening, abscess, and atrophy of the brain, and other conditions of the tissue connected with disordered states of nutrition. This disorder, however, is not necessarily the effect of congestion, or organic alterations in the optic nerve or thalamus. Andral relates the particulars of several instances of disease of the *cerebellum*, accompanied by a complete loss of vision. This distinguished pathologist, when referring to these cases, says, "I am unable to account for the phenomenon. In two out of twelve cases of softening of the cerebellar lobes, blindness existed on the side of the body opposite the lesion."[1]

The organic diseases within the cranium, which occasionally produce amaurosis, are such as result from inflammation, softening (acute and chronic), serous effusion, induration, abscesses of various kinds, tumors, tuberculous formations, adipose tumors, flesh-like tumors, tumors of a fibro-cartilaginous nature, bony and calcareous concretions, hygromatous tumors, cysts containing a serous or albuminous fluid, hydatids, fungus hæmatodes, melanosis, hæmatomatous tumors, disease of the bloodvessels, aneurismal tumors, thickening of the membranes, depositions of matter between their laminæ; dense tumors of a uniform whitish or ash color, and exhibiting the appearance and properties of coagulated albumen, which are most frequently attached to the dura mater; diseases of the cranial bones, osteosa coma, exostosis, &c.

In an amaurotic boy, who was attacked by mania a short time before his death, Beer found a considerable spicula at the side of the *sella turcica* which had penetrated the optic nerve at the chiasma.

The most frequent cause of amaurosis is a sero-albuminous exudation, commonly the result of meningitis, taking place at the base of the brain compressing the chiasma of the optic nerve. The oculo motor nerve, from its close proximity, is generally involved in the disorder, so that convulsions or paralysis of the muscles of the eye are found to coexist.[2]

"Amaurosis from organic disease within the cranium is frequently complicated with epilepsy, apoplexy, paralysis, and affec-

[1] "Clinique Médicale." Andral.

[2] "A Manual of the Nervous Diseases of Man," by M. H. Romberg, M.D. Translated by E. H. Sleveking, M.D., vol. i, p. 232. London, 1853.

tions of the mental powers. It is remarkable that tumors, for example, will be found under the first class, unaccompanied by any remarkable symptoms, while under the second in the same situation, and of no larger size, they were associated with blindness, convulsions, or paralysis.

"It does not appear that these diversities depend either upon the size of the tumors, or, as far as we know at present, upon their particular structure. But these points remain to be investigated; particularly what diversity of symptoms is connected with the nature of the tumors, and especially with their characters as being tumors distinct from the cerebral mass, or as being indurations of the substance of the brain itself.[1]

"The loss of vision, which results from organic cerebral disease, more commonly affects one eye previously to, or independently of, the other; and if both are attacked, the amaurosis is more rapid in one than in the other, but frequently at the commencement of the disease the field of vision is not equally obscure."[2]

The patient complains of *muscæ volitantes*, scotoma, or sometimes there is increased sensibility to light with luminous spectra and contracted pupil. Not unfrequently objects appear distorted and confused with convulsive movements of the globe or eyelids. As the amaurosis becomes more complete, the vacant stare of the amaurotic patient is evidenced; the pupil becomes widely dilated and motionless, and the muscles convulsed. The eye usually appears on examination free from all organic change, and the retina, as far as can be ascertained, to be perfectly sound in its structure. But the appearance of the eye, and particularly of the pupil, is not to be depended upon, for, although it is usually dilated and immovable, the exceptions are too numerous to admit of its being considered as of uniform occurrence.[3]

Sudden loss of sight is occasionally premonitory of apoplexy. A locksmith experienced considerable vertigo for eight days. He then suddenly became blind. He remained in this state of vision for fifteen days, when he was seized with sudden deprivation of consciousness, followed by paralysis. His sight was gradually restored, but the hemiplegia continued.[4]

The impairment of vision which so often precedes apoplexy, may

[1] " Abercrombie on Diseases of the Brain," pp. 322, 323.
[2] Tyrrell, " Cyclopædia of Practical Surgery," vol. i, p. 94.
[3] "Copland's Medical Dictionary," vol. i, p. 56.   [4] Andral.

exist for some time without being recognized by the patient or his friends in consequence of the defect of sight being limited to one eye, the other compensating, as suggested by Dr. F. Devay (of Lyons), for the weakness of its fellow.

Total loss of sight, unassociated with other symptoms of brain disease, may exist for a long period antecedently to the manifestation of other symptoms of cerebral disorder.   Baron Hornestein, whose case is cited by Wepfer, became blind three weeks before he was seized with a fatal attack of apoplexy.[1]   Dr. Young lost the sight of one eye from tumor of the brain some time before he was aware of the fact.   It was not until he applied his eyes to a telescope, and found that the sight of *one* was entirely lost, that he became acquainted with the morbid state of his visual powers.

The amaurosis, so often associated with morbid states of the brain connected with apoplexy, occasionally continues after the patient recovers from the acute symptoms of the cerebral attack.

A gentleman, after an apoplectic seizure, lost his sight, and continued in a state of perfect blindness for about seven years. After that period, while one day out in his carriage, he suddenly recovered his sense of vision.   It was subsequently found that he had entirely retained his skill in drawing, for which he was previously much distinguished.

The late Dr. Gregory, of Edinburgh, was in the habit of mentioning in his lectures the case of Dr. Adam Ferguson, the celebrated historian, as affording one of the strongest illustrations he ever met with, of the benefit to be derived from an early attention to the incipient symptoms of cerebral plethora and apoplexy.   Dr. Ferguson experienced several attacks of temporary blindness some time before he had an attack of palsy; and he did not take these hints so readily as he should have done.   He observed that while he was delivering a lecture, his class and the papers before him would disappear, vanish from his sight, and reappear again in a few seconds.   He was a man of full habit; at one time corpulent and very ruddy, and, though by no means intemperate, he lived freely.   I say he did not attend to these admonitions, and at length, in the sixtieth year of his age, he suffered a decided shock of paralysis.   He recovered, however, and from that period, under the advice of his friend, Dr. Black, became a strict Pythagorean

---

[1] " Anatomica Apoplecticorum."

in his diet, eating nothing but vegetables, and drinking only water or milk. He got rid of every paralytic symptom, became even robust and muscular for a man of his time of life, and died in full possession of his mental faculties at the advanced age of ninety-three, upwards of thirty years after his first attack. Sir Walter Scott describes him as having been, "long after his eightieth year, one of the most striking old men it was possible to look at. His firm step and ruddy cheek contrasted agreeably and unexpectedly with his silver locks, and the dress which he usually wore, much resembling that of the Flemish peasant, gave an air of peculiarity to his whole figure. In his conversation, the mixture of original thinking with high moral feeling and extensive learning, his love of country, contempt of luxury, and especially the strong subjection of his passions and feelings to the dominion of his reason, made him, perhaps, the most striking example of the stoic philosopher which could be seen in modern days."[1]

"Amaurosis dependent upon vascular congestion is marked by some or all of the following symptoms: Dilated, sluggish or immovable pupil, ptosis or strabismus, and oblique or double vision of the affected eye; a preternatural action of the carotids, flushed face, sense of weight, pain or stricture of the scalp, lethargy, occasional tinnitus aurium, with greatly disordered and irritable stomach. The patient frequently complains, particularly in straining, stooping, or on first lying down, of seeing luminous sparks and flashes, and a reflection of one or more of the choroidal vessels, the visible pulsation of which is a cause of much distress to him."[2]

The following case is recorded by Dr. Wigan, and is illustrative of the benefit occasionally derived from subjecting cases of brain disease connected with morbid states of the vision to medical supervision: A gentleman had been under treatment about six months before for a severe attack of phrenitis, and had only been restored by the aid of very active remedies administered by a very judicious practitioner. I afterwards saw him in a state which was called perfect recovery. He had for some time resumed his active habits of business; but, although considering himself perfectly well, complained confidentially to me, that for some time he had been constantly arguing with himself on an increasing apathy towards his

[1] "Lectures on the Principles and Practice of Physic," by Dr. T. Watson. London, 1857. Vol. i, p. 527.
[2] "Diseases of the Eye," by B. Travers, F.R.S. 1825. P. 162.

wife—not physical apathy, quite the contrary—it was a strange disinclination to be in her society; he found himself frequenting the haunts of his former bachelor state against his intention, and almost against his will, yet received no gratification from any indulgences they afforded, and was constantly harassed by a feeling of remorse for neglecting the society of his wife, whom he had married from choice, whom he respected and thoroughly loved, and who was exceedingly tolerant of his indifference, from a belief that it was caused by pecuniary anxiety. I endeavored to convince him that it was a moral produced by a physical change, and that it would pass away with the consolidation of his health. He remained some time in this state, when he gradually began to see faces in the dark—afterwards in the daylight; groups of faces constantly changing their shape; sometimes a portion of one face would join itself to a portion of another face; sometimes parts of faces—eyes, noses, mouths, cheeks, and foreheads—would float about in vast numbers before him, and from time to time unite themselves in the most fantastic combinations. The whole occupied his mind, and rendered him incapable of continuous attention to any subject of importance requiring deep consideration. A large bleeding and a blister to the nape of the neck immediately restored him to vigorous health, and all his original delights in the society of his amiable and affectionate wife.[1]

HYPERÆSTHESIA, OR EXALTATION OF VISION.—A morbid exaltation of the sense of sight is occasionally observed among the premonitory symptoms of cerebral disease, the patient complaining either of an acute and sensitive condition of the retina, or of his abnormal expanded visual capabilities. A young gentleman, a few days before an attack of inflammation of the brain, had a painful condition of sight. If his eyes were exposed, even for a minute, to the light, he shrieked with pain. In another case the symptom was *precursory* of apoplexy for at least *ten* days. It was, however, associated with severe attacks of vertigo. Andral says, when alluding to this symptom of brain disease, " Cases have been observed in which, for a longer or shorter period before the attack, the sight has acquired an unusual degree of fineness."

The existence of important morbid visual phenomena, like those previously detailed, manifesting themselves prior to the occurrence

---

[1] "On the Duality of the Mind," by R. Wigan, M.D.

of hemorrhage, incontestably proves, as Andral sagaciously observes, that "BEFORE THE BLOOD IS EFFUSED, THERE IS ALREADY SOME MORBID ACTION, EITHER CONTINUOUS OR INTERMITTENT, IN THE BRAIN, OF WHICH IT WOULD BE IMPORTANT TO DETERMINE THE PRECISE NATURE."[1]   How significantly does this sagacious pathologist point out, in this passage, the necessity of carefully studying the *principiis obsta* of cerebral diseases!

In the following case, disease of the brain was first indicated by an acute condition of vision.   A painter, aged thirty-two, was admitted, in 1849, into the Hôtel Dieu, at Lyons.   This young man, who was possessed of some talent, had been gradually reduced to distress by political disturbances and other causes.   A year before entering the hospital, his sight, which was previously good, acquired greater development.   From his window, which opened into a very long street, he could distinguish objects and persons whom he could before neither distinguish nor even see.   This circumstance troubled him, and surprised those about him.   The exaltation of vision continued until August, 1848, when he was seized with violent continued pains in the right parietal region; at this time there was a slight weakness in the left arm.   The symptoms increased till March, 1849, when there was paralysis and contraction of the right arm, and blindness of the left eye.   When he entered the hospital in July, the following was his condition. There was almost profound stupor.   The paralyzed eye was almost completely covered by the upper eyelid, and there was paralysis, with contraction, of all the left side of the body.   There was complete loss of power over the sphincters.   He continued in this state until the beginning of September, when death ensued, preceded by symptoms of low fever.   The autopsy revealed partial circumscribed softening of the middle and upper part of the right hemisphere, for the extent of about two *centimètres*.   The convolutions were pale and puffy; the pulp was diffluent, and of a dirty gray color.

Dr. Brachet relates, when he was *interne* at the Bicêtre, in 1811, the *infirmier* of the surgical ward one day astonished him by the extent which his vision had acquired since the previous day.   The man could distinguish the most minute objects at an enormous distance.   Five hours afterwards he felt a slight head-

---

[1] Andral, "Clinique Médicale," tom. v.

ache, and in a few hours more was seized with apoplexy ("*une apoplexie fou droyante*"), and died the next night ! A recent coagulum was found in the right optic thalamus. The inflammation which had preceded this effusion had irritated by its proximity a part of the brain concerned in vision.

Dr. Hibbert, in his work on Spectral Illusions, makes particular mention of morbidly acute sensorial symptoms as connected with certain obscure conditions of brain disease. He observes, that, in particular forms of cerebral inflammation, the first symptoms evinced an increasing intensity of visual sensation. In the case of a lady, a patient of Dr. Good, there was an intolerable acuteness of hearing and vision, insomuch that the slightest light and sound, even the humming of a fly, became insupportable. Ideas, also, were rendered more vivid. But as the inflammation increased the acute sensibility to external impressions gradually diminished, whilst the recollected images of the mind assumed a most frightful reality. In an example which came under my own notice, the illusions of vision were so intense that although the patient closed his eyelids, he could not, even then, dispel the lively images of demons that haunted his bed. The sleep was, moreover, disturbed with the most horrible dreams.[1]

A single woman, of delicate frame, aged twenty-two, had been much afflicted with hysteria for more than three months. The paroxysms of the disease were often violent, accompanied frequently, but not constantly, with temporary delirium: so that the disease appeared to be well marked, never being preceded by any local irritation, of which the patient was conscious. During some of these attacks she was occasionally so much in possession of the faculties of the mind and of speech, as to be able to reply appositely to questions put to her by the attendants ; but of these

---

[1] The illustrious Goethe possessed the rare faculty of producing phantasms at will. He says: "When I closed my eyes and depressed my head, I could cause the image of a flower to appear in the middle of the field of vision ; this flower did not for a moment retain its first form, but unfolded itself, and developed from its interior, new flowers, formed of colored or sometimes green leaves. These were not natural flowers, but of fantastic forms, although symmetrical as the rosettes of sculptors. I was unable to fix any one form, but the development of new flowers continued as long as I desired it, without any variation in the rapidity of the changes. The same thing occurred when I figured to myself a variegated disk. The colored figures upon it underwent constant changes, which extended progressively from the centre towards the periphery, exactly like the changes in the modern kaleidoscope."

conversations she retained no recollection whatever after the termination of the attack.   Certain paroxysms were productive of convulsions so violent as to require coercion ; whilst others were attended merely with wild delirium.   In the latter, impressions made by surrounding objects upon the retina, were transmitted to the brain, as usual inverted, and were represented to the mind in that position so forcibly, that the young woman could not resist the impulse she felt to place the chairs in the room horizontally, lest they should fall, finding they would not stand on the other end.   She expressed her surprise, and laughed heartily, on seeing the attendants all standing, as she thought, upon their heads. The illusion immediately subsided with the fit, both lasting generally about an hour.   This, therefore, was not a singular occurrence in one particular fit, but recurred repeatedly.   The disease yielded, at length, to the ordinary treatment of hysteria, no defect either in the organ of vision, or the faculties of the mind, remaining.[1]

Romberg relates the particulars of the following case of hyperæsthesia of vision connected with disease of the *optic thalamus:* "A widow of eighty-five years of age, and of a robust constitution, was affected eight years previous to her death with cataract of both eyes.   She underwent an operation, which appeared at first to prove successful ; after a few months, however, her sight became impaired, the left bulb was atrophied, the right pupil closed, and the patient was only able to distinguish light from darkness.   At this time she first began to complain of seeing long rows of worms, strips of colored linen, or threads of worsted constantly passing upwards.   An artificial pupil was now made in the right eye. The phantasms ceased for a time, but returned after eight weeks ; first assuming the old shapes, and subsequently new ones.   High walls rose up before her, heavily-laden carts surrounded her, or human figures hovered about her, generally threatening and alarming, rarely with a friendly aspect.   These phenomena generally occurred only during the waking state ; they soon became so vivid, that the patient felt convinced of their real existence, and, though continuing in the full possession of her intellectual faculties, made defensive movements with her hands whilst conversing.   Her forehead was hot, the face much flushed, the pulse

---

[1] " Medical and Physical Journal," vol. xiv, p. 117.

full and hard, and there was a sense of anxiety and oppression which, with the other symptoms, became aggravated towards night. The phantasms continued with occasional remissions and exacerbations during six years, until death ensued. Fits of vertigo and unconsciousness supervened, associated with weakness, and subsequently with paralysis of the left arm; these recurred several times during the year without exerting any influence upon the visual phenomena. In the month of January, 1837, the patient was seized with a violent apoplectic attack, the symptoms of which were deep coma, continuing for four-and-twenty hours, stertorous breathing, slow, full pulse, paralysis of the left arm and leg, and involuntary discharges. She recovered also from this attack, and lived for a year and three months without further inconvenience.

On the 16th March, 1838, after feeling particularly well and happy during the previous day, she was seized during the night with another apoplectic attack, accompanied by complete hemiplegia of the right side. She died in the evening of the following day."

In the right hemisphere of the cerebrum, not far from the external edge of the posterior lobe and the surface, there was discovered a cavity of the size of a plum, invested with a reddish membrane, containing a small quantity of ochra fluid. There was fresh extravasation of blood in the middle and posterior lobe of the left hemisphere, near the *corpus striatum* and the *optic thalamus*. The latter was converted into a grayish pulp. The optic nerves and the chiasma were in a normal condition. An examination of the retina was not permitted.

DERANGEMENT, PERVERSION, OR ABERRATION OF SIGHT.— These morbid phenomena will be found more frequently symptomatic of disease of the brain than impairment, loss, or exaltation of the function of vision.

Such morbid states of the eyes vary from slight disturbances and irregularities of sight to actual illusions, *ocula spectra*, and phantasms. The physiognomy of the eye is peculiar in these cases of brain disease. This symptom should be accurately observed. The eyes present occasionally an unnatural brightness, and the vision an intensity of power, when the patient's attention is concentrated upon any object, or if engaged in exciting topics of conversation.

Again, in some conditions of cerebral disorder, the patient is conscious of an inability to fix his eyes for many minutes, continuously, upon any one point or object. There is an evident want of control over the sight, the vision ceasing to obey the mandates of volition. Occasionally, the patient exhibits a propensity to stare at objects; there is a fixed expression of the eyes associated with an apparent immobility of the pupil.

There is often observed in these cases what has been termed by Romberg, a destruction of the *motor parallelism* of the optic nerve; a deviation, in fact, from the optic axis.

I have been attending a case, with Dr. Birkett, of obscure cerebro-spinal disease, in which there exists a singular irregularity of vision, the effect, it is presumed, of atrophy and impaired nutrition of the brain, possibly of the *optic thalamus*. There never has been in this case any marked headache. The patient has, however, complained of mental confusion, want of confidence in himself, and of severe paroxysms of vertigo. He appears to have lost the controlling power over the lower extremities. He has had for some time an impairment of sensibility in two of the fingers of his left hand. His intellect appears unclouded. The eyes are peculiarly affected. There is a marked difference in the dilatation of the pupils. The left pupil is contracted, and the right dilated. The left eye appears to be atrophied, and has the appearance as if it were flat, sunk in its socket, and much smaller than the opposite one. The vision is also defective in each eye. With the left he has short, and with the right eye long sight.

In some forms of brain disease the accurate observer notices a peculiar expression of the eyes, similar to that seen in some cases of strabismus, but without the muscular affection upon which that affection depends. The patient stares as if he were under the influence of an optical illusion. There is in these cases, as Dr. F. Devay pertinently remarks, "*a want of parallelism in the organ of vision. The eyes are not in the axis of reason.*"[1]

[1] Dr. Mérier has lately called attention to a kind of trembling, oscillation, and vacillation of the ocular globes among the insane threatened with dementia. It is, says this practitioner, a kind of permanent and continual convulsion, in consequence of which the small lateral movements are confined to the ocular globes. Sometimes they work up and down, but the last movement is much more rare. The observations of Dr. Mérier have led to these conclusions: 1. That the exhibition of convulsive movements, laterally and up and down, which he has observed in a great number of patients, has always coincided with that period of the disorder marked by the

Portal predicated an attack of apoplexy in a gentleman (apparently in perfect health) from observing a slight fixedness of his left eye and a trifling weakness (incipient paralysis) on the same side of the body.

Previously to an apoplectic seizure, patients have been known to complain of objects appearing to be colored red. Others fancy that a line of a like tint borders all bodies, or complain of a sensation similar to that experienced by the eyes when they have been exposed for some time to a strong light. Objects appear as if they were dotted with black or red spots, or the patient imagines that a mist or thin veil intervenes between the eyes and the objects at which they are directed.

Meningitis, congestion, or cerebral hyperæmia, and other acute diseases of the brain are occasionally preceded by double vision, strabismus, and other derangements of sight. These are also the well-recognized premonitory symptoms of acute inflammation of the substance of the brain.

Andral had an opportunity of observing a person who for several years was constantly tormented by the imaginary sight of small bodies of different forms and colors dancing before his eyes. If he looked steadily at an object, he saw it dotted with red or black points. These *ocula spectra*, which were permanent, prevented his reading or writing. He did not complain of vertigo, or headache. The conjunctivæ were habitually congested, and he could not endure, without considerable suffering, a more than ordinary strong light.

Among the aberrations of the sense of sight precursory of cerebral disease are the following: Seeing objects cut in half, double vision, inversion of objects.[1] A lady who had complained of being

change from an acute to a chronic state: for example, in the transition from mania to dementia; 2. That the existence and persistence of these ocular movements among patients give to the prognosis a very great gravity, justifying the notion that the insane who were in a supposed favorable condition were already, or were about to become, *incurable.*

M. Morel (who refers to the previous facts), adds, that in these same patients the eye throws out an extraordinary and undefinable brilliancy; but this last phenomenon is scarcely ever remarked except during the period of transition. When dementia is confirmed, the eye is as it were extinct, and the gaze has that stupid and doltish expression quite in harmony with the weakness of the intellectual faculties.

[1] Dr. Wollaston relates that it twice occurred to him not to be able to see but on one side of the axis of vision. The first time the left side of each eye was affected; he saw but the half of a man's face or of any object he looked at; and in attempting to

out of health, of slight headache and partial deafness, found, in
the early part of one morning, that her sight was disordered.   In
attempting to read a book, she remarked that the printed letters
and sentences were running one into the other.   Subsequently the
page appeared as if a piece of finely glazed paper had been placed
over it, through which she was just able to discern the letters.   In
the afternoon of that day she had an attack of apoplexy which
ended fatally !

Vitiated perception is one of the common precursory symptoms
of apoplexy.   A lady of vigorous and cultivated understanding,
whom Dr. Cheyne attended, was menaced with apoplexy.   Previously to the attack, she complained of being annoyed by numerous
unusual appearances in luminous bodies ; the flame of a candle was
enlarged to the shape of a tulip, and with a red centre ; the moon
appeared oval with a central portion of a bright scarlet.   All
distant objects were hazy, yet she read and wrote without any
difficulty.

A gentleman complained a few hours before he was attacked
with paralysis, of his being able to recognize only half of everything
he saw.   If he looked at a person there appeared to be but one eye,
half of a nose, and mouth.   In another case every part of the
body was enveloped in a thick mist.   This was among the premonitory signs of a severe attack of phrenitis, and existed some days
before severe headache excited alarm as to the state of the brain.
When speaking of the affections of vision connected with cerebral
hemorrhage, Andral remarks, " Sight is sometimes, but not always,
disturbed.   We see individuals struck down with apoplexy and

---

read the name JOHNSON over a door, he saw only . . . . SON, the commencement
of the name being totally obliterated from his view ; the complaint was of short duration.   About nineteen years afterwards the visual phenomenon recurred ; this time
the right side of the eye, about three degrees from the centre of the retina, was affected,
and its duration was ten minutes.   Two analogous cases are also mentioned by Dr.
Wollaston.   Desmoulins states that M. Arago has experienced this affection of vision
three times : on the first two occasions objects situated to the right of the axis of vision
were invisible ; the third time he saw objects on the right only of this axis.   The
same author notices also the following remarkable case.   In consequence of a cerebral
fever, the external side of the left retina of M. de M—— became insensible : with
his eye he saw objects only situate to the left of the centre of vision, and, as at the
same time there was an outward deviation of the axis of this eye through a paralysis
of the nerve of the third pair, when he employed both eyes, he saw objects double ;
but, what was still more singular, the right eye being closed, he saw with the left eye
the objects removed from twenty to twenty-five degrees to the right of their real
position.

affected with paralysis and loss of sensation, where, nevertheless, consciousness and vision remain. Different sensations, resulting from disturbance of this function, are experienced by patients, who describe them in different ways; some say that they have motes before their eyes; others, they see the light as through a cloud, just as on the onset of cataract—yet here the crystalline lens is clear; others see various colors. Sometimes, those who at a later period are attacked with apoplexy, have the sight modified for a longer or shorter time before the attack, in such a manner that all objects appear double, a symptom which is sometimes transient, being present one day and not another. In other cases the loss of sight is nearly complete, but such cases are very rare. When the sight is lost, this may take place on one side or on both, and this blindness coincides with the loss of numerous other senses."[1]

Photopsia, or the appearance of luminous phenomena, objects in a state of ignition, or surrounded by a phosphorescent halo, are common incipient symptoms of acute disease of the brain.

The late Dr. James Johnson relates the particulars of an interesting case of the kind. "A distinguished artist for several years suffered from photopsia, to which afterwards headache and diminution of vision were added, terminating in complete blindness. Nevertheless the luminous phenomena continued night and day, occasionally assuming the appearance of angels with flaming swords, whose movements were apparently accompanied by an electric light. The forms, however, frequently varied. The mental powers of the individual remained unimpaired, and whenever he went out he was very attentive to everything that did not require eyesight. In the spring of 1835 he had an apoplectic seizure which deprived him of movement, consciousness, and speech. There was complete paralysis of the sphincters, and the pupils were dilated. He recovered from this condition, and after a few weeks was again able to go about the town and attend to his business. But the visual phenomena returned, and the sight was as painfully dazzling, and more continuously so than before. In the month of August an apoplectic attack occurred, and death ensued in three days. The right lateral ventricle of the brain was found after death to contain nearly three ounces of clear fluid.

[1] "Clinique."

The left was full of bladders resembling hydatids of various sizes, and containing fluids varying in consistency. This accumulation sprung from the floor of the ventricle by a kind of pedicle, and penetrated into all the recesses of the cavity, pushing its branches forwards so as to extend the thalamus of one side into the opposite half of the brain, destroying everything that opposed its passage. Both thalami optici were converted into a pulp, as well as the whole anterior lobe, which was so diffluent as scarcely to bear the slightest pressure. The optic nerves were compressed by the hydatids, so as to present a mere thready appearance. Pressure at the back of the neck caused great uneasiness, extending to the lower trunk and extremities. It was not pain, but a horrid feeling that was induced. This pervaded the whole frame, and it was only by the greatest entreaty that he could be induced to permit a repetition of the manual examination. The sensibility had now so much increased that simply touching was sufficient to renew these distressing sensations. A pint of blood was taken from the arm. During the operation the vision returned. He said he saw three women standing behind the gentleman who was bleeding him. Being asked were they as large as life, he replied. 'that they were rather low,' and pointed to the place where they stood. It was inquired, ' Had he ever seen them before ?' ' No.' ' Were they speaking to each other ?' ' No.' ' What were they doing ?' ' They were usually minding their business, but sometimes stopped to watch him, and kept their eyes fixed on his for some moments.' The sense of feeling was quite as much disturbed and illusive as that of sight, for in a few moments after he called out that he felt ' one of them thumping up against that part of the bed on which he lay ;' and presently again looked abruptly behind him, saying ' that somebody had hit him two or three times on the back.' All this was very different from the usual raving of the insane, as he scarcely felt the impression before he was himself aware of its being an illusion. In fact, his chief distress arose from the alarming nature of the disordered perceptions. ' Rid me of these sights and sounds,' was his entreaty, ' and get me some sleep, or I shall lose my senses !'

" Active purgatives were exhibited, after venesection was performed. Subsequently a blister was applied over the ninth dorsal vertebra with great benefit. He soon recovered under the continued use of gentle alterative aperients, combined with counter-irritation.

"He had a recurrence of the attack some months after in consequence of hard drinking, but though he complained more of the head, especially at the back of it, there was no material fulness or frequency of the pulse, or febrile irritation. He was relieved by purgatives and blistering, and was afterwards treated with camphor and other nervine medicines."

A nobleman, for some weeks previously to an attack of apoplexy, was subject to a curious phantasmal phenomenon. He, on several occasions during the day when suffering from acute headache, saw clearly a spectral image resembling himself. This form of hallucination is termed *deuteroscopia*. The phenomenon is considered of rare occurrence, even among the insane. Aristotle refers to this type of illusion in his essay, "*De Memoria et Reminiscentia*," but it is explained more at length in his Meteorology.

A certain Antipheron, Aristotle says, when he was walking, saw a phantasmal reflection of himself advancing towards him. A traveller who had passed a long time without sleeping, perceived one night his own image, which rode by his side. It imitated all his actions. The horseman having to cross a river, the phantom passed over it with him. Having arrived at a place where the mist was less thick, this curious apparition vanished. Goethe relates having had a similar hallucination. This form of hallucination is frequently observed during the delirium of typhoid fevers.[1]

Morel relates the case of a lady who was restored to health from a state of general paralysis. In the incipient phase of the disease, she affirmed that she constantly saw at the end of the garden a man without a head. When she directed her steps boldly towards the place where the apparition appeared to be, it immediately vanished. She said nothing about this phantom to her family, fearing that she would be thought insane. This patient observed, after her alleged restoration to reason, that the first trial she made of her intellectual powers whilst communing with herself, consisted in her occupying the place where the apparition formerly appeared. The absence or presence of the phantom ought to prove, she said, the validity of her cure.

In many cases the ocula spectra, illusions of visions and phantasms are supposed to be referable to spinal disease or irritation.

[1] "Anatomie Comparée du Système Nerveux," par Fr. Lenret and P. Gratiolet, Paris, 1857. P. 539.

I, however, suspect that when morbid psychical phenomena of this kind are present, the affection is to be viewed more as one of a cerebro-spinal character than as a disorder exclusively localized in the spinal column.

An instance occurred some years since of a young girl being haunted, whilst laboring under spinal irritation, by a spectral figure, which she described as standing by her bedside. She was frequently seized with fits of screaming as she fancied the phantom approached her. She kept her relatives in the greatest state of alarm and astonishment. A few active purgatives gave immediate and effectual relief. Dr. Griffin cites the particulars of two cases presenting singular phenomena.

A man, aged thirty-six, of a good constitution, but very intemperate habits, complained for some days of occasional pains in the stomach and arch of the colon, with costiveness, loss of appetite, and general nervous excitement. He had constant slight pain in the brow, with disturbance of vision, and extreme sensibility to noise, conjoined with a morbid state of exaltation of the senses. His eyes were suffused, tongue white, pulse about ninety. He had a pain in his chest, accompanied with great anxiety. His chief distress, however, arose from optical visions, with which he was continually troubled. Figures of persons, almost all of whom were wholly unknown to him, were frequently before him, sometimes so plain and distinct, that although his reason assured him they were mere illusions, he could scarcely avoid believing that they had an absolute existence. They were not always the same, nor always present, but went and came, renewing his anxiety and irritation of mind as often as they appeared. On examining the spine, tenderness was found at the three upper cervical vertebræ, pressure on any of them exciting much pain. The eighth, ninth, and tenth dorsal vertebræ, were excessively tender, the slightest pressure on any of them occasioning an exceedingly distressing sensation along the spine to the sacrum.

J. H., aged fifteen years, complained that, at night, he invariably became blind : he could not see the furniture or people about the room, when they were perfectly visible to every one else. The candle or fire-light appeared like a broad red haze, just distinguishable from darkness, but making nothing perceptible. He could perceive any dark object between him and the light, and no more. He was affected in this way for about a fortnight, and had a similar complaint a year ago, which continued a long time. There is great tenderness on pressing the second cervical vertebra. He perfectly recovered in less than forty-eight hours, by a small bleeding, an active calomel purgative, and a blister to the nape of the neck, and has since continued well.

In the following case the vision was affected in an extraordinary manner.

A young gentleman, aged seventeen, is frequently attacked with violent headache and sickness of stomach, which symptoms are always ushered in by indistinctness of vision. His first warning of the fit is a sudden appearance of something misty and tremulous before his eyes; soon afterwards he perceives only the vertical half of any object he looks at, and eventually the outlines fade away altogether into thick darkness. This almost total blindness continues generally for a very short period; the thick dark mist gradually clears off, and the forms of everything around him are again distinctly observed. He is then instantly seized with intense headache, chiefly affecting the forehead, usually so dreadful in its nature, and accompanied by such distressing nausea or sickness, that he says he could scarcely live if it lasted a second day. He commonly finds relief by lying down: the pain is thus more easily endured, and the paroxysm is shorter, terminating in four or five hours, when it might otherwise continue for twenty. Instead of pain, a deep lethargy sometimes supervenes on the affection of vision, during which he lies as in heavy slumber, but frightfully conscious of time passing, and of terrific sights and sounds crowding upon his imagination. He awakes out of this state of mind in a state of temporary delirium; does not know for some time where he is, or what has happened, and speaks incoherently. Even after the subsidence of the headache, although there is much less confusion of mind than after the lethargy, the memory is always very imperfect for some hours. He cannot recollect the words he wishes to make use of, but employs others wholly inapplicable in their stead; and of this mistake he is always conscious at the moment. To these attacks he has been subject for about two years, but in their intervals he has sometimes been affected in a very different way. He awakes suddenly out of his sleep at night in dreadful apprehension, for which he cannot account. There is a continued crowding and rushing of ideas through his mind. He feels as if everything he did, and all that was done about him, passed over with a frightful and hurried rapidity. This at•last wears away, and is generally, even from the first, more or less under the influence of his will; an effort to check the current of his ideas, and divert it into another direction, frequently proving successful.

On examination, there was found great tenderness of the second cervical and of the seventh or eighth dorsal vertebræ. When this last was slightly pressed upon, he felt a horrible sensation shoot through his whole frame. It was quite indescribable, and nearly made him faint. He expressed the greatest apprehension at the thought of the pressure being repeated, and had a disagreeable feeling in his back for the entire day afterwards.[1]

STRABISMUS.—This is occasionally observed among the early signs of disease of the brain, particularly in the cerebral affections of children; and, if present, should be carefully noted. A slight squint in the eye has occasionally been found precursory of an attack of apoplexy, and is often diagnostic of the commencement of effusion on the brain.

A gentleman, who had complained for a few days of headache and depression of spirits, was observed, whilst at dinner, to have strabismus. A few minutes subsequently, he dropped down in a fit of apoplexy. Illustrations of a similar character could be cited, in which other forms of acute brain disease have been ushered in by this symptom.

DOUBLE VISION.—I have not yet spoken of this perversion of sight. It is one of the most important precursory symptoms of disease of the brain. This sign of cerebral disease is of great practical value and diagnostic significance, and never should escape attentive observation. It is often the first indication of acute mischief originating in the brain, and occasionally in the obscure cerebral diseases of children it constitutes an important diagnostic sign. This aberration of vision is occasionally symptomatic of gastric and hepatic disorder, but when associated with persistent or paroxysmal attacks of headache, lowness of spirits, morbid conditions of the *sensorial* or *motorial* powers, we cannot be too closely observant of the state of the patient's brain.

Attacks of apoplexy, paralysis, cerebritis, and meningitis have often been preceded by double vision. Dr. Watson relates the

[1] *Vide* "On Functional Disorders of the Spinal Cord," by W. L. D. Griffin, M.D.

following case in point: "Dr. Gregory was acquainted with a sportsman who, one day when out shooting, disputed with his gamekeeper as to the number of dogs they had in the field. He asked how he came to bring so many as eight dogs with him. The servant assured him there were but four, and then the gentleman became at once aware of his situation, mounted his horse, and rode home. He had not been long in the house when he was attacked by apoplexy, and died."

MORBID PHENOMENA OF HEARING.—This sense is variously affected in different morbid states of the brain and disordered conditions of the cerebral circulation. In some cases there is observed, in connection with subtle changes of structure within the cranium, complete loss of hearing. In other instances, this special sense becomes obtuse. In some patients it is perverted, and in particular forms of disease of the brain an exalted condition, or hyperæsthesia of the faculty, is developed.

Occasionally, among the incipient symptoms of cerebral disease, there is a sudden paralysis of the auditory nerve, destroying all sense of sound. These extreme cases are not, however, of common occurrence. The symptoms most generally noticed in the insidious affections of the brain, in relation to the faculty of hearing, are either a gradual, progressive impairment, or obtuseness of the sense, or an intensely morbid exaltation and aberration of the faculty.

A disordered state of hearing is one of the most frequent symptoms attendant upon those extremely dangerous affections of the internal structure of the ear involving the bones, membranes, and ultimately the brain itself, which are so frequently preceded, for a length of time, by a chronic purulent discharge from the external meatus, known by the name of otorrhœa, and often connected with chronic meningitis, or cerebral suppurative inflammation.

In the incipient stage of certain affections of the brain the hearing often becomes painfully acute. The faintest whisper reverberates through the ear like the noise of thunder, and conversations that are taking place in remote parts of the house are clearly and distinctly heard by the patient whilst in this state of auricular hyperæsthesia.

It is extraordinary how acute the sense of hearing occasionally becomes in certain forms of delirium. I was informed by a distinguished living physician that he was able, when in a state of cerebral exaltation, whilst occupying a room at the top of the house, to hear with remarkable clearness the conversation taking place in the kitchen. I have witnessed some remarkable instances of this phenomenon in the early as well as advanced stages of brain disease.

Dr. Elliotson attended a gentleman, about forty years of age, who had suddenly an attack of hemiplegia, and whilst in bed he heard the least sound at the bottom of the house with an acuteness which surprised him; and could tell the hour by a watch placed on a table at such a distance from his bed as to have rendered it impossible for him to distinguish the hands when he was in health.

A patient, for nearly a week previously to an attack of inflammation of the brain, complained to those immediately about him of great exaltation of the sense of hearing. In another case, for · few hours prior to an apoplectic seizure, the patient remarked his son that, when in a distant part of the house, he could, and. fact, did hear distinctly a conversation that was taking plac the dining-room at a time when no one else could distinguisl sound of human voices!

I have often witnessed in the brain affections of children ticularly in scrofulous diseases of this organ and its investing membranes, a sudden acuteness of this sense preceding the manifestation of more formidable and fatal cerebral symptoms.

Insanity is occasionally ushered in by hyperæsthesia of hearing. This is not an unfrequent symptom of approaching mental derangement. In the premonitory stage the patient often complains of great sensorial activity. He sees what no other person is able to recognize; smells offensive and disagreeable odors not recognized by those near him, and hears noises and voices appreciable only by himself. This condition of disordered acuteness of the senses is often witnessed for some time previously to the patient manifesting any observable *alienation* of intellect characterized by illusions or hallucinations.

When the mind is losing its balance in the incipient stage of insanity the patient will be heard to ask rather anxiously to those about him, " Did *you* not speak?" "Did *you* hear a voice?" "I thought," repeats the patient earnestly, " I heard some person calling *my* name." "Surely there *must* be some one in the room or outside the door addressing *me*." Such were the nervous ejaculations of a patient to his wife three or four days prior to an attack of furious delirium, associated with frightful hallucinations, resulting unhappily in suicide.

A lady, a fortnight before her mind was considered to be deranged, was in the habit of waking her husband several times during the night, imagining that she heard the voices of persons in the room or in some part of the house. On one or two occasions she declared that she distinctly recognized the voice of her mother (who was then in New Zealand) calling her by name, and begging her, in accents of the deepest distress, to come to her. The patient insisted upon getting up and examining the whole of the house before she would be persuaded her mother was not there. At this time no one suspected that these were incipient symptoms insanity.

These illusions of hearing often lead to a sad sacrifice of life, sionally impelling its unhappy victim to the commission of murder and suicide. Under the irresistible influence of an nary voice, many a patient is driven to acts of violence and ide. Occasionally, the illusions of hearing are of a double ter, that is, the patient is subject to the influence of *two voices*, a good and a bad voice; one inciting him to sacrifice life, e other a restraining voice, begging and imploring the patient not to yield to his dangerously insane impulses. "My bad voices urge, my good voices restrain me," was the remark of a patient who believed himself to be demoniacally possessed. "I should have destroyed myself long ago," said an insane person to Dr. Morel, "or I should have killed somebody else, if the voice of my good angel had not begged and encouraged me to suffer."

Patients are often seen contending with these antagonistic illusions, or "double voice," as Morel designates the phenomenon. In one ear the most frightfully obscene ideas are suggested; whilst at the same moment, in the opposite one, sentiments of the greatest purity will be whispered to the disordered imagination of the sufferer. These antagonistic and opposing illusions lead to fearful contests, and produce a sad amount of mental agony. "Which voice ought I to obey?" said a delicate and sensitive-minded patient to me one day after a fit of hysterico-maniacal excitement. "I am urged by persons that address me on my right side to utter blasphemous and indecent expressions, and to commit acts the most repugnant and repulsive to my nature; whilst in the opposite ear I clearly recognize a tender voice (conscience ?) beseeching me not to yield to the fearful temptations of Satan, but to battle with his vile and wicked suggestions." Another patient was urged by a voice to destroy himself. He was commanded to cut his throat. The words, " blood," " blood," " blood," were repeated with terrible emphasis, and in rapid succession to him ; and on more than one occasion he was discovered with a razor in his possession, seriously contemplating an act of self-destruction. This gentleman was subject to the influence of the double voice, for at times when the word " blood" was ringing awfully in his ear, and an " air-drawn dagger" stained with gore, glittered before his eyes, there stood, as he imagined, on the opposite side of his body a good spirit whispering to him texts of Scripture, repeating verses of hymns applicable to his then state of mind, and imploring him, in most affectionate and touching language, not to eternally damn his soul by destroying his own life.

MORBID PHENOMENA OF TASTE, TOUCH, AND SMELL.—These senses exhibit, occasionally, at the commencement of cerebral disease, evidence of impairment, exaltation, and perversion. Prior to the development of the more characteristic symptoms of disease of the brain, the patient complains of a morbid condition of taste, of abnormal states of the tactile sensibility, and of perversion of the sense of smell. In all affections of the brain and mind associated with derangement of the digestive organs, the latter sense is observed to be greatly affected; but there is no special and characteristic symptom in connection with either of them pathognomonic of the commencement of organic disease of the brain.

The insane, in the incipient stage of their malady, are often heard to complain of being exposed to the influence of most offensive and noxious smells. The predominant odors noticed by patients in the early period of their mental alienation are those of sulphur and putrid bodies.

A lady declared that her inside was in a state of putrefaction, a fact she recognized by a particular exhalation from her body for some months before her intellect was palpably deranged. She was frequently heard to complain of the offensive odor, but no one suspected her mind to be in the slightest degree affected, until one morning she left home before breakfast, and going to a neighboring police-station, accused herself of having committed a serious criminal offence.

The tactile sensibility is frequently observed to be disordered in the early stage of paralysis. The patient will be heard to complain of a feeling of numbness or want of sensation in the ramifications of the nerves at the tips of the fingers. This condition of anæsthesia often extends to the fingers, and sometimes to the whole of the hand. I have known this local impairment of sensibility to exist for many months previously to the recognition of more decided manifestation of disease of the brain. This lesion of sensation often precedes attacks of general paralysis. Professor Simpson, of Edinburgh, has alluded to the morbid phenomenon. Patients suffering from incipient general paralysis, he says, often complain of their fingers "feeling like sausages."[1] A tailor who died of this disease, lost all sensation at the tips of his fingers for twelve months previously to any suspicion existing as to the healthy state of his brain. He was unable to work with his needle, as he never knew, owing to the anæsthesia, when he had it between his fingers.

I have referred in a previous part of this volume to the loss of sensation that occasionally occurs at the peripheral terminations of the nerves in the incipient stage of paralysis. Dr. Todd cites a case of hemiplegia that commenced six months prior to admission into King's College Hospital, with a sensation of tingling and pricking in both hands, and a considerable amount of numbness about both elbows, just as if the ulnar nerve had been jarred, or, in the patient's own words, as if he had struck his funny-bone. Accompanying these symptoms there was a sensation of heat in the forearms, and he soon became unable to button his clothes or pick up any small object with his right hand.

Occasionally, the sensation at the tips of the fingers will be observed in a state of great exaltation. A morbid irritation in this part of the hand often coexists with insanity, as well as with other types of nervous disorder. The habit of biting the nails to the quick, and gnawing the tips of the fingers is very common among the insane. In many cases of mental exaltation, irritation, hysteria, and anxiety, unassociated with insanity, there is often manifested a morbid degree of exalted tactile insensibility. This local hyperæsthesia is occasionally observed among the incipient symp-

---

[1] During a discussion at the "Medico-Chirurgical Society of Edinburgh," on a paper read by Dr. David Skae on "General Paralysis of the Insane," Feb. 1, 1860.

toms of mental derangement. A lady who has had several attacks
of insanity, is annoyed by an intense irritation at the ends of the
fingers, for some weeks previously to positive alienation of mind
exhibiting itself. Her family are able to predicate the approach
of the paroxysms of insanity by this symptom. It is difficult to
explain physiologically or pathologically the relation between certain cerebral and mental disorders and this type of exalted local
sensibility.

CHAPTER XXIII.

THE phenomena of sleep are so closely identified with, and so intimately dependent upon, the state of the brain, that the varied affections of the sensorium (functional as well as organic) are usually accompanied by some deviation from a normal state of this important function.

The morbid affections of sleep will be considered in the following order :—

    a. A State of Sleeplessness, or Insomnia.
    β. An Abnormal Disposition to Excess of Sleep.
    γ. Morbid Phenomena of Dreaming.

The first division of the subject embraces the many gradations of insomnia, ranging from a simple state of restlessness, to a disturbed, eccentric, irregular, cerebral repose (*pavores, jactatio*), and unrefreshing condition of slumber, to a state of positive *insomnia,* or sleeplessness.

The second section of the subject will embody a brief analysis of certain morbid dispositions to excess of sleep, designated, according to the extent of the symptoms, by the nosological phrases *sopor, coma, carus, lethargus.*

There is no symptom, when viewed in relation to the health of the brain and mind, that requires more careful and unremitting attention than that of insomnia, or wakefulness. It is one of the most constant concomitants of some types of incipient brain disease, and in many cases *a certain forerunner of insanity !*

It is an admitted axiom in medicine, that the brain cannot be in a healthy condition whilst a state of sleeplessness exists. Sound, continuous, unbroken, regular, and uninterrupted sleep are essential to the preservation of the mental and bodily health. Any interference with this important function or state of cerebral rest, seriously damages the health of both body and mind.

We cannot too zealously guard against, or too anxiously watch for, the first approaches of this characteristic symptom of incipient brain and mental disorder. Persons predisposed to attacks of cerebral disease and morbid affections of the mind, ought never to permit a condition of sleeplessness, or even a state of disturbed and broken rest, to continue for many consecutive nights, without seriously considering their state of bodily, cerebral, and mental health.

In the premonitory stage of some forms of acute insanity, and particularly of delirium tremens, the patient is in a constant state of sleeplessness by night and restlessness by day. His repose, at first, is broken and disturbed. He slumbers lightly, and has only snatches of sleep. If asleep, the slightest noise or ruffle of the bedclothes awakens him ; and when suddenly aroused, *he looks like a person whose eyes had never been closed in sleep.* This is a characteristic and significant symptom of the *insomnia of incipient insanity.*

In conditions of healthy sleep the vital energy or nerve-force is supposed to be reproduced, evolved, or regenerated in the vesicular neurine, and the individual commences his morning's work, whether it be of a mental or muscular character, with a renewed supply of the powers of life or nervous energy, sufficient to carry him successfully through the day's regular and appointed duties; but the partial and unhealthy snatches of repose obtained in certain states of brain disorder do not appear to refresh or invigorate the system. In this condition of cerebral activity, irritability, or disease, the gray matter of the brain is incapable of eliminating normal conditions of *nerve* or *vital* force.

A state of wakefulness is frequently consequent upon an unduly worked and agitated brain, and is often exhibited by persons of a nervous and excitable temperament, who have been subject to great anxiety, or whose intellects have been overwrought and unduly strained. When addressing himself to the importance of anticipating the first dawnings of the cerebral diseases of children, as well as those of adult age, Dr. Graves observes : " You will find in patients who are about to have cerebral symptoms a degree of restless anxiety, and a higher degree of energy, than accords with their condition. They either do not sleep at all, or their sleep is broken by startings and incoherent expressions. When a person is spoken to in this state, he answers in a perfectly rational manner; he will declare that he has little or no headache; and were the physician to be led away by a hasty review of his symptoms, would be very likely to overlook the state of the brain. If a close inquiry be made, it will be found that *the patient scarcely ever sleeps, or even dozes*—that he is irritable, excitable, frequently incoherent, and muttering to himself. Under such circumstances, although there is no remarkable heat of scalp, suffusion of the eye, or headache, the medical attendant must suspect the supervention of cerebral symptoms, particularly about the ninth or tenth day of the fever (for it is generally about this period that cerebral symptoms begin to manifest themselves); and whenever these premonitory indications are observed, the physician should not hesitate to take proper measures to anticipate the evil. In other cases, the encephalic symptoms are ushered in by drowsiness. The patient seems otherwise well, *but he sleeps too much*. About the ninth or tenth day he begins to rave, and exhibits undoubted proofs of congestion and excitement of the brain. To be put on our guard is to be armed in such cases."[1]

In some forms of cerebral irritation and capillary congestion the patient feels un intense and overpowering desire to sleep. *He experiences a heavy and drowsy sensation, but is unable to close his eyes in slumber for many minutes.* He often continues for hours in this state of semi-sleeplessness or morbid drowsiness, without actually sleeping or feeling at all refreshed. This condition of the brain, if permitted to continue for any lengthened period, is productive of much, and often fatal, mental and bodily mischief.

Cases of what may be termed idiopathic sleeplessness occasionally occur, in which the intellect is not (for a period) in the slightest degree disordered. Persons have been known to remain in this state of insomnia for several weeks, *never closing their eyes for five continuous minutes in sleep!* In one female patient the state of sleeplessness arose from a severe shock which she had received, consequent upon finding her husband, in the middle of the night, dead by her side, he having retired to bed apparently in excellent health. In these cases, the patients are seldom heard to complain

---

[1] "Clinical Medicine," by Dr. Graves.

of the want of sleep; they appear to experience none of the usual sensations of bodily and mental fatigue, physical uneasiness, and discomfort, which follow ordinary states of partial and incomplete repose.

Persons actively engaged in literary pursuits, and whose occupations absorb a large amount of nervous energy and energetic thought, are subject to conditions of insomnia. It is said that Paganini rarely slept, so entirely was his mind occupied, night and day, in his intense passion for music. Boerhaave is recorded not to have closed his eyes in sleep for a period of *six* weeks, in consequence of his brain being overwrought by intense thought on a profound subject of study.[1]

The insane are capable of sustaining, with apparent impunity and indifference, long-continued conditions of sleeplessness. The case is published of a deranged person who was not known to close his eyes in sleep for the period of *three* months! He was in the habit of walking long distances, greatly excited during the day, and at night he never ceased talking to imaginary persons. No form or dose of opium had any effect upon him. Dr. Wigan had a patient under his care who did not sleep for fifteen days. He was in the habit of getting up in the night, and tiring three horses with galloping, in the vain hope that excessive muscular fatigue might induce a disposition to sleep.

The pathological state of the brain may account for the condition of sleeplessness so often seen associated with insanity; but in many cases the insomnia connected with mental derangement arises from a complete absorption, abstraction, concentration of the thoughts and preoccupation of the mind, in some terrible and

[1] The question, how long a person can exist without sleep, is one oftener asked than answered, and the difficulties of answering the question by experiment would seem to leave it forever unsolved. A Chinese merchant had been convicted of murdering his wife, and was sentenced to die by being deprived of sleep. This painful mode of death was carried into execution under the following circumstances: The condemned was placed in prison under the care of three of the police guard, who relieved each other every alternate hour, and who prevented the prisoner from falling asleep night or day. He thus lived nineteen days without enjoying any sleep. At the commencement of the eighth day his sufferings were so intense that he implored the authorities to grant him the blessed opportunity of being strangulated, guillotined, burned to death, drowned, garotted, shot, quartered, blown up with gunpowder, or put to death in any conceivable way which their humanity or ferocity could invent. This will give a slight idea of the horrors of death from want of sleep.— *Semi-Monthly Medical News.* Louisville, 1859.

fearful form of illusion, or frightful type of hallucination, that has firmly seized upon the morbid imagination.

The snatches of transient repose which those so unhappily afflicted are able to obtain,

> " Are not sleep,
> But a continuance of enduring thought."

"Sleep is one of the functions which, among insane patients, undergoes the greatest changes. It is especially in the period of incubation of insanity that the absence of sleep presents itself as an important symptom. When I interrogate parents on the incipient phenomena of the disease of their relations, they never fail to inform me of the deprivation of sleep as one of the greatest sufferings that they have had to endure. One can with difficulty form an idea of the tenacity of sleeplessness in the incipient periods of insanity. The absence of a function so eminently reparative increases the conditions of irritability in which the insane are generally found ; and it ordinarily happens that in the confirmed stage of insanity, sleep is more and more disturbed. Complete sleep among the insane is seldom observed except in confirmed dementia, and in the condition of melancholy with stupor. Even in their convalescence, patients often complain of not being able to sleep. In all cases it is frequently interrupted.

"Incomplete sleep is the repose of one of these two orders of sense, and waking of the other ; it refreshes much less, but it satisfies nature more than entire sleep, and I know many men who have no other. Now, when one says that the insane do not sleep, perhaps it is better to say that they are always dreaming, except in their lucid intervals."[1]

I formerly attended a patient who rarely closed her eyes in sleep for ten consecutive minutes for nearly a year. Her existence under these circumstances was perfectly miraculous. The mind was tortured by the most horrible phantasy that ever racked a poor maniac's brain. She imagined she was the original serpent that tempted Eve to eat the forbidden fruit, and was to be punished for this great sin by being compelled to have scorpions, venomous snakes, and reptiles of every description about her person night and day. Whenever she retired to rest, she, in an agonizing tone

---

[1] Morel, p. 458.

of voice, begged, in most piteous terms, that the snakes might be taken from her bed. "I sleep upon scorpions, my bed is full of horrible reptiles, adders are in my pillow and clinging round my neck; for heaven's sake, I beseech,—I implore you,—to have compassion upon me, and rid me of this terrible affliction!" In language thus touching and affecting would this poor creature earnestly and affectionately appeal to every one who approached her.

No preparation or dose of opium, however strong, had any sedative effect upon her brain. She at one time had administered to her large and repeated quantities of the most potent and concentrated preparation of this drug without causing sleep, or even a condition analogous to it :—

> . . . . . . " Not poppy, nor mandragora,
> Nor all the drowsy syrups of the world,"

could, alas !

> " Medicine to a sweet sleep,"

that unhappy and perturbed mind, so fearfully was it shattered and shipwrecked! Her wailings of profound grief and frantic shrieks of wild and hopeless despair were occasionally heard in the dead of the night, towering loudly above the noisy tempest often raging without.

In some types of insanity the patient's mind is altogether absorbed in the contemplation of a frightful spectral illusion. Under these circumstances the unhappy sufferer is afraid to close his eyes in sleep, from an intense fear and dread that he will then fall an easy prey to the horrible phantasm which his morbid imagination has called into existence, and which he imagines follows him in all his movements. The patient so afflicted declares he will not sleep, and resolutely repudiates and perseveringly ignores all disposition to slumber. On many occasions he obstinately refuses to go to bed, or to place himself in a recumbent position. He will battle with his attendant if he attempts to confine him to bed. He insists on remaining in the chair, or standing in an erect position all night, and often determinately walks about the room when those near him are wrapt in profound repose. In these cases the hallucinations appear to be most exquisitely and acutely vivid when the patient is placed in a recumbent position, on account, it is conceived, of the mechanical facilities thus afforded for the blood gravitating freely to the head.

A gentleman who appeared free during the day from any acute hallucinations, never could lie on his back without being distressingly harassed by a number of frightful imps, whom he imagined to be dancing fantastically around him during the night. Under these circumstances, undisturbed sleep whilst in bed could never be obtained. He was in the habit of sleeping in an arm-chair for some time in consequence of these symptoms. He, however, eventually recovered, and has been for many years entirely free from all hallucinations. In cases similar to those previously narrated, the heart is occasionally found in an unhealthy state. Valvular disease of this organ is a common concomitant of disease of the brain associated with illusions or hallucinations.

When speaking of the attack of insanity with which Southey was afflicted previously to his death, Dr. Charles Mackay directs attention to the fact that the poet laureate's mental illness arose from the loss of sleep that he experienced during the time he was in close and affectionate attendance upon the sick bed of his wife. Dr. Mackay observes, alluding to a visit he had paid to Wordsworth, " I found the bard of the ' Excursion' walking in his garden when I arrived at the Mount; and long and fervently did I admire the beauty of the scene from the lawn before the window, and the calm philosophy and true love of nature that had led him to make choice of such a place, and kept him in such happy and such long seclusion from the busy world. The view of Windermere from his door was the finest I had yet seen; and at another part of his grounds, the view of Rydal water was combined with that of Windermere, forming, with Loughrigg in front, amid the encircling hills on every side, a landscape of extreme beauty. * * * In speaking of Southey, whose name is so intimately associated with his own, and whose friendship and society he enjoyed for so many years, he dwelt with much emphasis on the long-continued and systematic economy of his time, by which he was enabled to vary his studies from history to politics, from politics to poetry, and do more work in each than would have sufficed to make the reputation of half a dozen, even of inferior attainments. At the period of his death, and indeed long before, it was the general opinion that he had tasked his brain too severely by study; that his intellect had become overclouded from excess of mental toil,

and that he had labored 'not wisely but too well.' Mr. Wordsworth, however, upon my putting the question to him, denied that
such was the case.   Though Southey's labors were almost super-
human, and varied in a wonderful manner, they seemed, he said,
rather to refresh and strengthen, than to weary and weaken his
mind.   He fell a victim, not to literary toil, but to his strong
affection for his first wife, which led him night after night, when
his labors of the day were ended, to watch with sleepless anxiety
over her sick bed.   The strongest mind, as he observed, will ultimately give way under the long-continued deprivation of the natural refreshment of the body.   No brain can remain in permanent
health that has been overtasked by nightly vigils, still more than
by daily labor.   When such vigils are accompanied by the perpetually-recurring pain of beholding the sufferings of a beloved
object, and the as perpetually-recurring fear of losing it, they become doubly and trebly injurious ; and the labor that must be
done, becomes no longer the joy and solace that it used to be.   It
is transformed from a pleasure into a pain, from a friend into an
enemy, from a companion into a fearful monster, crying like the
daughter of the horse-leech, 'give! give!'   It is then that the fine
and delicate machinery of the mind is deranged.   It is then that
the 'sweet bells are jangled and out of tune,' that the light is extinguished, and the glory under a cloud, that Eternity may lift,
but not Time.   Such, it appears, was the case with the amiable
Southey; the grand, if not the great poet, the accomplished
scholar, and the estimable man in every relation of life."[1]

MORBID DISPOSITION TO EXCESS OF SLEEP.—This symptom
is frequently precursory of attacks of apoplexy, and often exists
in other forms of disease of the brain caused by the presence of
toxic agents in the blood.   A state of lethargic sleep is one of the
peculiar and well-marked signs of cerebral disorder consequent
upon functional derangement or chronic organic disease of the kidneys interfering with the free elimination of urea.   When this
poison is retained in the blood in consequence of the kidneys not
being in a condition to separate and eject it from the system, the
brain often becomes seriously involved.   I have seen renal delirium of a formidable character arise from this cause.[2]

[1] "The Scenery and Poetry of the English Lakes," by Charles Mackay, LL.D.
[2] Dr. Todd has given the following instructions for the detection of urea in the
brain after death, as well as for its discovery in the blood during life: "Take the

A gentleman, apparently in good health at the time, was observed for several days to be unusually lethargic. He was found on several occasions asleep during the day, and was with difficulty roused. He made no complaint of bodily indisposition, and beyond being less active in mind and indisposed to conversation, his wife recognized nothing in connection with his condition to awaken her apprehensions. On the fifth day from the development of the lethargy, he was seized with a sudden attack of vertigo, followed by headache. During the previous morning, whilst dressing, he had an apoplectic fit. He remained in a state of coma for five hours, but eventually recovered without having apparently sustained any serious cerebral damage.

An elderly lady left York in the month of June of last year in good health. During the journey to London, she complained of unusual drowsiness. It was with difficulty she could be kept awake. A few hours after her arrival at the hotel, she was found on the floor of her sitting-room in a state of apoplectic insensi-

serum from a good sized blister and evaporate it to dryness over a water-bath. The residue is to be extracted with alcohol, which is a ready solvent of urea. This alcoholic extract is then to be evaporated to dryness, and a little water added, so as to make a syrupy mass, which should be plunged into a freezing mixture, and a few drops of pure nitric acid added to it. If urea be present the characteristic crystals of nitrate of urea are soon found in the solution, and may be recognized either by the naked eye or by the microscope.

"Take about three-fourths of a whole brain and cut it up into small pieces. Then treat it with four successive portions of boiling distilled water, each portion, consisting of about ten ounces, being allowed to stand six or eight hours before the next is added. The brain while thus macerating should be frequently stirred and mashed about with a glass rod. The washings, after being poured off, are to be mixed together and filtered. The filtered aqueous extract so obtained must be evaporated to dryness over a water-bath, and the dry residue, after being powdered, is to be again treated with four successive portions of boiling distilled water, observing the same precautions as before. The washings, after being mixed together, as before, are to be filtered, and the clear solution evaporated to dryness over a water-bath, and after being thoroughly dried in a hot-water oven, the residue obtained in this manner should be finely powdered, and the powder boiled in five successive portions of ether. The ethereal extract so obtained should be evaporated to dryness at a low temperature, and then treated with a little tepid water, and allowed to get quite cold. It is then to be filtered through paper previously moistened with water, and the clear solution again evaporated to dryness at a low temperature, the extract procured in this way (which would contain all the urea present in the brain operated upon), is to be placed on a glass slide, treated with a drop of strong nitric acid, covered with a bit of thin glass, and allowed to stand a little time, and then examined under the microscope. A few crystals will then be seen, having all the characters of those of nitrate of urea."—*Clinical Lectures*, by Dr. Todd. 1859.

bility, from which she never completely rallied. In this case there was, with the extravasation of blood in the brain, long-existing cardiac disease,—valvular in its character.

MORBID PHENOMENA OF DREAMING.—The premonitory warnings of acute attacks of brain disease, as well as of insanity, occasionally occur during sleep. Patients have complained of being the subject of horrible nocturnal visions and of the severer forms of incubus, or nightmare, previously to attacks of apoplexy, cerebritis, and insanity. These are common premonitory symptoms of the brain affections in early life. Disturbed and frightful dreams often precede the ordinary indications of acute tubercular meningitis. A patient had, for a fortnight preceding an attack of apoplexy, a consecutive series of horrible dreams, in one of which he fancied that he was being scalped by Indians. Other patients have dreamt of falling down precipices, and of being torn to pieces by wild beasts. A gentleman dreamt that his house was in flames, and that he was gradually being consumed to a cinder. This dream occurred a few days before an attack of inflammation of the brain. A person prior to an attack of epilepsy, dreamt that he was severely lacerated by a tiger. Another epileptic patient, shortly before a seizure, fancied, during sleep, he was attacked by murderers, and that they were knocking his brains out with a hammer.

For some weeks previously to the manifestation of acute cerebral symptoms, patients have complained of being the subject of troubled and distressing hallucinations, occurring between sleeping and waking. A barrister, for some years before an attack of cerebral paralysis, was, as his wife informed me, in the habit of frequently awaking from sleep in a state of great alarm and terror, without being able satisfactorily to explain the reasons for his state of apprehension. This condition of mind was not apparently consequent upon a troubled dream, for he had no recollection of having been the subject of one. Cases are on record in which persons who have been attacked by epilepsy, paralysis, and apoplexy, have had for some period previously to their seizures, distinct recollection of dreaming of these affections; in fact, they appear to have had a morbid psychical *presentiment* of their particular disease as well as mode of death. Insanity is often preceded by disturbed sleep and frightful nocturnal visions. This abnormal condition of the mind during sleep cannot be too closely watched in all the acute cerebral diseases of children, as well as of adults, particularly in severe attacks of fever occurring in scrofulous constitutions.

Dr. Beddoes attended an epileptic patient whose first fit succeeded a dream, in which there had occurred the idea of his being crushed by an avalanche, which he had seen the day before.[1]

" Many patients, before becoming completely insane, have frightful dreams, and appear as if they were conscious of being on the eve of losing their reason. They often express this sad prognosis, and their anxiety is very great. They start up out of their sleep, pass the greater part of the night in walking about, complaining of suffering intolerable headaches. Some almost dread to go to sleep, so much are their dreams filled with horrible apparitions. In a book attributed to Hippocrates, there are, with regard to the symptomatology of dreaming, indications which are not without interest. Perhaps it is correct to say that, in our days of modern science, this element of diagnosis and prognosis has been too much neglected. Among other prognostications, noisy and animated dreams, according to the father of medicine, are the indication of a state of excitement of the nervous system. Quiet, soft dreams announce a favorable crisis in nervous fevers. Frightful dreams indicate a determination of blood to the head causing delirium. If a person

---

[1] " In certain respects, dreams ought to be attentively studied : natural instinct can, in certain cases, while inciting the imagination to certain ideas, induce useful dreams, containing salutary warnings. Aspasia thus learnt the simple remedy which restored her to health, and it is likewise in a dream that the physician Abin-Zoar had the revelation of a medicine by the aid of which he freed himself from severe ophthalmia. If one, in fact, notices the extreme facility with which the ideas, free from the chain of exterior impressions, associate themselves during sleep, one can conceive how, in the midst of a thousand strange combinations, luminous perceptions sometimes arise."

" One can explain in the same way the marvellous perspicuity of certain dreamers who, under one form or other, seem to foresee diseases of which the germ until then had been latent. Arnauld de Villeneuve dreamt one night that a black cat bit him on the side. The next day an anthrax appeared on the part bitten. A patient of Galen's dreamt that one of his limbs was changed into stone. Some days after, this leg was paralyzed. Such was also the case of the woman of whom Gunther has spoken; she dreamt that she was being beaten with a whip. In the morning she bore lesions like scars. Roger d'Oxteyn, knight of the company of Douglas, went to sleep in good health. Towards the middle of the night he saw in his dream a man infected with the plague, quite naked, who attacked him with fury, threw him on the ground after a desperate struggle, and holding him between his open thighs, vomited the plague into his mouth. Three days after he was seized with the plague, and died. Hippocrates remarks that dreams in which one sees black spectres are a bad omen."—*Anatomie Comparée du Système Nerveux*, &c., par Drs. Leuret et Gratiolet. Paris, 1839–1857.

sees in dreams frightful figures making grimaces, the person is
menaced with an intestinal malady, or an affection of the liver.
Diseases of the internal organs cause in dreaming painful sensations, which relate to the parts affected. Apoplexy is preceded
by dreams in which the person believes that he is in danger of
perishing. . . . . The nightmare announces the concentration
of blood in the great cavities of the chest. I mention these principal prognostics because the ordinary subject of complaints in
individuals destined to become insane are associated with sensations
of this kind."[1]

A gentleman who had previously manifested no appreciable
symptoms of mental disorder, or even of disturbed and anxious
thought, retired to bed apparently in a sane state of mind. Upon
rising in the morning, to the intense horror of his wife, he was
found to have lost his senses! He exhibited his insanity by asserting that he was going to be tried for an offence which he could not
clearly define, and of the nature of which he had no right conception. He declared that the officers of justice were in hot pursuit
of him; in fact, he maintained that they were actually in the
house. He begged and implored his wife to protect him. He
walked about the bedroom in a state of great agitation, apprehension, and alarm, stamping his feet and wringing his hands in the
wildest agony of despair. Upon inquiring into the history of the
case, his wife said, that she had not observed any symptom that
excited her suspicion as to the state of her husband's mind; but
upon being questioned very closely, she admitted that during the
previous night he appeared to have been under the influence of
what she considered to be the nightmare, or a frightful dream.
Whilst apparently asleep he cried out several times, evidently in
great distress of mind, "Don't come near me." "Take them
away." "Oh, save me, they are pursuing me!" It is singular
that in this case, the insanity which was clearly manifested in the
morning appeared like *a continuation of the same character and
train of perturbed thought that existed during his troubled sleep,*
when, according to the wife's account, he was evidently dreaming.

Pinel observes, "Ecstatic visions during the night often form
the prelude to paroxysms of maniacal devotion. It is also sometimes by enchanting dreams, and a supposed apparition of a beloved

---

[1] "Traité des Maladies Mentales," par le Docteur B. A. Morel. Paris, 1860.

object, that insanity from love breaks out with fury after longer or shorter intervals of reason and tranquillity."

I am indebted to a medical friend for the particulars of the following case : During the winter of 1849, he was called to see H. B., about five or six o'clock in the morning.   The patient was the wife of a tailor, and mother of three children.   At this time she was rather emaciated and debilitated in bodily health, and anæmic in appearance.   She was of religious turn of mind, and belonged to the Wesleyan persuasion.   On the morning of the narrator's visit, he found the woman in a state of great mental excitement, and under the influence of hallucinations.   She had gone to bed apparently well, but during the night was the subject of a vivid dream, imagining that she saw her sister, long since dead, and to whom she was very much attached, suffering the pains of hell.   When quite awake, no one could persuade her that she had been under the influence of an agitated dream.   She stoutly persisted in maintaining the reality of her vision.   During the whole of that day she was clearly insane ; but on the following morning the mind appeared to have recovered its balance.   She continued tolerably well mentally for four years, with the exception of her occasionally having moments of despondency, arising from real or fancied troubles.   At the end of the fifth year she gave birth to a child.   Seven months afterwards, she went to bed apparently as well as usual.   In the middle of the night she got up, without apparently knowing what she was doing, and cut her child's throat with a razor.   The wound, however, was not fatal.   When requested to explain why she had attempted the life of her child, she replied, that she had been ordered during the night to murder all her children, as well as herself.   When taken into custody, she expressed no regret for what she had done, but appeared to entertain a great fear of punishment. During the night of the murder, her husband states that she was unusually disturbed.   It is conceived that the hallucination which led to the commission of the murder occurred during a dream.   This woman was tried and acquitted on the ground of insanity, and is now confined in Stafford County Lunatic Asylum.

Suicide has been committed under analogous circumstances. A person, apparently well, has gone to bed without manifesting the slightest tendency to self-destruction, and being suddenly aroused from a frightful dream, has destroyed himself.

An old lady, residing in London, awoke in the middle of the night, went down stairs, and threw herself into a cistern of water, where she was found drowned. The suicide was supposed to be the result of certain mental impressions originating in the mind during a dream.

Dr. Pagan refers to the following interesting case, to prove that murder may be committed by a person when under the effects of a frightful vision :—

"Bernard Schedmaizig suddenly awoke at midnight; at the moment he saw a frightful phantom, or what his imagination represented as such—a fearful spectre! He twice called out, 'Who is that?' and, receiving no answer, and imagining that the phantom was advancing upon him, and having altogether lost his self-possession, he raised a hatchet which was beside him, and attacked the spectre, and it was found that he had murdered his wife."[1]

A peddler, who was in the habit of walking about the country, armed with a sword-stick, was awakened one evening while lying asleep on the high road by a man suddenly seizing him, and shaking him by the shoulders. The man, who was walking by with some companions, had done this out of a joke. The peddler suddenly awoke, drew his sword, and stabbed the man, who soon afterwards died. He was tried for manslaughter. His irresponsibility was strongly urged by his counsel, on the ground that he could not have been conscious of his act in the half waking state. This was strengthened by competent medical witnesses. He was, however, found guilty, and, I think, most unjustly punished.[2]

[1] "Medical Jurisprudence of Insanity," by Dr. Pagan. London, 1840.
[2] "Medico-Chirurgical Review."

CHAPTER XXIV.

MORBID PHENOMENA OF ORGANIC AND NUTRITIVE LIFE.

THIS division of the subject will be briefly considered in the following order :—

  a. Digestion and Assimilation.
  β. Circulation.
  γ. Respiration.
  δ. Generation.

DIGESTION AND ASSIMILATION.—Owing to the close and intimate sympathy existing between the brain, organs of digestion, and in fact the whole of the chylopoietic viscera, we are usually able to detect, in association with cerebral diseases, functional disturbances of the digestion and nutrition, often giving rise to serious complications. These symptoms, however, are often altogether overlooked, in consequence of their being masked by the more prominently developed signs of local head affection or psychical disorder.[1]

In the early stage of insanity, the stomach exhibits evidences of great functional derangement. The appetite fails, the powers of digestion become impaired, the secretions vitiated, the liver disordered, and the bowels act with great irregularity, or are obstinately costive. The gastric affection is recognized by fœtid breath, coated tongue, anorexia, sometimes amounting to loathing of food, deficient hepatic secretion, and great depression of spirits. The

---

[1] Willis, as quoted by Morel, says Dr. Griesinger, relates a remarkable case of a lady whose health had been injured by profound grief. One day, after having eaten a very indigestible cake, she was seized with a feeling of burning heat in the precordial region. There followed an instantaneous sensorial delirium. She imagined that the upper part of her body was on fire. She took a spring, and precipitated herself into the street, crying out that she was cursed by God, damned, and that she already was experiencing the punishments of hell. The same delirium was reproduced as soon as this lady experienced the same physical sensation.

patient complains of flatulence, cardialgia, and acidity of the stomach; occasionally there is extreme nausea, and often actual vomiting. The presence of constant sickness, when it cannot be clearly traced to an idiopathic affection of the uterus, kidney, or stomach, is significant of functional or organic disease of the brain, particularly when connected with headache, vertigo, and other indications of local cerebral disturbance. These symptoms will be considered more in detail in the succeeding chapter.

In tumors of the brain, the patient will be often heard to complain not only of irritability, but of a disposition to vomit. The nausea so induced in a remarkable manner resembles that preceding or accompanying sea-sickness. The patient is rarely, if ever, actually sick, but he constantly feels so at the stomach. This sensation of nausea is occasionally observed more prominently manifested on first rising in the morning. The patient, when washing, or whilst shaving, will be suddenly stopped by an inclination to vomit. A person who was troubled by this symptom, caused by a cerebral tumor, remarked that it appeared as if he were constantly rolling about in a boat at sea, or repeatedly under the influence of small doses of tartar-emetic or ipecacuanha. I have observed this symptom in some cases of abscess of the brain. A gentleman who died suddenly of this disease, was annoyed for some months previously to his decease by a troublesome and depressing sensation of nausea. For some time this symptom was supposed to arise from disordered state of the stomach, and he was treated for this affection. After examining the case several times, I diagnosed disease of the brain (tumor). There was associated with the nausea severe vertigo, and paroxysmal attacks (somewhat localized) of headache. The cerebral abscess was considered to be the effect of a severe injury inflicted upon the head by a fall from a horse, whilst hunting, ten years previously.

The sensation of nausea, not amounting to actual vomiting, is occasionally symptomatic of acute and chronic softening of the brain. It often indicates the commencement of inflammatory and congested encephalic conditions. In the obscure cerebral diseases of children, the presence of irritability of the stomach, clearly not connected with gastric or intestinal derangement, is an important diagnostic symptom.

Chronic disorders of the digestive organs frequently precede, are associated with, if they do not operate as the direct cause of, various types of mental derangement. A morbid state of the liver, stomach, and bowels, is seen prominently manifested in all forms and degrees of insanity. These gastric disturbances and visceral complications are often observed in an advanced position throughout the whole course of the malady. They give character and persistence to the mental impressions. In consequence of these physical derangements, patients are often led to believe that they have been or are being poisoned, and under such hallucinations obstinately refuse all nourishment. In such cases, there is generally found clear and unmistakable evidence of serious disorder of the stomach, disease of the liver, or chronic irritation of the mucous membrane of the bowels. The breath is fœtid, the tongue furred, the secretions vitiated, bowels inactive, and appetite either altogether lost or extremely vitiated. Under these circumstances, there is a positive loathing of food.

"The refusal to take nourishment," says M. Morel, "often depends upon a disordered condition of the digestive organs. The truly wonderful obstinacy with which certain insane persons refuse food is, however, most commonly caused by their delirious ideas, such as the fear of poison and a desire to die of hunger in obedience to an order given them by a superior power." M. Morel relates the case of a lady whom he had to feed for several weeks by means of the stomach-pump, who refused to eat voluntarily, under the influence of an illusion that the food placed before her was composed of the flesh of her murdered children!

"Some insane patients complain of a fire that devours them, and sometimes of an icy coldness which paralyzes the peristaltic action. They are subject to borborygmus and flatulence. All the phenomena that men enjoying their reason bring easily to a right interpretation, become among hypochondriacs the starting-point of the most strange illusions. They have in their intestines unclean animals who gnaw them; some even pretend to have neither stomach nor intestines. It seems to them that all they eat falls down a bottomless gulf. One patient imagines that she ought no longer to eat or speak. Her body no longer exists; it is one composed of shapeless fragments, which have no cohesion between them. Also her clothes are not attached to her person, and she constantly experiences a most painful sensation for a modest woman,—she believes that she is going to be exposed naked to public view."[1]

[1] Morel.

32

The presence of worms in the stomach and intestines often creates an uncontrollable indisposition for food. Chronic inflammation, and sometimes ulceration of the bowels, have been known to produce analogous symptoms.

The appetite is frequently seriously vitiated and depraved. In these cases the patient has a morbid craving, and never satisfied desire for food. His hunger cannot be appeased. After eating an enormous meal he will emphatically declare that he has been starved, or had supplied to him either the minimum amount of nutriment, or no food at all! A vitiation of the appetite is shown by the patient eating with an apparent relish or at least indifference, the most repulsive and disgusting matters. The sense of taste in these cases occasionally appears to be paralyzed.

In the incipient stage of insanity the assimilative functions are often seriously disordered. Hence the emaciation so often observed to accompany, not only the commencement of insanity, but of various organic diseases of the brain uncomplicated with aberration of mind.[1]

As the mental disorder advances, the function of assimilation is occasionly restored to a state of healthy action, and the patient not only gains flesh, but becomes *embonpoint*. This condition is often observed in chronic types of insanity, and in other cases where the patient is less sensitive to the destructive effect of his insane delusions. He ceases to be worried or vexed by his morbid ideas, and consequently an improvement in the digestion and nutrition takes place. If the mental does not proceed *pari passu* with the physical restoration to health, an unfavorable prognosis is generally entertained. But even under these discouraging conditions I have frequently seen patients recover.

MORBID PHENOMENA OF CIRCULATION, RESPIRATION, AND GENERATION.—Considering the close organic sympathy between the heart and brain, we should, *à priori*, infer that in all affections of the great nervous centre, the cardiac functions would almost invariably exhibit marked deviations from a normal state. In

---

[1] All disorders of the nervous system, particularly those implicating the intelligence, have a damaging influence upon the functions of *nutrition*. In cases of simple anxiety of mind, how often do we observe the general health to become seriously impaired, and the assimilative powers to be completely paralyzed. In the incipient stage of insanity the nutritive functions appear occasionally altogether suspended. The patient, long before attention is called to the state of the mind, loses flesh, and is occasionally reduced to a dangerous state of emaciation and inanition.

the writings of Morgagni, Baglivi, Lieutaud, and Corvisart, this subject is but cursorily referred to. Although the latter authority affirms that he has never seen an instance of apoplexy that can be clearly traced to cardiac disease, he is, nevertheless, of opinion that the cases recorded by Testa, Laurent, and the other writers previously mentioned, "*suffisent pour établir qu'une affection du cœur peut devenir la cause determinante de l'apoplexie.*" Richerand is said to be the first writer who pointed out pathologically the intimate connection between encephalic and cardiac disorders."

This distinguished physiologist says, "the dissection of patients who have died of apoplexy has proved to me that the excess of force in the left ventricle of the heart is a more powerfully predisposing cause of the disease than a large head and short neck— a state of body which is supposed by most physicians to indicate the apoplectiform conformation."[1]

In a Mémoire read by Richerand before the *Ecole de Médecine*, he refers to the case of the illustrious Cabanis, who died of apoplexy caused by, or associated with, disease of the heart. The autopsy of this distinguished philosopher revealed extensive cardiac disease. The left ventricle was enormously enlarged and hypertrophied. Eight ounces of blood were effused into the ventricles of the brain, and this effusion had been so violent, that the septum lucidum was torn through, and the surface of the thalami and corpora striata found rough and jagged. Malpighi and Ramazzini died of apoplectic attacks connected with hypertrophy of the heart.

More recently Lallemand, Broussais, Andral, Bouillaud, Bertin, and Rochoux have directed attention to this subject. MM. Bertin and Bouillaud remark that, "the majority of the patients in whom hypertrophy of the left ventricle of the heart is present, will be found to exhibit symptoms of cerebral congestion, and that many of them will fall victims of disease of the brain."[2] In our own country Drs. Hope, Copland, Watson, Wardrop, Bright, Burrows, and Bennett, have considered this subject at some length.[3]

Important as this subject is to the practical physician as well as physiologist, it is not my intention to go minutely into its analysis.

---

[1] "Nosographie Chirurgicale," vol. iii. [2] "Traité des Maladies du Cœur."
[3] "On Diseases of the Heart," by Dr. Hope. "Dictionary of Medicine," by Dr. Copland. Communication read at the College of Physicians, March 30, 1835, by Dr. Watson. "On Disease of the Heart," by Dr. Wardrop. "Medical Reports," by Dr. Bright. "Disorders of the Cerebral Circulation," by Dr. Burrows.

It is sufficient for my purpose to call attention to the fact, reserving for the succeeding volume any detailed remarks I may have to make in reference to the influence exercised by certain affections of the heart upon various functional and organic diseases of the brain.

There can be no doubt among those whose duty it is to investigate the disorders of the mind in all their numerous phases, that cardiac disease exercises a material influence over the psychical functions of the cerebrum. How common it is for the physician whilst performing his autopsies in acute and particularly chronic cases of insanity, to discover apparently long-existing organic disease of the heart, especially in its valvular structure. All writers on the subject of insanity have called attention to this fact.

M. Falret, of the Hospice de la Salpêtrière, has published the results of his dissections in ninety-two cases of chronic mania. In twenty of these there were "*des lésions diverses du cœur, coincidant avec des alterations chroniques du cerveau, ou des membranes cérébrales.*"

More recently, Morel, when referring to the connection between the central circulatory system and cerebral diseases, observes, "that the affections of the heart enter largely into the etiology of mental affections." A patient under his care, subject to maniacal paroxysms, imagined that he had confined in his chest an animal that was devouring his heart. After death, hypertrophy of this organ was discovered, with disease interfering with the free passage of the blood through the auriculo-ventricular orifice. These organic changes in the substance of the heart as well as in its valves, associated with insanity, give rise to great difficulty of respiration, headache, restlessness, insomnia, and severe paroxysms of irritability. These symptoms are often associated with great œdema of the extremities. Morel adds, "I have observed among such patients the periodical return of strange ideas, hypochondriacal sensations, and often special hallucinations, which arise with the increase of the impediment to the circulation and the cerebral congestion which is the consequence of it. These hallucinations are usually of a terrifying nature." "It is known," says M. Saucerotte, "what a powerful shock the beating of the arteries occasions to the encephalic mass, and one conceives, *à priori*, what disorder might be caused to the intelligence if they were repeated with abnormal frequency,

on the organ destined to elaborate the ideas.   We are bound also
to consider the effect thus produced in the physiological stimula-
tion and nutrition of the brain.   The blood, altered in its character, and hurried or impeded in its course through the cerebral
vessels, must produce profound modifications in the nervous tissue
of the organ of thought.''

In the early stage of insanity the pulse occasionally indicates
great activity of the centre of circulation, but more generally the
action of the heart is feeble, and the state of the pulse establishes
the presence of great vascular, vital, and nervous depression.
This condition of the radial artery is quite compatible with a considerable amount of acute mental agitation and muscular violence.

There is considerable difference in the action of the radial,
carotid, and temporal vessels, as well as in the intensity of the
pulsation of the ascending and descending aorta.   Jacobi has
called particular attention to this phenomenon, but the consideration of this important and interesting physiological and pathological subject must be deferred for another occasion.

RESPIRATION AND GENERATION.—There are no special morbid
conditions of the respiratory function which can be considered
symptomatic of incipient insanity, or as indicative of the commencement of organic disease of the brain.   The lungs are, no
doubt, in close organic sympathy with the brain, and in many
cases of mental alienation, the two organs in a marked manner
reciprocally influence each other.

The autopsies of the insane often reveal extensive disorganizations of the substance as well as investing membrane of the lungs,
which have · seriously complicated the psychical disorder, and in-
terfered with the satisfactory progress of the case.

The generative functions in some forms of cerebral disorder are
exalted.   In other states of the brain and nervous system, they
are perverted, impaired, or altogether paralyzed.   I have known
insanity, of a senile type, develope itself by a sudden and unnatural manifestation of virile inclination and capacity, at a
period of life when this function is generally considered to be in
a state of dormancy.   But this important subject, in all its numerous ramifications, physiological, pathological, and psychological,
will be analyzed *in extenso*, when I proceed to consider, in the
succeeding volume, the obscure diseases of the cerebrum, but
particularly the *cerebellum*, as influencing, directly and indirectly,
the reproductive organs.

CHAPTER XXV.

GENERAL PRINCIPLES OF CEREBRAL PATHOLOGY, DIAGNOSIS, TREATMENT, AND PROPHYLAXIS.

PATHOLOGY.—It was never my intention to enter, in this work, at any length into a consideration of the subject of cerebral and mental pathology. This vast and important field of scientific research must, as far as this treatise is concerned, be but cursorily examined, if not left altogether unexplored. This is unavoidable, considering the number of complex and disputed questions involved in its investigation.

The obscurity that envelopes the pathology of the brain, is admitted by every writer whose attention has been directed to its analysis. How vain and illusory would it be were I to attempt to embody in a few pages, anything approximating to an accurate conception of the numerous changes, functional and organic, which the brain, appendages, and vessels are susceptible of, and which are known to give rise to a variety of types of cerebral disease and mental disorder?

Let me briefly illustrate the difficulties of this subject. A gentleman, aged fifty-six, apparently in good health, and with, it is alleged, no constitutional predisposition to disease of the brain, was the subject of a violent mental shock. I purposely avoid going more into detail. Insanity in its most acute form developed itself. The mental excitement was of a most frightful and alarming character. There was nothing in the state of the pulse, condition of the carotids or temporal arteries, or in the action of the heart itself, to justify the conclusion that there was any great disturbance of the vascular system. The head was cool, the conjunctivæ presented a normal appearance, and the tongue was but slightly furred. A most careful examination was made with the view of discovering the existence of physical complications, but none were detected. His delusions consisted in a belief that he was surrounded by evil spirits, and that some of them were engaged in tearing him to pieces. He was treated by means of prolonged hot-baths, cathartics, and sedatives, but no persistent impression was made upon the malady. The evident vital depression that characterized the attack, clearly contra-indicated antiphlogistic remedies; in fact, so great was the debility, that wine and ammonia to a considerable extent were administered, with the view of sustaining life during the fearful paroxysms of maniacal excitement which so remarkably distinguished the mental disorder. He died, and a few hours afterwards a most careful *post-mortem* examination was made. To the astonishment of every one who was present, no disease was discovered in the brain. The cerebral substance was of normal consistence, the membranes enveloping the brain exhibited no structural change, and the numerous vessels ramifying through the organ, were free from disease as well as congestion. In general terms, the brain appeared to be in a healthy condition. The heart was unusually small and flabby; the liver, stomach, and bowels, presented no symptom of disease. In one of the kidneys there was evidence of the commencement of granular disease. We had no reason to suspect the presence of urea in the blood or in the substance of the brain, and therefore no analysis was made with a view to its detection.

A gentleman holding an official position in one of our colonial dependencies, came to England on sick leave. Whilst in this country he formed an unhappy attachment to a lady whom he afterwards found to be a married woman living separately from her husband. This discovery caused at the time considerable agitation, eventually resulting in great mental depression. This state of mind continued for four or five weeks, during which period it was necessary to have him watched with great care, with the view of preventing him from committing suicide. At the expiration of three months from the commencement of his illness, the character of the affliction entirely altered. He became violently and acutely excited; he required three attendants to be constantly with him, and these he frequently attacked with great furor, threatening to murder them. This condition of cerebral and mental exaltation was associated with great vital depression. The case bid defiance to all treatment. None of the usual remedies appeared to touch the malady. There was no particular variation in the symptoms up to the period of death. At the *post-mortem* examination the brain was carefully examined. It was in a perfectly bloodless or anæmic condition. I never saw a brain so pale and free from blood. No disease of importance was discovered in any other part of the body.

A gentleman, alleged to have been previously free from all symptoms of mental derangement, became much impressed on hearing an exciting sermon. Great mental excitement soon followed, ending in a furious attack of mania. There was no symptom in connection with the case, to justify the conclusion that there was activity of the circulation. The pulse was weak, and the action of the heart feeble. The case appeared in its principal features to resemble those previously detailed. After death I examined the brain in conjunction with Dr. W. O. Priestley, with whom I first saw the case in consultation. The substance as well as membranes of the brain were gorged with blood. The passive state of venous congestion that existed, gave a dark, and in fact, almost black appearance to the brain, as soon as the calvarium was removed. Beyond this engorgement of the cerebral vessels, no disease in the structure or membranes of the brain was discovered.

A lady, thirty-five years of age, became acutely insane a month after her confinement. She died. The *post-mortem* examination revealed no special organic change within the cranium, with this exception, that on the surface of the two hemispheres there appeared to be the smallest possible amount of turgescence, similar in character to a transient blush upon the cheek consequent upon some fugitive mental emotion.

A man, aged sixty-four, died laboring under symptoms characteristic of general paralysis. Neither the brain or membranes exhibited evidences of organic change. The surface of the two hemispheres appeared as if some water had been dashed over them.[1] This was the only appreciable cause for the severe cerebral disturbance which preceded for so many years the death of this patient.

A young gentleman had been subject, from an early period of his life, to epilepsy of varying degrees of frequency and severity. Many years back the fits appeared to occur less often, and were somewhat diminished in violence. At this time he discharged from

---

[1] This could not be considered as the effect of subarachnoid effusion. It was what Dr. Seymour terms a " watery brain."

his bowels an enormous tapeworm. The medical gentleman attending the patient at once exclaimed, "Here is the cause of the epilepsy!" and very reasonably inferred that the disease would immediately subside or be disarmed of its more formidable features. Contrary, however, to the expectation of every person acquainted with the facts of the case, the epileptic fits recurred with increased violence, and continued until the moment of death.

Reasoning, à priori, it was concluded that the brain would unquestionably manifest some unequivocal symptoms of organic change either in its substance or investing membranes. But such was not the case. Beyond an unusual firmness and consistence in the nervous tissue of the whole of the brain, not really amounting to induration, there was nothing within the cranium that could satisfactorily account for the great severity and long duration of the cerebral disorder.

I have designedly selected the preceding cases as illustrations of the difficulties that beset the efforts of the medical philosopher in his vain, and often illusory attempts, to unravel the obscurity enveloping the subject of cerebral pathology.

I have made no reference to cases of chronic organic encephalic disease of long duration, the existence of which was not suspected during life. I allude particularly to tumors and abscesses of the brain, which have produced serious disorganizations of structure, without apparently disturbing the special functions of the sensorium during life.

Let me cursorily glance at the pathology of the brain as elucidating the phenomena of incipient insanity. Is there any one condition of the encephalon, or its membranes, pathognomonic of mental derangement? It will be well to consider, before attempting to reply to this question, the variety of theories propounded by eminent and experienced pathologists, with the view of elucidating the cerebral or somatic origin of insanity. A short historical resumé of the kind proposed will enable the reader to appreciate the difficulties surrounding this important branch of pathological science.

Morgagni considered insanity to be more immediately connected with hardening and softening of the brain. Greding refers principally to thickening of the cranial bones, softening of the brain, and atrophy of the thalami. Broussais asserts that insanity is the result of irritation of the brain. Gall and Spurzheim attribute insanity to encephalitis, acute and chronic. Pinel considered mania to be the result of excessive exaltation of the nervous energy. He affirms that cerebral lesions are but the effect of the insanity, and are frequently altogether unobserved. He is also of opinion that insanity frequently arises from visceral complications. Delaye and Foville attribute alienation to inflammation of the superficies of the gray matter of the brain. Fodéré imputes insanity to an alteration of the vital principle. Defour endeavors to establish that the brain has directly no connection with insanity. According to his theory, alienation of mind is consequent upon some affection of the nervous ganglia of the abdomen. Leuret, Baillarger, and Boismont, appear to be of opinion that insanity does not arise from any specific disorganization of the brain or its membranes, but that, in all cases, cerebral disease of some kind exists. Grandchamp, Bayle, and Calmeil, are of opinion that the brain is always diseased in insanity. Rodriguez recognizes three kinds of disease of the brain which give rise to insanity, viz.: 1. Hypertrophic hardening. 2. Inflammatory hardening. 3. Atrophic, or serous hardening. The first and third class he believes generally affect the whole cerebral mass. The second is only partial in its operation, and is characterized by change of color. Rush, the distinguished American authority, traces insanity to a disordered state of the bloodvessels. Haslam refers principally, in his *post-mortem* data, to adhesions of the Pacchionian glands, alterations in the membranes of the brain, and softening of the cerebral pulp. Cox ascribes insanity to determination of blood to the head. Arnold and Parry trace insanity to determination of blood to the brain, or increased activity of the cerebral vessels. Cullen considered that insanity arose from some irregularity in the action of the brain or nervous system, and that, in the majority of cases, derangement was caused by cerebral excitement. Sir Alexander Crichton was of opinion that insanity was caused by a specific morbid action of the vessels which secrete the nervous fluid, affecting not only its quality but quantity.

It would be useless, and foreign to the design of this work, to proceed any further into the historical analysis of this subject. This matter will be considered at great length in a succeeding treatise.

The question more immediately in review is, whether there are any specific and clearly definable characteristic organic alterations

in the tissue of the encephalic mass, its membranes, osseous investment, bloodvessels, &c., invariably present in insanity, that can be
considered to stand in relation of cause and effect. If the substance of the brain be universally implicated in all cases of alienation of mind, is there any uniformity in the organic changes? If
insanity be, as many suppose, an inflammatory affection, what is
the precise nature and seat of the phlegmasia?

There can be no doubt entertained by those who have had practical opportunities of observing and treating the varied phenomena
of mental derangement, that in many instances the disease clearly
arises from a state of active capillary congestion on the surface of
the hemispherical ganglia, or in the vessels ramifying over the
membranes immediately in contact with them. Hence the great
relief so frequently obtained in certain types of acute incipient
insanity, by a judicious local abstraction of blood from the head.
No doubt there are many phases of morbid alienation of thought
not dependent upon an inflammatory, or even a congested state of
the brain, and which do not admit of antiphlogistic treatment.
Cases occur associated with wild, violent, and ungovernable excitement, and characterized by active delirium, apparently unconnected with any appreciable deviation from a normal state of the
skull, brain, meninges, or vessels. I have often been much surprised, when examining the heads of patients who have died from
the effects of acute insanity, with the remarkable absence of even
an approximation to an *adequate* physical cause for the fatal mental disorder.

Such types of insanity must either be connected with subtle
changes in the vesicular neurine, of which we at present have no
knowledge, and which are not even detectable by means of the
microscope, or arise from an altered condition of the blood, nerve
force, or chemical constituents of brain matter, of the nature of
which we are obliged to confess ourselves profoundly ignorant.

I am inclined to the opinion, that such forms of derangement of
mind when they cannot be traced to alterations of nervous *tissue*,
or to the influence of some destructive poison retained in the system and floating in the blood seriously damaging the nutrition of
the brain, may depend upon a disordered condition or altered action of the *psychical co-ordinating principle* evolved in the cerebrum, which (when the brain is free from a material change, and
the mind not disordered) preserves intact the unity of action and

normal balance of the intellectual powers. In an early part of this work I have termed this condition of mind a *choreic* phase of insanity. No doubt, in many cases of mental disorder, the encephalon is in a state of nervous irritation, innervation, hyperæmia (active and passive). In instances of intense exaltation of mind (resembling, in many of their features, violent and ungovernable passion), with or without aberration of the ideas, apparently untraceable to physical molecular alterations in the structure of the brain, its membranes, or to derangement in other organic portions of the body in intimate sympathy with the sensorium, the condition of the mind may be either one of cerebral irritation, or, if I may coin a phrase, psychical hyperæsthesia.

I designedly avoid entering into a consideration of these subtle changes in the gray matter of the brain, the effect of irritation, congestion, or inflammatory action, recognized by slight variations in the color or tint of the cineritious matter of the hemispheres, or to those organic alterations in the structure of the *dura mater*, *tunica arachnoidea*, or *pia mater*, as well as formation of adventitious membranes so often observed after death in cases of insanity. I also defer for subsequent consideration certain morbid conditions of the blood, diseases of the cerebral arteries (fatty degeneration), affections of the heart, liver, lungs, and kidneys, as well as visceral complications, so often seen in association with various types of mental alienation.

I have previously addressed myself briefly to the pathology of general paralysis, as well as to those conditions of the brain which usually accompany ordinary attacks of apoplexy, softening, and hemiplegia. In the former affection, the following pathological phenomena are generally more or less appreciable after death: Albuminous jelly-like effusion in the cavity of the arachnoid; false membranes on the convexity of hemispheres; suppurative meningitis; pus between the folds of the arachnoid and the pia mater, different from the ordinary character of pus (white, and composed of irregularly formed globules, smaller than those in pus detected in other parts of the body); hyperæmia of the brain; pulp red, injected, and slightly tumid, and when sliced small points of blood appearing; softening of brain, superficial or deeply seated, or partial diminution in the consistency of the gray matter of the hemispheres, appreciable by aid of the microscope; alterations in the color of the brain, varying from red, deep brown, pale green, and yellow ; induration of the brain ; organic alterations in the membranes of the brain, of the character of chronic meningitis ; subarachnoid effusion ; injected as well as indurated condition of the medullary portion of the brain ; effusion into the ventricles, delicate layers of coagulable lymph over the cineritious substance of the brain ; highly congested state of the cineritious neurine ; thickening, opacity, and engorgement of the meninges ; marble-like appearance of the white substance of the brain ; atrophy of the convolutions ; fatty degeneration of the cerebral vessels ; organic changes in the pons varolii and medulla oblongata ; œdematous state of the brain.

I do not propose to go at any length into a consideration of the pathology of apoplexy, hemiplegia, or what is termed red and white softening of the brain. All these organic affections are so closely and intimately allied, that it would be impossible to analyze one without reviewing the morbid phenomena characteristic of the other encephalic conditions.

Softening of the brain is frequently followed by apoplexy, and its sister affection, hemiplegia. The latter disorder, when consequent upon the rupture of one of the cerebral vessels (the effect of extravasation of blood), often gives rise (operating mechanically) to a pulpy disorganization of the brain immediately connected with and surrounding the clot.

In what may be termed idiopathic ramollissement the effect of disordered states of cerebral nutrition, termed gangrene of the brain, and occasionally in that type of pulpy disorganization the result of inflammation, acute and chronic, of the substance of the encephalon, the numerous vessels are often in a diseased condition, caused by a deposition of osseous matter on their internal coats, thus causing a mechanical interruption to the free admission and circulation of blood through the brain, and cutting off a proper supply of nutrient fluid to the encephalic mass.[1]

[1] " The deposits in the arteries produce a twofold influence upon the circulation,— by roughening the inner surface of the arterial channels they create a certain amount of direct obstacle to the flow of blood from the ventricle ; and by diminishing, or nearly destroying the elasticity of the arterial walls, they impair one of the most important forces by which the circulation is carried on in the arterial system. Thus the arteries, from being elastic yielding channels, with perfectly smooth inner surfaces, are changed into resisting inert tubes, with rough inner surfaces. It is plain, then, that under these circumstances, the heart has to encounter great obstacles, and to do a great deal more work than when the arteries are in their normal state. Hence the dilata-

If the cerebral vessels are not themselves diseased in the first instance, they often become so after being for some time imbedded in a mass of softened brain. The tissue of this organ often in cases of severe ramollissement is pulpy and diffluent in character, and of the consistence of cream.

When describing cases of hemiplegia occurring in the manner previously narrated, Dr. Todd remarks, "that the diseased blood-vessels lie in the midst of this pulpy mass without undergoing any further change; but sooner or later, under some mental emotion, or during some increased heart's action, depending either upon mental emotion, upon derangement of the digestive organs, some bodily exertion, or increased mental effort of any kind, the blood is sent with undue force or in unusual quantity into the vessels, and in consequence, the vascular canals in the pulpy portion of the cerebral tissue, being deprived of their usual support, give way, and blood is effused into the softened part of the brain, which it breaks up, and the more readily in consequence of its already diminished consistence. This is the rationale of the development of many an attack of apoplexy, from which the patient may or may not recover, according to the extent of the brain previously softened, and according to the amount of blood effused."[1]

In considering the subject of cerebral pathology very erroneous

tion caused by the obstacle to the free flow of the blood; and the hypertrophy, by the greater exercise and effort of the muscle of the heart. The increase of force is merely remedial, to meet the increase of obstacle, and is one of those beautiful instances of self-adaptation to change of circumstances with which the animal organism, especially the muscular system, so much abounds.

"As these deposits go on they impair the materials of the arteries of the brain; the degenerated walls of these vessels possess less strength, and are less able to support their contents. There is no undue determination of blood to the brain, but the reverse, for the blood that goes to the head has, in the erect posture, to be pumped up against the force of gravity; and therefore any obstacle in the course of the arteries would be more felt in this direction than in any other. It is a common notion that the hypertrophy of the heart gives rise to apoplexy by sending the blood with an undue impulse to the head; but for the correction of this error we need only remember that the additional force is merely such as is necessary for the exigencies of the circulation, and such as shall preserve the force of the blood's current as near as possible to the normal point, in spite of the existing obstruction. The actual force with which the blood circulates in the morbid arteries is, most probably, less than in health. The apoplexy is, in fact, due to the diseased state of the arteries, which renders their walls an inadequate support to their contents, and to the diseased state of brain, which imperfectly supports the arteries."—"Clinical Lectures," by Dr. Todd, p. 115.

[1] "Clinical Lectures on Paralysis, Disease of the Brain, and other Affections of the Nervous System," by R. B. Todd, M.D., F.R.S. London, 1854. P. 129.

conclusions would be arrived at, if the inquirer were to exclusively confine his attention to an examination of the contents of the cranium. Such a course of investigation would indeed lead him in pursuit of an *ignis fatuus*. Close and intimate is the sympathy, indissoluble and inseparable the connection, between the material instrument of thought and other vital and organic structures.

Hypertrophy, atrophy, and valvular disease of the heart; chronic irritation of the mucous membrane of the bowels and stomach (often the effect of protracted dyspepsia); morbid conditions of the blood; impaired powers of assimilation; pulmonary affections; hepatic disease (acute and chronic); nephritis, granular degeneration, or any other renal disorder interfering with the elimination of urea from the blood, play an important part in the pathology of cerebral and mental affections.

No analysis of the anatomical characteristics of the cerebral diseases previously referred to could be viewed as satisfactory or complete, that did not embrace a full consideration of the morbid conditions of other structures in close organic sympathy with the great nervous centre.

DIAGNOSIS.—By what general principles is the physician to be guided, when attempting accurately to diagnose between mental aberration and those abnormal states of thought, and erratic flights of fancy, which so closely resemble, in many of their modes of manifestation, alienation of reason? Is mental pathology a certain and exact science, and are its *data* so clearly established, and the conclusions deduced therefrom so accurately defined, as to enable the psychological physician to speak with authority and confidence of the actual presence of aberration in every case of suspected or alleged deviation from a healthy standard of intellect?

Is it possible clearly to discriminate eccentricity, vice, and crime from insanity, or to fully appreciate the precise position of the frontier that marks the boundary between extraordinary departures from ordinary modes of thought and conduct (consistent with sanity and responsibility of mind), and those deviations from states of thinking and action utterly irreconcilable with the hypothesis of mental soundness?

When does violent and ungovernable passion become symptomatic of psychical disorder, and what extent of brutality, prodigality, cruelty, parsimony, revenge, and jealousy is compatible with intellectual sanity? When does an idea which has acquired an influence over the imagination, obviously incommensurate with its value, cease to be healthy in its character, and become a monomaniacal conception ?

Admitting the difficulties that undoubtedly surround a solution of these subtle questions, I am, nevertheless, of opinion, that the carefully and cautiously observant and practically educated physician will encounter no *bonâ fide* impediment in his attempt to diagnose between actual disorder of the mind (insanity) and other states of intellect, emotion, and conduct, generally supposed to be allied to or confounded with it. The boundary line separating morbid from analogous states of thought, is no doubt occasionally obscure, faint, and shadowy, and cases occur which puzzle and confound the most sagacious and experienced psychologists.

I have elsewhere spoken of the impossibility of defining insanity, and pointed out briefly not only the rules that should guide the physician when called upon to investigate a subtle and complex case of morbid thought, but the serious error that would be committed if he, whilst making an analysis of such types of alleged mental unsoundness, were to restrict himself to a consideration of the then manifest state of intellect, utterly disregarding the normal psychical development and ordinary modes of thinking and action generally characteristic of the person whose sanity of mind and conduct is under his consideration.

As a general rule, derangement of mind, whether it consist in a vitiation of the mental, emotional, or moral psychical element, or exhibit itself in actions different from those generally considered to be the effect of a sane, well-governed, and rightly-balanced understanding, ordinarily manifests itself by a marked deviation from natural states of thought, and normal modes of conduct. I have entered at length into an analysis of this subject in a former part of this work, and to the remarks there made I refer the reader.

There are three affections of the cerebro-spinal system with which insanity is liable to be confounded, viz., 1. A state of depression, or hyperæsthesia of the nervous functions, generally designated nervous disorder; 2. Delirium tremens; 3. Ordinary attacks of congestion of the brain, meningitis, acute and chronic encephalitis.

It has been propounded as an axiom by a well-known English psychological authority, that all disorders of the nervous system are but *degrees* of insanity. If such a *dictum* were to be universally admitted and generally acted upon, how mischievous and sad would be the consequences! There is a vast amount of nervous derangement, of a very formidable and distressing character, which has no pathological connection with, or psychical relation to, mental derangement.

I have detailed in the chapter on the Morbid Phenomena of Conscious Insanity, several illustrations of this type of incipient alienation of thought. But this state of unhealthy apprehension of the approach of insanity very often exists as a *nervous disorder*, without being complicated with, or passing into a phase of, mental derangement. I have seen many remarkable examples of the kind in connection with various forms of acute hysteria.

There are other affections of the nervous system that resemble in many of their features mental alienation. In such cases there is often great emotional exaltation, perversion of the instincts, confusion of thought, exaggeration closely bordering on aberration of ideas, as well as great eccentricities of conduct. Such symptoms may exist independently of insanity, as a distinct type of nervous disorder. It is only when the mind exhibits signs of positive alienation, manifested by the presence of delusion associated with a paralysis of the controlling power (the will), that we can satisfactorily affirm that insanity, in the right acceptation of the term, has clearly and unmistakably exhibited itself. I do not affirm that a delusive impression is always appreciable in incipient or even in the more advanced forms of mental derangement, for there are many phases of alienation of mind, often leading to the most fatal results, where no apparently fixed false perception can be detected.

The experienced physician is not likely to confound delirium tremens, clearly the consequences of an excessive indulgence in, or the effect of a *sudden* abstraction of stimulants from the brain, with insanity. The acute accession of the delirium; remarkable insomnia which precedes its development, and continues through its course; peculiar muscular tremor; anxiety and distress of mind so characteristically marked in the physiognomy; the *fussy* and *busy* nature of the delirium; fumbling of the bed-clothes; extreme loquacity of the patient; peculiar sensorial illusions; suffused face; injected conjunctivæ; soft and feeble pulse; moist and creamy tongue; wild look of suspicion, terror, and alarm; clammy state of the skin, accompanied by a peculiar cutaneous

33

exhalation similar to that observed in rheumatism; great agitation of manner, and unceasing restlessness, are all specific and peculiar diagnostic features of this type of cerebro-mental disorder, clearly distinguishing it from insanity.

In considering the subject of cerebral congestion, it will be necessary to diagnose between active determination to, and arterial congestion of the brain, as well as to distinguish the latter condition from one of venous plethora. The ordinary symptoms of active determination are cephalalgia of an acute type, a feeling of tension, weight, or heaviness in the head, severe vertigo, aggravated whenever the patient stoops, suffusion of the face, injected conjunctivæ, distressing noises in the ears, sensorial hyperæsthesia, activity of the arterial circulation, recognized by undue action of the temporal and radial arteries, depression of spirits, apprehensions of an approaching calamity, optical illusions, increased temperature of the scalp, wakefulness, or disturbed sleep, accompanied with frightful dreams, sudden muscular twitchings, and spasmodic startings.

It is difficult to define when the preceding cerebral state of active determination passes into a condition of congestion. In the former affection there exists marked hyperæsthesia of the ordinary functions of the cerebrum, whereas in the state of hyperæmia, the symptoms indicate an opposite condition of the brain. This depression of the cerebral functions is marked by a sensation of dull, heavy weight in the head, seldom amounting to acute cephalalgia. The patient complains of vertigo and obtuseness of hearing. In many cases there is partial amaurosis. The intellectual faculties are in an inactive state. The memory is impaired, thoughts confused, and all the great functions of life are in a state of severe vital depression.

The insidious, slow, and progressive advance of insanity, exhibiting itself, in the majority of cases, by great singularity of conduct, delusive ideas, and clear deviations from normal modes of thinking and acting, as well as by an absence of the acute cerebral symptoms (except in cases of mania) that mark the condition of active determination and hyperæmia, will assist the practitioner in arriving at an accurate diagnosis. Again, insanity is easily distinguished from the acute symptoms of meningitis and cerebritis. These inflammatory affections are accompanied by severe cephalalgia, occasionally fugitive in its character, sense of weight and fulness in the head, flushing of the face, heat of the scalp, lethargy, attacks of vertigo, exaltation of the sense of hearing, seeing, and smelling, optical illusions, tinnitus aurium, injected conjunctivæ, full and laborious pulse, sudden startings during heavy sleep, as if the patient were alarmed by a frightful dream, bowels obstinately constipated, pupil contracted, skin dry and parched, and the mental condition alternating between delirious excitement and depression.   With the preceding symptoms there will occasionally be great irritability of the stomach, sometimes amounting to actual vomiting. Inflammation of the membranes and substance of the brain (affections very difficult to distinguish from each other) is often complicated with delirium (different in its character from the delusions and hallucinations of insanity) as well as with convulsions.

Lallemand professed to be able to diagnose between meningitis and inflammation of the substance of the brain, by means of lesions of the functions of the *muscular* system, which accompany, he affirms, almost exclusively, the former cerebral condition ; but, according to his own admission, the two types of inflammatory disease very frequently blend with, and are not easily to be distinguished from, the other.

The premonitory symptoms of inflammatory affections of the brain are essentially dissimilar from those that precede attacks of mental derangement. For some period before the invasion of the acute cerebral disease, the patient complains of rarely being free from some degree of headache, either continued, fugitive, fixed, or deep-seated in its character. These degrees of cephalalgia, Dr. Crawford says, are accompanied by pain, numbness, weakness, and a sensation of creeping and tingling in one of the extremities, or in one-half of the body. These sensations may be confined to one portion of the body, and the numbness and loss of power is often restricted to one finger, or to one set of muscles.[1] In the

---

[1] The isolated attacks of anæsthesia, occurring particularly in the fingers, that so often precede attacks of cerebro-spinal disease, did not escape the acute observation of Galen. " Pausanius the sophist," says this illustrious authority, " whilst making a voyage from Syria to Rome, experienced a loss of feeling in the two last fingers and on one side of the middle finger of his left hand. Under injudicious treatment the insensibility of the affected part became permanent. I made inquiries into his condition, and learned, among other things, that during the voyage he had fallen from his chair, and struck with force the upper part of his back. The contusion was soon cured, but a numbness of the fingers supervened. I immediately advised that the

early stage of inflammation of the brain the speech is occasionally affected. There is a degree of hesitation, stuttering, or indistinctness of pronunciation. The patient complains of drowsiness, languor, and depression of spirits.

The practitioner will encounter but few difficulties in diagnosing between progressive general paralysis, ordinary attacks of encephalic softening (white and red), paraplegia, hemiplegia, cerebral abscesses, and various kinds of tumor of the brain.

I have, in the preceding pages, in the chapters on the Morbid Phenomena of Intelligence, Motion, Sensation, and Speech, described so fully the subtle advance of general paralysis, that it will be unnecessary for me here to recapitulate the description there given of the incipient as well as diagnostic symptoms of this obscure and generally fatal type of cerebral disease.

Dr. Skae has, in a recent communication to one of the learned medical societies, so admirably delineated the steady and treacherous advance of this affection, that I offer no apology for quoting somewhat in detail, his account of its premonitory and diagnostic signs.

The most significant, and generally, but not always, the first symptom of general paralysis is, according to Dr. Skae, a peculiar impairment of the power of *articulation*. The patient speaks thick, mumbles certain words, like a person who is slightly intoxicated.

" Accompanying this affection of the speech there is (I think always) a peculiar expression of the countenance, very difficult to describe, but so peculiar and so easy to recognize, when frequently seen, and so very characteristic of the disease, that any one who has had a few years' experience among the insane could pronounce upon the existence of general paralysis from the aspect of the face alone. The face is characterized by a general hebetude or want of expression—a heaviness of the features;—the eyes have a vacant and absent expression, the pupils being often unequally dilated ; the angles of the mouth are sluggish in their movements, the risor and levator anguli oris muscles not appearing to act at all;—the mouth opens and shuts in a piece, as it were, without any

same remedies which had been applied to the fingers should be directed to the part that had been first injured, viz., the spinal cord, and my patient speedily recovered the entire use of his left hand."—From a paper in " L'Expérience," communicated by M. Dubois d'Amiens, " On the writings of Galen."

play of the lips indicative of the sentimens and passions.   Not
unfrequently the face trembles before speaking, as if the person
were about to cry.

"When the tongue is protruded, it is done without any marked
deviation to one side, as in palsy, at least rarely; but it often
wavers from side to side, as if beyond control; and, in the more
advanced stages, the patient is unable, by an effort of the will, to
protrude it at all, but simply opens his mouth, when asked to show
his tongue.   The pulse of the general paralytic is more commonly
feeble and easily compressed; the extremities cold and livid, and
every indication exists of a weak and languid circulation.

"The affection of the speech which I have described, gradually
increases during the progress of the disease, until, in its latter
stages, the speech becomes almost entirely inarticulate and unintelligible.

"At some period of the disease the powers of locomotion appear
to be impaired, and the gait is unsteady.   This affection sometimes
precedes, but more generally succeeds, the impaired articulation.
In some cases I have known the unsteady walking precede for
some *years* the affection of the speech or the symptoms of insanity,
and the disease appeared to creep slowly upwards from the lower
part of the spinal cord, as it were, to the central organ of the
nervous system.   Generally, however, the impaired locomotion
succeeds the impaired speech.

"This affection of the lower limbs, which certainly generally
precedes any affection of the upper extremities, is very different
from the affection of the limbs in ordinary palsy.   And this is one
of the features of the malady which has not, I think, been sufficiently distinguished.   There is no dragging of the limbs, as in
hemiplegia; there is no loss of muscular power; no *palsy*, in the
ordinary sense of the term, in the limbs at all.   There is an impairment in the power of *directing* the movements of the limbs,
an inability to control their co-ordinate action.   The result of
this is, that the person walks unsteadily, widens his base of support, and sways from side to side like a drunken man.   In well-
pronounced cases, especially in those where the so-called paralysis
has long preceded the mental affection, he rises slowly from his
seat, balances himself, and begins to walk, very wide in the gyves,
fixing his eye sometimes on the object towards which he is tend-
ing, and making for it as steadily as he can.   In such cases, if

the individual is made to close his eyes, it often happens that he
cannot balance himself, and with difficulty saves himself from falling: he walks up a stair with comparative ease and comfort,
because he has some object before his eyes to guide him; but he
goes down stairs with fear and difficulty, because there is nothing
before him on which he can fix his eye. This is the most exaggerated or fully-developed form of the paralytic condition; but it is
seldom seen, in the early stages at least, of the disease which I
am describing, so strongly marked. Very often it is hardly observable, consisting merely of a slight widening of the limbs, and
a rolling or shambling, and somewhat unsteady gait; in fact, the
affection of the speech is not more truly like that of drunkenness
than that of the locomotive powers; they are both the result of
the loss or impairment of that power by means of which we regulate and control the co-ordinate action of our voluntary muscles:
and may exist, in ever varying degree, from the slightest appreciable thickness of speech or unsteadiness of walking, up to total
loss of articulate speech or the power of walking.

" In *ordinary palsy*, the nervous connection between the muscles
of the palsied part and the organ of volition is, as it were, cut off
entirely, and the individual can no longer, by an effort of the will,
make the palsied muscles act; he cannot lift his arm, or close his
hand, or draw up his limb. Or, it may be, he conveys a feeble
and imperfect volition to the part (if the palsy is incomplete or
passing off), and the hand is grasped feebly, or the limb is slowly
and with difficulty drawn up. In the so-called paralysis of the
general paralytic, on the other hand, there appears to be no *stoppage* of the nervous connection or electric current between the
organ of volition and the affected parts; but the volition is *irregularly* conveyed and *distributed*. The person cannot *control* and
direct his movements perfectly and *consentaneously*, just as a
drunken man sees double, because he cannot make his eyes converge upon a given object; or walks unsteadily, because he cannot
direct and regulate the harmonious movements of his limbs. In
these movements of the general paralytic or drunken man, there
is no *palsy*, in the ordinary sense of the term; the person affected
will run, or dance, or kick, as actively and violently as ever, but
his movements are irregular, and not always those desired or
willed. In fact, they resemble in kind, although very much modified in degree, the movements of *chorea*, in which the patient in

vain attempts to steady his hand or carry it to his mouth. I am anxious to enforce these distinctions, because I think they have not hitherto been recognized, and because the name of this affection is apt to mislead as to their nature.

" Dr. Reynolds corroborates my statements, by pointing out as a means of diagnosis, between general paralysis and wasting palsy, that in general paralysis the muscles contract readily under the stimulus of galvanism, while in wasting palsy they do not. In wasting palsy, in fact, the contractility of the muscular fibre is impaired or lost, while in general paralysis it still remains unimpaired.[1]

" This impairment of the muscular movement gradually increases and extends, the speech becomes more and more inarticulate, the locomotion more and more unsteady, until at last scarcely a word can be distinguished, and the patient cannot rise or cross the room without being assisted.

" The progress of these changes, however, varies very much in different cases; sometimes, for example, the speech is very little affected, hardly appreciably so, until a very advanced stage of the disease. In other cases it varies, being at times much more perceptible than at others. In the same way, the impairment of the locomotive powers in some cases is far from being obvious, even towards the latter stages of the disease; and in others, it is at times more perceptible than it is in general. In all cases, however, I think there is enough evidence left, either from one of these sources or the other, taken in connection with the state of the pupils, the expression of the face, and the action of the facial muscles, to make the physiognomy of the case diagnostic to an experienced observer."[2]

Although this disease very closely resembles, in its incipient manifestations as well as in its more mature stage of development, ordinary attacks of softening (such a disorganization of the cerebral matter being frequently found after death from general paralysis), it is, nevertheless, considered by pathologists as an affection *sui generis*, and distinct in its nature from that of ramollissement. The morbid changes, chronic in their character, discovered in the membranes of the brain, gray matter of its convolutions (indicated

[1] On Wasting Palsy.
[2] *Vide* " Edinburgh Medical Journal," for April, 1860, No. 4, vol. iii.

by changes of color), as well as alterations in the medullary or conducting portion of the encephalic structure, undoubtedly lead to this conclusion.

Are there any pathognomonic or diagnostic symptoms by which we are able unerringly to detect in all cases the commencement of an attack of softening of the brain? I am, from a close observation of the phenomena of this disease, obliged to answer the question in the negative. In some cases where I felt justified in predicating a state of pulpy degeneration of the brain, no such pathological change was discovered after death. Nevertheless, in a vast number of instances, the indications of softening are clearly and unmistakably manifested.

There are two principal forms of ramollissement of the brain ; viz., *red* or inflammatory, *white* or non-inflammatory. This affection of the brain admits, however, of other divisions and subdivisions, but it is my intention only to describe cursorily the symptoms of the two leading forms of softening. This important subject will be fully considered in all its details in the succeeding volume.

The premonitory stage of acute softening is not well or distinctly marked. Many of the symptoms manifested at this period of the disease closely resemble the incipient signs of cerebral hemorrhage and paralysis, such as headache, vertigo, muscular debility, loss of sensibility in some part of the body, tinnitus aurium, formications, a sensation of weight, or slight symptoms of hemiplegia on one side of the body, muscular tremors, tetanic spasm, occasionally resembling a stiffness or rigidity of one of the limbs, slight palsy of one of the eyelids, strabismus, defective articulation, misplacement of words, with marked changes in the physiognomy, the expression being that of "astonishment, stupor, indifference, or imbecility." The eyes are sometimes brilliant and staring, and at other times dull and without expression. The face is occasionally suffused, indicating a state of cerebral sanguineous congestion.

Durand-Fardel says, that a remarkable and striking symptom, frequently observed in acute softening, is an increased secretion from the mouth and eye. This is especially remarked with old people, in whom this viscid secretion dries, and forms hard masses on the edge of the eyelids, which irritate the eyes, whilst an abundant glairy fluid drops from the mouth, or, when more viscid, adheres to the tongue and palate, forming a thick yellowish crust, which is reproduced as soon as removed. A remarkable fact connected with these increased secretions, says Fardel, is that, if a partial cerebral amendment takes place, the discharge of itself ceases, but reappears as soon as the acute softening progresses.

In acute softening the patient often complains of optical illusions, and of impaired powers of deglutition. But the principal diagnostic symptoms are undoubtedly cephalalgia, more or less persistent and acute in its character, vertigo, affections of the speech, marked symptoms of paralysis of the palpebræ, face, or one side of the body, associated with muscular debility, loss of memory, irritability of temper, occasional attacks of epilepsy, and a muddled and confused state of the intellect. The spirits are sometimes depressed and occasionally excited. The pupils are often contracted, but as frequently dilated.

In chronic, white, or non-inflammatory conditions of softening, the premonitory symptoms very closely resemble those previously described as characteristic of acute types of this disease, but materially varying in severity. I have described in the chapters on Impairment of the Intelligence, including the Morbid Phenomena of Attention, Volition, Emotion, and Memory, the principal psychical symptoms indicative of the commencement of this form of cerebral degeneration or disorganization.

It will be unnecessary for me more than briefly to recapitulate what I have previously described as the psychical evidences of white softening. I refer principally, first, to a confusion and then to a gradual impairment of the intelligence, showing itself in defective powers of attention, enfeebled memory, infirmity of purpose, vacillation of will, and a general sluggishness, apathy, and subsequently imbecility of intellect. Associated with these mental symptoms, there are cephalalgia, obscure, but often obvious changes in the sensor and motor powers (hyperæsthesia and often partial paralysis). I have described these insidious and subtle lesions when analyzing the morbid phenomena of motion, sensation, and speech.

In cerebral tumors and abscesses of the brain there are not generally detected in the early stage any well-marked diagnostic symptoms. In these types of organic disease of the brain, headache, often localized, is generally present, but often intermittent or paroxysmal in its character. If cephalalgia should not be present the patient will complain of sensations of vertigo, tinnitus aurium, defective memory, and occasionally of confusion of intellect; but I have observed in several cases of tumor and abscess of the brain, an absence of acute local pain, or even uneasiness in the head.   In all cases of suspected organic disease of this kind, it is important to inquire minutely into the antecedents of the patient.   In many of these affections it will be found that blows have been inflicted upon the cranium many years previously to the appearance of cerebral symptoms.   Abscess of the brain is often associated with chronic purulent discharge from the internal ear. Under these circumstances persistent headache, vertigo, distressing noises in the ear and head, and pain upon pressure over the mastoid process, are important diagnostic signs.

I have, in a former part of this work, addressed myself to a consideration of two important general symptoms usually indicative of organic disease of the brain, viz., headache and sickness of the stomach.   Cerebral cephalalgia may be confounded with hemicrania, nervous, neuralgic, gastric, and rheumatic headache.   In cerebral headache the pain may be either acute, lancinating, throbbing, or obtuse.   The intensity of the suffering of inflammatory headache is occasionally so great that the patient is obliged to remain for a considerable time in one position, the slightest motion aggravating the pain to perfect torture.   The patient, says Dr. Abercrombie, cannot generally bear a warm room, the noise of company, or even the exertion of cheerful conversation, without feeling greatly distressed and the headache being increased.   There is also connected with this type of cephalalgia, intolerance of light, and, in fact, in many cases great sensorial acuteness.   In this type of headache, says Romberg, the pain "is generally characterized by the following peculiarities: it is permanently confined to a larger or smaller portion of the cranium.   There is a sensation of pressure, tension, or pulsation, or the pain has a shooting, tearing, or rolling character.   It varies in intensity, and is excited and exalted by bodily or mental fatigue, movement of the head, elevated temperature, highly spiced food, and long and sound sleep.   The pain is relieved by raising the head or by assuming the erect position, or resting the head firmly against something; it possesses a remittent character.   There are intervals, but during the intermissions the health is impaired.   Spasmodic action or paralysis, generally confined to one side of the face or trunk, supervenes, or the organ of sense becomes afflicted with anæsthesia, and delirium follows. The pain abates and ceases altogether as the paralysis and sopor advance.

"It is a matter of much difficulty to define these features with accuracy sufficient for the purposes of diagnosis, as the organ is withdrawn from examination by a rigid osseous case; still one means of approach has been overlooked, which we ought certainly to avail ourselves of. It is a fact that during every vigorous and long-continued act of expiration the brain is elevated, the cerebellum being pressed against the tentorium, the cerebrum against the cranial bones. We may easily convince ourselves of the latter by placing the hand upon the fontanelle of a child while it is crying. The old surgeons, acting upon a knowledge of this circumstance, recommended to their patients who suffered from penetrating wounds of the cranium, to cough violently, or to sneeze, in order to promote the discharge of blood or pus.

"We may, therefore, employ continued expiration, or holding the breathing during expiration, in cerebral diseases, especially if it affects the surface, as a sort of substitute for the external pressure which we so frequently have recourse to in the exploration of the abdomen or thorax.

"The patients alluded to generally complain of the headache being brought on by straining in defecation. For the purposes of diagnosis, we may cause the patient to imitate this effort by holding the breath for some time during expiration, while the abdominal muscles are contracted. This at once brings on the pain, or if it were present, increases it to the utmost. The same occurs in screaming, coughing, and vomiting. Similar experiments may be instituted during inspiration, during which the brain falls and approaches the basis of the skull.[1] We may thus obtain some information on the diseases affecting the base of the cerebrum and cerebellum.

"We are more in the habit of using the influence of position

---

[1] Ravina found that during inspiration he was able to introduce a quill between the skull and the brain of a pointer. On placing a cork cylinder divided into degrees upon the brain, it sank during ordinary inspiration one line, during strong inspiration three lines. If a cylindrical glass tube filled with water was placed upon the brain, the fluid disappeared during inspiration and returned discolored with blood on expiration.—See Lund: "Physiologische Resultate der Vivisectionen neuerer Zeit," p. 149: and the still more recent experiments of Dr. Ecker, in "Physiologische Untersuchungen über die Bewegungen des Gehirns und Rückenmarks," 1843, pp. 27–102, and pp. 112–122.

and movement of the head as the means of diagnosis. Swinging the head from side to side, stooping down, rising rapidly from the horizontal to an erect position, are apt to produce and augment the pain.

"The modifications and relations of cephalalgia to definite diseases of the brain, are important in a diagnostic point of view. Before investigating them, it is necessary to point out that, in order to determine the existence of the pain in these diseases, it is even more necessary than in affections of other organs, to have an accurate history and a continued series of observations of the patient. This is necessary, not only on account of the longer intermissions, but also on account of the recurrence of pain when other symptoms, and especially paralysis, supervene, and on account of the loss of memory which ensues in many cases."[1]

The absence of well-marked symptoms of gastric disorder, such as furred tongue, loss of appetite, acidity of the stomach, flatulence, pain or uneasiness after eating, vitiated secretions, sluggish action of the liver as well as intestinal canal, will assist the physician in his diagnostic examination of a case of headache suspected to proceed from organic disease of the brain.

In cases of neuralgic and rheumatic cephalalgia, the pain will not be confined to the head, but will be felt in other parts of the body, particularly in certain conditions of the atmosphere and alternations of temperature.

In types of nervous headache, the pain is generally frontal, and often relieved by cheerful society, and when food and stimulants are administered. Attacks of this kind are seldom of long duration, whereas in cerebral headache, arising from softening, tumor, and abscess of the brain, the cephalalgia is, in acute cases, rarely absent. The pain, undoubtedly, in many instances intermits, but it is generally followed by, or associated with vertigo and distressing noises in the head, often compared to the roaring of the sea.

The headache symptomatic of the presence of tumors of the brain, Romberg affirms, is considerably diminished, if not in some cases altogether removed, by the accumulation of serum in the cavities and between the membranes of the brain, but the pain is aggravated when inflammation and softening occur in the immediate vicinity of the tumor. The headache that accompanies cancerous affections of the brain is generally acute and lancinating in its character. In abscesses of the brain it is generally paroxysmal.

[1] Romberg, p. 159.

I have previously referred to the intimate sympathy existing between the brain and the stomach, and to the frequent presence of nausea, gastric irritability, and actual vomiting, in many cases of obscure organic disease of the brain. Romberg has, with his usual perspicuity and accuracy, described the characteristic diagnostic symptoms, by means of which we are enabled to distinguish cerebral from idiopathic sickness of the stomach. They are as follows :—

1. " The influence of the position of the head; the vomiting is arrested in the horizontal, and recurs, and is frequently repeated in the erect position. It is also easily induced by movements of the head, by swinging, shaking, or stooping, or suddenly rising. 2. The prevailing absence of premonitory nausea. 3. The peculiar character of the act of vomiting; the contents of the stomach are ejected without fatigue or retching, as the milk is ejected by babies at the breast. 4. The complication with other phenomena, the more frequent of which are pain in the head, constipation, and the irregularity of the cardiac and radial pulse, which is increased during, and subsequent to the act of vomiting. The duration of the vomiting is limited in the inflammatory affections of the brain, meningitis, encephalitis, and acute hydrocephalus, to the first stages of the disease; and the prevailing rule is, that as the paralytic and comatose symptoms increase the vomiting remits and ceases."

TREATMENT AND PROPHYLAXIS.—In all acute affections of the brain and disorders of the mind the cure and life of the patient depend, 1. *Upon the speedy detection of incipient symptoms;* 2. *Upon the accuracy of the diagnosis formed as to the nature of the cerebral affection;* 3. *Upon the immediate application of remedial treatment.*

I propose, in the first instance, to consider briefly the general principles that should guide the practitioner in the treatment of incipient insanity.

The treatment of the early stage of insanity requires great delicacy, discrimination, and judgment. Under these circumstances, where the brain is in a morbid state of irritation, and the mind struggling between sanity and insanity, the person being conscious that his " wits" are beginning " to turn," the medical attendant should proceed cautiously and discreetly in his examination. If the patient be led to believe, from the conduct of the physician or from anything which falls from him, that derangement of mind is suspected, the most painful and disastrous consequences in all probability will ensue. In the early stages of insanity the patient's suspicions are morbidly excited. He has a dread of "going mad;" expresses a horror of such a calamity, and often most positively refuses to allow himself to be questioned on the subject of his mental health. Should the patient believe that he is imagined to be deranged, he will sometimes exhibit great violence and excitement.

If the practitioner proceeds judiciously in his inquiry, he may generally succeed in effecting his object without inducing the patient in the slightest degree to suspect the purport of his visit. In many cases the physician may administer remedial agents, and succeed in warding off an attack of acute insanity, without conveying to the mind of the patient an intimation of the suspicions which exist as to his state of mind. When a medical man is called in to a case of this description, it is his duty first to direct his observations to the state of the general health. He will almost invariably detect either hepatic, gastric, cardiac, renal, or intestinal disorder which may be irritating and sympathetically disordering the brain. By the timely use of appropriate remedies, these affections may speedily be removed.

It may occasionally be necessary to relieve the overloaded condition of the vessels of the brain. The patient often complains of severe headache, attended with an increase of temperature, for the relief of which the application of a few leeches, cold evaporating lotions, and ice to the head may be recommended. Great caution is, however, necessary in the use of depleting and antiphlogistic measures. Alas! how often have patients, who have been injudiciously treated by such means, sunk into incurable chronic melancholy. In *recent* attacks, occurring in young and plethoric subjects, when the symptoms are closely allied to inflammation of the brain, local bloodletting is often attended with the happiest results.

In considering the physical treatment of insanity, it is essentially necessary that we should clearly understand upon what pathological condition of brain the morbid state of the mind depends. I think it may be safely laid down, as a general principle, that the brain, in cases of mania, even of the most exalted kind, is not *necessarily* in a state of active congestion or inflammation. The character of insanity, the symptoms which usher it

in, and mark its progress, all unequivocally establish that alienation of mind frequently arises from a cerebral disorder, unaccompanied with vascular activity or turgescence.

In obscure and doubtful cases tartrate of antimony will be found
an excellent substitute for bleeding.   Violent maniacal excitement,
accompanied by every apparent indication of a high degree of
cerebral congestion and inflammation, will often yield to the administration of this drug.   The physician should begin with small
doses, and gradually increase them, until the patient is able to
take two or three grains without exciting actual vomiting.

On the subject of depletion in insanity Dr. Seymour observes :
" In the great majority of cases, the functions of the brain in
mental derangement are increased in force, while the circulation
is depressed, extremely quick and feeble, and the action of the
heart gives way to the smallest abstraction of blood ; and yet
these are often attended by raving delirium, great increase of
muscular force, and are, in fact, what are termed *high* cases.
The consequence of such practice is, either the more frequent
return of the high stage, or the patient sinks into one approaching idiotcy."

When bleeding is clearly inadmissible, cold applied to the head
will be found not only to diminish vascular excitement, but to
lessen powerfully the morbid sensitiveness of the cerebral organs.
Should there, however, exist a tendency to active plethora and
apoplexy, cold lotions and ice should be used with great caution.
The prolonged hot bath, in conjunction with the cold *douche*, will
often be found most efficacious in subduing maniacal excitement.
I have witnessed the mental perturbation of incipient insanity
frequently yield to this potent remedy.   The *douche* is to be used
when the patient is in the hot bath.

In the incipient, as well as in advanced stages of insanity, the
generally overloaded and inactive state of the bowels should be
relieved by means of purgatives.   Much caution, however, must
be observed in the use of aperient medicine.   Very frequently the
whole surface of the mucous membrane of the intestinal canal is
in a state of subacute inflammation.   This condition acts sympathetically upon the brain and nervous system, and aggravates the
mental irritation.   When this morbid state of the intestines is present, the use of aperients should be preceded by the application
of a few leeches (particularly if there be pain upon pressure), or

counter-irritants, to the neighborhood of the abdominal affection. In other cases of insanity, it will be necessary to exhibit drastic purgatives. Insanity has been known to yield to the steady and persevering use of cathartics. Hellebore had in ancient times the reputation of being a specific in cases of insanity. This drug was considered to operate powerfully in cleansing and invigorating the intellectual faculties. It is said that Carneades, the Academic, when preparing to refute the dogmas of the Stoics, went through a course of purgation by means of white hellebore. So celebrated was this medicinal agent as a mental remedy that the poets of antiquity have sung its virtues. Horace, in allusion to the "happy madman," says (I have quoted a portion of the original in a former part of this work)—

> " He, when his friends, at much expense and pains,
> Had amply purged with hellebore his brains,
> Came to himself—' Ah cruel friends !' he cried,
> ' Is this to save me ? Better far had died,
> Than thus be robbed of pleasure so refined,
> The dear delusion of a raptured mind.' "

Persius also refers to the fame which this medicine had acquired in cases of disordered mind. In his fourth satire he tells Nero that, instead of taking upon himself the great and weighty task of government, which required much experience and sound judgment, he ought to take the most powerful medicine to clear his understanding.

—" *Anticyras* melior sorbere meracas.'[1]

Melampus, the son of Amythaon, is said to have cured the daughters of Prœtus, king of Argos, of melancholy, by purging them with hellebore. According to the traditionary fable, Melampus had observed that the goats who fed on this plant were purged ; and having administered it to the king's daughters, who were wandering in the woods under the delusion that they were cows, he cured them, and received the hand of one of them in marriage, and a part of the kingdom of Argos as his reward.

[1] The islands of Anticyra were famous for producing hellebore. The above quotation from Persius has been thus translated by Dryden :—

> " Thou hast not strength such labors to sustain,
> Drink hellebore, my boy—drink deep, and purge thy brain."

In the treatment of incipient insanity, clearly unconnected with active head symptoms, there is no remedy which so effectually masters the disease as that of opium in one of its many formulæ. I am satisfied that a vast amount of mental derangement may be successfully treated in its early stage by the continuous and persevering administration of sedatives. When insanity is clearly associated with a depressed condition of the vital powers, evidenced by a weak pulse, feeble action of the heart, and general anæmic state of the system, the exhibition of the hydrochlorate, acetate, or muriate of morphia, *combined* with iron and quinine, will, in a great majority of cases, be found to act like a charm in arresting the progress of the mental malady.

In some forms of insanity, belladonna, conium, hydrocyanic acid, chloroform, Indian hemp, henbane, stramonium, and hops, may be administered with advantage. It is obvious that no particular instructions can be given for the administration of these remedial agents. Much must necessarily be left to the judgment of the practitioner, who should be directed in the application of sedatives by the peculiar circumstances of each individual case presented for his consideration. It will be occasionally found necessary to administer opium by what is termed the endermic method, as well as by enemata. In some cases of acute maniacal excitement, I have found great benefit from the careful use of chloroform by inhalation. In epileptic and other forms of delirium this anæsthetic agent may be occasionally used with much advantage. It will often be found beneficial in cases of acute mental excitement to give, in combination, digitalis and opium. I have known instances of active cerebral and mental disorder yield to this mode of treatment after other remedies have failed.

Before dismissing this part of the subject, I would make a few observations on the necessity of separating the patient from his friends and family in the incipient stage of insanity.

There cannot be two opinions among experienced medical men as to the propriety of occasionally recommending that a patient suffering from acute mental disorder should, immediately the malady manifests itself, be removed from all his former associations. As a *principle* of treatment, no sensible person will refuse his assent to such a course of procedure. The object of separation is to break through the morbid train of thought, and to place the patient at once within the range of efficient curative treatment. As long as he is surrounded by circumstances likely to encourage and give activity to his morbid suspicions and delusive ideas, all remedial efforts will be of little or no avail.

No physician would be justified in undertaking the treatment of a case of acute insanity without receiving from the friends and family of the invalid absolute and unconditional permission to isolate the patient completely from home and every circumstance with which he had been previously connected. The lunatic may fancy (and this is one of the peculiar features of the disease) that his family are conspiring against his life—he may imagine that his house is daily visited by persons engaged in devising schemes for depriving him of his life and property. The physician would exhibit great want of judgment if he were to lose valuable time by attempting to combat with the mental derangement under such unfavorable circumstances. In the majority of cases, it will be necessary to remove the patient from the sphere of his own circle, before any permanent advantage is likely to ensue from medical or moral treatment. Cases no doubt occasionally occur, in which the practitioner would not be justified in suggesting this course. When the prognosis is favorable and the attack of recent character evidently dependent upon *temporary* bodily conditions of ill-health, and the delusions of the patient unconnected with any member of the family, every effort should be made to grapple with the malady before separation from home is advised or carried into effect.

I have, in the chapter on the stage of consciousness referred to the distressing, blasphemous, and often obscene thoughts that occasionally occur in certain forms of nervous disorder and particular types of incipient insanity. It is possible in many cases, whilst such morbid ideas are transient impressions, to overpower, conquer, and dismiss them from the imagination by an indomitable and persevering effort of the will.

Alas! the unhappy sufferer is occasionally so fearfully under the dominion of morbid thoughts that he makes no effort to interfere with or dislodge them from their fortress. Instead of attempting to do so, he often appears to encourage their admission into, as well as to promote their unhealthy ascendency over his mind, exclaiming with the poet—

" Vapors, and clouds, and storms, be these my theme ;
 . . . . Welcome, kindred glooms,
Congenial horrors, hail !"

Mr. Spurgeon, when recounting an episode of his life connected with his conversion, says: " In the early days of my Christian career I was much troubled with wicked and blasphemous thoughts, which would force themselves into my mind when I fancied myself most ardently struggling with God in prayer. To such a degree was I under the influence of these terrible suggestions, that when they made an effort to rush to my lips I was obliged to put my hand to my mouth to prevent myself giving utterance to them. So greatly afflicted was I in this manner, that I consulted a venerable Christian friend respecting these wicked thoughts. He asked me whether they came into my mind in any consecutive form, or only by fits and starts. I replied that they came quite suddenly, and had nothing consecutive about them. ' Oh, then,' said my Christian friend, ' care nothing for these thoughts ; I know where they come from ; treat them as in Old England we used to treat vagrants, flog them well at the cart's tail, and send them home to their 'parish. These thoughts are suggested to your mind by Satan, who says to himself, " I am likely to lose this man, and I will make a desperate effort to keep him within my power." Flog them, I repeat, well, and send them home.' " I did," continues Mr. Spurgeon, " what my dear Christian counsellor advised, and conquered the enemy."

The power of self-control is, in many instances, weakened, or altogether lost, by a voluntary and criminal indulgence in a train of thought which it was the duty of the individual, in the *first* instance, to resolutely battle with, control, and subdue. Nervous disorders as well as insane delusive thoughts are thus often self-created. It may not be an easy task to subdue morbid suggestions, obtain a mastery over unhappy feelings, crush unnatural inclinations, destroy in their infancy the tyranny of unhealthy impulses, keep in subjection wicked, vicious, and criminal tendencies. The difficulty of obtaining such a dominion over the perturbed mind may be apparently insurmountable, nevertheless, a resolute and persevering exercise of the volitional power will, in many cases, effectually enable the patient to accomplish it.

> " Nemo adeo ferus est, ut non mitescere possit,
> Si modo culturæ patientem commodet aurem."—HOR.

Directly the will ceases to exercise controlling influence over the understanding and emotions, the intellect loses its healthy balancing power. A man indulges in a depraved course of conduct, harbors and encourages vicious ideas, his actions often corresponding with the unfortunate condition of his mind and feelings, until all power of volition becomes suspended, and he is actually reduced to a state of *quasi* lunacy. A person, perhaps for some real cause, feels a degree of animosity towards a particular individual who has injured him. Instead of making an effort to conquer this feeling, he allows—in fact, forces his mind to dwell upon it; the idea pursues him in all his walks, haunts him in his waking thoughts, and exercises a fearful ascendency over him during the darkness of the night. The mind eventually becomes so absorbed in the idea, that the bitter, angry feeling which, at the *first onset*, was insignificant and amenable to control, seizes hold of the mind, and influences and distorts every idea and action. The morbid soon becomes a deranged mind, the insanity manifesting itself in an exaggerated, extravagant, and perverted conception of a notion which had originally some semblance of truth for its foundation. The self-created delusive idea may thus obtain a fearful influence over the mind, and eventually lead to the commission of criminal acts.

If self-control is to be exercised with any great advantage, it must be practised in the incipient stages of disordered mind. At this period it is possible, even when insanity has begun to throw a dark shadow over the intellect, to subdue the morbid thoughts and perverted feelings, by a resolute and determined effort of the will.

> " Our remedies oft in ourselves do lie,
> Which we ascribe to Heaven ; the fated sky
> Gives us free scope ; only doth backward pull
> Our slow designs, when we ourselves are dull."

In many of these *quasi* morbid states of thought, or early scintillations of insanity, much benefit is often derived from the adoption of a course of remedial medical treatment. Happily we possess the means of invigorating the functions of the brain and nervous system, and thereby giving tone to the flagging and enfeebled efforts of the will. It would be most unwise, while struggling to keep in check unhealthy thoughts, to neglect a careful consideration of the state of the bodily health.

It will be impossible for me to enter, except in general terms, into a consideration of the treatment of incipient paralysis, apoplexy, softening of the brain, and other organic cerebral diseases, without anticipating what I shall have to advance in reference to this important subject in the succeeding work.

I am convinced from the number of cases of incipient organic disease of the brain which have come under my observation, that much may be effected by means of treatment in arresting the progress of these encephalic affections, provided they are brought at an early period of their development within the range of remedial treatment.

The abstraction of a small quantity of blood from the head, the administration of mercurial alteratives, a careful attention to the state of the secretions, skin, and renal·functions, combined with counter-irritation and an abstinence from all mental agitation and anxiety, will often be found of essential benefit in the incipient stages of apoplexy and paralysis. In a certain type of case connected with organic or functional disease of the heart, I have, after relieving the local head symptoms by means of cupping (wet and dry), leeches and blisters, found great benefit from a combined use of opium, digitalis, and iodide of potassium. Where there is laborious action of the heart consequent upon hypertrophy or valvular disease, the preceding formula almost invariably alleviates the cardiac as well as the head symptoms.

There are other types of incipient apoplexy and paralysis only to be successfully treated by means of tonics and stimulants. I have observed well-marked symptoms of apparently acute attacks of cerebral hemorrhage and paraplegia yield speedily to the administration of iron, quinine, and various preparations of zinc and copper.   In this anæmic class of case wine and good nourishment will also be indispensable.   The pulse is generally weak, action of the heart feeble, and the blood deficient in red globules. This is indicated by the pallor of the countenance and general state of anæmia.   The patient complains of great muscular debility and nervous depression.   Associated with the preceding symptoms, I have often observed signs of what was considered at the time to be *threatening* indications of apoplexy and paralysis.

In incipient general paralysis, I am of opinion that much benefit is to be derived from a persevering and continuous course of *tonic* treatment.   In this affection it will be found necessary, whilst building up the patient, and conserving his powers of life by means of iron, quinine, zinc, cod-liver oil, &c., to apply a seton or issue to the arm or nape of the neck.

In cases of this disease we occasionally observe symptoms of temporary congestion of the brain. For the relief of this complication I have generally applied one or two leeches to the schneiderian membrane with marked benefit. In some instances I have exhibited the various preparations of arsenic and copper with apparent advantage. In depressed conditions of the cerebral force, phosphorus, combined with minute doses of strychnine and cod-liver oil, may be administered.

In the treatment of incipient softening of the brain, it will be necessary, in the majority of cases, to give tonics and stimulants. I am satisfied of the possibility of arresting, in the early stages of softening, the progress of the cerebral disorganization by means of the treatment previously suggested. Much, however, will depend upon the characteristics of each individual case. In some patients it will be necessary to apply, even at the first onset of the disease, if the physician be fortunate enough to see the case in this early stage, counter-irritation to the neck, as well as to use dry cupping. In particular formations of the cranium, states of the heart and cerebral vessels, it will be necessary, whilst sustaining the powers of life by the therapeutic agents specified, to cautiously relieve local head symptoms by means of leeches. But antiphlogistic treatment will rarely be found necessary.

I need not, whilst advising a course of tonic treatment, associated with generous diet, and a liberal use of wine, &c., in cases of incipient softening of the brain, suggest the importance of carefully protecting the patient from mental labor, irritation, and anxiety. It will be useless to grapple by means of medicine with this serious cerebral disease, unless the mind is most scrupulously preserved from an undue exercise or strain of its powers.

It will often be found desirable to send the patient abroad, or to a remote part of the country, with the view of removing him from all temptation to work, or to advise a sea voyage after his state of general, mental, and cerebral health has been well analyzed and remedially treated.

I have on record the particulars of a number of cases of incipient softening of the brain which have been successfully cured by an adoption of these remedial means. It is impossible here to enter into details respecting the treatment of this important type of cerebral disease. I can only, in this work, deal with general

principles. Every case as it presents itself to the physician will
exhibit peculiar and characteristic idiosyncrasies, or morbid phenomena, requiring a modification of treatment, medical, moral,
and hygienic.

Do we estimate in a manner commensurate with its grave and
vital importance the necessity of watching, with the most scrupulous care, the cerebral symptoms that follow all mechanical injuries to the head ? I am satisfied that a vast amount of organic,
chronic, and incurable disease of the brain and disorder of the
mind can be directly traced to this cause.

In many cases, positive and undoubted evidences of disease of
the brain are present without exciting a suspicion as to the cerebral
origin of the affection, or character of the symptoms. A man
receives a blow upon the head. He may suffer from partial concussion of the brain, or be merely stunned. He recovers without
any apparent inconveniences from the injury, but subsequently
head symptoms exhibit themselves, clearly the consequence of the
injury which the brain has sustained many years previously !

I am satisfied that the importance of this subject cannot be
exaggerated. Repeatedly have I had cases of epilepsy bidding
defiance to all treatment, tumors, abscesses, cancer, softening of
the brain, as well as insanity in its more formidable types, under
my care, whose origin could unquestionably be traced back, for
varying periods of one, two, five, eight, ten, fifteen, and even
twenty years, to damage done to the delicate structure of the
brain by injuries inflicted upon the head !

In some instances accidents of the kind may not be followed by
serious results ; but in certain temperaments, conditions of bodily
health, and in particular predispositions, we may safely predicate
the development of chronic disease of the brain as the result of
neglected blows on the head. Injuries of this character occurring
to persons of a strumous habit, or to those suffering from long-
continued debilitating diseases, impaired and perverted nutrition,
overwrought and anxious minds, or inheriting a constitutional
liability to mental or cerebral disease, are frequently followed by
serious and often fatal results.

It is therefore highly necessary to keep a vigilant and watchful
eye upon those who have been exposed to accidents of this kind,
with a view of anticipating, if possible, the development of important cerebral symptoms. I am satisfied that we have it in our

power, by timely and judicious measures, to arrest the progress
of many of the organic affections of the brain originating from
mechanical causes, if the patient's condition immediately after the
injury be attended to, the state of his cerebral health for a time
carefully regarded, the incipient symptoms of brain disorder, when
they present themselves, recognized, and the patient immediately
subjected to prompt and appropriate treatment.

Softening of the brain, the formation of cerebral abscesses, the
slow growth of encephalic tumors, subtle degeneration of the nervous tissue in the form of cancerous growths (all the remote effects
of injuries to the head) are, in my opinion, *preventable* diseases of
the brain, if the unmistakable warnings afforded in the majority
of cases of their existence are not neglected, unrecognized, and
untreated.

A gentleman was actively engaged, apparently in excellent
health, in playing cricket. He suddenly complained of faintness,
he then began to vomit, and in a few seconds dropped down dead!
A *post-mortem* examination being made, the brain revealed the
existence of a chronic encysted abscess that had emptied itself into
one of the ventricles. It appeared that this gentleman had been
thrown from his horse *six* years previously whilst hunting, and
had suffered from partial concussion of the brain. He quite recovered from all the acute head symptoms, but two years after the
accident he complained of repeated headaches, not, however, of a
violent character, as well as of occasional loss of memory. These
symptoms, however, were of so trifling a character that he did not
consider it necessary to apply for medical advice. In this case
how much good might have been effected if the cerebral symptoms
had been at this time recognized, *and viewed in connection with
the injury of the head he had sustained two years previously!·*
Judicious treatment, adopted at this early period, would, in all
probability, have saved a valuable life.

A man, aged fifty-two, fell from the mainyard of a ship upon
the deck. He was removed to the cabin in a state of unconsciousness. In the course of the day he became sensible, and in about
a fortnight he was able to resume work. For *four* years this sea-
man never complained of any head symptoms. He continued
active in his habits, as well as intelligent in his conversation.
Five years after the accident he became subject to headaches of a
severe but paroxysmal type. These attacks were accompanied by

occasional acts of vomiting, coming on immediately after meals. At times he exhibited much depression of spirits. He was treated for what was considered to be a *gastric* affection, and appeared greatly to improve; the headache was less severe in character, and became more intermittent. In the sixth year from the accident the patient complained of numbness down the left side, and the headache returned with increased violence. It was still considered that all his symptoms proceeded from hepatic and gastric disorder, and nothing was done for the relief of the cerebral symptoms, beyond giving him occasional doses of blue pill, in combination with extract of rhubarb, mineral acids, and bitter infusions. In a few months from the appearance of the numbness, he became paralytic, and died in this state eight weeks subsequently. An encysted abscess was found after death in the left hemisphere of the brain.

A boy received a violent blow on the head from a cricket bat. He did not appear to suffer any inconveniences from the injury until *ten* or *eleven* years afterwards, when he became subject to paroxysmal attacks of headache, associated with extreme vertigo, clearly of an epileptic character. He eventually had a succession of severe attacks of epilepsy, which continued for a period of five years. He ultimately died in a violent epileptic paroxysm. An encysted abscess of the size of an egg was found in the cerebellum.

What course of treatment would I advise under these circumstances? In severe blows upon the head it is important to keep in check all tendency to cerebral congestion and inflammation in the portion of the brain immediately under the part of the scalp and skull that has been injured. By closely watching for *local* cerebral disorder, we may prevent those states of chronic irritation, congestion, and inflammation that so frequently induce disorganization of structure, in the form of tumors, softening, and abscesses. In the days of Pott, venesection was almost universally practised after the head had received a mechanical injury. This mode of treatment has, in modern times, been altogether exploded. In these cases the local abstraction of blood by means of leeches applied over, or in the immediate neighborhood of the injury, is decidedly advantageous in preventing the development of organic alterations in the brain. It will often be necessary also to give mercurials, and to apply cold evaporating lotions to the head.

I have, in some cases of severe cranial injury, applied a seton to the nape of the neck, as well as *issues in the scalp near the situation of the blow*, when I have had reason to believe that local, cerebral, and meningeal mischief existed. It may often be necessary, in particular diatheses, to sustain the vital powers by means of iron, quinine, stimulants, and generous diet, whilst the cerebral irritation and congestion is being attacked by the means suggested. I am satisfied that it is in our power to arrest the progress of the fatal cerebral disorganization that so often follows, after the lapse of years, injuries to the head, if we do not sleep at our posts, and are on the look-out for the first scintillations of brain disorder. It is our duty, under such circumstances, to watch for head symptoms. "It is not enough," as Dr. Graves remarks, when referring to the obscure cerebral affections observed in some cases of fever, "to treat them when they come, they MUST BE SEEN and MET COMING." Wise and sagacious counsel!

I have paid anxious attention to this subject, and, as the result of much experience, I am fully convinced that in many instances the advance of softening, tumors, and abscesses of the brain, has been checked by means of the local head, combined with the constitutional treatment previously referred to.

I have spoken of impairment of attention, the effect of certain morbid conditions of the cerebral health. Such cases of psychical debility are generally associated with a depressed state of the nerve and vital force, impoverished condition of the blood, and impaired state of the nutrition of the brain. A stimulating plan of treatment, generous diet, cod-liver oil, combined with the sulphate and valerianate of zinc, quinine, iron, and other blood tonics, are valuable remedies in these cases. In instances of impaired intelligence, associated with active head symptoms, vertigo, headache, &c., such as to justify the belief that capillary congestion exists, judicious local depletion and counter-irritation are often of much service. The abstraction of blood, however, is rarely necessary in these cerebro-psychical affections, and yet I have known patients to be greatly relieved by a modified course of antiphlogistic treatment. Minute doses of strychnine are occasionally indicated, and the various preparations of arsenic, with and without iron, and ammoniated solution of copper, I have found to afford considerable tone to the brain and mind, if judiciously administered. I am of opinion that the therapeutic value of arsenic and copper are not sufficiently appreciated in the affections of the brain and nervous system, particularly if associated with states of vital depression.

The faculty of attention, like that of memory, is susceptible of being greatly cultivated and strengthened by a regular and continuous exercise of its powers. Habits of slovenly thought and careless attention are easily formed, and, when once contracted, not easily combated. The effort to subject the attention to the controlling influences of the will may at first be difficult, but all obstacles will vanish before a steady and unrelaxed determination to conquer and bring into a state of subjugation the restive faculty. "When we turn," says Sir W. Hamilton, "for the first time, our view on any given object, a hundred other things still retain possession of our thoughts. Even when we are able, by an arduous exertion, to break loose from the matters which have previously engrossed us, or which every moment force themselves on our consideration, even when a resolute determination, or the attraction of the new object, has smoothed the way on which we are to travel, still the mind is continually perplexed by the glimmer of intrusive and distracting thoughts, which prevent it from placing that which should exclusively occupy its view in the full clearness of an undivided light. How great soever may be the interest which we take in the new object, it will, however, only be fully established as a favorite, when it has been fused into an integral part of the system of our previous knowledge, and of our established associations of thoughts, feelings, and desires. But this can only be accomplished by time and custom. Our imagination and our memory, to which we must resort for materials with which to illustrate and enliven our new study, accord us their aid unwillingly, and indeed only by compulsion. But if we are vigorous enough to pursue our course in spite of obstacles, every step as we advance will be found easier; the mind becomes more animated and energetic, the distractions gradually diminish, the attention is more exclusively concentrated upon its object, the kindred ideas flow with greater freedom and abundance, and afford an easier selection of what is suitable for illustration. At length our system of thought harmonizes with our pursuit. The whole man becomes, as it may be, philosopher, historian, or poet; he lives only in the trains of thought relating to this character. He now energizes freely, and consequently with pleasure, for pleasure is the reflex of unforced and unimpeded energy. All that is produced in this state of mind bears the stamp of excellence and perfection."[1]

I have yet to address myself to the treatment, medical and moral, of impairment and loss of memory. In such cases, clearly the effect of physical disease or irritation established in the brain, or in some part of the body closely sympathizing with this organ, no good will result from an attempt to strengthen or revivify this mental power, apart from a careful pathological investigation of the *cerebral* state of the patient, and the adoption of a mode of *physical* and *psychical* treatment suggested by such examination. In all acute affections of the brain damaging the memory, it is useless to battle with a *symptom*, to treat an *effect*, without carefully considering the *cause*. Great benefit occasionally results from the exhibition of stimulants in certain cases of impaired memory consequent upon an exhausted condition of the nerve and vital force.

In less acute conditions of defective memory, advantage undoubtedly accrues from judicious attempts on the part of the patient to revivify the faculty; but if these efforts should be succeeded (as is occasionally the case) by vertigo, headache, or other corporeal symptoms of distress, the mind should be left in a *passive* state, until the cerebral condition is such as to justify a repetition of the experiment. It occasionally occurs that a language, apparently forgotten, has been suddenly revived during the effort made to seize hold of and resuscitate past impressions. When making these efforts we should be careful not to strain the faculty beyond justifiable limits. How often the attempt to recall ideas to the mind is abortive? Under these circumstances, if the brain is permitted to be in a quiescent state, the ideas will frequently recur to the mind spontaneously. If I were permitted to theorize on the subject, I should be inclined to suggest, that the endeavor thus made to remember past impressions establishes a cerebral and psychical oscillating movement, which continues in the vesicular neurine of the brain after we cease to make any conscious effort to resuscitate apparently obliterated ideas.

Is not this hypothesis supported by the following fact? How often does it happen that all attempts to exercise the memory previously to retiring late at night to rest, are found to be nugatory; but how vivid and life-like are the ideas in the morning

---

[1] "Lectures on Metaphysics," by Sir W. Hamilton, Bart. Vol. i, p. 255.

following a state of brain activity, consequent upon a satisfactory amount of cerebral and psychical repose? Impressions which we were not conscious of effecting previously to sleep have undoubtedly been made upon the mind, and the oscillations or actions thus induced in the nerve vesicle have continued during the night, the mind being clearly and forcibly impinged with the ideas which we tried to stamp upon it on the previous evening.

During the stage of convalescence, and occasionally after recovery from attacks of insanity, I have known patients to complain of a distressing rapidity of thought, and of an acute sensitiveness to impressions, physical as well as moral, which have caused them at times great anxiety of mind. There has been a want of cerebral repose and mental quietude, of which the patient has been painfully conscious. The " tempest of the mind" having subsided, has left a slight ruffle on the surface of the waves which time and immunity from excitement only can subdue.

Dr. Abercrombie refers to a case related by Dr. Gregory, of a maniac who had been some time under his care, and had entirely recovered. For a week after his restoration to health, he was harassed, particularly during his dreams, by the same rapid and tumultuous thoughts, and the same violent emotions which had agitated him whilst insane.

A patient, who during his insanity imagined himself to be an exalted personage, told me, that for some months after his recovery he never could entirely dispossess his mind of the idea of his having acquired a certain degree of social elevation. He had no belief in his having obtained regal distinction, for this delusion no longer existed in his mind; but "I believed," to use his own words, "I was a *little* higher in rank than the class I legitimately belonged to."

In these cases there undoubtedly exists a cerebral action or oscillation, which continues after the balance of the mind has been restored. It is phenomena like these that render the stage of convalescence, perhaps, the most critical one to treat in cases of insanity.

There is no faculty of the mind so susceptible of being improved by moderate and regular exercise as that of the memory. It is said that Sir Isaac Newton, at one period of his life, entirely forgot the contents of his celebrated " Principia," in consequence of his neglecting to exercise the memory. The famous Mr. Hude spent

several years in close application to conic sections. Leibnitz, in
returning from his travels, called to see him, and expected to have
been highly entertained by conversing with him on the subject of
his studies. "Here," said Mr. Hude, sighing, "look at this manuscript; I have forgotten everything in it since I became burgo-
master of Amsterdam."

Lord Bacon is of opinion that the memory is not strengthened
by repeated efforts to fix certain ideas on the mind; in other
words, that if a passage which we wish to recollect is carefully
read *ten*, it is more likely to be remembered than if it were read
twenty times, provided an effort be made to *recite the words* after
each reading. "*Quæ expectantur et attentionem excitant, melius
hærent quam quæ prætervolant. Itaque si scriptum aliquod vicies
perlegeris, non tam facile illud memoriter disces, quam si illud legas
decies, tentando interim illud recitare et ubi deficit memoria, inspi-
ciendo librum.*"[1]

Dr. Rush suggests some valuable rules for the treatment of impaired loss of memory. The mental remedies for loss or decay of
memory should be, says this authority, a "frequent repetition of
what we wish to remember. The benefits of this practice are
strikingly illustrated in the history of a London printer, who after
working seven years in composing the Bible, was able to repeat
every chapter and verse in it by memory. The advantage of this
mode of strengthening the memory is seen in persons who repeat
questions or whole sentences that are proposed to them before they
can answer them. The door of the mind in such people requires
two knocks before it can be opened, one by the person who asks,
and the other by the person who answers the questions; or, to speak
more simply, the mind requires a double impression from words
before it is able to convert them into thoughts. Again, calling in
the aid of two or more of the senses to assist in the retention of
knowledge, is found beneficial in cases of impaired memory. It
is said that we seldom forget what we have handled, or tasted, seen
or heard. The eyes assist the ears, and the ears the eyes. Children
and the vulgar, whose memories are alike weak, are unable to
retain what they read unless they receive it at the same time
through their eyes and ears; hence their practice of reading, when
alone, with an audible voice. In some cases they are unable to
remember even their own thoughts without rendering them audible;

[1] "Nov. Org." lib. ii, aph. 26.

hence we so often hear them talking to themselves. The same thing is observed in the low and chronic state of insanity, partially from the same cause. Where the eyes and ears cannot both be employed in acquiring knowledge, the use of the ears should be preferred.

"Julius Cæsar says the reason why the ancient Druids did not commit their instructions to writing was, that their pupils might, by receiving them through their ears, more easily acquire, and more durably retain them in their memories. The ear is less apt to be distracted than the eye by the obtrusion of surrounding objects, the one being more constant than the other. The mind, moreover, is more concentrated in hearing than in seeing. The truth of these remarks is confirmed by few of the sayings or songs learned by the ear only, and in the nursery, being ever forgotten. The memory is improved by exercise. Its low state among savages is occasioned by the small number of objects upon which they exercise it. The memory is aided in hearing and after reading by shutting the eyes. In this way Mr. Woodfall received and retained the speeches of the members of the British Parliament until he committed them to paper, after which he published and forgot them. The memory is restored and strengthened by means of association. The principal circumstances which influence this operation of the mind are time, place, pleasure, pain, sounds, words, letters, habit, and interest. Ideas, and even words that have been forgotten, are often recalled by conversation upon subjects that are related to them. This is effected by some incidental word or idea awakening, by association, the word or idea we wish to revive in our minds. Dr. Van Rohr, a Danish physician, who visited Philadelphia in the year 1798, informed me that he could at any time excite the remembrance of words by committing two or three lines of poetry to memory. Singing aids the memory in acquiring a knowledge of words, and of the ideas connected with them. A song is always learned sooner than the same number of words not set to music.[1] Reading or repeating what we wish to

[1] " I remember having seen, while six months in the service of MM. Pariset and Mitivié, an insane woman, whose ideas were so incoherent that, though always speaking, she did not associate two syllables capable of composing a word. However, when she sang, which she did willingly when the example was set, she repeated very clearly not only the air but the words. Thus the memory, unfaithful in cases where the words were ideas, became clear and precise when the words were songs."—(Gratiolet.)

commit to memory the last thing before we go to bed impresses ideas on the mind."[1]

The habit of keeping a commonplace book for the purpose of dotting down occurrences, thoughts, or passages from books, with the view of fixing them strongly on the recollection, is thought by some to be injurious instead of beneficial to the mind.   Undoubtedly such would be the result, if the memoranda so recorded were not repeatedly brought under the cognizance of the intellect, and past impressions thus reproduced to the mind and impressed on the memory.   It is not judicious, however, to rely too implicitly upon such a mode of refreshing and invigorating this faculty.

Montaigne frequently complains in his writings of a loss of memory.   He cites many extraordinary instances of his ignorance in regard to some of the ordinary topics of information.   It is obvious, however, to any one who reads his works with attention, that this ignorance did not proceed from an original defect of memory, but from the singular or whimsical direction which his curiosity had taken at an early period of life.   " I can do nothing," says he, " without my memorandum-book, and so great is my difficulty in remembering proper names, that I am forced to call my domestic servants by their offices.   I am ignorant of the greater number of our coins in use ; of the difference of one grain from another, both in the earth and in the granary ; what use leaven is of in making bread, and why wine must stand some time in the vat before it ferments."   Yet the same author seems evidently, from his writings, to have had his memory wonderfully stored with an infinite variety of apophthegms, and of historical passages which had impressed his imagination, and to have been familiarly acquainted, not only with the names, but with the absurd and exploded opinions of the ancient philosophers.

In several cases that have come under my observation, the memory has become impaired in consequence of an undue straining of the faculty in early life.   I once saw a youth who eventually sank into a condition of imbecility, caused (as was alleged by medical attendants of the patient's family) by severe and prolonged exercise of the memory.

It is with the memory as with the other intellectual faculties, the amount of strain to which it is subjected should have an equi-

[1] " Medical Inquiries and Observations upon the Diseases of the Mind," by B. Rush, M.D.   Philadelphia, 1855.   P. 281.

table relation to its condition of connate or *normal* vigor. It would be manifestly unphilosophical to subject all memories to the same degree of pressure, or to imagine that because a few minds are capable of committing expeditiously and accurately to memory, within a prescribed period, a certain degree of knowledge, that every intellect is competent, with facility, to execute a similar task.   There are as great differences in the *mental* as in the *physical* capacities of children. It is consequently absurd to deal with them *en masse*, as if the human mind were a mere machine, capable, without scientific discrimination, of the same amount of sustained intellectual labor and rapid progress.   It is undoubtedly an important element in education to carefully, steadily invigorate and discipline the memory in early life; but in effecting this most desirable object, it is our duty to avoid mistaking *natural* mental dulness for culpable idleness, and *organic* cerebral incapacity for criminal indifference to intellectual culture and educational advancement.

When speaking of the injurious effects of overstraining the memory in early life, it has been observed, "The faculty of memory is much too hardly pressed by the practice of some schools. It is a great temptation to a schoolmaster, who may be overworked or indolently inclined, to have recourse to long repetition tasks, because it economizes his own time.   It keeps a whole class actively employed, and costs him a very little time to hear what it has cost them a very long time, comparatively, to learn.   This is a very different thing from laboring *with* boys, and patiently solving their difficulties.[1]

"I am quite aware that this exercise, in its degree, is very useful; that to commit passages to memory in a language conduces to a thorough acquaintance with it, and a power of composing in it.   But this is carried beyond all bounds in some schools. In that in which I was educated, it was the custom, once a year, that boys in the middle and lower classes should repeat all the Latin and Greek poetry they had learned in the year, with such addition to it of fresh matter as each boy could accomplish.   So much did our place in the school depend on success in this, and so severe was the rivalry, that although we were then only about fourteen years of age, the usual quantity for the boys to repeat

[1] "Mental Vigor; its attainment impeded by Errors in Education," by the Rev. H. Fearon, B.D. London, 1859.

35

was from six to eight thousand lines, which we did in eight different lessons, and it took about a week to hear us. One boy, in my year, construed and repeated the enormous quantity of fourteen thousand lines of Homer, Horace, and Virgil; I heard him say it. The master dodged him about very much, but he scarcely ever missed a single word. One wonders in what chamber of the brain it could possibly have been stowed away!

"Now I do not think that this excessive strain on the mnemonic faculty is calculated to strengthen it; nor do I believe that this or any other faculty ought to be so severely pressed. I have a lively recollection of the long-sustained exertion it required; how, week after week, we rose early, and late took rest, in our anxiety to outstrip others, upon which our station in the school, and, I may say, the *bread* of many of us depended. This custom is, I hope, now, though not given up, modified. Boys ought to be rather repressed than encouraged in such a trial. Do not send them out into the world with minds overweighted, and with things which, after all, are, in such an excess, not needed. Education, as a rule, ought to be directed more to what elicits thought than what merely encourages memory. Feats of repetition are but poor offerings to the goddess of wisdom,—rendering unto Minerva, as it were, only a lip service."[1]

[1] "Children are made to fill their heads with words, or are severely punished, and by these means become dull, heavy, and stupid, because, instead of cultivating their reason, their masters seem to aim at fatiguing and weakening their memory by their over-exertions. Instead of teaching children to consider and examine a thing, in order to understand it, these masters oblige them to pronounce it fifteen or twenty times, with a view to imprint it on their memory. Boerhaave styled this a piteous mode of instruction. Baron Haller observes, that the truth of this is but too palpable, because, instead of enabling them to analyze a compound idea, and making them feel the due value of the simple ideas it includes, they teach them only the syllables and words that express them, and thus add obstacle after obstacle to the improvement of the understanding.

"This absurd method, which is so generally adopted, makes all the knowledge of children consist not in the understanding, as it ought to do, but in memory. This seems to be the reason why so many young people who have shone at school make so diminutive a figure when they launch into the world. As the chief object of their studies was to load their memories with things which, as they never understood, were soon forgotten, so they find themselves incapable of observing or judging, and in general of thinking, because in their younger days they had never been taught to think for themselves.

"Baron Van Swieten tells us he has seen children of the most promising dispositions rendered stupid, and even epileptic, through the mismanagement of their masters."—*Zimmerman's Experience in Physic.*

I should regret if, in the preceding observations, I were to convey the impression that I estimated lightly the benefit to be derived from a steady and persevering cultivation of the memory in early life. It is, in every point of view, most essential that this faculty should be carefully developed, disciplined, and invigorated during the scholastic training which most boys intended for the universities, and subsequently for political and professional life, have to undergo. The knowledge then acquired is seldom if ever obliterated, except by disease, from the mind. How much of the pure, refined, and elevated mental enjoyment in which we luxuriously revel in after years is to be traced to that period when we were compelled to commit to memory, often as a task, but more frequently as a part of the regular curriculum of the school, long and brilliant passages from illustrious classical authors? Do we ever regret, when our bark is being tossed upon the noisy and tempestuous ocean of life, having had to go through such an intellectual ordeal? Is not the mind thus stored with an imperishable knowledge of passages from the poets, orators, and historians of antiquity, full of elevated thoughts, profound wisdom, exquisite imagery, noble and magnanimous sentiments?

It would be absurd to undervalue a system of educational discipline productive of so many obvious advantages. My animadversions are directed against the too *exclusive* cultivation, as well as undue *straining* of the memory, forgetting, as I think we sometimes do, that there are higher and more exalted mental faculties that require to be carefully expanded and fortified, before the mind is fitted to enter into the great arena of life, and qualified to contend successfully in its many battles, struggles, and trials.

Before concluding this chapter, I would briefly address myself to the consideration of two important questions intimately connected with the very interesting facts previously discussed in this volume, viz. :

1. *At what particular period of life does the intellect begin to decline, and when, as a general rule, is first observed the commencement of an insenescence of the intellectual principle?*

2. *Is great strength of memory often associated with limited powers of judgment and reasoning, and conjoined with a low order of intelligence?*

"In old persons," says Cabanis, "the feebleness of the brain, and of those functions which originate therein, gives to their determination the same mobility, the same characteristic uncertainty which they possess during childhood; in fact, the two conditions closely resemble each other." The Professor of Physiology at the University of Montpelier, Dr. Lordat, denies the truth of this aphorism, and terms it a "popular delusion." This able physiologist and philosopher maintains that it is the *vital*, not the *intellectual* principle that is seen to wane as old age throws its autumnal tinge over the green foliage of life. "It is not true," he says, "that the intellect becomes weaker after the vital force has passed its culminating point. The understanding acquires more strength during the first half of that period which is designated as old age. It is impossible," he says, "to assign any period of existence at which the reasoning power suffers deterioration." Numerous illustrations are adduced for the purpose of establishing that senescence of the intelligence is not isochronous with that of the vital force.

The conversation of the celebrated composer, Cherubini, at the age of eighty, is said to have been as brilliant as during the meridian of his existence. Gosse composed a *Te Deum* at the age of seventy-eight. Corneille, when seventy years of age, exhibited no decay of intellect, judging from his poetic address to the king. M. des Quensounnières, the accomplished poet, at the advanced age of one hundred and sixteen, was full of vivacity, and fully capable of sustaining a lively and intelligent conversation. M. Leroy, of Rambouillet, at the age of one hundred, composed a remarkably beautiful and spirited poem. Abbé Taublet, when speaking of the intellect of Fontenelle when far advanced in life, says, "His intellectual faculties, with the exception of a slight defect of memory, had preserved their integrity in spite of corporeal debility. His thoughts were elevated, his expressions finished, his answers quick and to the point, his reasoning powers accurate and profound." Cardinal de Fleury was Prime Minister of France from the age of seventy to ninety. At the age of eighty, Fontenelle asked permission, on the ground of physical infirmity, to retire from the post of perpetual secretary of the Academy of Sciences. The prime minister refused his request. Three years subsequently, Fontenelle again expressed a wish to resign office. "You are an indolent, lazy fellow," writes the Cardinal; "but I suppose we must occasionally indulge such characters." Voltaire, when at the age of eighty-four, came to Paris, agreeably to his own language, "*to seek a triumph and to find a tomb.*" Richelieu died at the age of ninety-three, full of mental vigor. A few minutes before his death, his daughter-in-law, wishing to encourage him, said, "You are not so ill as you would wish us to believe; your countenance is charming." "What!" said he, with the utmost vivacity, and full of wit and humor, "*has my face been converted into a mirror?*"[1]

Mr. Waller wrote, when he was past eighty, a poem, entitled "A Presage of the Ruin of the Turkish Empire, presented to his Majesty King James II, on his birthday." . . . "Poetry had been the supreme delight of his youth, and he refreshed his old age with the same cordial; and it cannot be denied that whatever traces of decay may appear in his later compositions, yet Longinus's observation of Homer is justly applied to our poet, it was the old age of Mr. Waller. Could it be supposed that the verses he wrote on the Earl of Roscommon's translation of Horace's Art of Poetry were the composition of a man twelve years beyond his grand climacteric? for he was then seventy-five. Even at this advanced age, he continued to write with beauty and spirit. Not many years after this, he turned his muse, as became his age, towards heaven, for which flight his soul had evidently been preparing. And though his Divine Poems were written at fourscore and after, yet the same elevation and fire, though with a little fainter flame, glows in them as in his earlier productions. He intended to crown all his labors with the poem, ' of the last verses in the book,' which can never be too much admired, so natural are the images, so lively the representation of old age, so feelingly does the author speak of its infirmities, and all is so poetical!"[2]

John Maplesoft was a learned physician and pious divine. He was born June 16, 1631. . . He was one of the Directors of Greenwich Hospital. In 1707, he was chosen President of Sion College, having been a benefactor both to that building and library. He continued to preach in his church of St. Laurence Jewry (where he was also Thursday lecturer) till he was past eighty years of age; and when he thought of retiring, he printed a book, entitled, *The Principles and Duties of the Christian Religion*, a copy of which

---

[1] Vide "Lectures on Mental Dynamics," by Professor Lordat. Translated by Dr. Speers for the *Psychological Journal*.

[2] "Biographia Britannica."

he sent to every house in his parish. He died in the ninety-first year of his age.[1]

Titian, the greatest painter of the Venetian school, and the founder of the true principles of coloring, continued to exercise his art until 1576, when he died of the plague at Venice, in the ninety-sixth year of his age. Soon after 1553 (at the age of seventy-three or seventy-six) he painted, at Innspruck, the portraits of Ferdinand, king of the Romans, his queen, and all his family, in one picture, which is said to have been his masterpiece. Benjamin West, the historical painter, was born in 1738, and in 1814 (aged seventy-six) exhibited a picture of "Christ rejected by the Jewish High-priest," one of his best works; and in 1817 (aged seventy-nine) he painted his picture of "Death on the Pale Horse." He died at the age of eighty-two, in full mental vigor. Fontenelle wrote his "Elements of the Geometry of Infinites," in 1727, at the age of seventy.

Richard Cumberland, Bishop of Peterborough, was born July 15, 1632. When Dr. Wilkins had published his Coptic Testament, he made a present of a copy to his lordship, who sat down to study it when he was past eighty-three. At this advanced age he mastered the language, and went through great part of this version, and would often give excellent hints and remarks as he proceeded in reading it. At length, in the autumn of the year 1718, he was struck with palsy, from which he never recovered.[2]

Handel's last appearance in public was on the 6th of April, 1759. He then had reached the advanced age of seventy-five. After that period his faculties rapidly declined; and it was evident he had not long to live. Of this he was himself fully aware, and prepared to meet his end with a resignation and composure based upon a sincere belief in the doctrines of Christianity. As the close of his life approached, he signified a fervent wish that he might expire on Good Friday, and it is singular that he breathed his last on that day.

Ben Jonson died in 1637, aged sixty-three. He composed, literally on his death-bed, that exquisite fragment of a pastoral drama, the "Sad Shepherd," which in beauty and freshness of conception and treatment, is the most youthful of all his works. Sir Isaac Newton died in 1727, aged eighty-four. About a month

---

[1] "Biographia Britannica."   [2] Ibid.

previously to his death he presided, with great ability and unimpaired intellect, at the Royal Society.   Locke died in 1704, aged seventy-three.   Some of his last compositions, which were written shortly before his death, and published with his posthumous papers, were, A Discourse on Miracles, and Paraphrases, with Notes of the Epistles of St. Paul.   These works evidence no decadence in his powerful intellect.   Dr. Johnson died in 1784, aged seventy-five. He published his last work, "The Lives of the English Poets," only three years before his death.   His last hours were employed in adjusting his worldly concerns, with composure and exactness, as one who was fully conscious that he was soon to render his last account to God.   His intellect was powerful and clear to the last. Whilst dying, he repeated the Lord's Prayer in the Latin language. Bacon died in 1625, aged sixty-seven, and retained to the last his love for science.   Shortly before his death, he was driving in the neighborhood of Highgate; the day was cold, and the snow lay on the ground.   It had previously occurred to him that snow might be used for the purpose of preserving animal substances from putrefaction, and determined to try the experiment, he descended from his carriage, entered a cottage, and purchased a fowl, which with his own hands he stuffed with snow; in doing this he was seized with a sudden cold, which terminated fatally after suffering for a week.

Chaucer died at the age of seventy-two.   During his retirement in 1391, and up to the time of his death, with an intellect in full vigor, he was employed in writing his learned treatise on the "*Astrolabe*," for the use of his son, a boy ten years old.   Sir E. Coke died at the advanced age of eighty-two.   He spent his last days, in full intellectual vigor, in revising his numerous works. He died, repeating with his last breath, "Thy kingdom come. Thy will be done."

Lord Eldon died at the age of eighty-six.   He remained in the full enjoyment of his mental powers until shortly before his death, when, although his mind on the whole was clear and correct, yet he formed on some subjects erroneous impressions; and his pleasantry, though it very visibly waned, yet sparkled forth from time to time so as to recall its former brilliancy.

Lord Kenyon died at the age of seventy.   He retained to the last his mental powers.   Gratefully expressing, with his last breath, his sense of the many blessings he had enjoyed, and his

resignation to the will of God. Lord Hardwicke died at the age
of seventy-three. He resigned the Great Seal in 1754; but he
still continued to serve the public in a more private station with
an unimpaired vigor of mind, which he enjoyed even under a long
indisposition, until his death. Lord Stowell died at the advanced
age of ninety. His mind was vigorous until within two years of
his death. Bolingbroke died at the age of seventy-three. His
intellect was powerful to the last.

Sir Isaac Newton published the third edition of his great work,
the "*Principia*," in February or March, 1726, with a new preface
by the author, dated January 12, 1725–6, at the age of 83–4.[1]

The illustrious Lord Mansfield died at the advanced age of
eighty-nine, in full and unclouded vigor of intellect. "So completely," says his noble biographer, "had he retained his mental
faculties, that only a few days before his last illness his niece,
Lady Anne Laving, in his hearing asked a gentleman what was
the meaning of the word 'psephismata,' in Mr. Burke's book on
the French Revolution? and the answer being that it must be a
misprint for 'sophismata,' the old Westminster scholar said, 'No;
psephismata is right;' and he not only explained the meaning of
the word with critical accuracy, but quoted off-hand a long passage
from Demosthenes to illustrate it. On the day of his death, in
the year 1793, he desired to be taken up and carried to his chair,
but he soon wished again to be in bed, and said, 'Let me sleep!—
let me sleep!' It might have been expected that in the wandering of his thoughts which followed, he might have conceived himself in some of the most exciting scenes of his past life, and that
he might have addressed some taunt to Lord Chatham respecting
the action for damages to be brought against the House of Commons; or, like Lord Tenterden, he might have desired the jury to
consider whether the publication and the inuendoes were proved on
a trial for libel, cautioning them to leave the question of *libel or
no-libel* for the court. But he never spoke more. On his return
to bed he breathed freely and softly like a child, and with as calm
and serene a countenance as in his best health, though apparently
ever after void of consciousness. . . . . He had entered his
eighty-ninth year. When he had a visit from Dr. Turton, his
physician, he thus broke off a discussion respecting his symptoms:

[1] "Brewster's Life of Sir I. Newton."

'Instead of dwelling on an old man's pulse, let me ask you, dear Doctor, what you think of this wonderful French Revolution ?' Dr. Turton. 'It is more material to know what your lordship thinks of it.' Lord Mansfield. 'My dear Turton, how can two reasonable men think differently on the subject ? A nation which for more than twelve centuries has made a conspicuous figure in the annals of Europe ; a nation where the polite arts first flourished in the northern hemisphere, and found an asylum against the barbarous incursions of the Goths and Vandals ; a nation whose philosophers and men of science cherished and improved civilization, and grafted on the feudal system the best of all systems, their laws respecting the descents and various modifications of territorial property : to think that a nation like this should not, in the course of so many centuries, have learned something worth preserving, should not have hit upon some little code of laws, or a few principles sufficient to form one ! Idiots ! who instead of retaining what was valuable, sound, and energetic in their constitution, have at once sunk into barbarity, lost sight of first principles, and brought forward a farrago of laws fit for Botany Bay ! It is euough to fill the mind with astonishment and abhorrence ! A constitution !—a constitution like this may survive that of an OLD MAN, but nothing less than a miracle can protect and transmit it down to posterity.' Horrors broke out and succeeded each other even more rapidly than he had anticipated ; and old as he was he lived to hear the news that, every vestige of liberty being extinguished in France, the reign of Terror was inundating the country with blood, and Louis XVI, the constitutional king, was executed on the scaffold as a malefactor."[1]

I now proceed to a brief consideration of the question, whether there is any truth in the popular notion that great vigor of memory is often associated with limited powers of judgment, defective reasoning, and circumscribed reflective faculties ; in other words, conjoined with a low order of intelligence. Do facts establish such an hypothesis or justify the axiom, "*beati memoria, expectantes judicium?*"

If we based our conclusions upon *à priori* reasoning, we might, upon a superficial examination of the question, be disposed to answer the interrogatory in the affirmative. The faculty of

---

[1] Campbell's " Lives of the Lord Chief Justices," vol. ii, p. 558.

memory is in its fundamental features an automatic or involuntary power. The mental process involved in the reception of ideas is in itself a simple and elementary one, not necessarily calling into action any complex intellectual operations. The majority of our ideas enter the mind whilst it is in a passive state. Little or no mental effort is required in order to grasp or receive the myriads of impressions that are momentarily forcing an admission into the mind. It is true that many of our ideas are the result of an active state of the intelligence. Among such are those which Locke designates as ideas of reflection, as contradistinguished from those of sensation. Whilst endeavoring to comprehend a subtle and profoundly philosophical process of reasoning, the mind is in the highest state of activity, with the view of seizing hold and retaining the ideas embodied in the argument immediately suggested to consciousness. In order to effect this object a great and sustained effort of thought is required, and the more important faculties of the understanding are unavoidably called into active exercise. But to reproduce the ideas so imbibed, a voluntary act of the mind, termed recollection or reminiscence, is only necessary, that is, supposing the ideas do not occur to the mind as a spontaneous act of suggestion.

It requires no obvious exercise of thought or severe course of reasoning to enable us to recall to the mind, when once thoroughly comprehended, the leading principles embodied in Paley's "Evidences," Butler's "Analogy," Newton's "Principia," or Kant's "Pure Reason." They are indelibly (presupposing a healthy state of the brain and intellect) impressed upon the mind of every educated man conversant with these branches of literature, and are easily made objects of consciousness by an effort of the will. Considered metaphysically, the memory, although a most important faculty, is not one of a high intellectual character. How different is the memory in this respect from the more exalted faculties of reason and judgment!

If my argument be tenable, we can easily understand the proposition, that great vigor of memory is not *necessarily* associated with superior powers of judgment or strength of reasoning capacity. Hence an active state of this faculty may coexist with an intellect generally defective in its organization; in other words, with a mind but partially and imperfectly developed in its higher manifestations.

Many facts have been cited to establish, that extraordinary powers of memory are often allied to an enfeebled condition of the other mental faculties, amounting occasionally to imbecility.[1] Men possessing but limited intellectual endowments have been favored with most retentive memories. Idiots have exhibited the faculty of retention to a remarkable extent, and men of very limited and circumscribed powers of reasoning and of most defective judgment have had memories distinguished for their tenacity. I do not question the accuracy of this statement; but what does it demonstrate? Let me consider for a moment the converse of the preceding proposition.

Do we not often witness mental powers of a high order, great manifestations of intellectual vigor, extraordinary reasoning and reflective faculties, combined with great strength of memory? Dr. Johnson, the gigantic character of whose intellect no one can question, was remarkable for the wonderful accuracy of his memory. He never forgot anything that he had seen, heard, or read. He often gave his intimate friends evidence of his wonderful capacity of retaining knowledge. Edmund Burke, of transcendent genius, was also noted for having great powers of retention. Clarendon, celebrated for his "History of the Rebellion," Gibbon, the immortal author of the "Decline and Fall," Locke, the celebrated metaphysician, and Archbishop Tillotson, were all distinguished for having great strength of memory. When alluding to this subject, Sir W. Hamilton observes, "For intellectual power of the highest order none were distinguished above Grotius and Pascal, and Grotius and Pascal forgot nothing they had ever read or thought. Leibnitz and Euler were not less celebrated for their intelligence than for their memory, and both could repeat the whole of the '*Æneid*.' Donnellus knew the '*Corpus Juris*' by heart, and yet he was one of the profoundest and most original speculators in jurisprudence. Muratori, though not a genius of the very highest order, was still a man of great ability and judgment, and so powerful was his retention, that in making quota-

---

[1] " There was," says the Rev. Henry Fearon, "a man in my father's parish who could remember the day when every person had been buried in the parish for thirty-five years, and could repeat with unvarying accuracy the name and age of the deceased, and the mourners at the funeral. But he was a complete fool. Out of the line of burials he had not one idea, could not give an intelligible reply to a single question, nor be trusted even to feed himself."—(*On " Mental Vigor*," &c.)

tions he had only to read his passages, put the books in their places, and then to write out from memory the words. Ben Jonson tells us that he could repeat all he had ever written, and whole books that he had read. Themistocles could call by their names the 20,000 citizens of Athens. Cyrus is reported to have known the name of every soldier in his army. Hortensius, after Cicero, the greatest orator of Rome, after sitting a whole day at a public sale, correctly enunciated from memory all the things sold, their prices, and the names of their purchasers. Niebuhr, the historian of Rome, was not less distinguished for his memory than his acuteness. In his youth he was employed in one of the public offices of Denmark. Part of a book of accounts having been destroyed, he restored it by an effort of memory. Sir James Mackintosh, Dugald Stewart, and Dr. Gregory, are examples of great talent united with great memory."

Seneca confessed that he had a miraculous memory, not only " to receive but to hold." " I myself," says Ben Jonson, " could, in in my youth, have repeated all that ever I had made, and so continued till I was past forty ; since, it is much decayed in me. Yet I can repeat the whole books that I have read, and *poems* of some selected friends which I have liked to charge my memory with. It was wont to be faithful to me, but shaken with *age* now, and *sloth* (which weakens the strongest abilities), it may perform somewhat, but cannot promise much."

The facts previously referred to are susceptible at least of two important conclusions : 1. That an active and vigorous condition of the mental faculties is compatible with old age. 2. That a continuous and often laborious exercise of the mind is not only consistent with a state of mental health, but is apparently productive of longevity.

In the succeeding volume this subject will be still further considered, when I address myself to the effects of an undue straining or exercise of the mind upon the mental and bodily health.

In glancing retrospectively over the preceding pages, I am conscious of having omitted a detailed reference to what many may conceive to be an important section of the subject I have had under consideration. I allude to the moral treatment of incipient types of insanity, as well as to the special duties devolving upon those legally intrusted with the medical, mental, and social management of the insane.

I designedly defer for another work any detailed exposition of my views on the first part of this subject. My sentiments on the latter important topic are fully expressed in a Presidential address I had the honor of delivering to a section of the profession officially connected with the management of public and private institutions for the treatment of the insane, and from that discourse I quote the subjoined passage :—

How noble is the study in which the psychological physician is engaged!   How important the duties that devolve upon him! How solemnly responsible is his position!   Is it possible to exaggerate or over-estimate his character, influence, importance, usefulness, and dignity!   What profound and accurate knowledge of the mind in its normal state is required before the physician is fitted successfully to investigate, unravel, and treat remedially its deviations from a healthy standard!   How intimate must be his acquaintance with the phenomena of thought, and with the nature and operations of the passions!   How exact should be his notions of the instinctive and perceptive faculties before he is fully qualified to appreciate subtle, morbid, psychical conditions!

The physician should entertain right notions of his duty and position ; he should encourage elevated, lofty thoughts and grand conceptions of his honorable vocation ; he should impress repeatedly, earnestly, and emphatically upon his own as well as upon the minds of all engaged in the same holy work the significant fact, that they are occupied in the study and treatment of a class of diseases affecting the very source, spring, and fountain of that principle which in its healthy operations alone can bring them into remote proximity to DEITY—that the physician has to deal with the spiritual part of man's complex nature, with that which elevates him in the scale of created excellences, and places him high on the pedestal among the great, good, and wise of this world.   But his solemn functions expand in interest, gravity, grandeur, and importance, as he reflects that it is HUMAN MIND prostrated, perverted, and often crushed by disease with which the practical physician has to deal ; that he has placed under our care a class of the afflicted human family, reduced by the inscrutable decrees of Providence to the most humiliating and helpless position to which a rational being can fall ; that it is his duty to witness the sad wreck of great and noble minds, and to sigh over the decay of exalted genius.

Like the historian and antiquarian wandering with a sad heart over ground made classical and memorable in the story of great men, and in the annals of heroic deeds, surveying with painful interest the crumbling ruins of ancient temples, viewing with subdued emotion the almost extinguished remains of proud imperial cities, consecrated by the genius of men renowned in the world's history as statesmen, scholars, artists, philosophers, and poets, so it is the duty of the mental physician to wander through the sad ruins of still greater temples than any that were in ancient days raised to the honor of an unseen DEITY. It is his distressing province to witness great and good intellects, proud, elevated understandings, levelled to the earth, crumbling like dust in the balance, under the dire influence of disease.

Survey that old man crouched in the corner of the room, with his face buried in his hands. He is indifferent to all that is passing around him; he heeds not the voice of man or woman; he delights not in the carolling of birds, or in the sweet music of the rippling brooks. The gentle wind of heaven, playing its sweetest melody as it rushes through the greenwood, awakens to his mind no consciousness of nature's charms. Speak to him in terms of endearment and affection; bring before him the glowing and impassioned images of the past. He elevates himself, gazes listlessly and mechanically at you, 'makes no sign,' and, dropping his poor head, buries it in his bosom, and sinks into his former state of moody melancholy abstraction. This man's oratory charmed the senate; the magic of his eloquence held thousands in a state of breathless admiration; his influence was commanding, his sagacity and judgment eminently acute and profound. View him as he is fallen from his high and honorable estate! Listen to the sweet and gentle voice of yonder woman, upon whose head scarcely eighteen summer suns have shed their genial warmth and influence. How merrily she dances over the greensward! How touchingly she warbles, like Ophelia, in her delirium, snatches of song! What a pitiful spectacle of a sweet mind lying in beautiful fragments before us! Look! she has decked herself with a spring garland. Now she holds herself perfectly erect, and walks with queenly majesty. Approach and accost her; she exclaims, "Yes, he will come; he promised to be here; where are the guests? where's the ring? where's my wedding dress—my orange blossoms?" Suddenly her mind is overshadowed, and her face assumes an expression of deep, choking, and bitter anguish—she alternately sobs and laughs —is gay and sad, cheerful and melancholy—

> " Thought and affliction, passion, hell itself,
>   She turns to favor and to prettiness."

Speak again to her, and another change takes place in the spirit of her dream. Like her sad prototype, the sweetest creation of Shakspeare's immortal genius, she plaintively sings—

> " He is dead and gone, lady,
>   He is dead and gone ;
>   At his head a green grass turf,
>   At his heels a stone."

Her history is soon told. Deep and absorbing passion, elevated hopes, bright, sunny, and fanciful dreams of the future—DEATH, with all its fictitious trappings, sad and solemn mockery of woe— seared affections, a broken heart, and a disordered brain ! .

The two illustrations I have cited are faithful and truthful out- lines of a type of case that must have come under the notice of those engaged in the treatment of the insane. How keenly cases like these tear the heartstrings asunder, and call into active ope- ration all the kindly sympathies of our nature.

The physician cannot too frequently allow his mind to dwell upon the peculiar state of those reduced by insanity to a condition of utter and childish helplessness. In other classes of disease, in which the psychical functions of the brain remain intact, the in- valid, even while suffering the most acute and agonizing pain, bodily distress, and physical prostration, is in a state to appreciate his actual relations with those around him—he feels sensitively the exhibition of tender sympathy—he properly estimates the care and attention bestowed upon his case, and recognizes the skill of his faithful medical adviser. Alas ! how different are the feelings and thoughts of many of the insane ! In this class of affections the kindness, sympathy, skill, unremitting assiduity and attention of the physician, are often not outwardly or manifestly appreciated. He has, in many cases, to pursue his holy work without the exhibition of the slightest apparent consciousness, on the part of the patient, of his efforts to assuage his anguish, and mitigate his condition of mental disease and bodily suffering. Nevertheless, it is his sacred duty, even where, as is occasionally the case, his actions are greatly misconstrued and perverted by those to whose relief he is administering, to unflaggingly persevere in his efforts to carry out a curative process of treatment. The poor, unhappy invalid, may believe that his physician is acting the part of a bitter foe. This ought not to excite any feeling but that of the most profound love and sympathy. If the patient's language be offensive and repulsive—if he be guilty of any acts of violence towards those in attendance upon him, the physician should never for a moment lose sight of the fact, that the unhappy affliction has, to a degree, destroyed the patient's free-will; and that he, for a time, has ceased to be a responsible being. It would be cruel, whilst such a condition of mind exists, to treat him otherwise than as a person deprived by disease of the power of complete self-government and moral control. Let me earnestly and affectionately urge upon all engaged in the treatment of the insane, the importance of never losing sight of the fact, that even in the worst types of mental disease there are some salient and bright spots upon which the physician may act, and against which may be directed his most potent curative agents. How true it is that

> " There is some soul of goodness in things evil,
>   Would men observingly distil it out."

The more formidable, apparently hopeless and incurable types of mental derangement admit, if not of cure, at least of considerable alleviation and mitigation. It is always in our power to materially add to the physical and social comforts of even the worst class of insane patients. We undoubtedly possess the means of materially modifying (if we cannot entirely re-establish the mental equilibrium) the more unfavorable and distressing forms of insanity, rendering the violent and turbulent tractable and amenable to discipline, the dangerous harmless, the noisy quiet, the dirty cleanly in their habits, and the melancholy, to an extent, cheerful and happy. It is possible, by a careful study of the bodily and mental idiosyncrasies of each individual case, and by an unremitting attention to dietetic and hygienic regimen, as well as by a persevering, unflagging, and assiduous administration of physical and moral remedies for their relief, to

> " Pluck from the memory a rooted sorrow," &c.

The spirit of love, tender sympathy, Christian benevolence, unwearying kindness, and warm affection, should influence every thought, look, and action of those engaged in the responsible treatment of the insane. It is the special province of the psychological physician to

> "Fetter strong madness in a *silken* thread,
> Charm ache with air, and agony with words."

What a holy, honorable, and sacred occupation is that in which he has the privilege of being engaged! Angelic spirits might well envy him the ennobling and exalted pleasures incidental to his mission of benevolence, love, and charity.

36

INDEX.

THE END.

wherever necessary. It has now been issued regularly for more than FORTY years, and it has been under the control of the present editor for more than a quarter of a century. Throughout this long period, it has maintained its position in the highest rank of medical periodicals both at home and abroad, and has received the cordial support of the entire profession in this country. Its list of Collaborators will be found to contain a large number of the most distinguished names of the profession in every section of the United States, rendering the department devoted to

ORIGINAL COMMUNICATIONS

full of varied and important matter, of great interest to all practitioners.

As the aim of the Journal, however, is to combine the advantages presented by all the different varieties of periodicals, in its

REVIEW DEPARTMENT

will be found extended and impartial reviews of all important new works, presenting subjects of novelty and interest, together with very numerous

BIBLIOGRAPHICAL NOTICES,

including nearly all the medical publications of the day, both in this country and Great Britain, with a choice selection of the more important continental works. This is followed by the

QUARTERLY SUMMARY,

being a very full and complete abstract, methodically arranged, of the

IMPROVEMENTS AND DISCOVERIES IN THE MEDICAL SCIENCES.

This department of the Journal, so important to the practising physician, is the object of especial care on the part of the editor. It is classified and arranged under different heads, thus facilitating the researches of the reader in pursuit of particular subjects, and will be found to present a very full and accurate digest of all observations, discoveries, and inventions recorded in every branch of medical science. The very extensive arrangements of the publishers are such as to afford to the editor complete materials for this purpose, as he not only regularly receives

ALL THE AMERICAN MEDICAL AND SCIENTIFIC PERIODICALS,

but also twenty or thirty of the more important Journals issued in Great Britain and on the Continent, thus enabling him to present in a convenient compass a thorough and complete abstract of everything interesting or important to the physician occurring in any part of the civilized world.

To their old subscribers, many of whom have been on their list for twenty or thirty years, the publishers feel that no promises for the future are necessary; but those who may desire for the first time to subscribe, can rest assured that no exertion will be spared to maintain the Journal in the high position which it has occupied for so long a period.

———

By reference to the terms it will be seen that, in addition to this large amount of valuable and practical information on every branch of medical science, the subscriber, by paying in advance, becomes entitled, without further charge, to

THE MEDICAL NEWS AND LIBRARY,

a monthly periodical of thirty-two large octavo pages. Its "NEWS DEPARTMENT" presents the current information of the day, while the "LIBRARY DEPARTMENT" is devoted to presenting standard works on various branches of medicine. Within a few years, subscribers have thus received, without expense, many works of the highest character and practical value, such as "Watson's Practice," "Todd and Bowman's Physiology," "Malgaigne's Surgery," "West on Children," "West on Females, Part I.," "Habershon on the Alimentary Canal," &c.

While the work at present appearing in its columns is

CLINICAL LECTURES ON THE DISEASES OF WOMEN.
By Professor J. Y. SIMPSON, of Edinburgh.

WITH NUMEROUS HANDSOME ILLUSTRATIONS.

These Lectures, published in England under the supervision of the Author, carry with them all the weight of his wide experience and distinguished reputation. Their eminently practical nature, and the importance of the subject treated, cannot fail to render them in the highest degree satisfactory to subscribers, who can thus secure them without cost. These Lectures are continued in the "News" for 1862.

———

It will thus be seen that for the small sum of FIVE DOLLARS, paid in advance, the subscriber will obtain a Quarterly and a Monthly periodical,

EMBRACING NEARLY SIXTEEN HUNDRED LARGE OCTAVO PAGES.

Those subscribers who do not pay in advance will bear in mind that their subscription of Five Dollars will entitle them to the Journal only, without the News, and that they will be at the expense of their own postage on the receipt of each number. The advantage of a remittance when ordering the Journal will thus be apparent.

Remittances of subscriptions can be mailed at our risk, when a certificate is taken from the Postmaster that the money is duly inclosed and forwarded.

Address   BLANCHARD & LEA, PHILADELPHIA.

BUMSTEAD (FREEMAN J.) M. D.,
Lecturer on Venereal Diseases at the College of Physicians and Surgeons, New York, &c.

HE PATHOLOGY AND TREATMENT OF VENEREAL DISEASES,
including the results of recent investigations upon the subject. With illustrations on wood. In one very hand-ome octavo volume, of nearly 700 pages, extra cloth; $3 75. (*Now Ready.*)

The object of the author has been to prepare a complete work, which should present the results the most recent researches and modern experience on all branches of the subject, with special ference to the wants of the practitioner, theoretical disquisitions being rendered subordinate to actical utility. To show the thoroughness of the outline which is thus filled up, a condensed nop-is of the contents is subjoined.

CONTENTS.

TRODUCTION.
ART 1.—GONORRHŒA AND ITS COMPLICATIONS.—CHAPTER I. Urethral Gonorrhœa in the Male.
II. Gleet III. Balanitis. IV Phymosis. V. Paraphymosis. VI. Swelled Testicle. VII. Inflammation of the Pro-tate. VIII. Inflammation of tne Bladder. IX. Gonorrhœa in Women. X. Gonorrhœal Ophthalmia. XI. Gonorrhœal Rheumatism. XII. Vegetations. XIII. Stricture of the Urethra.
ART II.—THE CHANCROID AND ITS COMPLICATIONS: SYPHILIS.—CHAP. I. Introductory remarks. II. Chancres. III. Affections of the Lymphatic Vessels and Ganglia attendant upon Primary Sores. IV. General Syphilis—Introductory remarks. V. Treatment of Syphilis. VI. Syphilitic Fever—State of the Blood—Affections of Lymphatic Ganglia. VII. Syphilitic Affections of the Skin VIII Syphilitic Alopecia, Onychia, and Paronychia. IX. Mucous Patches. X. Gummy Tumors. XI Syphilitic Affections of Mucous Membranes. XII. Syphilitic Affections of the Eye. XIII. Syphilitic Affections of the Ear. XIV. Syphilitic Orchitis. XV. Syphilitic Affections of the Muscles and Tendons. XVI. Syphilitic Affections of the Nervous System. XVII. Syphilitic Affections of the Periosteum and Bones. XVIII. Congenital Syphilis.

BARCLAY (A. W.), M. D.,
Assistant Physician to St. George's Hospital, &c.

A MANUAL OF MEDICAL DIAGNOSIS; being an Analysis of the Signs and Symptoms of Disease. In one neat octavo volume, extra cloth, of 424 pages. $2 00. (*Lately issued.*)

The task of composing such a work is neither an easy nor a light one; but Dr. Barclay has performed in a manner which meets our most unqualified approbation. He is no mere theorist; he knows his work thoroughly, and in attempting to perform it, is not exceeded his powers.—*British Med. Journal.*

We venture to predict that the work will be deservedly popular, and soon become, like Watson's Practice, an indispensable necessity to the practitioner.—*N. A. Med Journal.*

An inestimable work of reference for the young practitioner and student.—*Nashville Med. Journal.*

We hope the volume will have an extensive circulation, not among students of medicine only, but practitioners also. They will never regret a faithful study of its pages.—*Cincinnati Lancet.*

An important acquisition to medical literature. It is a work of high merit, both from the vast importance of the subject upon which it treats, and also from the real ability displayed in its elaboration. In conclusion, let us bespeak for this volume that attention of every student of our art which it so richly deserves – that place in every medical library which it can so well adorn.—*Peninsular Medical Journal.*

BARLOW (GEORGE H.), M. D.
Physician to Guy's Hospital, London, &c.

A MANUAL OF THE PRACTICE OF MEDICINE. With Additions by D. F. CONDIE, M. D., author of "A Practical Treatise on Diseases of Children," &c. In one handsome octavo volume, leather, of over 600 pages. $2 75.

We recommend Dr. Barlow's Manual in the warmest manner as a most valuable vade-mecum. We ave had frequent occasion to consult it, and have und it clear, concise, practical, and sound. It is minently a practical work, containing all that is essential, and avoiding useless theoretical discussion. The work supplies what has been for some me wanting, a manual of practice based upon modern discoveries in pathology and rational views of eatment of disease. It is especially intended for e use of students and junior practitioners, but it

will be found hardly less useful to the experienced physician. The American editor has added to the work three chapters—on Cholera Infantum, Yellow Fever, and Cerebro-spinal Meningitis. These additions, the two first of which are indispensable to a work on practice destined for the profession in this country, are executed with great judgment and fidelity, by Dr. Condie, who has also succeeded happily in imitating the conciseness and clearness of style which are such agreeable characteristics of the original book.—*Boston Med. and Surg. Journal.*

BARTLETT (ELISHA), M. D.

HE HISTORY, DIAGNOSIS, AND TREATMENT OF THE FEVERS OF THE UNITED STATES. A new and revised edition. By ALONZO CLARK, M. D., Prof. of Pathology and Practical Medicine in the N. Y. College of Physicians and Surgeons, &c. In one octavo volume, of six hundred pages, extra cloth. Price $3 00.

It is a work of great practical value and interest, containing much that is new relative to the several iseases of which it treats, and, with the additions f the editor, is fully up to the times. The distinctive features of the different forms of fever are plainly nd forcibly portrayed, and the lines of demarcation arefully and accurately drawn, and to the American practitioner is a more valuable and safe guide an any work on fever extant —*Ohio Med. and urg Journal.*

This excellent monograph on febrile disease, has

stood deservedly high since its first publication. It will be seen that it has now reached its fourth edition under the supervision of Prof. A. Clark, a gentleman who, from the nature of his studies and pursuits, is well calculated to appreciate and discuss the many intricate and difficult questions in pathology. His annotations add much to the interest of the work, and have brought it well up to the condition of the science as it exists at the present day in regard to this class of diseases.—*Southern Med. and Surg. Journal.*

BARWELL (RICHARD,) F. R. C. S.,
Assistant Surgeon Charing Cross Hospital, &c.

A TREATISE ON DISEASES OF THE JOINTS. Illustrated with engravings on wood. In one very handsome octavo volume, of about 500 pages, extra cloth; $3 00. (*Now Ready.*)

"A treatise on Diseases of the Joints equal to, or rather beyond the current knowledge of the day, has long been required—my professional brethren must judge whether the ensuing pages may supply the deficiency No author is fit to estimate his own work at the moment of its completion, but it may be permitted me to say that the study of joint diseases has very much occupied my attention, even from my studentship, and that for the last six or eight years my devotion to that subject has been almost unremitting. . . . . The real weight of my work has been at the bedside, and the greatest labor devoted to interpreting symptoms and remedying their cause."—AUTHOR'S PREFACE.

At the outset we may state that the work is worthy of much praise, and bears evidence of much thoughtful and careful inquiry, and here and there of no slight originality. We have already carried this notice further than we intended to do, but not to the extent the work deserves. We can only add, that the perusal of it has afforded us great pleasure. The author has evidently worked very hard at his subject, and his investigations into the Physiology and Pathology of Joints have been carried on in a manner which entitles him to be listened to with attention and respect. We must not omit to mention the very admirable plates with which the volume is enriched. We seldom meet with such striking and faithful delineations of disease.—*London Med. Times and Gazette*, Feb. 9, 1861.

We cannot take leave, however, of Mr. Barwell, without congratulating him on the interesting amount of information which he has compressed into his book. The work appears to us calculated to be of much use to the practising surgeon who may be in want of a treatise on diseases of the joints, and at the same time one which contains the latest information on articular affections and the operations for their cure.—*Dublin Med. Press*, Feb. 27, 1861.

This volume will be welcomed, both by the pathologist and the surgeon, as being the record of much honest research and careful investigation into the nature and treatment of a most important class of disorders. We cannot conclude this notice of a valuable and useful book without calling attention to the amount of *bonâ fide* work it contains. In the present day of universal book-making, it is no slight matter for a volume to show laborious investigation, and at the same time original thought, on the part of its author, whom we may congratulate on the successful completion of his arduous task.—*London Lancet*, March 9, 1861.

CARPENTER (WILLIAM B.), M. D., F. R. S., &c.,
Examiner in Physiology and Comparative Anatomy in the University of London.

PRINCIPLES OF HUMAN PHYSIOLOGY; with their chief applications to Psychology, Pathology, Therapeutics, Hygiene, and Forensic Medicine. A new American, from the last and revised London edition. With nearly three hundred illustrations. Edited, with additions, by FRANCIS GURNEY SMITH, M. D., Professor of the Institutes of Medicine in the Pennsylvania Medical College, &c. In one very large and beautiful octavo volume, of about nine hundred large pages, handsomely printed and strongly bound in leather, with raised bands. $4 25.

In the preparation of this new edition, the author has spared no labor to render it, as heretofore, a complete and lucid exposition of the most advanced condition of its important subject. The amount of the additions required to effect this object thoroughly, joined to the former large size of the volume, presenting objections arising from the unwieldy bulk of the work, he has omitted all those portions not bearing directly upon HUMAN PHYSIOLOGY, designing to incorporate them in his forthcoming Treatise on GENERAL PHYSIOLOGY. As a full and accurate text-book on the Physiology of Man, the work in its present condition therefore presents even greater claims upon the student and physician than those which have heretofore won for it the very wide and distinguished favor which it has so long enjoyed. The additions of Prof. Smith will be found to supply whatever may have been wanting to the American student, while the introduction of many new illustrations, and the most careful mechanical execution, render the volume one of the most attractive as yet issued.

For upwards of thirteen years Dr. Carpenter's work has been considered by the profession generally, both in this country and England, as the most valuable compendium on the subject of physiology in our language. This distinction it owes to the high attainments and unwearied industry of its accomplished author. The present edition (which, like the last American one, was prepared by the author himself), is the result of such extensive revision, that it may almost be considered a new work. We need hardly say, in concluding this brief notice, that while the work is indispensable to every student of medicine in this country, it will amply repay the practitioner for its perusal by the interest and value of its contents.—*Boston Med. and Surg. Journal*.

This is a standard work—the text-book used by all medical students who read the English language. It has passed through several editions in order to keep pace with the rapidly growing science of Physiology. Nothing need be said in its praise, for its merits are universally known; we have nothing to say of its defects, for they only appear where the science of which it treats is incomplete.—*Western Lancet*.

The most complete exposition of physiology which any language can at present give.—*Brit. and For. Med.-Chirurg. Review*.

The greatest, the most reliable, and the best book on the subject which we know of in the English language.—*Stethoscope*.

To eulogize this great work would be superfluous. We should observe, however, that in this edition the author has remodelled a large portion of the former, and the editor has added much matter of interest, especially in the form of illustrations. We may confidently recommend it as the most complete work on Human Physiology in our language.—*Southern Med. and Surg. Journal*.

The most complete work on the science in our language.—*Am. Med. Journal*.

The most complete work now extant in our language.—*N. O. Med. Register*.

The best text-book in the language on this extensive subject.—*London Med. Times*.

A complete cyclopædia of this branch of science.—*N. Y. Med. Times*.

The profession of this country, and perhaps also of Europe, have anxiously and for some time awaited the announcement of this new edition of Carpenter's Human Physiology. His former editions have for many years been almost the only text-book on Physiology in all our medical schools, and its circulation among the profession has been unsurpassed by any work in any department of medical science. It is quite unnecessary for us to speak of this work as its merits would justify. The mere announcement of its appearance will afford the highest pleasure to every student of Physiology, while its perusal will be of infinite service in advancing physiological science.—*Ohio Med. and Surg. Journ.*

CARPENTER (WILLIAM B.), M. D., F. R. S.,
Examiner in Physiology and Comparative Anatomy in the University of London.

HE MICROSCOPE AND ITS REVELATIONS. With an Appendix containing the Applications of the Microscope to Clinical Medicine, &c. By F. G. SMITH, M. D. Illustrated by four hundred and thirty-four beautiful engravings on wood. In one large and very handsome octavo volume, of 724 pages, extra cloth, $4 00; leather, $4 50.

Dr. Carpenter's position as a microscopist and physiologist, and his great experience as a teacher, minently qualify him to produce what has long been wanted—a good text-book on the practical se of the microscope. In the present volume his object has been, as stated in his Preface, " to ombine, within a moderate compass, that information with regard to the use of his ' tools,' which most essential to the working micro-copist, with such an account of the objects best fitted for is study, as might qualify him to comprehend what he observes, and might thus prepare him to encfit science, whilst expanding and refreshing his own mind " That he has succeeded in accomiishing this, no one acquainted with his previous labors can doubt.

The great importance of the microscope as a means of diagnosis, and the number of microscoists who are also physicians, have induced the American publishers, with the author's approval, to dd an Appendix, carefully prepared by Professor Smith, on the applications of the instrument to iinical medicine, together with an account of American Microscopes, their modifications and ccesories. This portion of the work is illustrated with nearly one hundred wood-cuts, and, it is oped, will adapt the volume more particularly to the use of the American student.

Those who are acquainted with Dr. Carpenter's revious writings on Animal and Vegetable Physiogy, will fully understand how vast a store of knowsdge he is able to bring to bear upon so comprehensive a subject as the revelations of the microscope; nd even those who have no previous acquaintance vith the construction or uses of this instrument, vill find abundance of information conveyed in clear nd simple language.—*Med. Times and Gazette*.

Although originally not intended as a strictly

medical work, the additions by Prof. Smith give it a positive claim upon the profession, for which we doubt not he will receive their sincere thanks. Indeed, we know not where the student of medicine will find such a complete and satisfactory collection of microscopic facts bearing upon physiology and practical medicine as is contained in Prof. Smith's appendix; and this of itself, it seems to us, is fully worth the cost of the volume.—*Louisville Medical Review*.

BY THE SAME AUTHOR.

ELEMENTS (OR MANUAL) OF PHYSIOLOGY, INCLUDING PHYSIOLOGICAL ANATOMY. Second American, from a new and revised London edition. With one hundred and ninety illustrations. In one very handsome octavo volume, leather. pp. 566. $3 00.

In publishing the first edition of this work, its title was altered from that of the London volume, by the substitution of the word " Elements" for that of " Manual," and with the author's sanction he title of " Elements" is still retained as being more expressive of the scope of the treatise.

To say that it is the best manual of Physiology now before the public, would not do sufficient justice o the author.—*Buffalo Medical Journal*.

In his former works it would seem that he had ixhausted the subject of Physiology. In the present, ie gives the essence, as it were, of the whole.—*N. Y. Journal of Medicine*.

Those who have occasion for an elementary treatise on Physiology, cannot do better than to possess themselves of the manual of Dr. Carpenter.—*Medical Examiner*.

The best and most complete exposé of modern Physiology, in one volume, extant in the English language.—*St. Louis Medical Journal*.

BY THE SAME AUTHOR.

PRINCIPLES OF COMPARATIVE PHYSIOLOGY. New American, from the Fourth and Revised London edition. In one large and handsome octavo volume, with over three hundred beautiful illustrations. pp. 752. Extra cloth, $4 80; leather, raised bands, $5 25.

This book should not only be read but thoroughly studied by every member of the profession. None are too wise or old, to be benefited thereby. But especially to the younger class would we cordially commend it as best fitted of any work in the English anguage to qualify them for the reception and comprehension of those truths which are daily being developed in physiology.—*Medical Counsellor*.

Without pretending to it, it is an encyclopedia of the subject, accurate and complete in all respects— a truthful reflection of the advanced state at which the science has now arrived.—*Dublin Quarterly Journal of Medical Science*.

A truly magnificent work—in itself a perfect physiological study.—*Ranking's Abstract*.

This work stands without its fellow. It is one few men in Europe could have undertaken; it is one

no man, we believe, could have brought to so successful an issue as Dr. Carpenter. It required for its production a physiologist at once deeply read in the labors of others, capable of taking a general, critical, and unprejudiced view of those labors, and of combining the varied, heterogeneous materials at his disposal, so as to form an harmonious whole. We feel that this abstract can give the reader a very imperfect idea of the fulness of this work, and no idea of its unity, of the admirable manner in which material has been brought, from the most various sources, to conduce to its completeness, of the lucidity of the reasoning it contains, or of the clearness of language in which the whole is clothed. Not the profession only, but the scientific world at large, must feel deeply indebted to Dr. Carpenter for this great work. It must, indeed, add largely even to his high reputation.—*Medical Times*.

BY THE SAME AUTHOR. (*Preparing.*)

PRINCIPLES OF GENERAL PHYSIOLOGY, INCLUDING ORGANIC CHEMISTRY AND HISTOLOGY. With a General Sketch of the Vegetable and Animal Kingdom. In one large and very handsome octavo volume, with several hundred illustrations.

BY THE SAME AUTHOR.

A PRIZE ESSAY ON THE USE OF ALCOHOLIC LIQUORS IN HEALTH AND DISEASE. New edition, with a Preface by D. F. CONDIE, M. D., and explanations of scientific words. In one neat 12mo. volume, extra cloth. pp. 178. 50 cents.

CONDIE (D. F.), M. D., &c.

A PRACTICAL TREATISE ON THE DISEASES OF CHILDREN. Fifth edition, revised and augmented. In one large volume, 8vo., leather, of over 750 pages. $3 25. (*Just Issued*, 1859.)

In presenting a new and revised edition of this favorite work, the publishers have only to state that the author has endeavored to render it in every respect "a complete and faithful exposition of the pathology and therapeutics of the maladies incident to the earlier stages of existence—a full and exact account of the diseases of infancy and childhood." To accomplish this he has subjected the whole work to a careful and thorough revision, rewriting a considerable portion, and adding several new chapters. In this manner it is hoped that any deficiencies which may have previously existed have been supplied, that the recent labors of practitioners and observers have been thoroughly incorporated, and that in every point the work will be found to maintain the high reputation it has enjoyed as a complete and thoroughly practical book of reference in infantile affections.

A few notices of previous editions are subjoined.

Dr. Condie's scholarship, acumen, industry, and practical sense are manifested in this, as in all his numerous contributions to science.—*Dr. Holmes's Report to the American Medical Association.*

Taken as a whole, in our judgment, Dr. Condie's Treatise is the one from the perusal of which the practitioner in this country will rise with the greatest satisfaction.—*Western Journal of Medicine and Surgery.*

One of the best works upon the Diseases of Children in the English language.—*Western Lancet.*

We feel assured from actual experience that no physician's library can be complete without a copy of this work.—*N. Y. Journal of Medicine.*

A veritable pædiatric encyclopædia, and an honor to American medical literature.—*Ohio Medical and Surgical Journal.*

We feel persuaded that the American medical profession will soon regard it not only as a very good, but as the VERY BEST "Practical Treatise on the Diseases of Children."—*American Medical Journal.*

In the department of infantile therapeutics, the work of Dr. Condie is considered one of the best which has been published in the English language.—*The Stethoscope.*

We pronounced the first edition to be the best work on the diseases of children in the English language, and, notwithstanding all that has been published, we still regard it in that light.—*Medical Examiner.*

The value of works by native authors on the diseases which the physician is called upon to combat, will be appreciated by all; and the work of Dr. Condie has gained for itself the character of a safe guide for students, and a useful work for consultation by those engaged in practice.—*N. Y. Med Times.*

This is the fourth edition of this deservedly popular treatise. During the interval since the last edition, it has been subjected to a thorough revision by the author; and all new observations in the pathology and therapeutics of children have been included in the present volume. As we said before, we do not know of a better book on diseases of children, and to a large part of its recommendations we yield an unhesitating concurrence.—*Buffalo Med. Journal.*

Perhaps the most full and complete work now before the profession of the United States; indeed, we may say in the English language. It is vastly superior to most of its predecessors.—*Transylvania Med. Journal*

CHRISTISON (ROBERT), M. D., V. P. R. S. E., &c.

A DISPENSATORY; or, Commentary on the Pharmacopœias of Great Britain and the United States; comprising the Natural History, Description, Chemistry, Pharmacy, Actions, Uses, and Doses of the Articles of the Materia Medica. Second edition, revised and improved, with a Supplement containing the most important New Remedies. With copious Additions, and two hundred and thirteen large wood-engravings. By R. EGLESFELD GRIFFITH, M. D. In one very large and handsome octavo volume, leather, raised bands, of over 1000 pages. $3 50.

COOPER (BRANSBY B.), F. R. S.

LECTURES ON THE PRINCIPLES AND PRACTICE OF SURGERY. In one very large octavo volume, extra cloth, of 750 pages. $3 00.

COOPER ON DISLOCATIONS AND FRACTURES OF THE JOINTS.—Edited by BRANSBY B. COOPER, F. R. S., &c. With additional Observations by Prof. J. C. WARREN. A new American edition. In one handsome octavo volume, extra cloth, of about 500 pages, with numerous illustrations on wood. $3 25.

COOPER ON THE ANATOMY AND DISEASES OF THE BREAST, with twenty-five Miscellaneous and Surgical Papers. One large volume, imperial 8vo., extra cloth, with 252 figures, on 36 plates. $2 50.

COOPER ON THE STRUCTURE AND DISEASES OF THE TESTIS, AND ON THE THYMUS GLAND. One vol. imperial 8vo., extra cloth, with 177 figures on 29 plates. $2 00.

COPLAND ON THE CAUSES, NATURE, AND TREATMENT OF PALSY AND APOPLEXY. In one volume, royal 12mo., extra cloth. pp. 326. 60 cents.

CLYMER ON FEVERS; THEIR DIAGNOSIS, PATHOLOGY, AND TREATMENT. In one octavo volume, leather, of 600 pages. $1 50.

COLOMBAT DE L'ISERE ON THE DISEASES OF FEMALES, and on the special Hygiene of their Sex. Translated, with many Notes and Additions, by C. D. MEIGS, M. D. Second edition, revised and improved. In one large volume, octavo, leather, with numerous wood-cuts. pp. 720. $3 50.

CARSON (JOSEPH), M. D.,
Professor of Materia Medica and Pharmacy in the University of Pennsylvania.

SYNOPSIS OF THE COURSE OF LECTURES ON MATERIA MEDICA AND PHARMACY, delivered in the University of Pennsylvania. Second and revised edition. In one very neat octavo volume, extra cloth, of 208 pages. $1 50.

CURLING (T. B.), F. R. S.
Surgeon to the London Hospital, President of the Hunterian Society, &c.

A PRACTICAL TREATISE ON DISEASES OF THE TESTIS, SPERMATIC CORD, AND SCROTUM. Second American, from the second and enlarged English edition. In one handsome octavo volume, extra cloth, with numerous illustrations. pp. 420. $2 00.

CHURCHILL (FLEETWOOD), M.D., M.R.I.A.

ƒN THE THEORY AND PRACTICE OF MIDWIFERY. A new American from the fourth revised and enlarged London edition. With Notes and Additions, by D. Francis Condie, M. D., author of a "Practical Treatise on the Diseases of Children," &c. With 194 illustrations In one very handsome octavo volume, leather, of nearly 700 large pages. $3 50. (*Just Issued.*)

This work has been so long an established favorite, both as a text-book for the learner and as a reliable aid in consultation for the practitioner, that in presenting a new edition it is only necessary to call attention to the very extended improvements which it has received Having had the benefit of two revisions by the author since the last American reprint, it has been materially enlarged, and Dr. Churchill's well-known conscientious industry is a guarantee that every portion has been thoroughly brought up with the latest results of European investigation in all departments of the science and art of obstetrics. The recent date of the last Dublin edition has not left much of novelty for the American editor to introduce, but he has endeavored to insert whatever has since appeared, together with such matters as his experience has shown him would be desirable for the American student, including a large number of illustrations. With the sanction of the author he has added in the form of an appendix, some chapters from a little "Manual for Midwives and Nurses," recently issued by Dr. Churchill, believing that the details there presented can hardly fail to prove of advantage to the junior practitioner. The result of all these additions is that the work now contains fully one-half more matter than the last American edition, with nearly one-half more illustrations, so that notwithstanding the use of a smaller type, the volume contains almost two hundred pages more than before.

No effort has been spared to secure an improvement in the mechanical execution of the work equal to that which the text has received, and the volume is confidently presented as one of the handsomest that has thus far been laid before the American profession; while the very low price at which it is offered should secure for it a place in every lecture-room and on every office table.

A better book in which to learn these important points we have not met than Dr. Churchill's. Every page of it is full of instruction; the opinion of all writers of authority is given on questions of difficulty, as well as the directions and advice of the learned author himself, to which he adds the result of statistical inquiry, putting statistics in their proper place and giving them their due weight, and no more. We have never read a book more free from professional jealousy than Dr. Churchill's. It appears to be written with the true design of a book on medicine, viz: to give all that is known on the subject of which he treats, both theoretically and practically, and to advance such opinions of his own as he believes will benefit medical science, and insure the safety of the patient. We have said enough to convey to the profession that this book of Dr. Churchill's is admirably suited for a book of reference for the practitioner, as well as a text-book for the student, and we hope it may be extensively purchased amongst our readers. To them we most strongly recommend it.—*Dublin Medical Press*, June 20, 1860.

To bestow praise on a book that has received such marked approbation would be superfluous. We need only say, therefore, that if the first edition was thought worthy of a favorable reception by the medical public, we can confidently affirm that this will be found much more so. The lecturer, the practitioner, and the student, may all have recourse to its pages, and derive from their perusal much interest and instruction in everything relating to theoretical and practical midwifery.—*Dublin Quarterly Journal of Medical Science.*

A work of very great merit, and such as we can confidently recommend to the study of every obstetric practitioner.—*London Medical Gazette.*

This is certainly the most perfect system extant. It is the best adapted for the purposes of a text-book, and that which he whose necessities confine him to one book, should select in preference to all others.—*Southern Medical and Surgical Journal.*

The most popular work on midwifery ever issued from the American press.—*Charleston Med. Journal.*

Were we reduced to the necessity of having but one work on midwifery, and *permitted to choose*, we would unhesitatingly take Churchill.—*Western Med. and Surg. Journal.*

It is impossible to conceive a more useful and elegant manual than Dr. Churchill's Practice of Midwifery.—*Provincial Medical Journal.*

Certainly, in our opinion, the very best work on the subject which exists.—*N. Y. Annalist.*

No work holds a higher position, or is more deserving of being placed in the hands of the tyro, the advanced student, or the practitioner.—*Medical Examiner.*

Previous editions, under the editorial supervision of Prof R. M. Huston, have been received with marked favor, and they deserved it; but this, reprinted from a very late Dublin edition, carefully revised and brought up by the author to the present time, does present an unusually accurate and able exposition of every important particular embraced in the department of midwifery. * * The clearness, directness, and precision of its teachings, together with the great amount of statistical research which its text exhibits, have served to place it already in the foremost rank of works in this department of remedial science.—*N. O. Med. and Surg. Journal.*

In our opinion, it forms one of the best if not the very best text-book and epitome of obstetric science which we at present possess in the English language.—*Monthly Journal of Medical Science.*

The clearness and precision of style in which it is written, and the great amount of statistical research which it contains, have served to place it in the first rank of works in the department of medical science.—*N. Y. Journal of Medicine.*

Few treatises will be found better adapted as a text-book for the student, or as a manual for the frequent consultation of the young practitioner.—*American Medical Journal.*

BY THE SAME AUTHOR. (*Lately Published.*)

ON THE DISEASES OF INFANTS AND CHILDREN. Second American Edition, revised and enlarged by the author. Edited, with Notes, by W. V. Keating, M. D. In one large and handsome volume, extra cloth, of over 700 pages. $3 00, or in leather, $3 25.

In preparing this work a second time for the American profession, the author has spared no labor in giving it a very thorough revision, introducing several new chapters, and rewriting others, while every portion of the volume has been subjected to a severe scrutiny. The efforts of the American editor have been directed to supplying such information relative to matters peculiar to this country as might have escaped the attention of the author, and the whole may, therefore, be safely pronounced one of the most complete works on the subject accessible to the American Profession. By an alteration in the size of the page, these very extensive additions have been accommodated without unduly increasing the size of the work.

BY THE SAME AUTHOR.

ESSAYS ON THE PUERPERAL FEVER, AND OTHER DISEASES PECULIAR TO WOMEN. Selected from the writings of British Authors previous to the close of the Eighteenth Century. In one neat octavo volume, extra cloth, of about 450 pages. $2 50.

CHURCHILL (FLEETWOOD), M. D., M. R. I. A., &c.
ON THE DISEASES OF WOMEN; including those of Pregnancy and Child-bed. A new American edition, revised by the Author. With Notes and Additions, by D FRAN-CIS CONDIE, M. D., author of "A Practical Treatise on the Diseases of Children." With nume-rous illustrations. In one large and handsome octavo volume, leather, of 768 pages. $3 00.

This edition of Dr. Churchill's very popular treatise may almost be termed a new work, so thoroughly has he revised it in every portion. It will be found greatly enlarged, and completely brought up to the most recent condition of the subject, while the very handsome series of illustra-tions introduced, representing such pathological conditions as can be accurately portrayed, present a novel feature, and afford valuable assistance to the young practitioner. Such additions as ap-peared desirable for the American student have been made by the editor, Dr. Condie, while a marked improvement in the mechanical execution keeps pace with the advance in all other respects which the volume has undergone, while the price has been kept at the former very moderate rate.

It comprises, unquestionably, one of the most ex-act and comprehensive expositions of the present state of medical knowledge in respect to the diseases of women that has yet been published.—*Am. Journ. Med. Sciences.*

This work is the most reliable which we possess on this subject; and is deservedly popular with the profession.—*Charleston Med. Journal*, July, 1857.

We know of no author who deserves that appro-bation, on "the diseases of females," to the same

extent that Dr. Churchill does. His, indeed, is the only thorough treatise we know of on the subject; and it may be commended to practitioners and stu-dents as a masterpiece in its particular department. —*The Western Journal of Medicine and Surgery.*

As a comprehensive manual for students, or a work of reference for practitioners, it surpasses any other that has ever issued on the same subject from the British press.—*Dublin Quart. Journal.*

DICKSON (S. H.), M. D.,
Professor of Practice of Medicine in the Jefferson Medical College, Philadelphia.

ELEMENTS OF MEDICINE; a Compendious View of Pathology and Thera-peutics, or the History and Treatment of Diseases. Second edition, revised. In one large and handsome octavo volume, of 750 pages, leather. $3 75. (*Just Issued.*)

The steady demand which has so soon exhausted the first edition of this work, sufficiently shows that the author was not mistaken in supposing that a volume of this character was needed—an elementary manual of practice, which should present the leading principles of medicine with the practical results, in a condensed and perspicuous manner. Disencumbered of unnecessary detail and fruitless speculations, it embodies what is most requisite for the student to learn, and at the same time what the active practitioner wants when obliged, in the daily calls of his profession, to refresh his memory on special points. The clear and attractive style of the author renders the whole easy of comprehension, while his long experience gives to his teachings an authority every-where acknowledged. Few physicians, indeed, have had wider opportunities for observation and experience, and few, perhaps, have used them to better purpose. As the result of a long life de-voted to study and practice, the present edition, revised and brought up to the date of publication, will doubtless maintain the reputation already acquired as a condensed and convenient American text-book on the Practice of Medicine.

DRUITT (ROBERT), M. R. C. S., &c.
THE PRINCIPLES AND PRACTICE OF MODERN SURGERY. A new and revised American from the eighth enlarged and improved London edition. Illustrated with four hundred and thirty-two wood-engravings. In one very handsomely printed octavo volume, leather, of nearly 700 large pages. $3 50. (*Just Issued.*)

A work which like DRUITT'S SURGERY has for so many years maintained the position of a lead-ing favorite with all classes of the profession, needs no special recommendation to attract attention to a revised edition. It is only necessary to state that the author has spared no pains to keep the work up to its well earned reputation of presenting in a small and convenient compass the latest condition of every department of surgery, considered both as a science and as an art; and that the services of a competent American editor have been employed to introduce whatever novelties may have escaped the author's attention, or may prove of service to the American practitioner. As several editions have appeared in London since the issue of the last American reprint, the volume has had the benefit of repeated revisions by the author, resulting in a very thorough alteration and improvement. The extent of these additions may be estimated from the fact that it now contains about one-third more matter than the previous American edition, and that notwithstanding the adoption of a smaller type, the pages have been increased by about one hundred, while nearly two hundred and fifty wood-cuts have been added to the former list of illustrations.

A marked improvement will also be perceived in the mechanical and artistical execution of the work, which, printed in the best style, on new type, and fine paper, leaves little to be desired as regards external finish; while at the very low price affixed it will be found one of the cheapest volumes accessible to the profession.

This popular volume, now a most comprehensive work on surgery, has undergone many corrections, improvements, and additions, and the principles and the practice of the art have been brought down to the latest record and observation. Of the operations in surgery it is impossible to speak too highly. The descriptions are so clear and concise, and the illus-trations so accurate and numerous, that the student can have no difficulty, with instrument in hand, and book by his side, over the dead body, in obtaining a proper knowledge and sufficient tact in this much neglected department of medical education.—*British and Foreign Medico-Chirurg. Review*, Jan. 1960.

In the present edition the author has entirely re-written many of the chapters, and has incorporated the various improvements and additions in modern surgery. On carefully going over it, we find that

nothing of real practical importance has been omit-ted; it presents a faithful epitome of everything re-lating to surgery up to the present hour. It is de-servedly a popular manual, both with the student and practitioner.—*London Lancet*, Nov. 19, 1859.

In closing this brief notice, we recommend as cor-dially as ever this most useful and comprehensive hand-book. It must prove a vast assistance, not only to the student of surgery, but also to the busy practitioner who may not have the leisure to devote himself to the study of more lengthy volumes.— *London Med. Times and Gazette*, Oct. 22, 1859.

In a word, this eighth edition of Dr. Druitt's Manual of Surgery is all that the surgical student or practitioner could desire. — *Dublin Quarterly Journal of Med. Sciences*, Nov. 1859.

DALTON, JR. (J. C.), M. D.
Professor of Physiology in the College of Physicians, New York.

A TREATISE ON HUMAN PHYSIOLOGY, designed for the use of Students and Practitioners of Medicine. Second edition, revised and enlarged, with two hundred and seventy-one illustrations on wood. In one very beautiful octavo volume, of 700 pages, extra cloth, $4 00; leather, raised bands, $4 50. (*Just Issued*, 1861.)

The general favor which has so soon exhausted an edition of this work has afforded the author an opportunity in its revision of supplying the deficiencies which existed in the former volume. This has caused the insertion of two new chapters—one on the Special Senses, the other on Imbibition, Exhalation, and the Functions of the Lymphatic System—besides numerous additions of smaller amount scattered through the work, and a general revision designed to bring it thoroughly up to the present condition of the science with regard to all points which may be considered as definitely settled. A number of new illustrations has been introduced, and the work, it is hoped, in its improved form, may continue to command the confidence of those for whose use it is intended

It will be seen, therefore, that Dr. Dalton's best efforts have been directed towards perfecting his work. The additions are marked by the same features which characterize the remainder of the volume, and render it by far the most desirable text-book on physiology to place in the hands of the student which, so far as we are aware, exists in the English language, or perhaps in any other. We therefore have no hesitation in recommending Dr. Dalton's book for the classes for which it is intended, satisfied as we are that it is better adapted to their use than any other work of the kind to which they have access.—*American Journal of the Med. Sciences*, April, 1861.

It is, therefore, no disparagement to the many books upon physiology, most excellent in their day, to say that Dalton's is the only one that gives us the science as it was known to the best philosophers throughout the world, at the beginning of the current year. It states in comprehensive but concise diction, the facts established by experiment, or other method of demonstration, and details, in an understandable manner, how it is done, but abstains from the discussion of unsettled or theoretical points. Herein it is unique; and these characteristics render it a text-book without a rival, for those who desire to study physiological science as it is known to its most successful cultivators. And it is physiology thus presented that lies at the foundation of correct pathological knowledge; and this in turn is the basis of rational therapeutics; so that pathology, in fact, becomes of prime importance in the proper discharge of our every-day practical duties.—*Cincinnati Lancet*, May, 1861.

Dr. Dalton needs no word of praise from us. He is universally recognized as among the first, if not the very first, of American physiologists now living. The first edition of his admirable work appeared but two years since, and the advance of science, his own original views and experiments, together with a desire to supply what he considered some deficiencies in the first edition, have already made the present one a necessity, and it will no doubt be even more eagerly sought for than the first. That it is not merely a reprint, will be seen from the author's statement of the following principal additions and alterations which he has made. The present, like the first edition, is printed in the highest style of the printer's art, and the illustrations are truly admirable for their clearness in expressing exactly what their author intended.—*Boston Medical and Surgical Journal*, March 28, 1861.

It is unnecessary to give a detail of the additions; suffice it to say, that they are numerous and important, and such as will render the work still more valuable and acceptable to the profession as a learned and original treatise on this all-important branch of medicine. All that was said in commendation of the getting up of the first edition, and the superior style of the illustrations, apply with equal force to this. No better work on physiology can be placed in the hand of the student.—*St. Louis Medical and Surgical Journal*, May, 1861.

These additions, while testifying to the learning and industry of the author, render the book exceedingly useful, as the most complete exposé of a science, of which Dr. Dalton is doubtless the ablest representative on this side of the Atlantic.—*New Orleans Med. Times*, May, 1861.

A second edition of this deservedly popular work having been called for in the short space of two years, the author has supplied deficiencies, which existed in the former volume, and has thus more completely fulfilled his design of presenting to the profession a reliable and precise text-book, and one which we consider the best outline on the subject of which it treats, in any language.—*N. American Medico-Chirurg. Review*, May, 1861.

DUNGLISON, FORBES, TWEEDIE, AND CONOLLY.

THE CYCLOPÆDIA OF PRACTICAL MEDICINE: comprising Treatises on the Nature and Treatment of Diseases, Materia Medica, and Therapeutics, Diseases of Women and Children, Medical Jurisprudence, &c. &c. In four large super-royal octavo volumes, of 3254 double-columned pages, strongly and handsomely bound, with raised bands. $12 00.

** This work contains no less than four hundred and eighteen distinct treatises, contributed by sixty-eight distinguished physicians, rendering it a complete library of reference for the country practitioner.

The most complete work on Practical Medicine extant; or, at least, in our language.—*Buffalo Medical and Surgical Journal.*

For reference, it is above all price to every practitioner.—*Western Lancet.*

One of the most valuable medical publications of the day—as a work of reference it is invaluable.—*Western Journal of Medicine and Surgery.*

It has been to us, both as learner and teacher, a work for ready and frequent reference, one in which modern English medicine is exhibited in the most advantageous light.—*Medical Examiner.*

The editors are practitioners of established reputation, and the list of contributors embraces many of the most eminent professors and teachers of London, Edinburgh, Dublin, and Glasgow. It is, indeed, the great merit of this work that the principal articles have been furnished by practitioners who have not only devoted especial attention to the diseases about which they have written, but have also enjoyed opportunities for an extensive practical acquaintance with them, and whose reputation carries the assurance of their competency justly to appreciate the opinions of others, while it stamps their own doctrines with high and just authority.—*American Medical Journal.*

DEWEES'S COMPREHENSIVE SYSTEM OF MIDWIFERY. Illustrated by occasional cases and many engravings. Twelfth edition, with the author's last improvements and corrections In one octavo volume, extra cloth, of 600 pages. $3 50.

DEWEES'S TREATISE ON THE PHYSICAL AND MEDICAL TREATMENT OF CHILDREN. The last edition. In one volume, octavo, extra cloth, 548 pages. $2 80

DEWEES'S TREATISE ON THE DISEASES OF FEMALES. Tenth edition. In one volume, octavo extra cloth, 532 pages, with plates. $3 00

DUNGLISON (ROBLEY), M. D.,
Professor of Institutes of Medicine in the Jefferson Medical College, Philadelphia.
NEW AND ENLARGED EDITION.

MEDICAL LEXICON; a Dictionary of Medical Science, containing a concise Explanation of the various Subjects and Terms of Anatomy, Physiology, Pathology, Hygiene, Therapeutics Pharmacology, Pharmacy, Surgery, Obstetrics, Medical Jurisprudence, Dentistry, &c. Notices of Climate and of Mineral Waters; Formulæ for Officinal, Empirical, and Dietetic Preparations, &c. With French and other Synonymes. Revised and very greatly enlarged. In one very large and handsome octavo volume, of 992 double-columned pages, in small type; strongly bound in leather, with raised bands. Price $4 00.

Especial care has been devoted in the preparation of this edition to render it in every respect worthy a continuance of the very remarkable favor which it has hitherto enjoyed. The rapid sale of FIFTEEN large editions, and the constantly increasing demand, show that it is regarded by the profession as the standard authority. Stimulated by this fact, the author has endeavored in the present revision to introduce whatever might be necessary "to make it a satisfactory and desirable—if not indispensable—lexicon, in which the student may search without disappointment for every term that has been legitimated in the nomenclature of the science." To accomplish this, large additions have been found requisite, and the extent of the author's labors may be estimated from the fact that about SIX THOUSAND subjects and terms have been introduced throughout, rendering the whole number of definitions about SIXTY THOUSAND, to accommodate which, the number of pages has been increased by nearly a hundred, notwithstanding an enlargement in the size of the page. The medical press, both in this country and in England, has pronounced the work indispensable to all medical students and practitioners, and the present improved edition will not lose that enviable reputation.

The publishers have endeavored to render the mechanical execution worthy of a volume of such universal use in daily reference. The greatest care has been exercised to obtain the typographical accuracy so necessary in a work of the kind. By the small but exceedingly clear type employed, an immense amount of matter is condensed in its thousand ample pages, while the binding will be found strong and durable. With all these improvements and enlargements, the price has been kept at the former very moderate rate, placing it within the reach of all.

This work, the appearance of the fifteenth edition of which, it has become our duty and pleasure to announce, is perhaps the most stupendous monument of labor and erudition in medical literature. One would hardly suppose after constant use of the preceding editions, where we have never failed to find a sufficiently full explanation of every medical term, that in this edition "*about six thousand subjects and terms have been added*," with a careful revision and correction of the entire work. It is only necessary to announce the advent of this edition to make it occupy the place of the preceding one on the table of every medical man, as it is without doubt the best and most comprehensive work of the kind which has ever appeared.—*Buffalo Med. Journ.*, Jan. 1858.

The work is a monument of patient research, skilful judgment, and vast physical labor, that will perpetuate the name of the author more effectually than any possible device of stone or metal. Dr. Dunglison deserves the thanks not only of the American profession, but of the whole medical world.—*North Am. Medico-Chir. Review*, Jan. 1858.

A Medical Dictionary better adapted for the wants of the profession than any other with which we are acquainted, and of a character which places it far above comparison and competition.—*Am. Journ. Med. Sciences*, Jan. 1858.

We need only say, that the addition of 6,000 new terms, with their accompanying definitions, may be said to constitute a new work, by itself. We have examined the Dictionary attentively, and are most happy to pronounce it unrivalled of its kind. The erudition displayed, and the extraordinary industry which must have been demanded, in its preparation and perfection, redound to the lasting credit of its author, and have furnished us with a volume indispensable at the present day, to all who would find themselves au niveau with the highest standards of medical information.—*Boston Medical and Surgical Journal*, Dec. 31, 1857.

Good lexicons and encyclopedic works generally, are the most labor-saving contrivances which literary men enjoy; and the labor which is required to produce them in the perfect manner of this example is something appalling to contemplate. The author tells us in his preface that he has added about six thousand terms and subjects to this edition, which, before, was considered universally as the best work of the kind in any language.—*Silliman's Journal*, March, 1858.

He has razed his gigantic structure to the foundations, and remodelled and reconstructed the entire pile. No less than *six thousand* additional subjects and terms are illustrated and analyzed in this new edition, swelling the grand aggregate to beyond sixty thousand! Thus is placed before the profession a complete and thorough exponent of medical terminology, without rival or possibility of rivalry.—*Nashville Journ. of Med. and Surg.*, Jan. 1858.

It is universally acknowledged, we believe, that this work is incomparably the best and most complete Medical Lexicon in the English language. The amount of labor which the distinguished author has bestowed upon it is truly wonderful, and the learning and research displayed in its preparation are equally remarkable. Comment and commendation are unnecessary, as no one at the present day thinks of purchasing any other Medical Dictionary than this.—*St. Louis Med. and Surg. Journ.*, Jan. 1858.

It is the foundation stone of a good medical library, and should always be included in the first list of books purchased by the medical student.—*Am. Med. Monthly*, Jan. 1858.

A very perfect work of the kind, undoubtedly the most perfect in the English language.—*Med. and Surg. Reporter*, Jan. 1858.

It is now emphatically *the* Medical Dictionary of the English language, and for it there is no substitute.—*N. H. Med. Journ.*, Jan. 1858.

It is scarcely necessary to remark that any medical library wanting a copy of Dunglison's Lexicon must be imperfect.—*Cin. Lancet*, Jan. 1858.

We have ever considered it the best authority published, and the present edition we may safely say has no equal in the world.—*Peninsular Med. Journal*, Jan. 1858.

The most complete authority on the subject to be found in any language.—*Va. Med. Journal*, Feb. 58.

BY THE SAME AUTHOR.

THE PRACTICE OF MEDICINE. A Treatise on Special Pathology and Therapeutics. Third Edition. In two large octavo volumes, leather, of 1,500 pages. $6 25.

DUNGLISON (ROBLEY), M. D.,
Professor of Institutes of Medicine in the Jefferson Medical College, Philadelphia.

HUMAN PHYSIOLOGY. Eighth edition. Thoroughly revised and extensively modified and enlarged, with five hundred and thirty-two illustrations. In two large and handsomely printed octavo volumes, leather, of about 1500 pages. $7 00.

In revising this work for its eighth appearance, the author has spared no labor to render it worthy a continuance of the very great favor which has been extended to it by the profession. The whole contents have been rearranged, and to a great extent remodelled; the investigations which of late years have been so numerous and so important, have been carefully examined and incorporated, and the work in every respect has been brought up to a level with the present state of the subject. The object of the author has been to render it a concise but comprehensive treatise, containing the whole body of physiological science, to which the student and man of science can at all times refer with the certainty of finding whatever they are in search of, fully presented in all its aspects; and on no former edition has the author bestowed more labor to secure this result.

We believe that it can truly be said, no more complete repertory of facts upon the subject treated, can anywhere be found. The author has, moreover, that enviable tact at description and that facility and ease of expression which render him peculiarly acceptable to the casual, or the studious reader. This faculty, so requisite in setting forth many graver and less attractive subjects, lends additional charms to one always fascinating.—*Boston Med. and Surg. Journal.*

The most complete and satisfactory system of Physiology in the English language.—*Amer. Med Journal.*

The best work of the kind in the English language.—*Silliman's Journal.*

The present edition the author has made a perfect mirror of the science as it is at the present hour As a work upon physiology proper, the science of the functions performed by the body, the student will find it all he wishes.—*Nashville Journ. of Med*

That he has succeeded, most admirably succeeded in his purpose, is apparent from the appearance of an eighth edition. It is now the great encyclopædia on the subject, and worthy of a place in every physician's library.—*Western Lancet.*

BY THE SAME AUTHOR. (*A new edition.*)

GENERAL THERAPEUTICS AND MATERIA MEDICA; adapted for a Medical Text-book. With Indexes of Remedies and of Diseases and their Remedies. SIXTH EDITION, revised and improved. With one hundred and ninety-three illustrations. In two large and handsomely printed octavo vols., leather, of about 1100 pages. $6 00.

In announcing a new edition of Dr. Dunglison's General Therapeutics and Materia Medica, we have no words of commendation to bestow upon a work whose merits have been heretofore so often and so justly extolled. It must not be supposed, however, that the present is a mere reprint of the previous edition; the character of the author for laborious research, judicious analysis, and clearness of expression, is fully sustained by the numerous additions he has made to the work, and the careful revision to which he has subjected the whole.—*N. A. Medico-Chir. Review,* Jan. 1858.

The work will, we have little doubt, be bought and read by the majority of medical students; its size, arrangement, and reliability recommend it to all; no one, we venture to predict, will study it without profit, and there are few to whom it will not be in some measure useful as a work of reference. The young practitioner, more especially, will find the copious indexes appended to this edition of great assistance in the selection and preparation of suitable formulæ.—*Charleston Med. Journ. and Review,* Jan. 1858.

BY THE SAME AUTHOR. (*A new Edition.*)

NEW REMEDIES, WITH FORMULÆ FOR THEIR PREPARATION AND ADMINISTRATION. Seventh edition, with extensive Additions. In one very large octavo volume, leather, of 770 pages. $3 75.

Another edition of the "New Remedies" having been called for, the author has endeavored to add everything of moment that has appeared since the publication of the last edition.

The articles treated of in the former editions will be found to have undergone considerable expansion in this, in order that the author might be enabled to introduce, as far as practicable, the results of the subsequent experience of others, as well as of his own observation and reflection; and to make the work still more deserving of the extended circulation with which the preceding editions have been favored by the profession. By an enlargement of the page, the numerous additions have been incorporated without greatly increasing the bulk of the volume.—*Preface.*

One of the most useful of the author's works.—*Southern Medical and Surgical Journal.*

This elaborate and useful volume should be found in every medical library, for as a book of reference, for physicians, it is unsurpassed by any other work in existence, and the double index for diseases and for remedies, will be found greatly to enhance its value.—*New York Med. Gazette.*

The great learning of the author, and his remarkable industry in pushing his researches into every source whence information is derivable, have enabled him to throw together an extensive mass of facts and statements, accompanied by full reference to authorities; which last feature renders the work practically valuable to investigators who desire to examine the original papers.—*The American Journal of Pharmacy.*

ELLIS (BENJAMIN), M. D.

THE MEDICAL FORMULARY: being a Collection of Prescriptions, derived from the writings and practice of many of the most eminent physicians of America and Europe. Together with the usual Dietetic Preparations and Antidotes for Poisons. To which is added an Appendix, on the Endermic use of Medicines, and on the use of Ether and Chloroform The whole accompanied with a few brief Pharmaceutic and Medical Observations. Eleventh edition, revised and much extended by ROBERT P. THOMAS, M. D., Professor of Materia Medica in the Philadelphia College of Pharmacy. (*Preparing.*)

ERICHSEN (JOHN),
Professor of Surgery in University College, London, &c.

THE SCIENCE AND ART OF SURGERY; BEING A TREATISE ON SURGICAL
INJURIES, DISEASES, AND OPERATIONS. New and improved American, from the second enlarged and carefully revised London edition. Illustrated with over four hundred engravings on wood. In one large and handsome octavo volume, of one thousand closely printed pages, leather, raised bands. $4 50. (*Just Issued.*)

The very distinguished favor with which this work has been received on both sides of the Atlantic has stimulated the author to render it even more worthy of the position which it has so rapidly attained as a standard authority. Every portion has been carefully revised, numerous additions have been made, and the most watchful care has been exercised to render it a complete exponent of the most advanced condition of surgical science. In this manner the work has been enlarged by about a hundred pages, while the series of engravings has been increased by more than a hundred, rendering it one of the most thoroughly illustrated volumes before the profession. The additions of the author having rendered unnecessary most of the notes of the former American editor, but little has been added in this country; some few notes and occasional illustrations have, however, been introduced to elucidate American modes of practice.

It is, in our humble judgment, decidedly the best book of the kind in the English language. Strange that just such books are not oftener produced by public teachers of surgery in this country and Great Britain. Indeed, it is a matter of great astonishment, but no less true than astonishing, that of the many works on surgery republished in this country within the last fifteen or twenty years as text-books for medical students, this is the only one that even approximates to the fulfilment of the peculiar wants of young men just entering upon the study of this branch of the profession.—*Western Jour. of Med. and Surgery.*

Its value is greatly enhanced by a very copious well-arranged index. We regard this as one of the most valuable contributions to modern surgery. To one entering his novitiate of practice, we regard it the most serviceable guide which he can consult. He will find a fulness of detail loading him through every

step of the operation, and not deserting him until the final issue of the case is decided.—*Stethoscope.*

Embracing, as will be perceived, the whole surgical domain, and each division of itself almost complete and perfect, each chapter full and explicit, each subject faithfully exhibited, we can only express our estimate of it in the aggregate. We consider it an excellent contribution to surgery, as probably the best single volume now extant on the subject, and with great pleasure we add it to our text-books.—*Nashville Journal of Medicine and Surgery.*

Prof. Erichsen's work, for its size, has not been surpassed; his nine hundred and eight pages, profusely illustrated, are rich in physiological, pathological, and operative suggestions, doctrines, details, and processes; and will prove a reliable resource for information, both to physician and surgeon, in the hour of peril.—*N. O. Med. and Surg. Journal.*

FLINT (AUSTIN), M. D.,
Professor of the Theory and Practice of Medicine in the University of Louisville, &c.

PHYSICAL EXPLORATION AND DIAGNOSIS OF DISEASES AFFECT-
ING THE RESPIRATORY ORGANS. In one large and handsome octavo volume, extra cloth, 636 pages. $3 00.

We regard it, in point both of arrangement and of the marked ability of its treatment of the subjects, as destined to take the first rank in works of this class. So far as our information extends, it has at present no equal. To the practitioner, as well as the student, it will be invaluable in clearing up the diagnosis of doubtful cases, and in shedding light upon difficult phenomena.—*Buffalo Med. Journal.*

A work of original observation of the highest merit. We recommend the treatise to every one who wishes to become a correct auscultator. Based to a very large extent upon cases numerically examined, it carries the evidence of careful study and discrimination upon every page. It does credit to the author, and, through him, to the profession in this country. It is, what we cannot call every book upon auscultation, a readable book.—*Am. Jour. Med. Sciences.*

BY THE SAME AUTHOR. (*Now Ready.*)

A PRACTICAL TREATISE ON THE DIAGNOSIS, PATHOLOGY, AND
TREATMENT OF DISEASES OF THE HEART. In one neat octavo volume, of about 500 pages, extra cloth. $2 75.

We do not know that Dr. Flint has written anything which is not first rate; but this, his latest contribution to medical literature, in our opinion, surpasses all the others. The work is most comprehensive in its scope, and most sound in the views it enunciates. The descriptions are clear and methodical; the statements are substantiated by facts, and are made with such simplicity and sincerity, that without them they would carry conviction. The style is admirably clear, direct, and free from dryness. With Dr. Walshe's excellent treatise before us, we have no hesitation in saying that Dr. Flint's book is the best work on the heart in the English language —*Boston Med. and Surg. Journal.*

We have thus endeavored to present our readers with a fair analysis of this remarkable work. Preferring to employ the very words of the distinguished author, wherever it was possible, we have essayed to condense into the briefest space a general view of his observations and suggestions, and to direct the attention of our brethren to the abounding stores of valuable matter here collected and arranged for their use and instruction. No medical library will here after be considered complete without this volume; and we trust it will promptly find its way into the hands of every American student and physician.— *N. Am. Med. Chir. Review.*

This last work of Prof. Flint will add much to his previous well-earned celebrity, as a writer of

great force and beauty, and, with his previous work, places him at the head of American writers upon diseases of the chest. We have adopted his work upon the heart as a text-book, believing it to be more valuable for that purpose than any work of the kind that has yet appeared.—*Nashville Med. Journ.*

With more than pleasure do we hail the advent of this work, for it fills a wide gap on the list of text-books for our schools, and is, for the practitioner, the most valuable practical work of its kind.—*N. O. Med. News.*

In regard to the merits of the work, we have no hesitation in pronouncing it full, accurate, and judicious. Considering the present state of science, such a work was much needed. It should be in the hands of every practitioner.—*Chicago Med. Journal.*

But there are very trivial spots, and in no wise prevent us from declaring our most hearty approval of the author's ability, industry, and conscientiousness.—*Dublin Quarterly Journal of Med. Sciences.*

He has labored on with the same industry and care, and his place among the *first* authors of our country is becoming fully established. To this end, the work whose title is given above, contributes in no small degree. Our space will not admit of an extended analysis, and we will close this brief notice by commending it without reserve to every class of readers in the profession.—*Peninsular Med. Journ.*

FOWNES (GEORGE), PH. D., &c.

A MANUAL OF ELEMENTARY CHEMISTRY; Theoretical and Practical.
From the seventh revised and corrected London edition. With one hundred and ninety-seven illustrations. Edited by ROBERT BRIDGES, M. D. In one large royal 12mo volume, of 600 pages. In leather, $1 65; extra cloth, $1 50. (*Just Issued.*)

The death of the author having placed the editorial care of this work in the practised hands of Drs. Bence Jones and A. W. Hoffman, everything has been done in its revision which experience could suggest to keep it on a level with the rapid advance of chemical science. The additions requisite to this purpose have necessitated an enlargement of the page, notwithstanding which the work has been increased by about fifty pages. At the same time every care has been used to maintain its distinctive character as a condensed manual for the student, divested of all unnecessary detail or mere theoretical speculation. The additions have, of course, been mainly in the department of Organic Chemistry, which has made such rapid progress within the last few years, but yet equal attention has been bestowed on the other branches of the subject—Chemical Physics and Inorganic Chemistry—to present all investigations and discoveries of importance, and to keep up the reputation of the volume as a complete manual of the whole science, admirably adapted for the learner. By the use of a small but exceedingly clear type the matter of a large octavo is compressed within the convenient and portable limits of a moderate sized duodecimo, and at the very low price affixed, it is offered as one of the cheapest volumes before the profession.

Dr Fownes' excellent work has been universally recognized everywhere in his own and this country, as the best elementary treatise on chemistry in the English tongue, and is very generally adopted, we believe, as the standard text book in all ur colleges, both literary and scientific.—*Charleston Med Journ. and Review.*

A standard manual, which has long enjoyed the reputation of embodying much knowledge in a small space. The author has achieved the difficult task of condensation with masterly tact. His book is concise without being dry, and brief without being too dogmatical or general.—*Virginia Med. and Surgical Journal.*

The work of Dr. Fownes has long been before the public, and its merits have been fully appreciated as the best text-book on chemistry now in existence. We do not, of course, place it in a rank superior to the works of Brande, Graham, Turner, Gregory, or Gmelin, but we say that, as a work for students, it is preferable to any of them.—*London Journal of Medicine.*

A work well adapted to the wants of the student It is an excellent exposition of the chief doctrines and facts of modern chemistry. The size of the work, and still more the condensed yet perspicuous style in which it is written, absolve it from the charges very properly urged against most manuals termed popular.—*Edinburgh Journal of Medical Science*

FISKE FUND PRIZE ESSAYS — THE EFFECTS OF CLIMATE ON TUBERCULOUS DISEASE. By EDWIN LEE, M.R.C S, London, and THE INFLUENCE OF PREGNANCY ON THE DEVELOPMENT OF TUBERCLES By

EDWARD WARREN, M.D, of Edenton, N.C. Together in one neat 8vo volume, extra cloth. $1 00. FRICK ON RENAL AFFECTIONS; their Diagnosis and Pathology. With illustrations. One volume, royal 12mo., extra cloth 75 cents

FERGUSSON (WILLIAM), F. R. S.,
Professor of Surgery in King's College, London, &c.

A SYSTEM OF PRACTICAL SURGERY. Fourth American, from the third and enlarged London edition. In one large and beautifully printed octavo volume, of about 700 pages, with 393 handsome illustrations, leather. $3 00.

GRAHAM (THOMAS), F. R. S.

THE ELEMENTS OF INORGANIC CHEMISTRY, including the Applications of the Science in the Arts. New and much enlarged edition, by HENRY WATTS and ROBERT BRIDGES, M. D. Complete in one large and handsome octavo volume, of over 800 very large pages, with two hundred and thirty-two wood-cuts, extra cloth. $4 00.
* Part II., completing the work from p. 431 to end, with Index, Title Matter, &c., may be had separate, cloth backs and paper sides. Price $2 50.

From Prof. E. N. Horsford, Harvard College.
It has, in its earlier and less perfect editions, been familiar to me, and the excellence of its plan and the clearness and completeness of its discussions, have long been my admiration.

No reader of English works on this science can

afford to be without this edition of Prof. Graham's Elements.—*Silliman's Journal,* March, 1858.

From Prof. Wolcott Gibbs, N. Y. Free Academy.
The work is an admirable one in all respects, and its republication here cannot fail to exert a positive influence upon the progress of science in this country.

GRIFFITH (ROBERT E.), M. D., &c.

A UNIVERSAL FORMULARY, containing the methods of Preparing and Administering Officinal and other Medicines. The whole adapted to Physicians and Pharmaceutists. SECOND EDITION, thoroughly revised, with numerous additions, by ROBERT P. THOMAS. M. D., Professor of Materia Medica in the Philadelphia College of Pharmacy. In one large and handsome octavo volume, extra cloth, of 650 pages, double columns. $3 00; or in sheep, $3 25.

"It was a work requiring much perseverance, and when published was looked upon as by far the best work of its kind that had issued from the American press. Prof Thomas has certainly "improved," as well as added to this Formulary, and has rendered it additionally deserving of the confidence of pharmaceutists and physicians.—*Am. Journal of Pharmacy.*

We are happy to announce a new and improved edition of this, one of the most valuable and useful works that have emanated from an American pen. It would do credit to any country, and will be found of daily usefulness to practitioners of medicine; it is better adapted to their purposes than the dispensatories.—*Southern Med. and Surg. Journal.*

It is one of the most useful books a country practitioner can possibly have.—*Medical Chronicle.*

This is a work of six hundred and fifty one pages, embracing all on the subject of preparing and administering medicines that can be desired by the physician and pharmaceutist.—*Western Lancet.*

The amount of useful, every-day matter, for a practicing physician, is really immense.—*Boston Med and Surg. Journal.*

This edition has been greatly improved by the revision and ample additions of Dr Thomas, and it now, we believe, one of the most complete works of its kind in any language. The additions amount to about seventy pages, and no effort has been spared to include in them all the recent improvements A work of this kind appears to us indispensable to the physician, and there is none we can more cordially recommend. *N Y Journal of Medicine.*

GROSS (SAMUEL D.), M. D.,

Professor of Surgery in the Jefferson Medical College of Philadelphia, &c.

Enlarged Edition—Now Ready, January, 1862.

A SYSTEM OF SURGERY: Pathological, Diagnostic, Therapeutic, and Operative. Illustrated by TWELVE HUNDRED AND TWENTY-SEVEN ENGRAVINGS. Second edition, much enlarged and carefully revised. In two large and beautifully printed octavo volumes, of about twenty-two hundred pages; strongly bound in leather, with raised bands. Price $12.

The exhaustion in little more than two years of a large edition of so elaborate and comprehensive a work as this is the best evidence that the author was not mistaken in his estimate of the want which existed of a complete American System of Surgery, presenting the science in all its necessary details and in all its branches. That he has succeeded in the attempt to supply this want is shown not only by the rapid sale of the work, but also by the very favorable manner in which it has been received by the organs of the profession in this country and in Europe, and by the fact that a translation is now preparing in Holland—a mark of appreciation not often bestowed on any scientific work so extended in size

The author has not been insensible to the kindness thus bestowed upon his labors, and in revising the work for a new edition he has spared no pains to render it worthy of the favor with which it has been received. Every portion has been subjected to close examination and revision; any deficiencies apparent have been supplied, and the results of recent progress in the science and art of surgery have been everywhere introduced; while the series of illustrations has been enlarged by the addition of nearly three hundred wood-cuts, rendering it one of the most thoroughly illustrated works ever laid before the profession. To accommodate these very extensive additions, the work has been printed upon a smaller type, so that notwithstanding the very large increase in the matter and value of the book, its size is more convenient and less cumbrous than before. Every care has been taken in the printing to render the typographical execution unexceptionable, and it is confidently presented as a work in every way worthy of a place in even the most limited library of the p actitioner or student.

A few testimonials of the value of the former edition are appended.

Has Dr. Gross satisfactorily fulfilled this object? A careful perusal of his volumes enables us to give an answer in the affirmative. Not only has he given to the reader an elaborate and well-written account of his own vast experience, but he has not failed to embody in his pages the opinions and practice of surgeons in this and other countries of Europe. The result has been a work of such completeness, that it has no superior in the systematic treatises on surgery which have emanated from English or Continental authors. It has been justly objected that these have been far from complete in many essential particulars, many of them having been deficient in some of the most important points which should characterize such works. Some of them have been elaborate—too elaborate—with respect to certain diseases, while they have merely glanced at, or given an unsatisfactory account of, others equally important to the surgeon. Dr. Gross has avoided this error, and has produced the most complete work that has yet issued from the press on the science and practice of surgery. It is not, strictly speaking, a Dictionary of Surgery, but it gives to the reader all the information that he may require for his treatment of surgical diseases. Having said so much, it might appear superfluous to add another word; but it is only due to Dr. Gross to state that he has embraced the opportunity of transferring to his pages a vast number of engravings from English and other authors, illustrative of the pathology and treatment of surgical diseases. To these are added several hundred original wood-cuts. The work altogether commends itself to the attention of British surgeons, from whom it cannot fail to meet with extensive patronage.—*London Lancet*, Sept. 1, 1860.

Of Dr. Gross's treatise on Surgery we can say no more than that it is the most elaborate and complete work on this branch of the healing art which has ever been published in any country. A systematic work, it admits of no analytical review; but, did our space permit, we should gladly give some extracts from it, to enable our readers to judge of the classical style of the author, and the exhausting way in which each subject is treated.—*Dublin Quarterly Journal of Med. Science.*

The work is so superior to its predecessors in matter and extent, as well as in illustrations and style of publication, that we can honestly recommend it as the best work of the kind to be taken home by the young practitioner.—*Am. Med. Journ.*

With pleasure we record the completion of this long-anticipated work. The reputation which the author has for many years sustained, both as a surgeon and as a writer, had prepared us to expect a treatise of great excellence and originality; but we confess we were by no means prepared for the work which is before us—the most complete treatise upon surgery ever published, either in this or any other country, and we might, perhaps, safely say, the most original. There is no subject belonging properly to surgery which has not received from the author a due share of attention. Dr. Gross has supplied a want in surgical literature which has long been felt by practitioners; he has furnished us with a complete practical treatise upon surgery in all its departments As Americans, we are proud of the achievement; as surgeons, we are most sincerely thankful to him for his extraordinary labors in our behalf.—*N. Y. Monthly Review and Buffalo Med. Journal.*

BY THE SAME AUTHOR.

ELEMENTS OF PATHOLOGICAL ANATOMY. Third edition, thoroughly revised and greatly improved. In one large and very handsome octavo volume, with about three hundred and fifty beautiful illustrations, of which a large number are from original drawings. Price in extra cloth, $4 75; leather, raised bands, $5 25. (*Lately Published.*)

The very rapid advances in the Science of Pathological Anatomy during the last few years have rendered essential a thorough modification of this work, with a view of making it a correct exponent of the present state of the subject. The very careful manner in which this task has been executed, and the amount of alteration which it has undergone, have enabled the author to say that "with the many changes and improvements now introduced, the work may be regarded almost as a new treatise," while the efforts of the author have been seconded as regards the mechanical execution of the volume, rendering it one of the handsomest productions of the American press.

We most sincerely congratulate the author on the successful manner in which he has accomplished his proposed object. His book is most admirably calculated to fill up a blank which has long been felt to exist in this department of medical literature, and as such must become very widely circulated amongst all classes of the profession.— *Dublin Quarterly Journ. of Med. Science*, Nov. 1857.

We have been favorably impressed with the general manner in which Dr Gross has executed his task of affording a comprehensive digest of the present state of the literature of Pathological Anatomy, and have much pleasure in recommending his work to our readers, as we believe one well deserving of diligent perusal and careful study.—*Montreal Med. Chron.*, Sept. 1857.

BY THE SAME AUTHOR.

A PRACTICAL TREATISE ON FOREIGN BODIES IN THE AIR-PASSAGES. In one handsome octavo volume, extra cloth, with illustrations. pp. 468. $2 75.

GROSS (SAMUEL D.), M. D.,
Professor of Surgery in the Jefferson Medical College of Philadelphia, &c.

PRACTICAL TREATISE ON THE DISEASES, INJURIES, AND MALFORMATIONS OF THE URINARY BLADDER, THE PROSTATE GLAND, AND THE URETHRA.
Second Edition, revised and much enlarged, with one hundred and eighty-four illustrations. In one large and very handsome octavo volume, of over nine hundred pages. In leather, raised bands, $5 25; extra cloth, $4 75.

Philosophical in ts design, methodical in its arrangement, ample and sound in its practical details, easy in truth be said to leave scarcely anything to desired on so important a subject.—*Boston Med. and Surg Journal*

Whoever will peruse the vast amount of valuable ractical information it contains, will, we think,

agree with us, that there is no work in the English language which can make any just pretensions to be its equal.—*N. Y. Journal of Medicine*

A volume replete with truths and principles of the utmost value in the investigation of these diseases.—*American Medical Journal*.

GRAY (HENRY), F. R. S.,
Lecturer on Anatomy at St. George's Hospital, London, &c.

ANATOMY, DESCRIPTIVE AND SURGICAL.
The Drawings by H. V. CARTER, M D., late Demonstrator on Anatomy at St. George's Hospital; the Dissections jointly by the AUTHOR and Dr. CARTER. Second American, from the second revised and improved London edition In one magnificent imperial octavo volume, of over 800 pages, with 388 large and elaborate engravings on wood. Price in extra cloth, $6 25; leather, raised bands, $7 00. (*Now Ready*, 1862.)

The speedy exhaustion of a large edition of this work is sufficient evidence that its plan and execution have been found to present superior practical advantages in facilitating the study of Anatomy. In presenting it to the profession a second time, the author has availed himself of the opportunity to supply any deficiencies which experience in its use had shown to exist, and to correct any errors of detail, to which the first edition of a scientific work on so extensive and complicated a science is liable. These improvements have resulted in some increase in the size of the volume, while twenty-six new wood-cuts have been added to the beautiful series of illustrations which form so distinctive a feature of the work. The American edition has been passed through the press under the supervision of a competent professional man, who has taken every care to render it in all respects accurate, and it is now presented, without any increase of price, as fitted to maintain and extend the popularity which it has everywhere acquired

With little trouble, the busy practitioner whose knowledge of anatomy may have become obscured by want of practice, may now resuscitate his former anatomical lore, and be ready for any emergency It is in this class of individuals, and not to the student alone, that this work will ultimately tend to be of most incalculable advantage, and we feel satisfied that the library of the medical man will soon be considered incomplete in which a copy of this work does not exist.—*Madras Quarterly Journal of Med. Science*, July, 1861.

This edition is much improved and enlarged, and contains several new illustrations by Dr. Westmacott. The volume is a complete companion to the dissecting-room, and saves the necessity of the student possessing a variety of "Manuals."—*The London Lancet*, Feb. 9, 1861.

The work before us is one entitled to the highest praise, and we accordingly welcome it as a valuable addition to medical literature. Intermediate in fulness of detail between the treatises of S iar pey and of Wilson, its characteristic merit lies in the number and excellence of the engravings it contains. Most of these are original, of much larger than ordinary size, and admirably executed. The various parts are also let ered after the plan adopted in Holden's Osteology. It would be difficult to over-estimate the advantages offered by this mode of pictorial illus ration Bones, ligaments, muscles, bloodvessels, and nerves are each in turn figured, and marked with their appropriate names; thus enabling the student to comprehend, at a glance, what would otherwise often be ignored, or at any rate, acquired only by prolonged and irksome application. In conclusion, we heartily commend the work of Mr. Gray to the attention of the medical profession, feeling certain that it should be regarded as one of the most valuable contributions ever made to educational literature —*N. Y. Monthly Review*, Dec 1859.

In this view, we regard the work of Mr Gray as far better adapted to the wants of the profession, and especially of the student, than any treatise on anatomy yet published in this country. It is destined, we believe, to supersede all others, both as a manual of dissections, and a standard of reference to the student of general or relative anatomy. — *N. Y. Journal of Medicine*, Nov. 1859

For this truly admirable work the profession is indebted to the distinguished author of "Gray on the Spleen." The vacancy it fills has been long felt

to exist in this country. Mr Gray writes throughout with both branches of his subject in view. His description of each particular part is followed by a notice of its relations to t e parts with which it is connected, and this, too, sufficiently ample for all the purposes of the operative surgeon. After describing the bones and muscles, he gives a concise statement of the fractures to which the bones of the extremities are most liable, together with the amount and direction of the displacement to which the fragments are subjected by muscular action. The section on arteries is remarkably full and accurate. Not only is the surgical anatomy given to every important vessel, with directions for its ligation, but at the end of the description of each arterial trunk we have a useful summary of the irregularities which may occur in its origin, course, and termination.—*N. A. Med. Chir. Review*, Mar. 1859.

Mr. Gray's book, in excellency of arrangement and completeness of execution, exceeds any work on anatomy hitherto published in the English language, affording a complete view of the structure of the human body, with especial reference to practical surgery. Thus the volume constitutes a perfect book of reference for the practitioner, demanding a place in even the most limited library of the physician or surgeon, and a work of necessity for the student to fix in his mind what he has learned by the dissecting knife from the book of nature.—*The Dublin Quarterly Journal of Med. Sciences*, Nov. 1858.

In our judgment, the mode of illustration adopted in the present volume cannot but present many advantages to the student of anatomy. To the zealous disciple of Vesalius, earnestly desirous of real improvement, the book will certainly be of immense value; but, at the same time, we must also confess that to those simply desirous of "cramming" it will be an undoubted godsend. The peculiar value of Mr. Gray's mode of illustration is nowhere more markedly evident than in the chapter on osteology, and especially in those portions which treat of the bones of the head and of their development. The study of these parts is thus made one of comparative ease, if not of positive pleasure; and those bugbears of the student, the temporal and sphenoid bones, are shorn of half their terrors. It is, in our estimation, an admirable and complete text-book for the student, and a useful work of reference for the practitioner; its pictorial character forming a novel element, to which we have already sufficiently alluded.—*Am. Journ. Med. Sci.*, July, 1859.

GIBSON'S INSTITUTES AND PRACTICE OF SURGERY. Eighth edition, improved and 'al tered. With thirty-four plates. In two handsome octavo volumes, containing about 1,000 pages, leather, raised bands. $6 50

GARDNER'S MEDICAL CHEMISTRY, for the use of Students and the Profession. In one royal 12mo. vol., cloth, pp. 396, with wood cuts. $1.

GLUGE'S ATLAS OF PATHOLOGICAL HISTOLOGY. Translated, with Notes and Addi-

tions. by JOSEPH LEIDY, M. D. In one volume, very large imperial quarto, extra cloth, with 320 copper plate figures, plain and colored. $5 00.

HUGHES' INTRODUCTION TO THE PRACTICE OF AUSCULTATION AND OTHER MODES OF PHYSICAL DIAGNOSIS IN DISEASES OF THE LUNGS AND HEART. Second edition 1 vol. royal 12mo., sm. cloth, pp. 304. $1 00.

HAMILTON (FRANK H.), M. D.,
Professor of Surgery in the Long Island College Hospital.

A PRACTICAL TREATISE ON FRACTURES AND DISLOCATIONS. In
one large and handsome octavo volume, of over 750 pages, with 289 illustrations. $4 25. (*Now Ready*, January, 1860.)

Among the many good workers at surgery of whom America may now boast 1 ot the least is Frank Hastings Hamilton; and the volume before us is (we say it with a pang of wounded patriotism) the best and handiest book on the subject in the English language. It is in vain to attempt a review of it; nearly as vain to seek for any one, either of commission or omission. We have seen no work on practical surgery which we would sooner recommend to our brother surgeons, especially those of "the services," or those whose practice lies in districts where a man has necessarily to rely on his own unaided resources. The practitioner will find in it directions for nearly every possible accident, easily found and comprehended; and much pleasant reading for him to muse over in the after consideration of his cases.—*Edinburgh Med. Journ* Feb 1861.

This is a valuable contribution to the surgery of most important affections, and is the more welcome, inasmuch as at the present time we do not possess a single complete treatise on Fractures and Dislocations in the English language. It has remained for our American brother to produce a complete treatise upon the subject, and bring together in a convenient form those alterations and improvements that have been made from time to time in the treatment of these affections. One great and valuable feature in the work before us is the fact that it comprises all the improvements introduced into the practice of both English and American surgery, and though far from omitting mention of our continental neighbors, the author by no means encourages the notion—but too prevalent in some quarters—that nothing is good unless imported from France or Germany. The latter half of the work is devoted to the consideration of the various dislocations and their appropriate treatment, and its merit is fully equal to that of the preceding portion.—*The London Lancet*, May 5, 1860.

It is emphatically *the* book upon the subjects of which it treats, and we cannot doubt that it will continue so to be for an indefinite period of time. When we say, however, that we believe it will at once take its place as the best book for consultation by the practitioner; and that it will form the most complete, available, and reliable guide in emergencies of every nature connected with its subjects; and also that the student of surgery may make it his text-book with entire confidence, and with pleasure also, from its agreeable and easy style—we think our own

opinion may be gathered as to its value.—*Boston Medical and Surgical Journal*, March 1, 1860.

The work is concise, judicious, and accurate, and adapted to the wants of the student, practitioner, and investigator, honorable to the author and to the profession.—*Chicago Med. Journal*, March, 1860.

We regard this work as an honor not only to its author, but to the profession of our country. Were we to review it thoroughly, we could not convey to the mind of the reader more forcibly our honest opinion expressed in the few words—we think it the best book of the kind extant. Every man interested in surgery will soon have this work on his desk. He who does not, will be the loser.—*New Orleans Medical News*, March, 1860.

Now that it is before us, we feel bound to say that much as was expected from it, and onerous as was the undertaking, it has surpassed expectation, and achieved more than was pledged in its behalf; for its title does not express in full the richness of its contents. On the whole, we are prouder of this work than of any which has for years emanated from the American medical press; its sale will certainly be very large in this country, and we anticipate its eliciting much attention in Europe.—*Nashville Medical Record*, Mar. 1860.

Every surgeon, young and old, should possess himself of it, and give it a careful perusal, in doing which he will be richly repaid.—*St. Louis Med. and Surg. Journal*, March, 1860.

Dr. Hamilton is fortunate in having succeeded in filling the void, so long felt, with what cannot fail to be at once accepted as a model monograph in some respects, and a work of classical authority. We sincerely congratulate the profession of the United States on the appearance of such a publication from one of their number. We have reason to be proud of it as an original work, both in a literary and scientific point of view, and to esteem it as a valuable guide in a most difficult and important branch of study and practice. On every account, therefore, we hope that it may soon be widely known abroad as an evidence of genuine progress on this side of the Atlantic, and further, that it may be still more widely known at home as an authoritative teacher from which every one may profitably learn, and as affording an example of honest, well-directed, and untiring industry in authorship which every surgeon may emulate.—*Am. Med. Journal*, April, 1860.

HOBLYN (RICHARD D.), M. D.

A DICTIONARY OF THE TERMS USED IN MEDICINE AND THE
COLLATERAL SCIENCES. A new American edition. Revised, with numerous Additions, by ISAAC HAYS, M. D., editor of the "American Journal of the Medical Sciences." In one large royal 12mo. volume, leather, of over 500 double columned pages. $1 50.

To both practitioner and student, we recommend this dictionary as being convenient in size, accurate in definition, and sufficiently full and complete for ordinary consultation.—*Charleston Med. Journ.*

We know of no dictionary better arranged and adapted. It is not encumbered with the obsolete terms of a bygone age, but it contains all that are now in

use; embracing every department of medical science down to the very latest date.—*Western Lancet.*

Hoblyn's Dictionary has long been a favorite with us. It is the best book of definitions we have, and ought always to be upon the student's table.—*Southern Med. and Surg. Journal.*

HOLLAND'S MEDICAL NOTES AND REFLECTIONS. From the third London edition. In one handsome octavo volume, extra cloth. $3.

HORNER'S SPECIAL ANATOMY AND HIS-

TOLOGY. Eighth edition. Extensively revised and modified. In two large octavo volumes, extra cloth, of more than 1000 pages, with over 300 illustrations. $6 00.

HODGE (HUGH L.), M. D.,
Professor of Midwifery and the Diseases of Women and Children in the University of Pennsylvania, &c.

ON DISEASES PECULIAR TO WOMEN, including Displacements of the Uterus. With original illustrations. In one beautifully printed octavo volume, of nearly 500 pages, extra cloth. $3 25. (*Now Ready.*)

We will say at once that the work fulfils its object capitally well; and we will moreover venture the assertion that it will inaugurate an improved practice throughout this whole country. The secrets of the author's success are so clearly revealed that the attentive student cannot fail to insure a goodly portion of similar success in his own practice. It is a credit to *all* medical literature; and we add, that the physician who does not place it in his library, and who does not faithfully con its pages, will lose a vast deal of knowledge that would be most useful to himself and beneficial to his patients. *It is a practical work of the highest order of merit; and it will take rank as such immediately.—Maryland and Virginia Medical Journal,* Feb. 1861.

This contribution towards the elucidation of the pathology and treatment of some of the diseases peculiar to women, cannot fail to meet with a favorable reception from the medical profession. The character of the particular maladies of which the work before us treats; their frequency, variety, and obscurity; the amount of malaise and even of actual suffering by which they are invariably attended; their obstinacy, the difficulty with which they are overcome, and their disposition again and again to recur—these, taken in connection with the entire competency of the author to render a correct account of their nature, their causes, and their appro-priate management—his ample experience, his matured judgment, and his perfect conscientiousness—invest this publication with an interest and value to which few of the medical treatises of a recent date can lay a stronger, if, perchance, an equal claim.—*Am. Journ. Med. Sciences*, Jan. 1861.

Indeed, although no part of the volume is not eminently deserving of perusal and study, we think that the nine chapters devoted to this subject, are especially so, and we know of no more valuable monograph upon the symptoms, prognosis, and management of these annoying maladies than is constituted by this part of the work. We cannot but regard it as one of the most original and most practical works of the day; one which every accoucheur and physician should most carefully read; for we are persuaded that he will arise from its perusal with new ideas, which will induct him into a more rational practice in regard to many a suffering female, who may have placed her health in his hands.—*British American Journal*, Feb. 1861.

Of the many excellences of the work we will not speak at length. We advise all who would acquire a knowledge of the proper management of the maladies of which it treats, to study it with care. The second part is of itself a most valuable contribution to the practice of our art.—*Am. Med. Monthly and New York Review*, Feb. 1861.

The illustrations, which are all original, are drawn to a uniform scale of one-half the natural size.

HABERSHON (S. O.), M. D.,
Assistant Physician to and Lecturer on Materia Medica and Therapeutics at Guy's Hospital, &c.

PATHOLOGICAL AND PRACTICAL OBSERVATIONS ON DISEASES OF THE ALIMENTARY CANAL, ŒSOPHAGUS, STOMACH, CÆCUM, AND INTESTINES. With illustrations on wood. In one handsome octavo volume of 312 pages, extra cloth $1 75. (*Now Ready.*)

JONES (T. WHARTON), F. R. S.,
Professor of Ophthalmic Medicine and Surgery in University College, London, &c.

THE PRINCIPLES AND PRACTICE OF OPHTHALMIC MEDICINE AND SURGERY. With one hundred and ten illustrations. Second American from the second and revised London edition, with additions by EDWARD HARTSHORNE, M. D., Surgeon to Wills' Hospital, &c. In one large, handsome royal 12mo. volume, extra cloth, of 500 pages. $1 50.

JONES (C. HANDFIELD), F. R. S., & EDWARD H. SIEVEKING, M.D.,
Assistant Physicians and Lecturers in St. Mary's Hospital, London.

A MANUAL OF PATHOLOGICAL ANATOMY. First American Edition, Revised. With three hundred and ninety-seven handsome wood engravings. In one large and beautiful octavo volume of nearly 750 pages, leather. $3 75.

As a concise text-book, containing, in a condensed form, a complete outline of what is known in the domain of Pathological Anatomy, it is perhaps the best work in the English language. Its great merit consists in its completeness and brevity, and in this respect it supplies a great desideratum in our literature. Heretofore the student of pathology was obliged to glean from a great number of monographs, and the field was so extensive that but few cultivated it with any degree of success. As a simple work of reference, therefore, it is of great value to the student of pathological anatomy, and should be in every physician's library.—*Western Lancet.*

KIRKES (WILLIAM SENHOUSE), M. D.,
Demonstrator of Morbid Anatomy at St. Bartholomew's Hospital, &c.

A MANUAL OF PHYSIOLOGY. A new American, from the third and improved London edition. With two hundred illustrations. In one large and handsome royal 12mo. volume, leather. pp. 586. $2 00. (*Lately Published.*)

This is a new and very much improved edition of Dr. Kirkes' well-known Handbook of Physiology. It combines conciseness with completeness, and is, therefore, admirably adapted for consultation by the busy practitioner.—*Dublin Quarterly Journal.*

One of the very best handbooks of Physiology we possess—presenting just such an outline of the science as the student requires during his attendance upon a course of lectures, or for reference whilst preparing for examination.—*Am. Medical Journal.*

Its excellence is in its compactness, its clearness, and its carefully cited authorities. It is the most convenient of text-books. These gentlemen, Messrs. Kirkes and Paget, have the gift of telling us what we want to know, without thinking it necessary to tell us all they know.—*Boston Med. and Surg. Journal.*

For the student beginning this study, and the practitioner who has but leisure to refresh his memory, this book is invaluable, as it contains all that it is important to know.—*Charleston Med. Journal.*

KNAPP'S TECHNOLOGY; or, Chemistry applied to the Arts and to Manufactures. Edited by Dr. RONALDS, Dr. RICHARDSON, and Prof. W. R. JOHNSON. In two handsome 8vo. vols., with about 500 wood engravings. $6 00.

LAYCOCK'S LECTURES ON THE PRINCI- PLES AND METHODS OF MEDICAL OB- SERVATION AND RESEARCH. For th- Use of Advanced Students and Junior Practitioners. In one royal 12mo. volume, extra cloth. Price $1.

LALLEMAND AND WILSON.

A PRACTICAL TREATISE ON THE CAUSES, SYMPTOMS, AND TREATMENT OF SPERMATORRHŒA. By M. LALLEMAND. Translated and edited by HENRY J MCDOUGALL. Third American edition. To which is added —— ON DISEASES OF THE VESICULÆ SEMINALES; AND THEIR ASSOCIATED ORGANS. With special refer- ence to the Morbid Secretions of the Prostatic and Urethral Mucous Membrane. By MARRIS WILSON, M. D. In one neat octavo volume, of about 400 pp., extra cloth. $2 00. *(Just Issued.)*

LA ROCHE (R.), M. D., &c.

YELLOW FEVER, considered in its Historical, Pathological, Etiological, and Therapeutical Relations. Including a Sketch of the Disease as it has occurred in Philadelphia from 1699 to 1854, with an examination of the connections between it and the fevers known under the same name in other parts of temperate as well as in tropical regions. In two large and handsome octavo volumes of nearly 1500 pages, extra cloth. $7 00.

From Professor S. H. Dickson, Charleston, S. C., September 18, 1855.

A monument of intelligent and well applied re- search, almost without example. It is, indeed, in itself, a large library, and is destined to constitute the special resort as a book of reference, in the subject of which it treats, to all future time.

We have not time at present, engaged as we are, by day and by night, in the work of combating this very disease, now prevailing in our city, to do more than give this cursory notice of what we consider as undoubtedly the most able and erudite medical publication our country has yet produced But in view of the startling fact, that this, the most malig-

nant and unmanageable disease of modern times, has for several years been prevailing in our country to a greater extent than ever before; that it is no longer confined to either large or small cities, but penetrates country villages, plantations, and farm- houses; that it is treated with scarcely better suc- cess now than thirty, or forty years ago; that there is vast mischief done by ignorant pretenders to know- ledge in regard to the disease, and in view of the pro- bability that a majority of southern physicians will be called upon to treat the disease, we trust that this able and comprehensive treatise will be very gene- rally read in the south.—*Memphis Med Recorder.*

BY THE SAME AUTHOR.

PNEUMONIA; its Supposed Connection, Pathological and Etiological, with Au- tumnal Fevers, including an Inquiry into the Existence and Morbid Agency of Malaria. In one handsome octavo volume, extra cloth, of 500 pages. $3 00.

LAWRENCE (W.), F. R. S., &c.

A TREATISE ON DISEASES OF THE EYE. A new edition, edited, with numerous additions, and 243 illustrations, by ISAAC HAYS. M. D., Surgeon to Will's Hospi- tal, &c. In one very large and handsome octavo volume, of 950 pages, strongly bound in leather with raised bands. $5 00.

LUDLOW (J. L.), M. D.

A MANUAL OF EXAMINATIONS upon Anatomy, Physiology, Surgery, Practice of Medicine, Obstetrics, Materia Medica, Chemistry, Pharmacy, and Therapeutics. To which is added a Medical Formulary. Third edition, thoroughly revised and greatly extended and enlarged. With 370 illustrations. In one handsome royal 12mo. volume, leather, of 816 large pages $2 50.

We know of no better companion for the student during the hours spent in the lecture room, or to re- fresh, at a glance, his memory of the various topics

crammed into his head by the various professors to whom he is compelled to listen.—*Western Lancet,* May. 1857.

LEHMANN (C. G.)

PHYSIOLOGICAL CHEMISTRY. Translated from the second edition by GEORGE E. DAY, M. D., F. R. S., &c., edited by R. E. ROGERS, M. D., Professor of Chemistry in the Medical Department of the University of Pennsylvania, with illustrations selected from Funke's Atlas of Physiological Chemistry, and an Appendix of plates. Complete in two large and handsome octavo volumes, extra cloth, containing 1200 pages, with nearly two hundred illus- trations. $6 00.

The work of Lehmann stands unrivalled as the most comprehensive book of reference and informa- tion extant on every branch of the subject on which it treats.—*Edinburgh Journal of Medical Science.*

The most important contribution as yet made to Physiological Chemistry.—*Am. Journal Med. Sci- ences,* Jan. 1856.

BY THE SAME AUTHOR. *(Lately Published.)*

MANUAL OF CHEMICAL PHYSIOLOGY. Translated from the German, with Notes and Additions, by J. CHESTON MORRIS, M. D., with an Introductory Essay on Vital Force, by Professor SAMUEL JACKSON, M. D., of the University of Pennsylvania. With illus- trations on wood. In one very handsome octavo volume, extra cloth, of 336 pages. $2 25.

From Prof. Jackson's Introductory Essay.

In adopting the handbook of Dr. Lehmann as a manual of Organic Chemistry for the use of the students of the University, and in recommending his original work of PHYSIOLOGICAL CHEMISTRY for their more mature studies, the high value of his researches, and the great weight of his autho- rity in that important department of medical science are fully recognized.

LYONS (ROBERT D.), K. C. C.,
Late Pathologist in-chief to the British Army in the Crimea, &c.

A TREATISE ON FEVER; or. selections from a course of Lectures on Fever. Being part of a course of Theory and Practice of Medicine. In one neat octavo volume, of 362 pages, extra cloth; $2 00. (*Now Ready.*)

From the Author's Preface.

" I am induced to publish this work on Fever with a view to bring within the reach of the student and junior practitioner, in a convenient form, the more recent results of inquiries into the Pathology and Therapeutics of this formidable class of diseases.

" The works of the great writers on Fever are so numerous, and in the present day are scattered in so many languages, that they are difficult of access, not only to students but also to practitioners. I shall deem myself fortunate if I can in any measure supply the want which is felt in this respect.

We have great pleasure in recommending Dr. Lyons' work on *Fever* to the attention of the profession. It is a work which cannot fail to enhance the author's previous well-earned reputation, as a diligent, careful, and accurate observer.—*British Med. Journal*, March 2, 1861.

Taken as a whole we can recommend it in the highest terms as well worthy the careful perusal and study of every student and practitioner of medi-

cine. We consider the work a most valuable addition to medical literature, and one destined to wield no little influence over the mind of the profession —*Med and Surg. Reporter*, May 4, 1861.

This is an admirable work upon the most remarkable and most important class of diseases to which mankind are liable.—*Med. Journ of N. Carolina*, May, 1861.

MEIGS (CHARLES D.), M. D.,
Professor of Obstetrics, &c. in the Jefferson Medical College, Philadelphia.

OBSTETRICS: THE SCIENCE AND THE ART. Third edition, revised and improved. With one hundred and twenty-nine illustrations. In one beautifully printed octavo volume, leather, of seven hundred and fifty-two large pages. $3 75.

Though the work has received only five pages of enlargement, its chapters throughout wear the impress of careful revision. Expunging and rewriting, remodelling its sentences, with occasional new material, all evince a lively desire that it shall deserve to be regarded as improved in *manner* as well as *matter*. In the *matter*, every stroke of the pen has increased the value of the book, both in expungings and additions —*Western Lancet*, Jan. 1857.

The best American work on Midwifery that is accessible to the student and practitioner—*N. W. Med. and Surg. Journal*, Jan. 1857.

This is a standard work by a great American Obstetrician. It is the third and last edition, and, in the language of the preface, the author has "brought the subject up to the latest dates of real improvement in our art and Science."—*Nashville Journ. of Med. and Surg.*, May, 1857.

BY THE SAME AUTHOR. (*Just Issued.*)

WOMAN: HER DISEASES AND THEIR REMEDIES. A Series of Lectures to his Class. Fourth and Improved edition. In one large and beautifully printed octavo volume, leather, of over 700 pages. $3 60.

In other respects, in our estimation, too much cannot be said in praise of this work. It abounds with beautiful passages, and for conciseness, for originality, and for all that is commendable in a work on the diseases of females, it is not excelled, and probably not equalled in the English language. On the whole, we know of no work on the diseases of women which we can so cordially commend to the student and practitioner as the one before us.—*Ohio Med. and Surg. Journal.*

The body of the book is worthy of attentive consideration, and is evidently the production of a clever, thoughtful, and sagacious physician. Dr. Meigs's letters on the diseases of the external organs, contain many interesting and rare cases, and many instructive observations. We take our leave of Dr. Meigs, with a high opinion of his talents and originality.—*The British and Foreign Medico-Chirurgical Review.*

Every chapter is replete with practical instruction, and bears the impress of being the composition of an acute and experienced mind. There is a terseness, and at the same time an accuracy in his description of symptoms, and in the rules for diagnosis,

which cannot fail to recommend the volume to the attention of the reader.—*Ranking's Abstract.*

It contains a vast amount of practical knowledge, by one who has accurately observed and retained the experience of many years.—*Dublin Quarterly Journal.*

Full of important matter, conveyed in a ready and agreeable manner.—*St. Louis Med. and Surg. Jour.*

There is an off-hand fervor, a glow, and a warm-heartedness infecting the effort of Dr. Meigs, which is entirely captivating, and which absolutely hurries the reader through from beginning to end. Besides, the book teems with solid instruction, and it shows the very highest evidence of ability, viz., the clearness with which the information is presented. We know of no better test of one's understanding a subject than the evidence of the power of lucidly explaining it. The most elementary, as well as the obscurest subjects, under the pencil of Prof. Meigs, are isolated and made to stand out in such bold relief, as to produce distinct impressions upon the mind and memory of the reader.—*The Charleston Med. Journal.*

BY THE SAME AUTHOR.

ON THE NATURE, SIGNS, AND TREATMENT OF CHILDBED FEVER. In a Series of Letters addressed to the Students of his Class. In one handsome octavo volume, extra cloth, of 365 pages. $2 50.

The instructive and interesting author of this work, whose previous labors have placed his countrymen under deep and abiding obligations, again challenges their admiration in the fresh and vigorous, attractive and racy pages before us. It is a de-

lectable book. * * * This treatise upon childbed fevers will have an extensive sale, being destined, as it deserves, to find a place in the library of every practitioner who scorns toing in the rear.—*Nashville Journal of Medicine and Surgery.*

BY THE SAME AUTHOR; WITH COLORED PLATES.

A TREATISE ON ACUTE AND CHRONIC DISEASES OF THE NECK OF THE UTERUS. With numerous plates, drawn and colored from nature in the highest style of art. In one handsome octavo volume, extra cloth. $4 50.

MACLISE (JOSEPH), SURGEON.

SURGICAL ANATOMY. Forming one volume, very large imperial quarto. With sixty-eight large and splendid Plates, drawn in the best style and beautifully colored. Containing one hundred and ninety Figures, many of them the size of life. Together with copious and explanatory letter-press. Strongly and handsomely bound in extra cloth, being one of the cheapest and best executed Surgical works as yet issued in this country. $11 00.

** The size of this work prevents its transmission through the post-office as a whole, but those who desire to have copies forwarded by mail, can receive them in five parts, done up in stout wrappers. Price $9 00.

One of the greatest artistic triumphs of the age in Surgical Anatomy.—*British American Medical Journal.*

No practitioner whose means will admit should fail to possess it.—*Ranking's Abstract.*

Too much cannot be said in its praise; indeed, we have not language to do it justice.—*Ohio Medical and Surgical Journal.*

The most accurately engraved and beautifully colored plates we have ever seen in an American book—one of the best and cheapest surgical works ever published.—*Buffalo Medical Journal.*

It is very rare that so elegantly printed, so well illustrated, and so useful a work, is offered at so moderate a price.—*Charleston Medical Journal.*

Its plates can boast a superiority which places them almost beyond the reach of competition.—*Medical Examiner.*

Country practitioners will find these plates of immense value.—*N. Y. Medical Gazette.*

A work which has no parallel in point of accuracy and cheapness in the English language.—*N. Y. Journal of Medicine.*

We are extremely gratified to announce to the profession the completion of this truly magnificent work, which, as a whole, certainly stands unrivalled, both for accuracy of drawing, beauty of coloring, and all the requisite explanations of the subject in hand.—*The New Orleans Medical and Surgical Journal.*

This is by far the ablest work on Surgical Anatomy that has come under our observation. We know of no other work that would justify a student, in any degree, for neglect of actual dissection. In those sudden emergencies that so often arise, and which require the instantaneous command of minute anatomical knowledge, a work of this kind keeps the details of the dissecting-room perpetually fresh in the memory.—*The Western Journal of Medicine and Surgery.*

MILLER (HENRY), M. D.,
Professor of Obstetrics and Diseases of Women and Children in the University of Louisville.

PRINCIPLES AND PRACTICE OF OBSTETRICS, &c.; including the Treatment of Chronic Inflammation of the Cervix and Body of the Uterus considered as a frequent cause of Abortion. With about one hundred illustrations on wood. In one very handsome octavo volume, of over 600 pages. (*Lately Published.*) $3 75.

We congratulate the author that the task is done. We congratulate him that he has given to the medical public a work which will secure for him a high and permanent position among the standard authorities on the principles and practice of obstetrics. Congratulations are not less due to the medical profession of this country, on the acquisition of a treatise embodying the results of the studies, reflections, and experience of Prof. Miller. Few men, if any, in this country, are more competent than he to write on this department of medicine. Engaged for thirty-five years in an extended practice of obstetrics, for many years a teacher of this branch of instruction in one of the largest of our institutions, a diligent student as well as a careful observer, an original and independent thinker, wedded to no hobbies, ever ready to consider without prejudice new views, and to adopt innovations if they are really improvements, and withal a clear, agreeable writer, a practical treatise from his pen could not fail to possess great value.—*Buffalo Med Journal.*

In fact, this volume must take its place among the standard systematic treatises on obstetrics; a position to which its merits justly entitle it. The style is such that the descriptionsare clear, and each subject is discussed and elucidated with due regard to its practical bearings, which cannot fail to make it acceptable and valuable to both students and practitioners. We cannot, however, close this brief notice without congratulating the author and the profession on the production of such an excellent treatise. The author is a western man of whom we feel proud, and we cannot but think that his book will find many readers and warm admirers wherever obstetrics is taught and studied as a science and an art.—*The Cincinnati Lancet and Observer.*

A most respectable and valuable addition to our home medical literature, and one reflecting credit alike on the author and the institution to which he is attached. The student will find in this work a most useful guide to his studies; the country practitioner, rusty in his reading, can obtain from its pages a fair résumé of the modern literature of the science; and we hope to see this American production generally consulted by the profession.—*Va. Med. Journal.*

MACKENZIE (W.), M. D.,
Surgeon Oculist in Scotland in ordinary to Her Majesty, &c. &c.

A PRACTICAL TREATISE ON DISEASES AND INJURIES OF THE EYE. To which is prefixed an Anatomical Introduction explanatory of a Horizontal Section of the Human Eyeball, by THOMAS WHARTON JONES, F. R. S. From the Fourth Revised and Enlarged London Edition. With Notes and Additions by ADDINELL HEWSON, M. D., Surgeon to Wills Hospital, &c. &c. In one very large and handsome octavo volume, leather, raised bands, with plates and numerous wood-cuts. $5 25.

The treatise of Dr. Mackenzie indisputably holds the first place, and forms, in respect of learning and research, an Encyclopædia unequalled in extent by any other work of the kind, either English or foreign.—*Dixon on Diseases of the Eye.*

Few modern books on any department of medicine or surgery have met with such extended circulation, or have procured for their authors a like amount of European celebrity. The immense research which it displayed, the thorough acquaintance with the subject, practically as well as theoretically, and the able manner in which the author's stores of learning and experience were rendered available for general use, at once procured for the first edition, as well on the continent as in this country, that high position as a standard work which each successive edition has more firmly established. We consider it the duty of every one who has the love of his profession and the welfare of his patient at heart, to make himself familiar with this the most complete work in the English language upon the diseases of the eye.—*Med. Times and Gazette.*

MAYNE'S DISPENSATORY AND THERAPEUTICAL REMEMBRANCER. With every Practical Formula contained in the three British Pharmacopœias. Edited, with the addition of the Formulæ of the U. S. Pharmacopœia, by R. E. GRIFFITH, M. D 1 12mo. vol. ex. cl., 300 pp. 75 c.

MALGAIGNE'S OPERATIVE SURGERY, based on Normal and Pathological Anatomy. Translated from the French by FREDERICK BRITTAN, A. B., M. D. With numerous illustrations on wood. In one handsome octavo volume, extra cloth, of nearly six hundred pages. $2 25.

MILLER (JAMES), F. R. S. E.,
Professor of Surgery in the University of Edinburgh, &c.

PRINCIPLES OF SURGERY. Fourth American, from the third and revised Edinburgh edition. In one large and very beautiful volume, leather, of 700 pages, with two hundred and forty illustrations on wood. $3 75.

The work of Mr. Miller is too well and too favorably known among us, as one of our best text-books, to render any further notice of it necessary than the announcement of a new edition, the *fourth* in our country, a proof of its extensive circulation among us. As a concise and reliable exposition of the science of modern surgery, it stands deservedly high—we know not its superior.—*Boston Med. and Surg. Journal.*

The work takes rank with Watson's Practice of Physic; it certainly does not fall behind that great work in soundness of principle or depth of reasoning and research. No physician who values his reputation, or seeks the interests of his clients, can acquit himself before his God and the world without making himself familiar with the sound and philosophical views developed in the foregoing book.—*New Orleans Med. and Surg. Journal.*

BY THE SAME AUTHOR. (*Just Issued.*)

THE PRACTICE OF SURGERY. Fourth American from the last Edinburgh edition. Revised by the American editor. Illustrated by three hundred and sixty-four engravings on wood. In one large octavo volume, leather, of nearly 700 pages. $3 75.

No encomium of ours could add to the popularity of Miller's Surgery. Its reputation in this country is unsurpassed by that of any other work, and, when taken in connection with the author's *Principles of Surgery*, constitutes a whole, without reference to which no conscientious surgeon would be willing to practice his art.—*Southern Med. and Surg. Journal*

It is seldom that two volumes have ever made so profound an impression in so short a time as the "Principles" and the "Practice" of Surgery by Mr. Miller—or so richly merited the reputation they have acquired. The author is an eminently sensible, practical, and well-informed man, who knows exactly what he is talking about and exactly how to talk it.—*Kentucky Medical Recorder.*

By the almost unanimous voice of the profession,

his works, both on the principles and practice of surgery have been assigned the highest rank. If we were limited to but one work on surgery, that one should be Miller's, as we regard it as superior to all others.—*St. Louis Med. and Surg. Journal.*

The author has in this and his "Principles," presented to the profession one of the most complete and reliable systems of Surgery extant. His style of writing is original, impressive, and engaging, energetic, concise, and lucid. Few have the faculty of condensing so much in small space, and at the same time so persistently holding the attention. Whether as a text-book for students or a book of reference for practitioners, it cannot be too strongly recommended.—*Southern Journal of Med. and Physical Sciences.*

MORLAND (W. W.), M. D.,
Fellow of the Massachusetts Medical Society, &c.

DISEASES OF THE URINARY ORGANS; a Compendium of their Diagnosis, Pathology, and Treatment. With illustrations. In one large and handsome octavo volume, of about 600 pages, extra cloth. (*Just Issued.*) $3 50.

Taken as a whole, we can recommend Dr. Morland's compendium as a very desirable addition to the library of every medical or surgical practitioner.—*Brit and For. Med.-Chir. Rev.*, April, 1859.

Every medical practitioner whose attention has been to any extent attracted towards the class of diseases to which this treatise relates, must have often and surely experienced the want of some full, yet concise recent compendium to which he could

refer. This desideratum has been supplied by Dr. Morland, and it has been ably done. He has placed before us a full, judicious, and reliable digest. Each subject is treated with sufficient minuteness, yet in a succinct, narrational style, such as to render the work one of great interest, and one which will prove in the highest degree useful to the general practitioner.—*N. Y. Journ. of Medicine.*

BY THE SAME AUTHOR —(*Now Ready.*)

THE MORBID EFFECTS OF THE RETENTION IN THE BLOOD OF THE ELEMENTS OF THE URINARY SECRETION. Being the Dissertation to which the Fiske Fund Prize was awarded, July 11, 1861. In one small octavo volume, 83 pages, extra cloth. 75 cents.

MONTGOMERY (W. F.), M. D., M. R. I. A., &c.,
Professor of Midwifery in the King and Queen's College of Physicians in Ireland, &c.

AN EXPOSITION OF THE SIGNS AND SYMPTOMS OF PREGNANCY. With some other Papers on Subjects connected with Midwifery. From the second and enlarged English edition. With two exquisite colored plates, and numerous wood-cuts. In one very handsome octavo volume, extra cloth, of nearly 600 pages. (*Lately Published.*) $3 75.

A book unusually rich in practical suggestions.—*Am. Journal Med. Sciences*, Jan. 1857.

These several subjects so interesting in themselves, and so important, every one of them, to the most delicate and precious of social relations, controlling often the honour and domestic peace of a family, the legitimacy of offspring, or the life of its parent, are all treated with an elegance of diction, fulness of illustrations, acuteness and justice of reasoning, unparalleled in obstetrics, and unsurpassed in medicine, the reader's interest can never flag, so

fresh, and vigorous, and classical is our author's style; and one forgets, in the renewed charm of every page, that it, and every line, and every word has been weighed and reweighed through years of preparation; that this is of all others the book of Obstetric Law, on each of its several topics; on all points connected with pregnancy, to be everywhere received as a manual of special jurisprudence, at once announcing fact, affording argument, establishing precedent, and governing alike the juryman, advocate, and judge.— *N. A. Med.-Chir. Review.*

MOHR (FRANCIS), PH. D., AND REDWOOD (THEOPHILUS).

PRACTICAL PHARMACY. Comprising the Arrangements, Apparatus, and Manipulations of the Pharmaceutical Shop and Laboratory. Edited, with extensive Additions, by Prof. WILLIAM PROCTER, of the Philadelphia College of Pharmacy. In one handsomely printed octavo volume, extra cloth, of 570 pages, with over 500 engravings on wood. $2 75.

NEILL (JOHN), M. D.,
Surgeon to the Pennsylvania Hospital,&c.; and

FRANCIS GURNEY SMITH, M. D.,
Professor of Institutes of Medicine in the Pennsylvania Medical College.

AN ANALYTICAL COMPENDIUM OF THE VARIOUS BRANCHES

OF MEDICAL SCIENCE; for the Use and Examination of Students. A new edition, revised and improved. In one very large and handsomely printed royal 12mo. volume, of about one thousand pages, with 374 wood-cuts. Strongly bound in leather, with raised bands. $3 00.

The very flattering reception which has been accorded to this work, and the high estimate placed upon it by the profession, as evinced by the constant and increasing demand which has rapidly exhausted two large editions, have stimulated the authors to render the volume in its present revision more worthy of the success which has attended it. It has accordingly been thoroughly examined, and such errors as had on former occasions escaped observation have been corrected, and whatever additions were necessary to maintain it on a level with the advance of science have been introduced. The extended series of illustrations has been still further increased and much improved, while, by a slight enlargement of the page, these various additions have been incorporated without increasing the bulk of the volume.

The work is, therefore, again presented as eminently worthy of the favor with which it has hitherto been received. As a book for daily reference by the student requiring a guide to his more elaborate text-books, as a manual for preceptors desiring to stimulate their students by frequent and accurate examination, or as a source from which the practitioners of older date may easily and cheaply acquire a knowledge of the changes and improvement in professional science, its reputation is permanently established.

The best work of the kind with which we are acquainted.—*Med. Examiner.*

Having made free use of this volume in our examinations of pupils, we can speak from experience in recommending it as an admirable compend for students, and as especially useful to preceptors who examine their pupils. It will save the teacher much labor by enabling him readily to recall all of the points upon which his pupils should be examined. A work of this sort should be in the hands of every one who takes pupils into his office with a view of examining them; and this is unquestionably the best of its class.—*Transylvania Med. Journal*

In the rapid course of lectures, where work for

the students is heavy, and review necessary for an examination, a compend is not only valuable, but it is almost a *sine qua non*. The one before us is, in most of the divisions, the most unexceptionable of all books of the kind that we know of. The newest and soundest doctrines and the latest improvements and discoveries are explicitly, though concisely, laid before the student. There is a class to whom we very sincerely commend this cheap book as worth its weight in silver—that class is the graduates in medicine of more than ten years' standing, who have not studied medicine since. They will perhaps find out from it that the science is not exactly now what it was when they left it off.—*The Stethoscope*

NELIGAN (J. MOORE), M. D., M. R. I. A., &c.
(A splendid work. Just Issued.)

ATLAS OF CUTANEOUS DISEASES.

In one beautiful quarto volume, extra cloth, with splendid colored plates, presenting nearly one hundred elaborate representations of disease. $4 50.

This beautiful volume is intended as a complete and accurate representation of all the varieties of Diseases of the Skin. While it can be consulted in conjunction with any work on Practice, it has especial reference to the author's "Treatise on Diseases of the Skin," so favorably received by the profession some years since. The publishers feel justified in saying that few more beautifully executed plates have ever been presented to the profession of this country.

Neligan's Atlas of Cutaneous Diseases supplies a long existent desideratum much felt by the largest class of our profession. It presents, in quarto size, 16 plates, each containing from 3 to 6 figures, and forming in all a total of 90 distinct representations of the different species of skin affections, grouped together in genera or families. The illustrations have been taken from nature, and have been copied with such fidelity that they present a striking picture of life; in which the reduced scale aptly serves to

give, at a *coup d'œil*, the remarkable peculiarities of each individual variety. And while thus the disease is rendered more definable, there is yet no loss of proportion incurred by the necessary concentration. Each figure is highly colored, and so truthful has the artist been that the most fastidious observer could not justly take exception to the correctness of the execution of the pictures under his scrutiny.—*Montreal Med. Chronicle.*

BY THE SAME AUTHOR.

A PRACTICAL TREATISE ON DISEASES OF THE SKIN.

Third American edition. In one neat royal 12mo. volume, extra cloth, of 334 pages. $1 00.

☞ The two volumes will be sent by mail on receipt of *Five Dollars.*

OWEN ON THE DIFFERENT FORMS OF THE SKELETON, AND OF THE TEETH.	One vol. royal 12mo., extra cloth with numerous illustrations. $1 25

PIRRIE (WILLIAM), F. R. S. E.,
Professor of Surgery in the University of Aberdeen.

THE PRINCIPLES AND PRACTICE OF SURGERY.

Edited by JOHN NEILL, M. D., Professor of Surgery in the Penna. Medical College, Surgeon to the Pennsylvania Hospital, &c. In one very handsome octavo volume, leather, of 780 pages, with 316 illustrations. $3 75.

We know of no other surgical work of a reasonable size, wherein there is so much theory and practice, or where subjects are more soundly or clearly taught.—*The Stethoscope.*

Prof. Pirrie, in the work before us, has elabo-

rately discussed the principles of surgery, and a safe and effectual practice predicated upon them. Perhaps no work upon this subject heretofore issued is so full upon the science of the art of surgery.—*Nashville Journal of Medicine and Surgery.*

PARRISH (EDWARD),
Lecturer on Practical Pharmacy and Materia Medica in the Pennsylvania Academy of Medicine, &c.

AN INTRODUCTION TO PRACTICAL PHARMACY. Designed as a Text-Book for the Student, and as a Guide for the Physician and Pharmaceutist. With many Formulæ and Prescriptions. Second edition, greatly enlarged and improved. In one handsome octavo volume of 720 pages, with several hundred Illustrations, extra cloth. $3 50. (*Just Issued.*)

During the short time in which this work has been before the profession, it has been received with very great favor, and in assuming the position of a standard authority, it has filled a vacancy which had been severely felt. Stimulated by this encouragement, the author, in availing himself of the opportunity of revision, has spared no pains to render it more worthy of the confidence bestowed upon it, and his assiduous labors have made it rather a new book than a new edition, many portions having been rewritten, and much new and important matter added. These alterations and improvements have been rendered necessary by the rapid progress made by pharmaceutical science during the last few years, and by the additional experience obtained in the practical use of the volume as a text-book and work of reference. To accommodate these improvements, the size of the page has been materially enlarged, and the number of pages considerably increased, presenting in all nearly *one-half more* matter than the last edition. The work is therefore now presented as a complete exponent of the subject in its most advanced condition. From the most ordinary matters in the dispensing office, to the most complicated details of the vegetable alkaloids, it is hoped that everything requisite to the practising physician, and to the apothecary, will be found fully and clearly set forth, and that the new matter alone will be worth more than the very moderate cost of the work to those who have been consulting the previous edition.

That Edward Parrish, in writing a book upon practical Pharmacy some few years ago—one eminently original and unique—did the medical and pharmaceutical professions a great and valuable service, no one, we think, who has had access to its pages will deny; doubly welcome, then, is this new edition, containing the added results of his recent and rich experience as an observer, teacher, and practical operator in the pharmaceutical laboratory. The excellent plan of the first is more thoroughly, and in detail, carried out in this edition.—*Peninsular Med. Journal,* Jan. 1860.

Of course, all apothecaries who have not already a copy of the first edition will procure one of this; it is, therefore, to physicians residing in the country and in small towns, who cannot avail themselves of the skill of an educated pharmaceutist, that we would especially commend this work. In it they will find all that they desire to know, and should know, but very little of which they do really know in reference to this important collateral branch of their profession; for it is a well established fact, that, in the education of physicians, while the science of medicine is generally well taught, very little attention is paid to the art of preparing them for use, and we know not how this defect can be so well remedied as by procuring and consulting Dr. Parrish's excellent work.—*St. Louis Med. Journal,* Jan 1860.

We know of no work on the subject which would be more indispensable to the physician or student desiring information on the subject of which it treats. With Griffith's "Medical Formulary" and this, the practising physician would be supplied with nearly or quite all the most useful information on the subject.—*Charleston Med. Jour. and Review,* Jan. 1860

PEASLEE (E. R.), M. D.,
Professor of Physiology and General Pathology in the New York Medical College.

HUMAN HISTOLOGY, in its relations to Anatomy, Physiology, and Pathology; for the use of Medical Students. With four hundred and thirty-four illustrations. In one handsome octavo volume, of over 600 pages. (*Lately Published.*) $3 75.

It embraces a library upon the topics discussed within itself, and is just what the teacher and learner need. Another advantage, by no means to be overlooked, everything of real value in the wide range which it embraces, is with great skill compressed into an octavo volume of but little more than six hundred pages. We have not only the whole subject of Histology, interesting in itself, ably and fully discussed, but what is of infinitely greater interest to the student, because of greater practical value, are its relations to Anatomy, Physiology, and Pathology, which are here fully and satisfactorily set forth.—*Nashville Journ. of Med. and Surgery.*

We would recommend it to the medical student and practitioner, as containing a summary of all that is known of the important subjects which it treats; of all that is contained in the great works of Simon and Lehmann, and the organic chemists in general. Master this one volume, we would say to the medical student and practitioner—master this book and you know all that is known of the great fundamental principles of medicine, and we have no hesitation in saying that it is an honor to the American medical profession that one of its members should have produced it.—*St. Louis Med. and Surg. Journal.*

PEREIRA (JONATHAN), M. D., F. R. S., AND L. S.
THE ELEMENTS OF MATERIA MEDICA AND THERAPEUTICS. Third American edition, enlarged and improved by the author; including Notices of most of the Medicinal Substances in use in the civilized world, and forming an Encyclopædia of Materia Medica. Edited, with Additions, by JOSEPH CARSON, M. D., Professor of Materia Medica and Pharmacy in the University of Pennsylvania. In two very large octavo volumes of 2100 pages, on small type, with about 500 illustrations on stone and wood, strongly bound in leather, with raised bands. $9 00.

*** Vol. II. will no longer be sold separate.

PARKER (LANGSTON),
Surgeon to the Queen's Hospital, Birmingham.

THE MODERN TREATMENT OF SYPHILITIC DISEASES, BOTH PRIMARY AND SECONDARY; comprising the Treatment of Constitutional and Confirmed Syphilis, by a safe and successful method. With numerous Cases, Formulæ, and Clinical Observations. From the Third and entirely rewritten London edition. In one neat octavo volume, extra cloth, of 316 pages. $1 75.

ROYLE'S MATERIA MEDICA AND THERAPEUTICS; including the Preparations of the Pharmacopœias of London, Edinburgh, Dublin, and of the United States. With many new medicines. Edited by JOSEPH CARSON, M. D. With ninety-eight illustrations. In one large octavo volume, extra cloth, of about 700 pages. $3 00.

RAMSBOTHAM (FRANCIS H.), M.D.

THE PRINCIPLES AND PRACTICE OF OBSTETRIC MEDICINE AND

SURGERY, in reference to the Process of Parturition. A new and enlarged edition, thoroughly revised by the Author. With Additions by W. V. KEATING, M. D., Professor of Obstetrics, &c., in the Jefferson Medical College, Philadelphia. In one large and handsome imperial octavo volume, of 650 pages, strongly bound in leather, with raised bands; with sixty-four beautiful Plates, and numerous Wood-cuts in the text, containing in all nearly 200 large and beautiful figures $5 00.

From Prof. Hodge, of the University of Pa.

To the American public, it is most valuable, from its intrinsic undoubted excellence, and as being the best authorized exponent of British Midwifery. Its circulation will, I trust, be extensive throughout our country.

It is unnecessary to say anything in regard to the utility of this work. It is already appreciated in our country for the value of the matter, the clearness of its style, and the fulness of its illustrations. To the physician's library it is indispensable, while to the student as a text-book, from which to extract the material for laying the foundation of an education on obstetrical science, it has no superior.—*Ohio Med and Surg. Journal.*

The publishers have secured its success by the

truly elegant style in which they have brought it out, excelling themselves in its production, especially in its plates. It is dedicated to Prof Meigs, and has the emphatic endorsement of Prof. Hodge, as the best exponent of British Midwifery. We know of no text-book which deserves in all respects to be more highly recommended to students, and we could wish to see it in the hands of every practitioner, for they will find it invaluable for reference.—*Med. Gazette.*

RICORD (P.), M.D.

A TREATISE ON THE VENEREAL DISEASE. By JOHN HUNTER, F.R.S.

With copious Additions, by PH. RICORD, M.D. Translated and Edited, with Notes, by FREEMAN J. BUMSTEAD M.D, Lecturer on Venereal at the College of Physicians and Surgeons, New York. Second edition, revised, containing a *résumé* of RICORD'S RECENT LECTURES ON CHANCRE. In one handsome octavo volume, extra cloth, of 550 pages, with eight plates. $3 25. (*Just Issued.*)

In revising this work, the editor has endeavored to introduce whatever matter of interest the recent investigations of syphilographers have added to our knowledge of the subject. The principal source from which this has been derived is the volume of "Lectures on Chancre," published a few months since by M. Ricord, which affords a large amount of new and instructive material on many controverted points. In the previous edition, M. Ricord's additions amounted to nearly one-third of the whole, and with the matter now introduced, the work may be considered to present his views and experience more thoroughly and completely than any other.

Every one will recognize the attractiveness and value which this work derives from thus presenting the opinions of these two masters side by side. But it must be admitted, that has made the fortune of the book, is the fact that it contains the "most complete embodiment of the veritable doctrines of the Hôpital du Midi," which has ever been made public. The doctrinal ideas of M. Ricord, ideas which, if not universally adopted, are incontestably dominant, have heretofore only been interpreted by more or less skilful

secretaries, sometimes accredited and sometimes not. In the notes to Hunter, the master substitutes himself for his interpreters, and gives his original thoughts to the world in a lucid and perfectly intelligible manner. In conclusion we can say that this is incontestably the best treatise on syphilis with which we are acquainted, and, as we do not often employ the phrase, we may be excused for expressing the hope that it may find a place in the library of every physician.— *Virginia Med. and Surg. Journal.*

BY THE SAME AUTHOR.

RICORD'S LETTERS ON SYPHILIS. Translated by W. P. LATTIMORE, M.D.

In one neat octavo volume, of 270 pages, extra cloth. $2 00.

SLADE (D. D.), M.D.

DIPHTHERIA; its Nature and Treatment, with an Account of the History of its

Prevalence in various countries. Being the Dissertation to which the Fiske Fund Prize was awarded, July 11, 1860. In one small octavo volume, extra cloth; 75 cents. (*Now Ready*, 1861.)

ROKITANSKY (CARL), M.D.,

Curator of the Imperial Pathological Museum, and Professor at the University of Vienna, &c.

A MANUAL OF PATHOLOGICAL ANATOMY. Four volumes, octavo,

bound in two, extra cloth, of about 1200 pages. Translated by W. E. SWAINE, EDWARD SIEVE-KING, C. H. MOORE, and G. E. DAY. $5 50.

The profession is too well acquainted with the reputation of Rokitansky's work to need our assurance that this is one of the most profound, thorough, and valuable books ever issued from the medical press. It is *sui generis*, and has no standard of comparison. It is only necessary to announce that it is issued in a form as cheap as is compatible with its size and preservation, and its sale follows as a matter of course. No library can be called complete without it.—*Buffalo Med. Journal.*

An attempt to give our readers any adequate idea of the vast amount of instruction accumulated in these volumes, would be feeble and hopeless. The effort of the distinguished author to concentrate in a small space his great fund of knowledge, has

so charged his text with valuable truths, that any attempt of a reviewer to epitomize is at once paralyzed, and must end in a failure.—*Western Lancet.*

As this is the highest source of knowledge upon the important subject of which it treats, no real student can afford to be without it. The American publishers have entitled themselves to the thanks of the profession of their country, for this timeous and beautiful edition.—*Nashville Journal of Medicine.*

As a book of reference, therefore, this work must prove of inestimable value, and we cannot too highly recommend it to the profession.—*Charleston Med. Journal and Review.*

This book is a necessity to every practitioner.— *Am. Med. Monthly.*

RIGBY (EDWARD), M.D.,

Senior Physician to the General Lying-in Hospital, &c.

A SYSTEM OF MIDWIFERY. With Notes and Additional Illustrations.

Second American Edition. One volume octavo, extra cloth, 422 pages. $2 50.

BY THE SAME AUTHOR. (*Lately Published.*)

ON THE CONSTITUTIONAL TREATMENT OF FEMALE DISEASES.

In one neat royal 12mo. volume, extra cloth, of about 250 pages. $1 00.

STILLÉ (ALFRED), M. D.

'HERAPEUTICS AND MATERIA MEDICA; a Systematic Treatise on the Action and Uses of Medicinal Agents, including their Description and History. In two large and handsome octavo volumes, of 1789 pages. (*Just Issued.*) $8 00.'

This work is designed especially for the student and practitioner of medicine. and treats the various articles of the Materia Medica from the point of view of the bed-side, and not of the shop or of the lecture-room. While thus endeavoring to give all practical information likely to be useful with respect to the employment of special remedies in special affections, and the results to be anticipated from their administration, a copious Index of Diseases and their Remedies renders the work eminently fitted for reference by showing at a glance the different means which have been employed, and enabling the practitioner to extend his resources in difficult cases with all that the experience of the profession has suggested.

Rarely, indeed, have we had submitted to us a work on medicine so ponderous in its dimensions as that now before us, and yet so fascinating in its contents. It is, therefore, with a peculiar gratification that we recognize in Dr. Stillé the possession of many of those more distinguished qualifications which entitle him to approbation, and which justify him in coming before his medical brethren as an instructor. A comprehensive knowledge, tested by a sound and penetrating judgment, joined to a love of progress—which a discriminating spirit of inquiry has tempered so as to accept nothing new because it is new, and abandon nothing old because it is old, but which estimates either according to its relations to a just logic and experience—manifests itself everywhere, and gives to the guidance of the author all the assurance of safety which the difficulties of his subject can allow. In conclusion, we earnestly advise our readers to ascertain for themselves, by a study of Dr. Stillé's volumes, the great value and interest of the stores of knowledge they present. We have pleasure in referring rather to the ample treasury of undoubted truths, the real and assured conquest of medicine, accumulated by Dr. Stillé in his pages; and commend the sum of his labors to the attention of our readers, as alike honorable to our science, and creditable to the zeal, the candor, and the judgment of him who has garnered the whole so carefully.—*Edinburgh Med. Journal.*

Our expectations of the value of this work were based on the well-known reputation and character of the author as a man of scholarly attainments, an elegant writer, a candid inquirer after truth, and a philosophical thinker; we knew that the task would be conscientiously performed, and that few, if any, among the distinguished medical teachers in this country are better qualified than he to prepare a systematic treatise on therapeutics in accordance with the present requirements of medical science. Our preliminary examination of the work has satis-

fied us that we were not mistaken in our anticipations.—*New Orleans Medical News*, March, 1860.

The most recent authority is the one last mentioned, Stillé. His great work on "Materia Medica und Therapeutics," published last year, in two octavo volumes, of some sixteen hundred pages, while it embodies the results of the labor of others up to the time of publication, is enriched with a great amount of original observation and research. We would draw attention, by the way, to the very convenient mode in which the *Index* is arranged in this work. There is first an "Index of Remedies;" next an "Index of Diseases and their Remedies." Such an arrangement of the Indices, in our opinion, greatly enhances the practical value of books of this kind. In tedious, obstinate cases of disease, where we have to try one remedy after another until our stock is pretty nearly exhausted, and we are almost driven to our wit's end, such an index as the second of the two just mentioned, is precisely what we want.—*London Med. Times and Gazette*, April, 1861.

We think this work will do much to obviate the reluctance to a thorough investigation of this branch of scientific study, for in the wide range of medical literature treasured in the English tongue, we shall hardly find a work written in a style more clear and simple, conveying forcibly the facts taught, and yet free from turgidity and redundancy. There is a fascination in its pages that will insure to it a wide popularity and attentive perusal, and a degree of usefulness not often attained through the influence of a single work. The author has much enhanced the practical utility of his book by passing briefly over the physical, botanical, and commercial history of medicines, and directing attention chiefly to their physiological action, and their application for the amelioration or cure of disease. He ignores hypothesis and theory which are so alluring to many medical writers, and so liable to lead them astray, and confines himself to such facts as have been tried in the crucible of experience.—*Chicago Medical Journal.*

SMITH (HENRY H.), M. D. AND HORNER (WILLIAM E.), M. D.

AN ANATOMICAL ATLAS, illustrative of the Structure of the Human Body. In one volume, large imperial octavo, extra cloth, with about six hundred and fifty beautiful figures. $3 00.

These figures are well selected, and present a complete and accurate representation of that wonderful fabric, the human body. The plan of this Atlas, which renders it so peculiarly convenient for the student, and its superb artistical execution, have been already pointed out. We must congratu-

late the student upon the completion of this Atlas; as it is the most convenient work of the kind that has yet appeared; and we must add, the very beautiful manner in which it is "got up" is so creditable to the country as to be flattering to our national pride.—*American Medical Journal.*

SHARPEY (WILLIAM), M. D., JONES QUAIN, M. D., AND RICHARD QUAIN, F. R. S., &c.

HUMAN ANATOMY. Revised, with Notes and Additions, by JOSEPH LEIDY, M. D., Professor of Anatomy in the University of Pennsylvania. Complete in two large octavo volumes, leather, of about thirteen hundred pages. Beautifully illustrated with over five hundred engravings on wood. $6 00.

SIMPSON (J. Y. , M. D.,
Professor of Midwifery, &c., in the University of Edinburgh, &c.

CLINICAL LECTURES ON THE DISEASES OF FEMALES. With numerous illustrations.

This valuable series of practical Lectures is now appearing in the "MEDICAL NEWS AND LIBRARY" for 1860, 1861, and 1862, and can thus be had without cost by subscribers to the "AMERICAN JOURNAL OF THE MEDICAL SCIENCES." See p. 2.

SOLLY ON THE HUMAN BRAIN; its Structure, Physiology, and Diseases. From the Second and much enlarged London edition. In one octavo volume, extra cloth, of 500 pages, with 120 wood-cuts. $2 00.

handsome octavo volume, extra cloth, of over 650 pages, with about one hundred wood-cuts. $3 25.
SIMON'S GENERAL PATHOLOGY, as conducive to the Establishment of Rational Principles for the prevention and Cure of Disease. In one

WATSON (THOMAS), M. D., &c.,
Late Physician to the Middlesex Hospital, &c.

LECTURES ON THE PRINCIPLES AND PRACTICE OF PHYSIC.

Delivered at King's College, London. A new American, from the last revised and enlarged English edition, with Additions, by D. FRANCIS CONDIE, M. D., author of "A Practical Treatise on the Diseases of Children," &c. With one hundred and eighty-five illustrations on wood. In one very large and handsome volume, imperial octavo, of over 1200 closely printed pages in small type; the whole strongly bound in leather, with raised bands. Price $4 25.

That the high reputation of this work might be fully maintained, the author has subjected it to a thorough revision; every portion has been examined with the aid of the most recent researches in pathology, and the results of modern investigations in both theoretical and practical subjects have been carefully weighed and embodied throughout its pages. The watchful scrutiny of the editor has likewise introduced whatever possesses immediate importance to the American physician in relation to diseases incident to our climate which are little known in England, as well as those points in which experience here has led to different modes of practice; and he has also added largely to the series of illustrations, believing that in this manner valuable assistance may be conveyed to the student in elucidating the text. The work will, therefore, be found thoroughly on a level with the most advanced state of medical science on both sides of the Atlantic.

The additions which the work has received are shown by the fact that notwithstanding an enlargement in the size of the page, more than two hundred additional pages have been necessary to accommodate the two large volumes of the London edition (which sells at ten dollars), within the compass of a single volume, and in its present form it contains the matter of at least three ordinary octavos. Believing it to be a work which should lie on the table of every physician, and be in the hands of every student, the publishers have put it at a price within the reach of all, making it one of the cheapest books as yet presented to the American profession, while at the same time the beauty of its mechanical execution renders it an exceedingly attractive volume.

The fourth edition now appears, so carefully revised, as to add considerably to the value of a book already acknowledged, wherever the English language is read, to be beyond all comparison the best systematic work on the Principles and Practice of Physic in the whole range of medical literature. Every lecture contains proof of the extreme anxiety of the author to keep pace with the advancing knowledge of the day, and to bring the results of the labors, not only of physicians, but of chemists and histologists, before his readers, wherever they can be turned to useful account. And this is done with such a cordial appreciation of the merit due to the industrious observer, such a generous desire to encourage younger and rising men, and such a candid acknowledgment of his own obligations to them, that one scarcely knows whether to admire most the pure, simple, forcible English—the vast amount of useful practical information condensed into the Lectures—or the manly, kind-hearted, unassuming character of the lecturer shining through his work.—*London Med. Times and Gazette.*

Thus these admirable volumes come before the profession in their fourth edition, abounding in those distinguished attributes of moderation, judgment, erudite cultivation, clearness, and eloquence, with which they were from the first invested, but yet richer than before in the results of more prolonged observation, and in the able appreciation of the latest advances in pathology and medicine by one of the most profound medical thinkers of the day.—*London Lancet.*

The lecturer's skill, his wisdom, his learning, are equalled by the ease of his graceful diction, his eloquence, and the far higher qualities of candor, of courtesy, of modesty, and of generous appreciation of merit in others. May he long remain to instruct us, and to enjoy, in the glorious sunset of his declining years, the honors, the confidence and love gained during his useful life.—*N. A. Med-Chir. Review.*

Watson's unrivalled, perhaps unapproachable work on Practice—the copious additions made to which (the fourth edition) have given it all the novelty and much of the interest of a new book.—*Charleston Med. Journal.*

Lecturers, practitioners, and students of medicine will equally hail the reappearance of the work of Dr. Watson in the form of a new—a fourth—edition. We merely do justice to our own feelings, and, we are sure, of the whole profession, if we thank him for having, in the trouble and turmoil of a large practice, made leisure to supply the hiatus caused by the exhaustion of the publisher's stock of the third edition, which has been severely felt for the last three years. For Dr. Watson has not merely caused the lectures to be reprinted, but scattered through the whole work we find additions or alterations which prove that the author has in every way sought to bring up his teaching to the level of his most recent acquisitions in science.—*Brit. and For. Medico-Chir. Review.*

WALSHE (W. H.), M. D.,
Professor of the Principles and Practice of Medicine in University College, London, &c.

A PRACTICAL TREATISE ON DISEASES OF THE LUNGS; including

the Principles of Physical Diagnosis. A new American, from the third revised and much enlarged London edition. In one vol. octavo, of 468 pages. (*Just Issued,* June, 1860.) $2 25.

The present edition has been carefully revised and much enlarged, and may be said in the main to be rewritten. Descriptions of several diseases, previously omitted, are now introduced; the causes and mode of production of the more important affections, so far as they possess direct practical significance, are succinctly inquired into; an effort has been made to bring the description of anatomical characters to the level of the wants of the practical physician; and the diagnosis and prognosis of each complaint are more completely considered. The sections on TREATMENT and the Appendix (concerning the influence of climate on pulmonary disorders), have, especially, been largely extended —*Author's Preface.*

*** In press, by the same author, a volume on Diseases of the Heart and Aorta, to match the above.

WILSON (ERASMUS), F. R. S.,
Lecturer on Anatomy, London.

THE DISSECTOR'S MANUAL; or, Practical and Surgical Anatomy. Third

American, from the last revised and enlarged English edition. Modified and rearranged, by WILLIAM HUNT, M. D., Demonstrator of Anatomy in the University of Pennsylvania. In one large and handsome royal 12mo. volume, leather, of 582 pages, with 154 illustrations. $2 00.

WINSLOW (FORBES), M. D., D. C. L., &c.

ON OBSCURE DISEASES OF THE BRAIN AND DISORDERS OF THE

MIND; their incipient Symptoms, Pathology, Diagnosis, Treatment, and Prophylaxis. In one handsome octavo volume, of nearly 600 pages. (*Just Issued.*) $3 00.

We close this brief and necessarily very imperfect notice of Dr. Winslow's great and classical work, by expressing our conviction that it is long since so important and beautifully written a volume has issued from the British medical press.—*Dublin Med. Press,* July 25, 1860.

We honestly believe this to be the best book of the season.—*Ranking's Abstract,* July, 1860.

It carried us back to our old days of novel reading, it kept us from our dinner, from our business, and from our slumbers; in short, we laid it down only when we had got to the end of the last paragraph, and even then turned back to the repe usal of several passages which we had marked as requiring further study. We have failed entirely in the above notice to give an adequate acknowledgment of the profit and pleasure with which we have perused the above work. We can only say to our readers, study it

yourselves; and we extend the invitation to unprofessional as well as professional men, believing that it contains matter deeply interesting not to physicians alone, but to all who appreciate the truth that "The proper study of mankind is man."—*Nashville Medical Record,* July, 1860.

The latter portion of Dr. Winslow's work is exclusively devoted to the consideration of Cerebral Pathology. It completely exhausts the subject, in the same manner as the previous seventeen chapters relating to morbid psychical phenomena left nothing unnoticed in reference to the mental symptoms pre-monitory of cerebral disease. It is impossible to overrate the benefits likely to result from a general perusal of Dr. Winslow's valuable and deeply interesting work.—*London Lancet,* June 23, 1860.

It contains an immense mass of information.—*Brit. and For. Med.-Chir. Review,* Oct. 1860.

WEST (CHARLES), M. D.,
Accoucheur to and Lecturer on Midwifery at St. Bartholomew's Hospital, Physician to the Hospital for Sick Children, &c.

LECTURES ON THE DISEASES OF WOMEN. Second American, from the

second London edition. In one handsome octavo volume, extra cloth, of about 500 pages; price $2 50. (*Now Ready,* July, 1861.)

✱ Gentlemen who received the first portion, as issued in the "Medical News and Library," can now complete their copies by procuring Part II, being page 309 to end, with Index, Title matter, &c., 8vo., cloth, price $1.

We must now conclude this hastily written sketch with the confident assurance to our readers that the work will well repay perusal. The conscientious, painstaking, practical physician is apparent on every page.—*N. Y. Journal of Medicine,* March, 1858.

We know of no treatise of the kind so complete and yet so compact.—*Chicago Med. Journal,* January, 1858.

A fairer, more honest, more earnest, and more reliable investigator of the many diseases of women and children is not to be found in any country.—*Southern Med. and Surg. Journal,* January 1858.

We gladly recommend his Lectures as in the highest degree instructive to all who are interested in obstetric practice.—*London Lancet.*

We have to say of it, briefly and decidedly, that it is the best work on the subject in any language; and that it stamps Dr. West as the *facile princeps* of British obstetric authors.—*Edinb. Med. Journ.*

As a writer, Dr. West stands, in our opinion, second only to Watson, the "Macaulay of Medicine;" he possesses that happy faculty of clothing instruction in easy garments; combining pleasure with profit, he leads his pupils, in spite of the ancient

proverb, along a royal road to learning. His work is one which will not satisfy the extreme on either side, but it is one that will please the great majority who are seeking truth, and one that will convince the student that he has committed himself to a candid, safe, and valuable guide. We anticipate with pleasure the appearance of the second part of the work, which, if it equals this part, will complete one of our very best volumes upon diseases of females.—*N. A. Med.-Chirurg. Review,* July, 1858.

Happy in his simplicity of manner, and moderate in his expression of opinion, the author is a sound reasoner and a good practitioner, and his book is worthy of the handsome garb in which it has appeared from the press of the Philadelphia publishers. —*Virginia Med. Journal.*

We must take leave of Dr. West's very useful work, with our commendation of the clearness of its style, and the industry and sobriety of judgment of which it gives evidence.—*London Med. Times and Gazette.*

Sound judgment and good sense pervade every chapter of the book. From its perusal we have derived unmixed satisfaction.—*Dublin Quart. Journ.*

BY THE SAME AUTHOR. (*Just Issued.*)

LECTURES ON THE DISEASES OF INFANCY AND CHILDHOOD.

Third American, from the fourth enlarged and improved London edition. In one handsome octavo volume, extra cloth, of about six hundred and fifty pages. $4 75.

The three former editions of the work now before us have placed the author in the foremost rank of those physicians who have devoted special attention to the diseases of early life. We attempt no analysis of this edition, but may refer the reader to some of the chapters to which the largest additions have been made—those on Diphtheria, Disorders of the Mind, and Idiocy, for instance—as a proof that the work is really a new edition; not a mere reprint. In its present shape it will be found of the greatest possible service in the every-day practice of nine-tenths of the profession.—*Med. Times and Gazette,* London, Dec. 10, 1859.

All things considered this book of Dr. West is by far the best treatise in our language upon such modifications of morbid action and disease as are within and when we have to deal with infancy and childhood. It is true that it confines itself to such disorders as come within the province of the physician, and even with respect to these it is unequal as regards minuteness of consideration, and some

diseases it omits to notice altogether. But those who know anything of the present condition of paediatrics will readily admit that it would be next to impossible to effect more, or effect it better, than the accoucheur of St. Bartholomew's has done in a single volume. The lecture (XVI.) upon Disorders of the Mind in children is an admirable specimen of the value of the later information conveyed in the Lectures of Dr. Charles West.—*London Lancet,* Oct. 24, 1859.

Since the appearance of the first edition, about eleven years ago, the experience of the author has doubled; so that, whereas the lectures at first were founded on six hundred observations, and our hundred and eighty dissections made among nearly fourteen thousand children, they now embody the results of nine hundred observations, and two hundred and eighty-eight post-mortem examinations made among nearly thirty thousand children, who, during the past twenty years, have been under his care.—*British Med. Journal,* Oct. 1, 1859.

BY THE SAME AUTHOR.

AN ENQUIRY INTO THE PATHOLOGICAL IMPORTANCE OF ULCER-

ATION OF THE OS UTERI. In one neat octavo volume, extra cloth. $1 00.

Lightning Source UK Ltd.
Milton Keynes UK
UKHW02f1030180618
324410UK00004B/699/P